# Trauma
# and
# Orthopedics

## Etiology, Diagnosis and Management

# Trauma and Orthopedics

## Etiology, Diagnosis and Management

**PS Kapoor**
MBBS, MS (Orthopedics), PCMS (Ex)

Senior Consultant Trauma and Orthopedic
Chandigarh Surgical Centre, Chandigarh
Amar Multispeciality Hospital, Mohali

*Former*

Chief Consultant and Head of Orthopedics, Derna, Libya
Senior Consultant Orthopedics
Fortis Heart Institute and Multispeciality Hospital, Mohali
Surgical Specialist (PCMS) ESI Hospital, Ludhiana

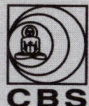

**CBS**

**CBS Publishers & Distributors** Pvt Ltd

New Delhi • Bengaluru • Chennai • Kochi • Kolkata • Mumbai
Hyderabad • Jharkhand • Nagpur • Patna • Pune • Uttarakhand

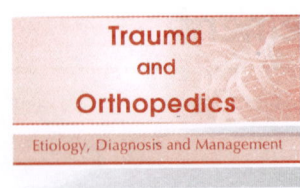

**Trauma and Orthopedics**

Etiology, Diagnosis and Management

**ISBN:** 978-93-86478-38-2

Copyright © Author and Publisher

**First Edition:** 2017

Published by Satish Kumar Jain and produced by Varun Jain for

**CBS Publishers & Distributors** Pvt Ltd

4819/XI Prahlad Street, 24 Ansari Road, Daryaganj, New Delhi 110 002, India.
Ph: 23289259, 23266861, 23266867  Website: www.cbspd.com
Fax: 011-23243014          e-mail: delhi@cbspd.com; cbspubs@airtelmail.in.
*Corporate Office:* 204 FIE, Industrial Area, Patparganj, Delhi 110 092

Ph: 4934 4934       Fax: 4934 4935    e-mail: publishing@cbspd.com; publicity@cbspd.com

**Branches**

• **Bengaluru:** Seema House 2975, 17th Cross, K.R. Road,
Banasankari 2nd Stage, Bengaluru 560 070, Karnataka
Ph: +91-80-26771678/79          Fax: +91-80-26771680          e-mail: bangalore@cbspd.com

• **Chennai:** 7, Subbaraya Street, Shenoy Nagar, Chennai 600 030, Tamil Nadu
Ph: +91-44-26680620, 26681266          Fax: +91-44-42032115          e-mail: chennai@cbspd.com

• **Kochi:** Ashana House, No. 39/1904, AM Thomas Road, Valanjambalam,
Ernakulam 682 016, Kochi, Kerala
Ph: +91-484-4059061-65          Fax: +91-484-4059065          e-mail: kochi@cbspd.com

• **Kolkata:** 6/B, Ground Floor, Rameswar Shaw Road, Kolkata-700 014, West Bengal
Ph: +91-33-22891126, 22891127, 22891128          e-mail: kolkata@cbspd.com

• **Mumbai:** 83-C, Dr E Moses Road, Worli, Mumbai-400018, Maharashtra
Ph: +91-22-24902340/41          Fax: +91-22-24902342          e-mail: mumbai@cbspd.com

*Representatives*

• **Hyderabad**  0-9885175004    • **Jharkhand**  0-9811541605    • **Nagpur**  0-9021734563
• **Patna**  0-9334159340    • **Pune**  0-9623451994    • **Uttarakhand**  0-9716462459

*Printed at* Rashtriya Printers, Dilshad Garden, Delhi, India

*to*

*the memory of
my father*

# Preface

This book has been written primarily for the medical student, medical officers and others, especially those working as a team in the department of trauma and orthopedics (T&O). Orthopedic trauma includes fractures and dislocations as well as musculoskeletal injuries to soft tissues including muscles, ligaments, tendons and nerves. Orthopedic trauma particularlly includes injuries to the upper limb (shoulder to hand), lower limb (hip to foot) and the spine. Orthopedic surgeons generally do not deal with injuries to the head, chest, abdomen and blood vessels. In case of a polytrauma patient, mostly caused by high velocity injuries like motor vehicle collisions or fall from a height, the orthopedic part of the patient's care is coordinated with other surgical specialties as appropriate usually in the department of A&E. Orthopedic trauma patients usually admitted via the department of A&E (emergency) or examined as an outpatient in a fracture clinic.

This book is intended to serve as a useful reference, on widely accepted techniques currently available for finding causes, clinical diagnosis, investigations, and management of acute trauma cases, and other common disorders. The contents of this book are presented as separate sections, anyone of which is complete in itself, for example management of trauma/disorders has been described fully — initial emergency treatment by the A&E staff, followed by further definitive treatment provided with the help of referred specialists in the department of T&O, depending on the infrastructure of the hospital.

Specific references are included as a guide to further study. Evaluation of new surgical/nonsurgical concepts and advances in determining causes, diagnosis, investigation and treatment has been a constant challenge. Orthopedics progress and space limitations are the deciding factors.

This book aims to guide the orthopedic surgeon who treats the patient in the A&E or T&O department or in a fracture clinic, on how to keep adequate records of history, physical examination, investigation, and management of cases. An attempt has been made to mention the trauma emergencies in the trauma section, and at the same time make mention of common orthopedic disorders in the orthopedic (elective) section, for which the patients visit the department of A&E, T&O and fracture clinic for consultation and treatment. Special mention has been made about examination and management of trauma cases on priority basis, especially while dealing with polytrauma emergencies.

Special chapters on management of fractures and dislocations, common orthopedic disorders are intended to serve as medically-oriented discussions of these fields with important clinical implications for the patient's care.

I have endeavored throughout to mention the authorities whose works I have made use of, but I should like to express here my appreciation of the fact that it is the work of others which gives this book any value it may have.

**PS Kapoor**

# Acknowledgments

I wish to express my appreciation to Miss Komal Kapoor, Miss Arshpreet Kaur and Ms Anju Malhotra for their skilful assistance with the manuscript and electronic information. Without their help the job would have been many times more difficult.

I would like to acknowledge the help received from Mr Jagdeep Kapoor and Ms Rita Kapoor, in form of useful suggestions and moral support. It is heartening to acknowledge the encouragement gained at each step by the sweet chatting with dearest Isaac.

I am indebted to Dr CN Malla, Dr Abha Gupta, Dr SK Madan, Dr Rajinder Singh, Dr HV Jindal, Dr S Saggar, Dr Vandhana Bhardwaj and Dr Vaneet Gupta, who have offered special suggestions, comments and corrections.

I am highly thankful to the management of British Library, and PGI, Chandigarh Library, for access to the medical books and journals.

Last, my sincere thanks are hereby extended to Mr SK Jain, Chairman & MANAGING DIRECTOR; Mr YN Arjuna, SENIOR VICE PRESIDENT, Publishing and Editorial; and other staff of CBS Publishers & Distributors, for their encouragement and generous help, and for the excellent work done in maintaining a good standard of print-production of the book.

**PS Kapoor**

# Contents

# Abbreviations

| | | | |
|---|---|---|---|
| A&E | Accident and emergency | CT | Computerised (axial) tomography |
| Ab | Antibody | CVA | Cerebrovascular accident |
| ABC | Airway, breathing, circulation | CXR | Chest X-ray |
| ABG | Arterial blood gases | D | Dimension |
| ACE | Angiotensin-converting enzyme | DIP | Distal interphalangeal joint |
| ACLS | Advanced cardiac life support | dL | Decilitre |
| ACTH | Adrenocorticotropic hormone | DLC | Differential leucocytic count |
| AKPOP | Above knee Plaster of Paris | DM | Diabetes mellitus |
| A-O (ASIF) | Association for the study of Internal Fixation | DPL | Diagnostic peritoneal lavage |
| APLS | Advanced pediatric (paediatric) life support | ECG | Electrocardiogram |
| AP | Anteroposterior | Echo | Echocardiogram |
| ASAP | As soon as possible | ED | Emergency department |
| ATLS | Advanced trauma life support | e.g. | For example |
| AXR | Abdominal X-ray | E.O.D. | Every other day (syn. alternate day) |
| b.d. (bd) | Bis die (twice daily) | esp. | Especially |
| b.i.w. | Twice a week | ESR | Erythrocyte sedimentation rate |
| BKPOP | Below knee Plaster of Paris | FB | Foreign body |
| BLS | Basic life support | FBC | Full blood count |
| BMJ | British medical journal | FH | Family history |
| BMT | Bone marrow transplant | G | Gauge |
| B/L | Bilateral | g | Gram (s) |
| BP | Blood pressure | GA | General anaesthesia |
| Ca | Carcinoma | GIT | Gastrointestinal tract |
| Ca$^+$ | Calcium | Hb | Hemoglobin (haemoglobin) |
| C1 | First cervical vertebra | HCO$_3$ | Bicarbonate |
| C2 | Second cervical vertebra | H$_2$CO$_3$ | Carbonate |
| C7 | Seventh cervical vertebra | Hg | Mercury |
| Cl | Chloride | HIV | Human immunodeficiency virus |
| C/I | Contraindication | hr | Hour |
| cm | Centimeter (s) | HRT | Hormone replacement therapy |
| CNS | Central nervous system | ICP | Intracranial pressure |
| CO$_2$ | Carbon dioxide | i.e. | That is |
| CPR | Cardiopulmonary resuscitation | IgA,G,E | Immunoglobulin A, G, E |
| CPAP | Continuous positive airways pressure | i.m. (IM) | Intramuscular |
| CRP | C-reactive protein | Inf | Inferior |
| CSF | Cerebrospinal fluid | IP | Interphalangeal |

| | | | | |
|---|---|---|---|---|
| Iu | International unit | PA | Posteroanterior |
| IV | Intravenous | PIP | Proximal interphalangeal |
| IVI | Intravenous infusion | PO | Per os (orally/by mouth) |
| IVP | Intravenous pyelography | POP | Plaster of Paris |
| IVU | Intravenous urogram | P/R | Per-rectum |
| JVP | Jugular venous pressure | PTA | Post-traumatic amnesia |
| K | Thousand | P/V | Per vaginum |
| K+ | Potassium | q.d.s.(qds) | Quater in die summendus (four times daily) |
| KCl | Potassium chloride | q.i.d. | Quarter in die (4 times a day) |
| kg | Kilogram | RA | Rheumatoid arthritis |
| kL | Kilolitre | RBC | Red blood cell |
| KUB | Kidneys, ureters, bladder | Rt | Right |
| L | Litre | s.c.(S/c) | Subcutaneously |
| LA | Local anaesthesia | SE (S/E) | Side-effect(s) |
| Lab | Laboratory | s | Second(s) |
| LAT | Lateral | SLR | Straight leg raising |
| LP | Lumbar puncture | Stat | Immediately |
| Lt | Left | STD | Sexually transmitted disease |
| max | Maximum | Sup | Superior |
| MC | Metacarpal | SXR | Skull X-ray |
| MCP | Metacarpophalangeal | TB | Tuberculosis |
| mEq/L | Millieqivalents per litre | t.i.d./t.d.s. | Ter in die sumendus (three times daily) |
| mg | Milligrams | THR | Total hip replacement |
| min | Minute/minutes | t.i.w. | Three times per week |
| mL | Millilitre | TKR | Total knee replacement |
| mm Hg | Millimetres of mercury | T&O | Trauma and orthopedics |
| mmol | Millimoles | u/U/IU | Unit |
| mU | Million units | UFH | Unfractionated heparin |
| MTP | Metatarsophalangeal | ug | Microgram |
| NG | Nasogastric | URC | Upper respiratory catarrh |
| NHS | National health service | UTI | Urinary tract infection |
| NSAIDs | Nonsteroidal anti-inflammatory drugs | USS | Ultrasound (ultrasonography) study |
| NVD | Nausea, vomiting, diarrhea | VDRL | Venereal diseases research laboratory |
| NWBPOP | Non-weight bearing plaster of Paris | WBC | White blood cell(s) |
| $O_2$ | Oxygen | WCC | White cell count |
| OA | Osteoarthritis | wk(s) | Week(s) |
| o.d. (od) | Omni die (once daily) | wt | Weight |
| OD | Overdose | X-match | Cross-match blood |
| OPD | Out-patients department | Yr(s) | Year(s) |
| ORIF | Open reduction and internal fixation | ZP | Zuelzer plating |

# Triage of Polytrauma Patient
## Triage of Medical/Surgical/Orthopedic Trauma Patient

Triage is a French word meaning sorting, selection, choice. It is the process of sorting patients based upon their requirement of immediate medical/surgical treatment as compared to their chance of benefiting from such care. Trauma patients visiting A&E are to be sorted immediately by an experienced triage staff on duty, in order to attend to serious patients on priority basis. A strategy must be driven for the detection of the highest risk group, in whom early intervention can improve outcome. This decision has to be based upon UK National Triage Scale considering the seriousness of illness/or injury.

**Table:** Triage of polytrauma patient

| National triage scale | Treatment acuity | Numeric code |
|---|---|---|
| Immediate resuscitation | Immediately | 1 |
| Very urgent | Within 10 mts. | 2 |
| Urgent | Within 60 mts. | 3 |
| Standard | Within 120 mts. | 4 |
| Non-urgent | Within 240 mts. | 5 |

(*Source*: UK National Triage Scale)

The A&E and T&O staff must have a clear knowledge of the benefit and harm of each therapy, allowing formulation of a simple approach to treatment selection base0d upon the disease/injury presentation. Properly attended/treated, acute emergency should have low hospital mortality, but if neglected/untreated, mortality is high. Proper history taking & investigations usually suffice for diagnosis. Careful surveillance and management by the A&E and referred T&O team, including invasive management in selected cases substantially reduce long-term risks. The clinical question is which patients with acute symptoms have a presentation benign enough to make discharge from the A&E or T&O department safe and appropriate.

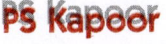

PS Kapoor

# SURGICAL TRAUMA

# 1

# Management of Surgical Trauma

## Management of multiple injuries
- Early trauma care
- Pre-hospital care (ambulance service)
- Trauma team
- Management in hospital (T&O)
- Assessment of injured patients
- Preliminary history and examination (primary survey)
- Detailed history and examination (secondary survey)

## Management of injuries
- Definitive care phase (management of specific injuries):
- Head injuries:
  - Scalp wounds
  - Head injuries
  - Brain injuries
  - Fractures of skull:
    - Fractures of vault of skull
    - Fractures of base of skull
- Intracranial hemorrhage:
  - Extradural hemorrhage
  - Subdural hemorrhage

## Chest injuries
- Thoracic injuries
- First aid treatment
- Local treatment (of complications)
- Fractured ribs
- Stove in chest
- Flail chest
- Traumatic pneumothorax
- Tension pneumothorax
- Traumatic hemothorax
- Lung injuries
- Chest wounds
- Thoracoabdominal wounds

**Abdominal injuries**
- Blunt injuries
- Perforated (rupture) injuries
- Shock

**Spine injuries**
- Anatomy of typical vertebra
- Spinal injuries:
  - Management of unstable fracture due to:
  - Flexion/rotation injuries
  - Sprains of spine
  - Dislocations
  - Fractures of spine
  - Fractures of spinous process
  - Fractures of transverse process
  - Fracture of lamina
  - Compression fractures of vertebral bodies
  - Collapse of the body and rarefaction
  - Cervical spine injuries
  - Fractures of thoracic and lumbar spine
  - Spinal cord injury
  - Cervical spine injury
  - Dorsal spine injury
  - Lumbar spine injury
  - Spinal cord lesions:
    - Cervical level
    - Dorsal level
    - Cauda equina
    - Spinal contusion
    - Management of spinal cord injuries
    - Management of complications

**Peripheral nerve injuries**
- Neurapraxia
- Axonotmesis
- Neurotmesis
- Brachial plexus injuries
- Complete brachial plexus injuries
- Incomplete brachial plexus injuries
- Upper lesion (Erb Duchen)
- Lower lesion (Klumpke)

**Limbs injuries**
- Management of fractures of the limbs.

## MANAGEMENT OF MULTIPLE INJURIES

### Trauma

The survival of a patient with multiple injuries, depends upon the judgment and planning of dealing surgeon, and readiness of hospital with adequate resuscitation facilities. Many improvements have been made in recent years, and subsequent development of Accident and Emergency (A&E) and Trauma and Orthopedic (T&O)

departments, for the management of Accident (multiple injuries) and Eemergency cases (medical/surgical).

## EARLY TRAUMA CARE

### Pre-hospital Care (Ambulance Service)

The management of patients with multiple injuries starts right from the site of accident. The ambulance attendants (professional staff members) are to be trained enough to bear the responsibility, until the patient reaches the hospital. The attendants record the site, date, and time of accident; position in which the patient was found, and whether conscious or unconscious, drunk or sober, apprehensive, hostile, or cooperative, and the amount of bleeding observed/assessed (at the site and from soaked clothes). Management of the injured (resuscitation measures) should start immediately in an orderly manner (ABC of trauma management), i.e. airway and cervical spine control, breathing care, control circulation, combat shock, splint fractured limbs. The attendant is responsible for the comfortable transportation of patient to the hospital, is to be trained enough and well versed with the resuscitation measures, that are continued uninterrupted until the patient reaches the A&E department, being informed in advance of the arrival of the injured patient.

## TRAUMAS AND ORTHOPEDIC DEPARTMENT

### Trauma Team

**Preplanning:** Usually accident and emergency (A&E) department or the trauma and orthopedic (T&O) receive a trauma call from the ambulance unit prior to arrival of a trauma/polytrauma case. The Accident and Emergency (A&E) and the trauma and orthopedics (T&O) teams consist of dedicated medical and nursing staff trained enough in trauma care and well versed with resuscitation), gets ready to receive the oncoming emergency, in the resuscitation chamber. In case of a polytrauma patient, mostly caused by the high velocity injuries like motor vehicle collisions (RSA), sports injuries, or fall from a height, the orthopedic part of the patient's care is coordinated with other surgical specialties as appropriate usually in the department of A&E. The team leader assigns tasks to the T&O staff, and may obtain help from concerned specialists if required. Care of the patient in the A&E/T&O requires the regular assessment and monitoring especially the trends. This based on physical examination and use of various monitoring equipment. However, the equipment are not a substitute for good clinical skills. In fact trauma and orthoperdics care is labor intensive. Record all the monitoring on a predesigned chart. The decision-making in the T&O should proceed in the continuous manner of evaluation, intervention, and re-evaluation. T&O should have access to well equipped laboratoty facilities. Quick diagnostic tests especially for estimation of glucose. electrolytes, proteins, blood counts, blood grouping, blood gas and cholesterol, etc. should be available. Portable X-ray unit, ultrasonography, and bone densitometry are desirable round the clock. Besides caring for the clinical disorder, proper attention should also be paid towards diet, sedation, and control of infection. Also mandatory to communicate regularly with the relatives/attendants and apprise them of patient's condition.

### Assessment of Injured Patient (Primary Survey) (Table 1.2)

Trauma (high velocity) is the commonest cause of death in the developed countries and one of the leading cause of deaths in the developing world; about third of these deaths occur from RSA.

**Trimodal death period (Table 1.1):** Trimodal death period—highest period of death occurs immediately or shortly post-trauma (caused by major head (brain) injury or hemorrhage; mostly unsalvageable; a second period of deaths (golden period) occurs couple of hrs. post-trauma (caused by airway, breathing or circulatory (ABC) disorders; the third period of deaths occur days/or weeks post initial trauma caused by infection or organ/s failure; aim in managing the trauma patients is to restore the anatomy and physiology (functions) ASAP—in order to prevent avoidable deaths and to keep late morbidity and mortality to a minimum.

## ADVANCED TRAUMA LIFE SUPPORT (ATLS)

### Triage (Priority of Treatment)

In the management of multiple injuries (as per guidelines of ATLS course) priority of treatment is directed to life-threatening conditions such as airway obstruction, shock, or external hemorrhage, even before a detailed examination begins.

### Aims of ATLS

- To provide an immediate treatment of patients with multiple injuries
- To standardize trauma resuscitation.

### Features of ATLS

- Frequent re-evaluation of patient's condition
- Response to treatment
- A deteriorating condition necessitates a re-evaluation and treatment of 'ABC'.

### Phases of ATLS

- Initial care
- Definitive care.

## INITIAL CARE (DIAGNOSIS AND MANAGEMENT OF LIFE-THREATENING ENTITIES)

### Preliminary (Brief) History)

Identification of a seriously injured patient relies on observation, history and physical examination (preliminary and detailed examination). At first contact (primary survey), the life-threatening entities, e.g. the ABC's (airway's patency and cervical spine control, adequacy of breathing and circulation) are quickly assessed. If there is an abnormality in anyone of these, life support/resuscitation must be initiated immediately, followed by a quick assessment of the other two parameters, e.g. the D&E (dysfunction of the CNS, i.e. conscious level and Exposure and environment). The finer points of history taking

| Table 1.1: Trimodal death period | |
|---|---|
| Period | Cause of death |
| Ist (Immediate/shortly post-trauma) | Head injury (Brain hemorrhage) |
| | Mostly brought dead on arrival |
| Golden hour (interval between 1st and 2nd periods) | Golden chance to save the patient with assessment and care (ASAP) |
| 2nd (couple of hrs. post-trauma) | ABC (Airway, breathing, circulatory) |
| 3rd (days/or weeks post-trauma) | Sepsis or multiple organs failure |

(secondary survey) including detailed examination may have to wait until later. Always suspect major injury in RSA and fall from a height.

### History of Accident

Inquire: From witnesses, ambulance crew, relatives or persons accompanying the patient:

- MOI: Was it vehicle accident or fall from a height?
- When, where and how did it happen? What happened next?
- Was it under influence of alcohol or drugs?
- Any seizure attack: pre/or post-accident?

## PRELIMINARY (BRIEF) EXAMINATION

### A. Airway Obstruction

| | |
|---|---|
| Etiology | Foreign bodies, blood, saliva, or vomitus. |
| | *Cervical spine injury with or without paralysis* |
| Diagnosis | Breathless or gasping, cyanosis |
| | Deformity |
| | Neck rigidity |
| | Local tenderness |
| | Paresis of arm and leg |
| | Movements—painful and restricted. |

### B. Breathing (Respiration) Disturbance

| | |
|---|---|
| Etiology | Head injury |
| | *Chest injuries* |
| | Fracure ribs |
| | Open chest wounds |
| | Hemothorax |
| | Tension pneumothorax |
| | Flail chest |
| | Cardiac tamponade. |
| Diagnosis | Breathless or gasping |
| | Chest pain |
| | Cyanotic or pale |
| | Tachycardia, hypotension |
| | X-Ray chest, head, cervical spine—cofirms clinical diagnosis. |

### C. Circulation Disturbance (Hemorrhage and Shock)

| | |
|---|---|
| Etiology | External or internal hemorrhage due to: Fracture pelvis, chest, and abdominal injuries. |
| Diagnosis | External hemorrhage is revealed type, while internal hemorrhage is concealed type. |
| Signs | Deep sighing respirations (air hunger) |
| | Restlessness, thirst, pallor |
| | Cold clammy skin—pallor or cyanotic |

Tachycardia, hypotension
Unconsciousness—in case of shock.

## D. Disability Syn. Dysfunction of the CNS (Assessment of Conscious Level)

Etiology          Trauma—head injury
                  Infection
                  Diabetes
                  Psychiatric—epilepsy
                  Alcohol abuse, drug abuse—opiates, poisons
                  Shock
Diagnosis         Assessment of conscious level made by AVPU system, i.e.
                  Alert
                  Response to verbal stimulus
                  Response pain
                  Unresponsive to any stimulus
                  Pupil—size and reaction.

## E. Exposure to Environment

With the consent and cooperation of patient/attendant, clothing be removed as per requirements for examination, in a warm and well lit examination room, but subsequently cover the patient as much as possible, in order to decrease the anxiety and to prevent excessive heat loss.

## F. Monitor Vital Signs

Pulse, BP, respiratory rate, temperature, ECG
Catheterization
IV lines,
Monitor input/output.

**Table 1.2:** Proforma for assessment of injured patients

SURNAME.......................... FIRST NAME...................... A&E No.................................

AGE/DOB...........................SEX...........................................................................

DATE.....................................

SON/DAUGHTER/WIFE of................... .........................TIME................................

OCCUPATION...................................................................TEL ...............................

ADDRESS..............................................................................................................

D.O.A ...........................................................................D.O.D..............................

DIAGNOSIS.............................................................................................................

A&E CONSULTANT/Dr.I/C ........................................................................................

**Complaints (Symptoms) and their duration:**

.............................................................................................................................
.............................................................................................................................
.............................................................................................................................

**Preliminary (Brief) History:**

..................................................................................................................................
..................................................................................................................................
..................................................................................................................................
..................................................................................................................................

**Preliminary (Brief) Examination:**

*Airway obstruction and cervical spine injury:*

Breathless ........................................... Gasping ..................... Cyanosis .......................

Foreign bodies ................. Blood ........... Saliva ......................... Vomitus........................

Neck rigidity ........................................... Tenderness ............................................

Deformity.........................................................................................................

Paresis of arm/& leg ............................. Movements...........................................

Breathing (Respiration) disturbance:

Respiration ........... Slow and shallow ........... Slow and deep ........... Noisy ..................

Pulse ...................... BP ......................................SBP .............................. DBP .......................

Temperature ......... Subnormal ..................... High (> 40 degree centigrade) ................

**Circulation disturbance (Hemorrhage and Shock):**

Respirations ............... Restlessness ................................ Thirst ...............................

Skin .......................... Cold clammy ...........................Pale ..................................

**Disability syn. Dysfunction of the CNS (assessment of conscious level):**

*Cconscious level made by AVPU system:*

Response .........Verbal stimulus .........Pain ................... Unresponsive ........... Pupil
..................................... Size ................... Reaction ...............................................

**Exposure:** (Expose the patient completely)

X-ray Cervical spine ........................ CXR ................. X-ray Pelvis ..............................

*Detailed history (Secondary survey):*

..................................................................................................................................
..................................................................................................................................

**Detailed examination:**

Head injuries:

*General physical examination:*

Position: ........... Lying flaccid .................. Curled up ................................................

Alert ................ Unconscious ................. Depth of unconsciousness...............................

Eyes: ................ Black eye ...................... Subconjunctival hemorrhage .........................

Pupil: ........... Dilated.......................... Pinpoint ..................... Equal ......................

Vision ......................................... Movements ...........................................

Reacting to light ............................. Not-reacting to light ..............................

Eyes: ............ Black eye ...................... Subconjunctival hemorrhage ........................

Pupil: ............ Dilated......................... Pinpoint ........................ Equal........................

Vision ................................. Movements ...............................................

Reacting to light .................................. Not-reacting to light ..............................................

Bleeding/or CSF: Nose .......................... Ear ............................................ Mouth...........................

Cranial nerves: Squint ........................... Facial palsy

Neck rigidity ......................................... Movements .....................................................

Limbs: Muscle power: RUL ........... LUL ............... RLL ............. LLL..............................

        Sensations: RUL ..................... LUL ............. RLL ............. LLL ....................

        Reflexes: RUL ....................... LUL ............. RLL ............. LLL ....................

**Local examination:** (Shave & clean the head)

Bruise ..........................Swelling ...............................Laceration ...........................................

Fracture .................... Simple ............................Compound ...........................................

**Chest injuries:**

General physical examination:

Position: Lying quite ........................ Retless .........................Dyspnea ................................
Cyanosis ..............................................................................................................................

Respiration: Abdominal ..................Thoracic ................... Movements ................................

Local examination:

Wound: Penetrating ........................ Swelling .....................Tenderness ...............................

Percussion: Resonant .....................Cardiac dullness .........................................................

Abdominal injuries:

General Physical Examination:

Position: Lying quite ............................. Restless .................................................................

Respiration: Air hunger .........................Movements ............................................................

Local examination:

Distension ....................................... Shifting dullness ..........................................................

Tenderness ...................................... Rigidity ......................................................................

Liver: Tenderness ............................... Shifting dullness...........................................................

Spleen: Ternderness ...........................Shifting dullness ........................................................

Kidney : Tenderness .......................... ...Shifting dullness ......................................................

Urinary bladder: Tenderness .................Shifting dullness .......................................................

Stomach: Distension .........................Shifting dullness .........................................................

Large intestine: Peritonitis ....................Surgical emphysema...................................................

Spinal injuries:

Spinal column injuries: Fractures ...........Fracture-dislocation ....................................................

Spinal cord injury: Paralysis .................................................................................................

Limbs injuries:

Deformity ..........................................Swelling ...................Shortening ...............................

Wounds ............................................Tenderness ..............Crepitus ..................................

Movements ....................................... Shortning .................Abnormal mobility ....................

Limbs: Muscle power: RUL .....................LUL .................LUL .................RLL ......... LLL...................

        Sensations: RUL .......................LUL ................ RLL ................ LLL ....................

        Reflexes: RUL .........................LUL ................RLL ................ LLL ......................

Investigations:

X-ray Skull ............................................. Chest ..............................................................
Abdomen ....................................... Pelvis ............................................................
Upper limb ................................. Lower limb ....................................................
Ultrasound ..............................................................................................................
MRI ........................................................................................................................
CT-Scan ..................................................................................................................
Color-Dopler ..........................................................................................................
BDM .......................................................................................................................
Biopsy ....................................................................................................................
FNAS .......................................................................................................................
Culture ...................................................................................................................
Specific investigations—as per presentation of each patient
Complete blood count (CBC) ..................................................................................
Serum proteins.......................................................................................................
Serum electrolytes..................................................................................................
Serum alkaline phosphatase....................................................................................
Blood cholesterol....................................................................................................
Blood sugar............................................................................................................
Blood grouping and cross matching..........................................................................
Blood urea..............................................................................................................
Urine analysis.........................................................................................................
ECG........................................................................................................................

(*Source*: Kaspoor's Accident and Emergency)

## MANAGEMENT OF LIFE-THREATENING ENTITIES (A, B, C)

### A. Airway Maintenance with Cervical Spine Control

Maintenance of free airway is strongly stressed upon and should take the top priority treatment, as a life saving measure. The treatment includes:

### Basic management

#### *Airway (with cervical spine control)*

Position of patient—supine, with tilting of head, and support of the jaw.

Immobilization of cervical spine—manually, sand bag, cervical collar.

**Caution:** Avoid tilting the head or moving the neck—in case of any suspicion of neck injury.

- Removal of foreign bodies, blood clots, saliva, and vomitus from the mouth and nose by suction or manually.

### Advanced Management

- Oxygen therapy—supply high flow oxygen by face mask. An apneic or hypoventilated patient requires bag and mask ventilation prior to the endotracheal intubation and IPPV.
- Endotracheal intubation.

### Surgical Management

- Cricothyroidotomy
- **Tracheostomy:** Indicated in head, chest, or upper abdomen injuries.

### B. Breathing (Respiration) and Ventilation Control

**Head injury:** May lead to cessation of central control of breathing.

**Management:** Described in appropriate section of head injury.

### Chest Injuries

a. **Open chest wounds:** May be simple or complicated, due to direct violence, e.g. stab, bullet, or bomb shell fragments.

 • *Contusion and laceration of lung*: Common in chest wounds.

   *Management:* To be covered with dressing pads and stitched later on, in order to prevent serious lesions like tension pneumothorax. An urgent surgical treatment is required after resuscitation.

   *Surgery:* Thoracotomy is indicated for uncontrollable bleeding.

b. **Flail chest:** Due to severe violence, resulting in a flaccid unstable chest wall showing paradoxical movement, which produces faulty ventilation with anoxia, whereas impaired coughing causes collection of bronchopulmonary secretions.

   *Management:* Oxygen, endotracheal intubation with positive pressure ventilation, deep breathing exercises, analgesics, antibiotics to prevent and control infection.

   *Surgery*: Urgent tracheostomy required—produces remarkable results.

c. **Traumatic pneumothorax:** Penetrating chest wounds/blunt injury may produce pneumothorax (air in pleural cavity).

   *Management*: Seal the wounds with dressing pad.

d. **Tension pneumothorax:** It is a life-threatening emergency.

   *Management*: Treated on priority basis by immediate decompression, i.e. plunging an aspirating needle into the pleural cavity (needle thoracocentesis) through 2nd intercostals space, at the midclavicular level, to relieve air under tension. It is followed by introducing a catheter (chest drain) through the 4th intercostal space, at the mid—axillary line and connected to the suction apparatus.

e. **Traumatic hemothorax:** Blood collects in the pleural cavity due to penetrating chest wounds, or from torn-heart, lungs, or blood vessels.

   *Management*: Seal the wounds with dressing pads; repeated aspirations, and if fails then, intercostals tube with water seal drainage is indicated. If the bleeding persists, then:

   *Surgery*: Thoracotomy is indicated.

f. **Fractured ribs:** Due to direct violence, resulting in isolated fracture of ribs, with/without any associated complication.

   *Management*: Treated by—analgesics, intercostal blocks, strapping.

g. **Stove in chest:** Due to severe violence, resulting in multiple rib fractures and indentation of the chest wall and distressing paradoxical chest movement.

   *Management*: Elevation of depressed chest wall by towel clips/or clamps round the ribs. Endotracheal intubation and positive pressure ventilation.

   *Surgery*: Tracheostomy—if required.

h. **Lung injuries:** Contusion injuries resolve spontaneously, whilst lacerated injuries may require repeated aspirations/thoracotomy.

   Antibiotics to prevent and control infection.

   Deep breathing exercises.

Thoracoabdominal wounds: Common in bomb blast injuries.

*Management*: Exploration to control bleeding.

Refer the patient to the surgical team.

## C. Circulation Disturbance (Hemorrhage and Shock) control

- **External hemorrhage:** Controlled by direct pressure, e.g. sterile dressings, covered with a compression bandage. Failure of this, may require a tourniquet (preferably a pneumatic).
- **Internal hemorrhage:** Occurs in fracture pelvis, chest, abdominal injuries.

### Management:

| | |
|---|---|
| General measures | Monitor pulse, BP, respiration, temperature, ECG |
| | Assess change in skin color, clamminess, conscious level |
| | IV fluids—adult 1 L of 0.9% saline children 20 mL/Kg |
| | Plasma expanders |
| | Blood grouping and cross matching |
| | Blood transfusion |
| | Catheterization |
| | Monitor input/output. |
| Hemothorax | Treated by repeated aspiration, catheterization, and if |

### Required

| | |
|---|---|
| Surgery: | Thoracotomy. |

### Abdominal hemorrhage

| | |
|---|---|
| Surgery | Laparotomy is to be performed as an emergency |
| Shock | Described in management of specific injuries Page 23. |

### Detailed History (Secondary Survey)

| | |
|---|---|
| History | Of circumstantial events/environment related to injury |
| | Of allergies |
| | Of drugs/alcohol abuse |
| | Of seizure |
| | Of previous illness |
| | Of last meal. |

### Detailed Examination

Includes a head to toe examination to identify other (specific) injuries. The patient is monitored throughout, and any deterioration necessitates a re-evaluation of 'ABC'.

| | |
|---|---|
| Head Injuries | General physical examination: |
| | Position—lying flaccid/or curled up |
| | Level of consciousness—depth of unconsciousness |
| | Respiration: |
| | Slow and shallow (concussion) |
| | Slow and deep, irregular, noisy (compression). |
| | *Eyes*: Black eye (local injury) or subconjunctival hemorrhage |
| | Pupil response |

Dilated, equal, reacting to light (concussion)
Dilated, fixed, not-reacting to light (compression)
Pinpoint, fixed, paralytic (hemorrhage).
Bleeding: Nose/ear/or mouth (# base of skull)
Hemoptysis

Temperature:  Subnormal (concussion)
                  Rises > 40 degree centigrade (hemorrhage).
Rigidity of neck: Due to meningeal irritation (hemorrhage)
Cranial nerves: Squint (injury 3rd/4th or 6th); facial palsy (7th nerve)
Muscle power of limbs: May be paralyzed
Reflexes
Local examination:
(Shave and clean the head)
Wound: Scalp/or head
Fracture: Depressed
Swelling: Hematoma
Rigidity of neck: Due to meningeal irritation (hemorrhage)
Cranial nerves: Squint (injury 3rd/4th or 6th); facial palsy (7th nerve)
Muscle power of limbs: May be paralyzed
Reflexes.

| | |
|---|---|
| Chest injuries | General physical examination:<br>Position: Lying quite/or restless and gasping<br>Dyspnea/or cyanosis<br>Respiration: Abdominal/or thoracic<br>Chest movements: Any restriction<br>Wound: Penetrating (pneumothorax, surgical emphysema)<br>Swelling: Surgical emphysema<br>Local examination:<br>Local tenderness<br>Percussion: Resonant (surgical emphysema, pneumothorax)<br>Cardiac dullness: Obliterated (pneumothorax)<br>Increased (hemothorax)<br>Crepitus audible. |
| Abdomen and perineum injuries | General physical examination:<br>Lying quite (peritonitis)<br>Restless (Hemorrhage)<br>Respiration: Air hunger (Hemorrhage)<br>Movements of abdominal wall: Abnormal<br>Local examination:<br>Distension<br>Local tenderness, rigidity, shifting dullness (as per seat of lesion)<br>Liver: Local tenderness, dullness—increased, shifting dullness<br>Spleen: Local ternderness, dullness—persistent over left side of abdomen, shifting dullness—over right side |

*Kidney*: Swelling (fullness), local tenderness, dullness—lateral to erector spinae

Urinary bladder: Swelling (fullness), local tenderness, shifting dullness

Stomach: Rigidity—board like, distension, shifting dullness

Large intestine: Peritonitis, surgical emphysema.

Spinal injuries:

- Spinal column injuries: Fractures, fracture-dislocation
- Spinal cord injury: Paralysis (meningeal hemorrhage).

Limbs injuries:

Any deformity, swelling, wounds

Local tenderness

Pitting edema

Muscle power, tone, reflexes, and sensations

Pulses: Peripheral

Joints: Movements

Shortning.

## Investigations

Specific investigations—as per presentation of each patient

Complete blood count (CBC)

Serum proteins

Serum electrolytes

Serum alkaline phosphatase

Blood cholesterol

Blood sugar

Blood grouping and cross matching

Blood urea

Urine analysis

ECG

X-ray of affected region (chest, skull, abdomen, pelvis, and limb)

Ultrasound—especially for abdominal injuries

CT scan and MRI

Angiography—indicated in pelvic injury, aortic injury

Echocardiography.

## II. Definitive Care (Management of Specific Injuries)

Preface        The doctor incharge should plan the line of treatment in consultation with other specialists involved in the management of various lesions. It may be possible to manage all the injuries simultaneously but at times, these lesions to be dealt with, on priority basis—in a definite sequence. Compound fractures should preferably be treated alongwith head, neck, or chest injuries. Operative treatment for simple fractures may better be postponed to a later stage. But it is better not to postpone the corrective orthopedic measures for more than a day or so, in the patients who appeared unlikely to recover from their associated injuries.

| | |
|---|---|
| **Head injuries** | Include scalp wounds and head injuries. |
| **Scalp injuries** | The scalp injuries bleed profusely, as the blood vessels of the scalp prevented from contraction due to firm adherence of vessel walls to the fibrous tissue of the scalp. |
| Anatomy | The scalp consists of five layers similar to that of palms of the hand and the soles of the feet; skin is firmly bound to the subjacent aponeurosis, by a densely fibrous tissue traversed by neurovascular structures, while palms and soles lie deep to the aponeurosis: |

- Skin: Denser than anywhere in the body; contains hairs and sebaceous glands.
- Dense connective tissue: Binds firmly skin and epicranius muscle to the underneath aponeurosis; very dense and fibrous embedded with nerves and vessels of scalp; vessels walls firmly anchored—tearing of that causes severe scalp bleeding.
- Aponeurosis of epicranius (occipitofrontalis) muscle: Muscular in front and behind, connected by galea aponeurotica (aponeurosis); scalp wounds fail to gape unless divided
- Loose connective tissue: Very tenuous; traversed by small veins connecting venous sinuses of the skull to the scalp veins; 1st three layers of scalp gets easily separated from pericranium through this plane
- Pericranium (periosteum of scalp): Loosely attached to skull bones except at the suture lines and temporal fossa.

| | |
|---|---|
| MOI | Direct violence—being hit by an object |
| | RSA. |
| Diagnosis | Bleeding scalp wound. |
| Management | Shaving of scalp and toilet of wound with antiseptic solutions |
| Local anesthesia | Inj. Xylocain 2%, local infiltration into the edges of the wound |
| | Debridement of the wound |
| | Apply artery forceps to the galea aponeurotica |
| | Stitching (interrupted stitches with black silk) of galea to galea and skin to skin |
| | Apply firm bandage |
| | Removal of stitches—after seven days. |

## Head Injuries

| | |
|---|---|
| | Include injury to skull, brain, intracerebral vessels, separately or collectively. |
| MOI | Direct violence |
| | RSA |
| | Fall from a height. |

## Fractures of Skull

| | |
|---|---|
| Types | Fractures of the vault and base of skull |

## Fractures of Vault

| | |
|---|---|
| MOI | Compression force—causes simple linear fissures |

Indentation force—causes simple or compound depressed fractures
Tangential force—causes compound fractures.

Pathogenesis (mechanism of injury)

- Compression force: Results in distortion of skull, while coming in contact with a hard flat surface, thereby causing displacement of brain, leading to severe cerebral injury.
- Indentation force: Blows from large objects cause closed depressed fracture, dura remains intact, while blows from small objects cause compound depressed fractures, tearing both dura and brain tissue.
- Tangential force: May tear apart a large segment of the bone, leaving dura matter intact. These are compound injuries, and injury to brain tissue is rare.

| | |
|---|---|
| Diagnosis | Simple depressed fractures are rare |
| | Swelling (hematoma) over the fracture site. |
| | Compound fractures of the vault are common, variable in severity and mostly fatal injuries. |
| | Hemiplegia may occur. |
| | Lacerated scalp wound sometimes conceal the extent of fracture. |
| Investigation | X-ray skull—AP and Lateral views to confirm the clinical diagnosis |
| | CT scanning—to rule out any brain injury. |
| Management | It is a serious emergency and requires urgent surgical treatment, until and unless the patient s condition warrants postponement |

*First aid treatment*:
Airway maintenance: By right posture.
Endotracheal intubation, suction, and if required—tracheostomy.

*Surgical treatment*:
Methods: Debridement of scalp wound and if required, extend the wound to expose fully the fracture.
Burr-hole surgery: To remove loose bone fragments, wound stitched in layers.
Reconstruction of skull defects—performed after an interval of 3–6 months period, by the use of plates, rib grafts, or acrylic inlay resin.

Refer: The patient to the surgical and neurosurgical team for surgery.

## Fractures of Base of Skull

| | |
|---|---|
| MOI | Compression force |
| | Indentation force |
| | Tangential force |
| Pathogenesis (mechanism of injury) | Fractures of base of skull are mostly produced by compression force and extension of fissures, extending from the vault fractures. The violent force extends into the weaker parts, e.g. middle ear fossae, air sinuses and finally into the foramina, exiting cranial nerves. Ring fracture occurs at the foramen magnum, by the indentation force of spinal column in |

headon collisions—car accidents. Mastoid process is fractured by a tangential force.

| | |
|---|---|
| Diagnosis | Discharge of blood, cerebrospinal fluid, or brain tissue. |

- Anterior fossa: Epistaxis—profuse and watery due to dilution with CSF or mixed with brain tissue.

  Subconjunctival hemorrhage

  Cranial nerves injury: 3rd, 4th or 6th nerve injury causing squint

- Middle fossa: Epistaxis—discharge blood mixed with CSF from the ear/or mouth

  Cranial nerves injury: Facial (7th) nerve injury causing facial paralysis, while injury to auditory (8th) nerve causes deafness.

- Posterior fossa: Swelling at the nape of neck due to collection of blood

  Cranial nerve injury: Injury to 9th, 10th, and 11th cranial nerves, injured at the jugular foramen.

| | |
|---|---|
| Investigation | X-ray Skull—to rule out an intracranial aerocoele. |
| Management | Patient to be propped up in the bed, to combat the escape of CSF from the nose/or ear |
| | Antibiotics |
| | Surgery: An early repair, to prevent occurrence of meningitis. |
| | **Refer:** The patient to the surgical and neurosurgical team. |

## Brain Injuries

| | |
|---|---|
| Pathogenesis (mechanism of injury) | In any brain injury, the mechanism of injury is the same, e.g. displacement and distortion of the brain tissues, occurring at the time of injury. Brain is suspended inside the skull by slings formed by the cerebral vessels, and floats in the CSF anteroposteriorly. Lateral displacement of the brain is restricted by the falx cerebri (septum). Hence any direct blow on the front or backside of the head causes displacement of brain, resulting in the brain damage especially brainstem. Lateral blow may fracture the skull, but not enough displacement to cause severe brain damage. |

## Types of Brain Injury

| | |
|---|---|
| Cerebral concussion | Displacement of brain tissues is slight. There is a transient loss of consciousness or amnesia, without any brain tissue damage. In majority of patients, the recovery is complete. |
| Cerebral | Displacement of brain tissues is severe, resulting in tearing of brain tissue, esp. brainstem. Loss of consciousness is prolonged and the recovery may be incomplete |
| Cerebral laceration | Displacement of brain tissues is more severe, resulting in more tearing of brain tissues. |
| Diagnosis | Posture: Lying flaccid—a serious entity |
| | Lying curled up—a nonserious entity |

- *Depth of consciousness*: Conscious or unconscious
- *Conscious*: History of prior unconsciousness—ICH
  Progressive deterioration of conscious level—brain compression
- *Unconscious*: History of prior consciousness—extradural hemorrhage
- Assessment of conscious level by:
  - Using Glasgow Coma Scale (GCS), i.e. by observing three types of responses: Eye opening, verbal and motor responses to the commands of speech and pain. Maximum score is 15. Any reduction in the score is an indication of a loss in the unconscious level. Alt:
    - Using AVPU system, i.e. alert, responds or unresponsive to the commands of vocal and painful stimuli.
- Bleeding from nose/ears/or mouth: In basal fracture of skull
- Vomiting
- Respiration:
  Rate: Slowed down
  Rhythm: Irregular
- Pulse:
  Rate: Tachycardia
  Rhythm: Thready
- BP: Hypotension followed by hypertension due to raised ICP.
- Pupil: size and reactions
- Eye movements
- Neck rigidity: May be due to cervical spine injury, or cerebral irritation
- Muscle power: Loss of muscle power (paresis)
- Reflexes: Absent
- Sensations: Loss of sensations.

**Investigations**  X-ray skull: AP and lateral views taken, to rule out any fracture, hemorrhage

CT scanning: To identify and define the brain injury, and intracranial hematoma

Lumbar puncture: Raised pressure in cerebral concussion. Blood stained cerebrospinal fluid—in cerebral laceration (subarachnoid hemorrhage).

**Management**  First aid treatment:

Airway maintenance: Endotracheal intubation, or tracheostomy

Oxygen supply

Protection of the cervical spine

Bleeding control

Correction of hypovolemia, and resuscitation

Correction of hypovolemia, and resuscitation

Drugs: Analgesics, antipyretics.

**Refer:** To neurosurgeon for persisting confusion, loss of consciousness, persisting coma, compound fractures, bleeding from nose/ears/or mouth.

### Definitive treatment

Continuous observation: Of the patient to detect onset of complications, e.g. edema or hemorrhage, and to treat accordingly.

Monitor: The pulse, BP, respiration, level of consciousness

Nursing care: To combat the neural lesion, by:

- Posture: Conscious patient—to be propped up, to relieve headache, while the unconscious patient—to be nursed on his/her side, to combat drowning of patient in his/her own secretions, e.g. saliva, blood, or vomitus.
- Repeated suctions to clear any secretions from throat or nose. Catheterization—to relieve a distended bladder

Drugs: The fewer the better.

- In a conscious patient asprin to relieve any headache
- In a serious patient IV aminophylline 250 mg for its vasodilatation action, i.e. enhances blood supply to the ischemic brainstem and improvement of respiration by dilatation of bronchi.

Hypothermia—use of ice bags/or cold sponging in brainstem lesions

Dehydration therapy—to relieve the high intracranial pressure, by use of 50 mL. of 50% sucrose IV slowly QDS.

Lumbar puncture—as a therapeutic measure to relieve high pressure. A clear fluid with high pressure is indication of extradural hemorrhage, while a bloodstained fluid with high pressure, indicates cerebral lacerations.

Surgical treatment: A deteriorating level of consciousness, with the development of paralysis, is indication of burr-hole exploration.

Refer: The patient to the surgical and neurosurgical team.

## Intracranial Hemorrhage

| Types | Extradural hemorrhage |
|---|---|
|  | Subdural hemorrhage |

## Extradural Hemorrhage (Middle Meningeal)

| MOI | Direct violence—blow from a stick, golf or cricket ball. |
|---|---|
| Mechanism of injury | Fracture of thin temporal bone, causing injury to the middle meningeal artery by the driven in dura. A short primary concussion occurs, followed by a lucid interval, e.g. intracranial hemorrhage collection and formation of a swelling underneath the temporal muscle. Finally there occurs cerebral compression esp. of brainstem. |
| Diagnosis | Swelling—temporal region |
|  | Confused, irritable |
|  | Drowsiness |
|  | Facial paralysis followed by paralysis of opposite arm and leg |
|  | Pupils—dilated. |
| Management | It is an emergency and needs urgent operation—burr-hole exploration to relieve pressure. |
|  | Refer: The patient to the surgical and neurosurgical team for surgery |

Method: A burr-hole or trephine opening is made, to open the skull. The bleeder point is usually seen over the dura, which is secured by ligature or coagulated with diathermy.

After care: Patient lying flat and carefully observed for improvement. If improvement is delayed or condition deteriorating then:

Lumbar puncture is indicated.

- Low pressure—Inj. Saline intrathecally, raises the pressure, and prevents coning formation of brainstem.

## Subdural Hemorrhage

| | |
|---|---|
| Preface | It is more common than extradural type of hemorrhage. |
| MOI | Direct violence |
| | RSA |
| | Fall from a height. |
| Mechanism of injury | Hemorrhage occurs due to rupture of connecting veins from cerebral hemispheres to the venous sinuses, due to displacement of brain esp. brainstem inside the skull. Usually the superior cerebral veins are injured, causing hemorrhage, resulting in pressure over the cerebral hemispheres, with fatal results. |
| Diagnosis | Headache |
| | Confusion |
| | Hemiplegia |
| | Coma |
| | Pupils—dilated. |
| Investigation | X-ray skull |
| | CT scan. |
| Management | Surgical treatment: |
| | Method: Burr-holes made—to expose the dura |
| | Opening of the subdural space, by incising the dura |
| | Drainage of blood and clots from subdural space |
| | After care: Patient lying flat with raised footend of bed to help in expansion of the brain. |
| Prognosis | The results are remarkable, if the surgery is performed before the formation of midbrain cone. |

**Refer:** The patient to the surgical and neurosurgical team for surgery.

## Chest injuries: Described in ATLS management

### Abdominal Injuries

| | |
|---|---|
| Types | Blunt injuries |
| | Perforated (rupture) injuries. |
| MOI | Direct violence—hitting with a stick/rod/stone, stabbing, gunshot RSA |
| | Fall from a height. |
| Diagnosis | Signs of abdominal injuries are usually concealed and may require repeated examinations |
| General S/S | Pain, local tenderness, abdominal rigidity, shifting dullness |
| | Liver dullness—abstinence |

| | |
|---|---|
| | Bruise over the abdominal wall or wound—may/or may not |
| | Internal hemorrhage—increasing pallor, restlessness, air-hunger, rising pulse, hypothermia, hypotension. |
| Local S/S | Liver—local tenderness, shifting dullness and increased area of liver dullness |
| | Spleen—local tenderness, muscle guard, shifting dullness, pain radiating to left shoulder |
| | Kidney—fullness, shifting dullness, tenderness, hematuria |
| | UB—local tenderness, shifting dullness, peritonitis |
| | Stomach and small intestine—pain over epigastrium, vomiting, hemoptysis, local tenderness, muscle guard, shifting dullness |
| | Large intestine—peritonitis, surgical emphysema. |
| Investigation | Ryle's tube aspiration |
| | Hemogram |
| | Blood grouping and cross matching |
| | Blood urea |
| | Serum electrolytes |
| | Serum proteins |
| | Urinalysis—catheterization to measure urine output |
| | P/R—may show bleeding or a hematoma (boggy swelling) |
| | P/V (if required as necessary)—may show bleeding |
| | X-ray pelvis—to rule out pelvic fractures |
| | CXR (sitting)—may show gas under the diaphragm |
| | Plain X-ray abdomen—may show loss of psoas shadow and gas in the peritoneum |
| | KUB |
| | IVU—in suspected renal injury |
| | Ultrasound—confirms diagnosis |
| | CT scan—confirms diagnosis but time consuming |
| | Diagnostic laparotomy |
| | Diagnostic laparoscopy. |
| Management | Emergency: |
| | Oxygen |
| | IV fluids—normal saline |
| | Blood transfusion |
| | Nasogastric (Ryle's) tube—for gastric aspiration |
| | Catheterization of bladder |
| Surgery | Laparotomy as an emergency procedure |
| | Aim: To control the hemorrhage |
| | Method: Repair: |
| | • Stomach: Repair of the perforation |
| | • Small intestine rupture: Simple closure of the perforation |
| | • Large intestine rupture: |
| |    – Exteriorization is procedure of choice |
| |    – Closure of perforation followed by colostomy |

- Mesentery laceration: Resection of lacerated portion
- Liver: Repair of the liver tear by mattress sutures parallel to tear
- Kidney rupture:
  - Repair of the perforation
  - Nephrectomy: Indicated in severely damaged kidney, provided the contralateral kidney is healthy
- Ureter rupture:
  - Ureteroureteric anastomosis for injury of one ureter
  - Nephrostomy (bilateral) for bilateral injury

Spleen rupture:
- Repair of perforation
- Spleenectomy.

Buttock rupture: That may occur due to turning of the seriously injured patient.
- Debidement: To be undertaken first, in order to avoid hypotension
**Refer:** The patient to the surgical team.

| | |
|---|---|
| **Shock** | **It is the effect of a threat to existence,** is a clinical state characterized by a sudden fall in the systolic blood pressure below 90 mm Hg. |
| **Etiology and mechanism:** | Variable, while the most important and consistent abnormality is the decreased circulating blood volume due to: <br> • External blood loss <br> • Internal hemorrhage into body cavities <br> • Extravasation of blood or plasma into damaged tissue due to trauma. |
| Pathogenesis | Hemorrhagic shock: <br> • Vasodilatation (loss of blood volume; low cardiac output; hypotension; impaired perfusion pressure of oxygen into tissues esp. brain and heart): followed by protective: <br> • Vasoconstriction (Nature's first aid): To maintain peripheral vascular resistance, arterial pressure, and the oxygen perfusion of the vital organs; persisting threat (unchecked or untreated) leading to anoxic brainstem and cardiac muscle; multiple organs failure; death. |
| Diagnosis | Restlessness <br> Respiration: Deep sighing (air hunger) <br> Skin: Cold, pale, sweating, empty veins <br> Thirst <br> Tinnitus <br> Eyes: Blindness <br> Pulse: Rate increased <br> Hypotension <br> Unconsciousness <br> Convulsions <br> Cardiac arrest <br> Death. |
| Management | Top priority (ASAP). <br> Aim: Removal of cause and replacement of blood volume (loss). |

Measures:

- Posture: Raising foot end of bed
- Oxygen (put patient on ventilator if available)
- Hemorrhage: Arrest of hemorrhage + blood transfusion
- Burns: Plasma transfusion + blood transfusion + dextran + antibiotics
- Analgesics: Morphia 10–15 mg IV or IM (to be avoided in head injury)
- Sedatives: Phenobarbitone IV in a frightened patient
- Vasoconstrictors to be given early, as given late may cause renal and hepatic failure:
  Drugs: Methedrine 15 mg + Noradrenaline 4 mg/L of IV fluid
  Hydrocortisone 100 mg may be added to IV fluid
- Immobilization of the injured limb

## Spinal Injuries: Described in Appropriate Chapter of Fractures

| | |
|---|---|
| Preface | Always consider the possibility of spinal injury while managing patients with: |
| | Major trauma: due to RSA/fall from height, |
| | Semi/unconsciousness, |
| | Neurological deficit. |
| | Sites: commonest sites: Cervical spine and dorsolumbar region. |
| | Types: Stable and unstable injuries: |
| | A. Stable injuries: |
| |   • Posterior ligament complex and neural arch intact |
| |   • Wedge (< 20) fractures—commonest thoracolumbar injuries |
| | B. Unstable injuries: |
| |   • Posterior ligament complex torn with/or without fracture of neural arch or facet joints |
| |   • Wedge (> 20 degree or collapse of anterior margin—less than half of the posterior margin) fractures. |
| MOI | Fall from a height |
| | Diving in shallow water |
| | Fall of heavy weight on the back |
| | RSA. |
| Mechanism of injury | Forces: Flexion, flexion rotation, hyperextension forces result in: Sprains, fractures, dislocations, fracture dislocations, and paraplegia, depending upon the violence. |
| **Management** | **Stable fractures:** |
| | Admit the patient |
| | Bedrest for 1/52 |
| | Analgesics |
| | Physiotherapy—extension exercises for 4–6/52 |
| | Allowed up and home at 4–6/52. |

**Unstable fractures with/or without neurological deficit:**

**First aid treatment:**

Airway maintenance: endotracheal intubation, or tracheostomy

Bleeding control

Drugs—Analgesics, antipyretics

Spinal immobilization:

- Apply skull traction, maintaining traction, neck is slowly extended.
- Support neck with sand bags/or apply a hard collar.
- Continue with traction.

Definitive treatment:

- Continuous observation—to detect onset of complications, e.g. cord damage, and to treat accordingly
- Monitor the pulse, BP, respiration
- Nursing care—to combat any neural lesion
- Catheterization—to relieve a distended bladder
- Dislocations/subluxation to be reduced by closed reduction (manipulation or traction) or by open reduction and internal fixation.

Surgical treatment: Refer the patient to the orthopedic and surgical team for surgery:

Surgery    Arthrodesis: If no neurological deficit.

If paraplegia: Then arthrodesis is not required.

After care: Apply a cervical collar after 4/52.

**Sprains of spine (Whiplash):**Described in appropriate Chapter of Fractures.

**Dislocations:**Described in appropriate Chapter of Fractures.

**Dislocation between atlas (C1) and axis (C2):**Described in appropriate Chapter of Fractures.

**Fractures of spine:**Described in appropriate Chapter of Fractures.

**Regional spine Injuries**

*Cervical spine injuries:* Described in appropriate Chapter of Fractures.

**Fractures of thoracic and lumbar spine:**Described in appropriate Chapter of Fractures.

**Spinal cord injury:**Described in appropriate Chapter of Fractures.

**Neurological assessment:**Described in appropriate Chapter of Fractures.

**Dorsal and lumbar injuries:**Described in appropriate Chapter of Fractures.

**Peripheral nerve injuries:**Described in appropriate Chapter of Peripheral Nerve Injuries.

**Brachial plexus injuries:**Described in appropriate Chapter of Fractures.

Described in appropriate Chapter of Peripheral Nerve Injuries.

**Upper lesion (Erb – Duchen):**Described in appropriate Chapter of Fractures.

Described in appropriate Chapter of Peripheral Nerve Injuries.

**Lower lesion (Klumpke)**

Described in appropriate Chapter of Fractures.

Described in appropriate Chapter of Peripheral Nerve Injuries.

## Management of Fractures of Limbs

**Preface**          In multiple injuries, it may be difficult to select particular methods of treatment, esp. in cases where multiple fractures occur in the same limb. It may be difficult to follow the principles of reduction and fixation.

**Management**       First aid treatment: Immobilization—by use of splints, or traction, to reduce pain and hemorrhage

Compound fractures—covered with sterile dressing pads, to prevent/control infection

Assessment-clinically and radiologically of fracture, e.g. site, pattern, displacement, angulation, rotation, and shortning to be noted

Recording of involvement of skin, nerves, and blood vessels.

### Local (definitive) treatment of fractures:

Principles:

- Reduction of fracture
- Immobilization (fixation)
- Rehabilitation.

### Reduction of fractures:

Anesthesia: Under general or local anesthesia reduction of displacement, angulation, or rotation of fragments is achieved.

Types: Closed or open reduction.

Methods: By traction force (manual)

- By manipulation with hands
- By continuous traction: skin or skeletal traction.

### Immobilization (fixation):

A. External fixation by:

- Splints: Thomas or Brawn splints
- Plaster of paris
- Traction: Fixed traction in a Thomas splint
- External fixators (Ilizarov).

B. Internal fixation by:

- Screws: Cortical and cancellous:
  - Self-tapping—Sherman and Lane
  - Require pretapping—AO series
- Plate and screws
- Intramedullary nailing
- Interlocking nailing
- Rush nails
- Tension wires, percutaneous wires
- Prosthesis, replacement arthroplasty.

### Rehabilitation:

Aim: To send back the patient to his/her work, at the earliest possible.

### Measures:

Physiotherapy

## Resuscitation in Trauma

MOI     Direct violence

       RSA

       Fall from height

       Sports injury

Management  Aim: As per dictum ABC:

       A. Airway and cervical spine control:

- Immobilize the cervical spine with a collar
- Head to be kept in neutral position
- Endotracheal intubation
- Cricothyroidotomy

       B. Breathing assessment/control

       C. Circulation control

- IV fluids
- Blood transfusion

       Drugs—described in appropriate section.

### Shock:

**Oxygen therapy**

**Morphia 10–15 mg. IV or IM (not s/c)**

**IV fluids**

**Blood transfusion/plasma transfusion**

**Hydrocortisone 100 mg IV**

**Methedrine IV.**

# 2

# Wounds

| | |
|---|---|
| **Definition** | It is defined as a break in the continuity of skin or mucous membrane, due to injury. It may be a cut, puncture, contusion (caused by a blow), abrasion (graze) or laceration (tear). Cuts tend to bleed. Puncture or stab wounds usually cause damage to internal organs with subsequent internal bleeding. |

## Classification

| | |
|---|---|
| Surgical | • Incised wounds<br>• Lacerated wounds<br>• Penetrating wounds<br>• Contused wounds<br>• Poisoned wounds<br>• Gunshot wounds |
| Medicolegal | Mechanical injuries:<br>• Abrasions<br>• Bruise or contusion<br>• Wounds: Incised, lacerated, penetrating, contused, poisoned, gunshot<br>• Closed injuries: Injuries to internal organs without any external injury |
| Burn injuries | • Burns<br>• Scalds<br>• Electricity and lightening injuries. |
| Pathological | • Mild/slight wounds<br>• Severe wounds<br>• Fatal/dangerous wounds<br>• Grievous wounds. |
| Age of the wounds | • Scabs formation: Within a day in case of abrasions<br>• Color changes: From the periphery 1–2 days in case of bruises<br>• Inflammation: Commences within 2–3 days in case of simple wounds<br>• Healing: Occurs within a week in case of scalp wounds<br>• Exudation of blood: Within 1–3 days in case of a fracture<br>• Granulation tissues: Appear after a week |

- Tooth injury: Bleeding stops within few hours. Cavity of the socket fills up within a week.

| | |
|---|---|
| Nature of wounds | Types: Accidental, suicidal or homicidal. |

Factors: Position, number, direction, circumstantial evidence

- Position: Suicidal wounds: Mostly found on the front and left side of the body, on account of easily accessible parts, e.g. left arm and left thigh. The direction of wound in case of upper limb is from above downwards and inwards, while in case of lower limb is from below up and inwards. The inflicted wounds are usually superficial ending in a tail and mostly parallel. Self-inflicted wounds are mostly made with malafide intentions (false charge of assault). A suicidal site may be homicidal but not the vice versa. In a case of suicide, the weapon is found grasped in the hand of victim on account of cadaveric spasm.

- Accidental wounds: Lacerated and contused wounds on the forehead are mostly accidental in nature. Wounds caused by RSA are very common these days.

- Homicidal wounds: May be found on any part of the body including on the part inaccessible to own's body, e.g. back. Deep stab wounds, lacerated and contused on the forehead, limbs and back are mostly homicidal. Severe incised wounds on the wrist, throat, breasts, genitals are mostly found to be homicidal. In case the right handed assailant attacks the victim from front, wounds are mostly inflicted on the left side of victim's body while a left handed assailant inflicts wounds on right side of victim's body. Gunshot wounds may be found on any part of the body, fired from a close or distant range. In homicidal case hair, cloth, etc. belonging to assailant may be found grasped in the victim's hand.

### Number:
- Suicidal wounds: Mostly multiple
- Accidental wounds: Mostly multiple
- Homicidal wounds: Mostly single.

### Direction:
- Suicidal wounds: Mostly directed from above downwards and inwards in case of upper parts of the body, while in case of lower parts of the body the direction is usually from below upwards and inwards. Suicidal stab and gunshot wounds on the cheat are usually from right to left direction.

- Accidental wounds: Mostly contused and lacerated and found on any part of the body, esp. on exposed parts. No particular direction is found in case of accident wound. Extensive body injuries (wounds) may occur in case of a fall from a height, e.g. shipyards, railway and in case of RSA.

- Homicidal wounds: Mostly multiple. Homicidal stab wounds are mostly from below upwards. They may have any direction and are mostly deep and extensive.

**Circumstantial evidence at site of accident:**

- Suicidal: Doors and windows found locked from inside, and in case the weapon found grasped in the victim's hand due to cadaveric spasm. Fingerprints of the victim on the weapon found near the body confirms the suicide. In case the body is found on a railway track without scratches and dragging marks may suggest suicide. In cut-throat wound, the hands may be found near the throat, outside the bed-sheets or blanket.
- Accidental: Doors and windows found locked from inside, and injuries might have occurred due to fall. In case the body is found on a railway track without scratches and dragging marks, may suggest accident.
- Homicidal: doors locked from outside may suggest homicide. The weapon is mostly not found on/or near the body. The weapon may be found distorted and may bear the fingerprints of the assailant and blood stains of the victim.
- Signs of struggle may be observed in the surroundings, i.e. bed, furniture, kitchenette, washroom. Footprints or finger marks of assailant/s may be observed. In cut-throat wound, the hands may be hidden under the bed sheets or blankets. Clothes of victim may be torn or stained with blood, mud or grease.

## INCISED WOUNDS

| | |
|---|---|
| Etiology | Injury by a sharp cutting instrument, e.g. knife, razor, safety razor/saw blades, sword, axe. |
| MOI | Direct trauma: Striking, sawing and drawing |
| Types | • Accidental: inflicted by razor, safety razor blades, knife, fish knife, on any part of the body esp. hands and fingers. Self-inflicted wounds are mostly slight in nature and found in accessible parts of the body. These are more or less parallel to each other and are mostly self-inflicted to blame someone with malafide intentions. |
| | • Suicidal: Wounds deeper at beginning and shallow at the end called tailing (scratch) inflicted by razor, knife, mostly self-inflicted on the wrists, throat, abdomen and chest. The tail reflects which hand been used. |
| | • Homicidal: Wounds of greater severity, inflicted by knife, razor blade, axe, sword or daos, mostly on the neck, chest, abdomen or head. The may also be seen on victim's hand or forearm, while attempting to ward off the attack. The tail reflects the relative positioning of the attacker and the victim. |
| Instruments | • Light cutting: Razor, knife—by means of striking, drawing or sawing |
| | • Heavy cutting: Swords, axes, choppers |
| | • Curved: Sickles, daos |
| PM findings | • Hemorrhage |
| | • Wound: |
| |    – Shape: Spindle |
| |    – Size: Length > breadth and depth |

        – Edges: Clean-cut, regular, everted, or irregular and inverted (neck and crotum)

        – Gaping: More in case of division of underneath muscles

| | |
|---|---|
| Medicolegal aspect | That whether the wounds are accidental, suicidal or homicidal |

## LACERATED WOUNDS

| | |
|---|---|
| Etiology | Inflicted by a hard and blunt instrument, e.g. swords, axes, daos and choppers. |
| MOI | Direct trauma: striking, tearing<br>RSA<br>Industrial accidents<br>Fall from a height on a sharp object |
| Types | • Accidental: Inflicted by fall from a height, RSA, on any part of the body esp. hands and fingers<br>• Suicidal: Wounds very rare, self-inflicted by lunatics on the wrists, throat, abdomen and chest<br>• Homicidal: Wounds of greater severity, inflicted by hard and blunt weapons, e.g. axe, sword or daos, mostly on the neck, chest, abdomen or head. |
| Instruments | • Hard and blunt: Swords, axes, choppers<br>• Curved: Sickles, daos |
| PM findings | • Hemorrhage < in an incised wound<br>• Wound:<br>  – Shape: Spindle<br>  – Size: Length > breadth and depth<br>  – Edges: Irregular, ragged and inverted |
| | Tissues: Torn and not cut as in incised wounds<br>• Bruises or contusions: Of adjacent parts<br>• Prone to infections, e.g. tetanus, gas gangrene, infective organisms. |
| Medicolegal aspect | • That whether the wounds are lacerated ones?<br>• That whether the wounds are accidental, suicidal or homicidal? |

## PENETRATING (PUNCTURED) WOUNDS

| | |
|---|---|
| Etiology | Inflicted by sharp pointed instruments, e.g. knives, daggers, swords, rifle bayonets, peck-axes, arrows, sickles broken glass pieces, nailings or sharp horns of wild animals. |
| MOI | Direct trauma: Striking, tearing<br>RSA<br>Industrial accidents<br>Fall from a height on a sharp object |
| Types | • Accidental: Inflicted by fall on a sharp projecting object, RSA, needle-pricks on any part of the body esp. hands and fingers<br>• Suicidal: Wounds very rare, self-inflicted by lunatics on the accessible parts of the body, e.g. wrists, throat, abdomen and chest |

|                    | • Homicidal: Wounds of greater severity, inflicted by on the neck, chest, abdomen or head. |

| PM findings | • Hemorrhage: External and internal |
| | • Wound: Notoriously deceptive. Penetrating wounds of the abdomen may be symptomless until internal hemorrhage or peritonitis reveals injured blood vessels or viscera. |
| | • Edges: Clean-cut or ragged and inverted at entrance and everted at exit site |
| | • Tissues: Torn and not cut as in incised wounds |
| | • Bruises or contusions of adjacent parts |
| Medicolegal aspect | • That whether the wounds are penetrating or punctured one? |
| | • That whether the wounds are accidental, suicidal or homicidal? |

## CONTUSED WOUNDS

| Etiology | RSA |
| --- | --- |
| MOI | Direct trauma: Striking |
| | RSA |
| | Industrial accidents |
| | Fall from a height |
| Types | • Accidental: Inflicted by fall from a height, RSA, on any part of the body esp. back and buttocks, hands and fingers |
| | • Suicidal: Wounds very rare, self-inflicted by jumping from a height, on the accessible parts of the body, e.g. wrists, throat, abdomen and chest |
| | • Homicidal: Wounds of greater severity, inflicted by on the neck, chest, abdomen or head |
| PM findings | • Hemorrhage |
| | • Wound: May be symptomless until internal hemorrhage or peritonitis reveals injured blood vessels, muscles or viscera. |
| | • Edges: Ragged and everted |
| | • Tissues: Pressed |
| | • Bruises or contusions of adjacent parts |
| Medicolegal aspect | • That whether the wounds are contused one? |
| | • That whether the wounds are accidental, suicidal or homicidal? |

## POISONED WOUNDS

| Etiology | Inflicted by bites of wasps or bees, dog, cat, horse, camel, jackal, snake or human beings. |
| --- | --- |
| Types | • Accidental: Common amongst picknickers inflicted by bites of wasps or bees, dog, cat, horse, camel, jackal, snake or human beings, on the exposed parts, e.g. face, neck, arms, legs |
| | • Suicidal: Self-inflicted by handling (disturbing) wasps, bees, dog, cat, horse, camel on the accessible (exposed) parts of the body, e.g. hands, fingers, arms, legs, face and neck |
| | • Homicidal: Inflicted by exposing (forcing) to poisonous snakes, scorpions, wasps, bees, ferocious dogs. |

| Cause of death | • Anaphylactic shock |
| --- | --- |
| | • Vasomotor collapse |
| PM findings | • Hemorrhage: External and internal |
| | • Wound: Notoriously deceptive. Penetrating wounds of the abdomen may be symptomless until internal hemorrhage or peritonitis reveals injured blood vessels or viscera. |
| | • Edges: Clean-cut or ragged and inverted at entrance and everted at exit site |
| | • Tissues: Torn and not cut as in incised wounds |
| | • Bruises or contusions of adjacent parts |
| Medicolegal aspect | • That whether the wounds are penetrating or punctured one? |
| | • That whether the wounds are accidental, suicidal or homicidal? |

## GUNSHOT WOUNDS

| Etiology | Inflicted by sharp projectiles discharged from firearms. |
| --- | --- |
| Motives | Suicidal: |
| | • Depression, feeling of shame, remorse, anger, failure in examination |
| | • Domestic conflicts |
| | • Disappointed love affairs |
| | • Insanity |
| | • Homicidal: |
| | ▪ Property disputes |
| | ▪ Disputable sexual affairs |
| | • Murder of wife for adultery or infidelity |
| | • Murder of a girl or young woman after rape |
| | • Murder of an elderly woman before rape |
| | • Murder of a woman followed by Necrophilia or Necrophagia (sexual perversions) |
| | • Murder of illegitimate newborn babies |
| | • Murder of newborn babies for inheritance. |
| MOI | Depends on: |
| | • Projectile's type: At the time of impact |
| | • Projectile's velocity: At the time of impact |
| | • Projectile's distance of the firearm from the victim at the moment of discharge |
| | • Projectile's angle: At which the projectile struck the body. |
| Types of projectiles | Round and cone shaped bullets. |
| | • Round bullets: Inflict greater damage, with bruising and lacerations of adjoining parts |
| | • Conical bullets: Inflict wounds of entry and exit, without any bruising or laceration. |
| Velocity of projectiles | |
| | • High and low velocity bullets. |
| | • High velocity bullets: Clean, circular, punched out opening at the entry, with splintering of the intervening bone |

Distance of projectiles

- Close to or at a distance from the victim's body.
- Close to body: At the entry, the adjacent area is lacerated and blackened, single entry
- At a distance: At the entry, no laceration or blackening of adjacent area
- 30 to 90 cm: Single entry, adjacent area blackened
- 180 cm: Central entry surrounded by multiple openings made by pellets
- 360 cm: Multiple openings made by pellets.

Angle of projectiles: Direct: inflict greater damage, while at angle inflict lesser damage.

Scattering of pellets: Depends on:

- Size of the firearm
- Distance of the firearm from the victim's body
- Powder's charging.

Types

- Accidental: Inflicted on any part of the body—self-inflicted always on front, but on any part of the body when inflicted by another person
- Suicidal: Wound self-inflicted on the accessible parts of the body, e.g. temple, inside the mouth, under the chin or chest, blackening of the adjacent area
- Homicidal: inflicted on any part of the body, multiple wounds of greater severity. Mostly the firearm is missing from the site of violence, and may be fired from a close or distance range.

Cause of death

- Hemorrhage: external (revealed) and internal (concealed)
- Shock
- Injury to vital organs, e.g. heart, lungs, liver, spleen, brain, blood vessels.

PM findings

- Case circumstances
- Nature of violence
- Hemorrhage—external and internal
- Wound:
  - Type: Accidental, suicidal or homicidal
  - Number: Single or multiple
  - Size: Length, breadth, depth and direction
  - Edges: Clean-cut or ragged and inverted at entrance and everted at exit site
  - Tissues: Torn and not cut as in incised wounds
  - Bruises or contusions of adjacent parts
  - Garments: Stained and torn

Antemortem vs postmortem wounds (Table 2.1).

## CIRCUMSTANTIAL EVIDENCE (CE)

Definition

It is defined as an important factor in determining the murderer, motive, victim, place of murder and the type of weapon used in the crime.

| Table 2.1: Antemortem vs postmortem wounds | | |
|---|---|---|
| | *Antemortem wounds* | *Postmortem wounds* |
| Hemorrhage | Severe—arteria | Slight—venous |
| Blood | Clotted | Not clotted |
| Wound | Edges—gape, stained | Edges—do not gape, not stained |
| Tissues | Inflammed | Noninflammed |

| | |
|---|---|
| Evidence | • Doors and windows found bolted/closed from inside: Suggestive of suicide |
| | • Doors and windows found bolted/closed from outside: Suggestive of homicide |
| | • Body found on railway tracks: Suggestive of accident, suicide or homicide |
| | • Weapon: Found near the body, may be bloodstained |
| | • Weapon: Not found near the body—suggestive of homicide. |
| Medicolegal aspect | • That whether the death sustained by firearm? |
| | • That whether the wounds are accidental, suicidal or homicidal? |
| | • That what about the age of the injury? |

# MEDICOLEGAL WOUNDS

## Mechanical Injuries

### Abrasions

| | |
|---|---|
| Definition | It is defined as an area on the surface of the skin, damaged or injured by being rubbed too hard. |
| Etiology | Direct violence: Finger nails or teeth bite |
| | RSA |
| PM findings | Bruise may be antemortem or postmortem: |
| | • Antemortem bruises: |
| | – Injured part swollen and discolored |
| | – Eextravasation of blood and infiltration in tissues. |
| | • Postmortem bruises: Injured part mostly not swollen and discoloured, even with major violence. |
| Medicolegal aspect | • That whether the abrasions are due to slight or major violence? |
| | • That whether the abrasions accidental, suicidal or homicidal? |

## BRUISE OR CONTUSION

| | |
|---|---|
| Definition | It is defined as surface discoloration and swelling resulting from a blow or pressure. Also being called contusion. Bruises are mostly simple wounds. |
| Etiology | Direct violence: Fist, blows or kicks: hit by a stick, brick or stone |
| | RSA |
| Pathogenesis | Lacerartion of soft tissues (subcutaneous tissues or blood vessels, etc.), leading to exravasation of blood. |

| Types | • Superficial bruise: Occurs at the seat of violence within a short-time of injury (few mts). It may appear much earlier if the skin involved is thin (eyelids, nipple, scrotum and back of hands). |
| | • Deep bruise: Occurs away from the seat of violence mostly after a period of few days. |
| | Examples: Black eye produced by a blow on the face or a fall on the vertex |
| Site and extent | Depend on: |
| | • Severity of violence |
| | • Vascularity of the injured part |
| | • Blood vessels: Arteriosclerosed vessels rupture easily |
| | • Looseness of adjoining tissues |
| Shape | Depends on shape of the used weapon: |
| | • Irregular—by a stone |
| | • Elongated—by a lathi/stick blow |
| | • Round—by a hammer strike |
| Age | Depends on color changes of the extravasated blood: |
| | • Red—immediately after the injury |
| | • Iolet/blue—3rd day |
| | • Green—5th day |
| | • Yellow—7th day |
| | • Gades away: 14th day |
| PM findings | • No signs of bleeding: dry surface |
| | • No signs of inflammation: no scab formation |
| Medicolegal aspect | • That whether the bruises are due to slight or major violence? |
| | • That whether the bruises are accidental, suicidal or homicidal? |
| | That whether the bruises are antemortem or postmortem? |

## Closed Wounds

| Definition | It is defined as an injury without any visible external wounds. |
| Etiology | Direct violence: Blows; hitting with a stick, base ball, mob lynching |
| | RSA |
| | Fall from height |
| Pathogenesis | Chest injuries: Heart and lungs injuries, due to fractured ribs or compression |
| | Abdomen injuries: Liver, spleen, kidneys |
| | Pelvis injuries: Urinary bladder, urethra, genitals injuries |
| | Spine injuries: PIVD, fracture dislocations of spine |
| | Limbs: Closed fractures, dislocations, sprains. |
| PM findings | • External examination: no visible external wounds. |
| | • Internal examination: |
| | Chest injury: Fractured ribs may be found, tearing heart or/and lungs |

**Abdomen injury:**
- Liver rupture: Commonest injury due to its large size and relatively unprotected
- Splenic rupture: Relatively unprotected, large size
- Kidneys: Target esp. In back injuries.

**Pelvis injury:**
- Urinary bladder: Injured esp. If full at the time of injury
- Urethra: Edematous
- Genitals: Edematous, hemorrhagic.

**Limbs injury:**
- Fractures, dislocations, swellings
- Spine injury: Fractured, dislocated or fracture-dislocation

Medicolegal aspect
- That whether the injuries are closed wounds, involving internal organs?
- That whether the injuries are accidental, suicidal or homicidal ?
- That whether injuries are the cause of death?

## BURNS AND SCALDS

Definition

Burns: It is defined as an area on the surface of the skin, damaged or injured by the dry heats—radient heat, a flame, electric current, acid/caustic throwing, or by friction, e.g. rubbing too hard of hands against hard/rough objects.

Scalds: It is defined as a burn caused by moist heats-hot liquid or steam.

Etiology
- Direct violence: Acid throwing, attack with a burning flame, gun-powder, coal-mines explosions
- Dry heat: Radiant heat, flame, electric current
- Wet heat—hot liquid or steam
- Occupation hazard: Rubbing too hard of hands against hard/rough objects, common in blacksmiths, farmers
- RSA.

Burns vs scalds (Table 2.2)

Grades

1st degree (slight): Redness alone

2nd degree (severe): Vesication alone

3rd degree (grievous): Destruction/death of the part.

Antemortem vs postmortem (burn injuries) Table (2.3).

**Table 2.2:** Burns vs scalds

|  | Burns | Scalds |
|---|---|---|
| Cause | Dry heats—flame, radiant heat, current | Moist heats—hot liquid, steam, electric |
| Blisters | Absent | Present |
| Singeing | Present | Absent of hairs |
| Skin | Bleaching or present scorching | Absent |
| Marks | Heat marks above and at site of heat application | Below and at site of heat application. Vesicles along line of liquid trickling |

| Table 2.3: Antemortem vs postmortem (burn injuries) | | |
|---|---|---|
| | *Antemortem* | *Postmortem* |
| Skin (line of redness | Present—encircling the injured (burnt) part | Absent |
| Vesication | Present—containing serous fluid. Base of vesication— red, inflamed, septic | Absent |
| Inflammation | Present | Absent |
| Internal organs | Congested, hemorrhagic | Roasted, smelly |
| Ulceration | Present | Absent |
| Mucous membranes | Bright red due to CO | Absent |

## PM Findings

**External appearance:**
- Clothings: To be removed with great caution and examined for evidence of acid, petrol, kerosene and any other combustible product
- Skin color: – Red produced by highly heated metallic object
  - White: Produced by the radiant heat
  - Black: Produced by gunpowder, coal mines explosions, kerosene oil
- Odor: Characteristic smell produced by kerosene oil
- No signs of bleeding: Dry surface
- No signs of inflammation: No scab formation
- Age: Ascertained from number of teeth and centers of ossification
- Identity (ID): Assisted by presence of foreign bodies, e.g. artificial tooth/teeth, jewelry, etc. In the ash leftover in extremely burnt bodies.

**Internal appearance:**
- Skull: May be fractured and burst open
- Brain and meninges: Inflamed and congested, extravasation of blood
- Neck: Larynx, trachea and bronchial tubes congested and frothy— asphyxia death
- Chest: Pleural congestion with serous effusion, lungs congested and Inflamed; heart filled with cherryred colored blood due to inhalation of $CO_2$.

Abdomen: Stomach and intestine inflamed, Peyer's patches ulcerated, hepatomegaly, splenomegaly, kidneys—signs of nephritis and hemorrhages.

**Medicolegal aspect:**
- That whether the burn injuries are accidental, suicidal or homicidal?
- That whether the burn injuries are antemortem or postmortem?

## ELECTRICITY AND LIGHTNING INJURIES

Definition      It is defined as an area on the surface of the skin, damaged or injured by the electric current (direct or alternating).

| Etiology | • Direct electric current—much less dangerous |
|---|---|
| | • Alternating current—more dangerous. |
| Grades | Flash (arcing) burns |
| | Flame (clotting) burns |
| | Direct heating. |
| Pathogenesis | Electrochemical cutaneous burns |
| PM findings | External appearance: |

- Clothings: To be removed with great caution and examined for evidence of electric shock
- Skin: Lesions—sharply demarcated, round or oval, grey inflammed areas, sloughing
- Odor: Absent
- No signs of bleeding: Dry surface
- Age: Ascertained from number of teeth and centers of ossification
- Identity (ID): Assisted by presence of foreign bodies, e.g. artificial tooth/teeth, jewelry, etc. In the ash leftover in extremely burnt bodies.

**Internal appearance:**
- Skull: May be fractured and burst open
- Brain and meninges: Inflamed and congested, extravasation of blood
- Neck: Larynx, trachea and bronchial tubes congested and frothy
- Chest: Pleural congestion with serous effusion, lungs congested and Inflamed; heart congested filled with blood
- Abdomen: Stomach and intestine inflamed, Peyer's patches ulcerated, hepatomegaly, splenomegaly, kidneys—signs of nephritis and hemorrhages.

**Medicolegal aspect:**
- That whether the death sustained by electric burns?
- That whether the burn injuries are accidental, suicidal or homicidal?
- That whether the burn injuries are antemortem or postmortem?

## PATHOLOGICAL WOUNDS

### Mild/Slight Wounds

| Definition | These are defined as wounds that heal in shorter time, without immobilizing a person from his/her work for > 2–3 weeks. |
|---|---|

### Severe Wounds

| Definition | These are defined as wounds that heal in longer time, thereby immobilizing a person for > 3 weeks. |
|---|---|

### Fatal/Dangerous Wounds

| Definition | These are defined as wounds that prove fatal due to the resulting serious complications, e.g. gas gangrene, tetanus, chest wounds (stab). |
|---|---|

### Grievous Wounds

| Definition | These are defined as wounds that cause a permanent damage, loss of a part, or immobilization for > 3 weeks. These wounds have the medicolegal importance. |
|---|---|

## REGIONAL WOUNDS

### Scalp Wounds

| | |
|---|---|
| Wounds | Abrasions, hematoma, contused, incised or lacerated. |
| MOI | • Fall on a hard object<br>• Direct violence: Severe blow on the head with a hard and blunt object, sharp cutting weapons. |
| Types | Suicidal, accidental or homicidal wounds. |
| Accidental | • Mode: Fall on a hard object<br>• Site: Usually top of the head<br>• Number: Usually single, occasionally multiple<br>• Depth: Usually deeper<br>• Blood trickling: Oozing<br>• Signs of struggle: Absent. |
| Suicidal | • Weapon: Usually found present at the site<br>• Site: Anyone (top, side, back or front)<br>• Number: Usually multiple severe wounds<br>• Depth: Abrasions, hematoma, contused, lacerated or incised wounds<br>• Blood trickling: Vertically down the back<br>• Signs of struggle: Usually absent<br>• Clothings: Usually stained with blood. |
| Homicidal | • Weapon: Usually heavy sharp cutting weapons, found absent from the crime<br>• Site: Usually on the top<br>• Number: Usually multiple severe lacerated or incised wounds<br>• Death: Usually instantaneous<br>• Blood trickling: Vertically down the back<br>• Signs of struggle: Usually visible<br>• Clothings: Usually stained with blood.<br>• Cause of death: Usually hemorrhage and/or brain injury. |
| Medicolegal aspect | • That whether the injuries are abrasions, hematoma, contused, incised or lacerated wounds?<br>• That whether the injuries are accidental, suicidal or homicidal?<br>• That whether injuries are the cause of death? |

## SKULL WOUNDS

| | |
|---|---|
| Wounds | Abrasions, hematoma, contused, incised or lacerated, fracture of skull. |
| MOI | • Fall on a hard object<br>• Direct violence: Severe blow on the head with a hard and blunt object, sharp cutting weapons |
| Types | Suicidal, accidental or homicidal wounds. |
| Accidental | • Mode: Fall on a hard object<br>• Site: Usually top of the head<br>• Number: Usually single, occasionally multiple<br>• Depth: Usually deeper<br>• Blood trickling: Oozing |

Suicidal
- Fracture: Usually found
- Signs of struggle: Absent.
- Weapon: Asually found present at the site
- Site: Anyone (top, side, back or front)
- Number: Usually multiple severe wounds
- Depth: Abrasions, hematoma, contused, lacerated or incised wounds
- Blood trickling: Vertically down the back
- Signs of struggle: Usually absent
- Clothings: Usually stained with blood.

Homicidal
- Weapon: Usually heavy sharp cutting weapons, found absent from the crime
- Site: Usually on the top
- Number: Usually multiple severe lacerated or incised wounds
- Death: Usually instantaneous
- Blood trickling: Vertically down the back
- Fracture: Closed or open, depressed or elevated, comminuted, bursting
- Signs of struggle: Usually visible
- Clothings: Usually stained with blood
- Cause of death: Usually hemorrhage and/or brain injury.

Medicolegal aspect
- That whether the injuries are abrasions, hematoma, contused, incised or lacerated, fracture of skull?
- That whether the injuries are accidental, suicidal or homicidal?
- That whether injuries are the cause of death?

## BRAIN WOUNDS

Wounds — Abrasions, hematoma, contused, incised or lacerated, fracture of skull.

MOI
- Fall on a hard object
- Direct violence: Severe blow on the head with a hard and blunt object, sharp cutting weapons
- RSA
- Sports injuries.

Types — Suicidal, accidental or homicidal wounds.

Accidental
- Mode: Fall on a hard object
- Site: Usually top of the head
- Number: Usually single, occasionally multiple
- Depth: Usually deeper
- Blood trickling: Oozing
- Fracture: Usually found
- Signs of struggle: Absent.

Suicidal
- Weapon: Usually found present at the site
- Site: Anyone (top, side, back or front)
- Number: Usually multiple severe wounds
- Depth: Abrasions, hematoma, contused, lacerated or incised wounds
- Blood trickling: Vertically down the back

Homicidal
- Signs of struggle: Usually absent
- Clothings: Usually stained with blood.
- Weapon: Usually heavy sharp cutting weapons, found absent from the crime
- Site: Usually on the top
- Number: Usually multiple severe lacerated or incised wounds
- Death: Usually instantaneous
- Blood trickling: Vertically down the back
- Fracture: Closed or open, depressed or elevated, comminuted, bursting
- Signs of struggle: Usually visible
- Clothings: Usually stained with blood
- Cause of death: Usually hemorrhage and/or brain injury.

Medicolegal aspect
- That whether the injuries are hematoma, contused, incised or lacerated, fracture of skull?
- That whether the injuries are accidental, suicidal or homicidal?
- That whether injuries are the cause of death?

## FACIAL WOUNDS

Wounds          Abrasions, hematoma, contused, incised or lacerated.

MOI
- RSA, fall downstairs
- Direct violence
- Severe blow on the face with fist, hitting with a hard and blunt object
- Dharp cutting weapons, gouging off the eyes with fingers or sharp objects
- Sports injury: boxing, martial arts.

Types
- Suicidal
- Accidental
- Homicidal wounds.

Accidental
- Mode: Fall on a hard object
- Site: Usually front—nose, lips, eyes, side ear
- Number: Usually single, occasionally multiple
- Depth: Usually deeper
- Blood trickling: Oozing
- Fracture: Usually found
- Signs of struggle: Absent.

Suicidal
- Weapon: Usually found present at the site
- Site: Anyone (front, or side)
- Number: Usually multiple severe wounds
- Depth: Abrasions, hematoma, contused, lacerated or incised wounds
- Blood trickling: Vertically down the cheek.
- Signs of struggle: Usually absent
- Clothings: Usually stained with blood.

Homicidal
- Weapon: Usually heavy sharp cutting weapons, found from the crime

- Site: Usually front or side
- Number: Usually multiple severe lacerated or incised wounds
- Death: Usually instantaneous
- Blood trickling: Vertically down the cheek
- Fracture: Nasal, orbital, maxilla, mandible, closed or open
- Signs of struggle: Usually visible
- Clothings: Usually stained with blood
- Cause of death: Usually hemorrhage and/or brain injury.

Medicolegal aspect
- That whether the injuries are abrasions, hematoma, contused, incised or lacerated, fracture of nose, mandible or maxilla?
- That whether the injuries are accidental, suicidal or homicidal?
- That whether injuries are the cause of death?

## NECK WOUNDS

Wounds
- Abrasions, hematoma, contused, incised or lacerated, fracture of spine

MOI
- RSA, fall on a hard object
- Direct violence: Severe blow on the neck with a hard and blunt object, sharp cutting weapons, judicial hanging or hanging by long dropping

Types
- Suicidal, accidental or homicidal wounds.

Accidental
- Mode: RSA, fall on a hard object
- Site: Usually lower part moreso on one side
- Number: Usually single, occasionally multiple
- Depth: Usually deeper
- Blood trickling: Oozing
- Fracture: Usually found
- Signs of struggle: Usually present.

Suicidal
- Weapon: Usually found present at the site
- Site: Anyone (top, side, back or front)
- Number: Usually multiple severe wounds
- Depth: Abrasions, hematoma, contused, lacerated or incised wounds
- Blood trickling: Vertically down the back
- Signs of struggle: Usually absent
- Clothings: Usually stained with blood.

Homicidal
- Weapon: Usually heavy sharp cutting weapons, found from the crime site
- Site: Usually front or sides
- Number: Usually multiple severe lacerated or incised wounds
- Death: Usually instantaneous
- Blood trickling: Vertically down the front, back or side.
- Fracture, fracture dislocation: Closed or open, comminuted, bursting
- Signs of struggle: Usually visible
- Clothings: Usually stained with blood.
- Cause of death: Usually from shock, syncope, asphyxia, hemorrhage, air embolism, pneumonia, and/or spinal cord injury.

| Medicolegal | • That whether the injuries are abrasions, hematoma, contused, aspect incised or lacerated, fracture of skull? |
|---|---|
| | • That whether the injuries are accidental, suicidal or homicidal? |
| | • That whether injuries are the cause of death? |

## CUT THROAT WOUNDS

| Dangers | Usually dangerous on account of involvement of adjoining unprotected vital structures. Main dangers are: |
|---|---|
| | • Hemorrhage from torn carotid artery and jugular veins |
| | • Asphyxia from torn larynx and trachea |
| | • Death: Occurs from asphyxia. |
| Types | Suicidal, accidental or homicidal wounds. |
| Suicidal | • Weapon: Usually sharp cutting weapons |
| | • Site: Above Pomum Adami |
| | • Direction: Usually with the head extended—more or less transverse |
| | • Position: Wound on the side of neck lies facing the hand used, e.g. on the right side when left hand used and vice versa |
| | • Number: Usually single, may be multiple—amongst these on may be the severe wound |
| | • Depth: Wound deeper at the start, but tails off at the end |
| | • Blood trickling: Vertically down the front or side of neck, in case of standing or sitting posture |
| | • Signs of struggle: Absent |
| | • Clothings: Usually intact. |
| Accidental | • Weapon: Usually sharp cut glass in case of RSA and fall from height over sharp object |
| | • Site: Not specific |
| | • Direction: Not particular |
| | • Number: Usually multiple |
| | • Depth: Usually deeper |
| | • Clothings: Usually torn and stained. |
| Homicidal | • Weapon: Usually heavy sharp cutting weapons, found absent from the crime |
| | • Site: Usually below Pomum Adami |
| | • Direction: From down upwards or horizontal |
| | • Position: Horizontal and from left to right by right handed assailant, while horizontal and from right to left by left handed assailant |
| | • Number: Usually multiple severe wounds dividing soft tissues up to vertebrae |
| | • Death: Usually instantaneous |
| | • Blood trickling: Vertically down the back |
| | • Signs of struggle: Usually visible |
| | • Clothings: Usually cuts in the clothing found. |
| Medicolegal aspect | • Cause of death: Usually from shock, syncope, asphyxia, hemorrhage, air embolism, pneumonia, and/or spinal cord injury. |

## SPINE AND SPINAL CORD WOUNDS

| | |
|---|---|
| Wounds | Abrasions, hematoma, contused, incised or lacerated, fracture of spine. |
| MOI | • RSA, fall on a hard object |
| | • Direct violence: Severe blow on the neck or lower back, with a hard and blunt object, sharp cutting weapons |
| Types | Suicidal, accidental or homicidal wounds. |
| Accidental | • Mode: Fall on a hard object |
| | • Site: Usually cervical, dorsolumbar or upper lumbar |
| | • Number: Usually single, occasionally multiple |
| | • Depth: Usually deeper |
| | • Blood trickling: Oozing |
| | • Fracture: Usually found |
| | • Signs of struggle: Absent. |
| Suicidal | • Weapon: Usually found present at the site |
| | • Site: Front or side |
| | • Number: Usually multiple severe wounds |
| | • Depth: Abrasions, hematoma, contused, lacerated or incised wounds |
| | • Blood trickling: Vertically down the front or back |
| | • Signs of struggle: Usually absent |
| | • Clothings: Usually stained with blood. |
| Homicidal | • Weapon: Usually heavy sharp cutting weapons, found absent from the crime |
| | • Site: Anywhere (back, side or front) |
| | • Number: Usually multiple severe lacerated or incised wounds |
| | • Death: Usually instantaneous |
| | • Blood trickling: Vertically down the back |
| | • Fracture, fracture dislocation: Closed or open, comminuted, bursting |
| | • Signs of struggle: Usually visible |
| | • Clothings: Usually stained with blood |
| | • Cause of death: Usually hemorrhage and/or cord injury. |
| Medicolegal aspect | • That whether the injuries are abrasions, hematoma, contused, incised or lacerated, fracture of spine? |
| | • That whether the injuries are accidental, suicidal or homicidal? |
| | • That whether injuries are the cause of death? |

## CHEST WOUNDS

| | |
|---|---|
| Wounds | Abrasions, bruises, contused, incised, penetrating or perforating, the lacerated, and rib fractures. |
| MOI | • RSA, fall from a height, fall of a heavy weight |
| | • Direct violence: Severe blow on the chest with fist or a hard and blunt object, stab wounds from sharp cutting weapons or broken ribs, bullet or explosive. |
| Types | Suicidal, accidental or homicidal wounds, simple or compound wounds. |
| Accidental | • Mode: RSA, fall from a height, fall of a heavy weight |
| | • Site: Usually front of the chest wall |

- Number: Usually single, occasionally multiple
- Depth: Usually deeper
- Blood trickling: Oozing
- Fracture: Ribs usually found
- Signs of struggle: Absent.

Suicidal
- Weapon: Usually found present at the site
- Site: Anyone (front, side or back)
- Number: Usually multiple severe wounds
- Depth: Abrasions, hematoma, contused, lacerated or incised wounds
- Blood trickling: Vertically down the front
- Signs of struggle: Usually absent
- Clothings: Usually stained with blood.

Homicidal
- Weapon: Usually heavy blunt or sharp cutting weapons, at the crime site
- Site: Usually the front
- Number: Usually multiple severe lacerated or incised wounds
- Death: Usually instantaneous
- Blood trickling: Vertically down the front
- Fracture: Closed or open, depressed or elevated, comminuted, bursting
- Signs of struggle: Usually visible
- Clothings: Usually stained with blood
- Cause of death: Usually hemorrhage, shock and cardiopulmonary failure.

Medicolegal aspect
- That whether the injuries are abrasions, hematoma, contused, incised or lacerated, fracture of ribs?
- That whether the injuries are accidental, suicidal or homicidal?
- That whether injuries are the cause of death?

## ABDOMEN WOUNDS

Wounds      Abrasions, bruises, contused, incised, penetrating or perforating, lacerated, and fracture pelvis.

MOI
- RSA, fall from a height, fall of a heavy weight
- Direct violence: Severe blow on the abdomen with a fist or hard and blunt object, sharp cutting weapons

Types
- Suicidal, accidental or homicidal wounds.
- Penetrating or nonpenetrating wounds

Accidental
- Mode: RSA, fall from a height, fall of a heavy weight
- Site: Usually front
- Number: Usually single, occasionally multiple
- Depth: Usually deeper
- Blood trickling: Oozing
- Fracture: Usually absent
- Signs of struggle: Absent.

Suicidal
- Weapon: Usually found from the crime site
- Site: Usually front

- Number: Usually multiple severe wounds
- Depth: Abrasions, hematoma, contused, lacerated or incised wounds
- Blood trickling: Vertically down the front
- Signs of struggle: Usually absent
- Clothings: Usually stained with blood.

**Homicidal**    Weapon: Usually heavy sharp cutting weapons, found absent from the crime

- Site: Usually on the top
- Number: Usually multiple severe lacerated or incised wounds
- Death: Usually instantaneous from penetrating wounds
- Blood trickling: Vertically down
- Fracture: Closed or open
- Signs of struggle: Usually visible
- Clothings: Usually stained with blood.
- Cause of death: Usually hemorrhage and/or brain injury.

**PM findings**    External appearance:

- Clothings: To be removed with great caution and examined for evidence of violence, staining with blood, semen, vomitus, etc.
- Skin: Coloration, dry or moistlesions, sloughing, etc. sloughing
- Odor: Present or absent
- Signs of bleeding: Present or absent
- Age: Ascertained from number of teeth and centres of ossification
- Identity (ID): Assisted by presence of foreign bodies, e.g. artificial tooth/teeth, jewelry, etc. In the ash leftover in extremely burnt bodies.

**Internal**    Skull:
**appearance**

- May be fractured—simple or compound, comminuted, depressed or raised, guttered or bursting
- Brain injury: Compressed, hemorrhage—extradural or subdural

**Brain and**
**meninges**

- Injuries: Lacerated, penetrating or perforating, incised wounds
- Hemorrhage: Extradural, subdural, and or intracerebral
- Compressed, inflamed and congested, extravasation of blood

**Face**

- Wounds: Bitting, cutting of nose, cheeks, lips, ears, lacerated or incised
- Teeth: Dislocated or uprooted

**Neck**

- Wounds: Abrasions or bruises (throttling), lacerated (judicial hanging or hanging) incised, punctured
- Larynx, trachea and bronchial tubes congested and frothy Spine and Spinal cord
- Fractures and fracture dislocations: Cervical, lower dorsal or dorso-lumbar
- Spinal cord injury: $C_2$—fatal due to injured medulla and cord.

**Chest**

- Heart: Penetrating or punctured (stabbing, bullet) wounds—fatal, congested

|  |  |
|---|---|
|  | • Ribs: Fractures |
|  | • Pleural congestion with serous effusion, lungs congested and inflamed. |
| Abdomen | • Wounds: Nonpenetrating (RSA, fall from a height) or penetraing (sharp cutting objects, tools, bullets) |
|  | • Extravasation of blood: May be present in the muscles or cellular tissues |
|  | • Rupturing of internal organs may be found. |

**Stomach**    MOI:
- Nonperforating: RSA, fall from a height, blow with a fist or a stick
- Perforating: Stab or gunshot wounds, fall from a height over a shar object, corrosive poisons—strong acids/alkalies.

Site: Usual sites are pyloric antrum, anterior surface near the lesser curvature

Rupture: Spontaneous

Death: Usually from shock, hemorrhage or peritonitis.

**Intestines**    MOI:
- Nonperforating: RSA, fall from a height, blow with a fist/a stick, kick
- Perforating: Stab or gunshot wounds, fall from a height over a sharp object, corrosive poisons—strong acids/alkalies.

Site: Usual sites are anterior surface of duodenum, jejunum and ileum

Rupture: Usually intra- or extraperitoneal

Death: Usually from shock, hemorrhage or peritonitis.

**Liver**    MOI:
- Nonperforating: RSA, fall from a height, blow with a fist or a stick
- Perforating: Stab or gunshot wounds, fall from a height over a sharp object, fractured ribs

Site: Usual sites are right lobe—outer surface and lower border

Rupture: Spontaneous

Death: Usually from shock, hemorrhage or peritonitis.

**Spleen**    MOI:
- Nonperforating: RSA, fall from a height, blow with a fist or a stick
- Perforating: Stab or gunshot wounds, fall from a height over a sharp object, diseased or enlarged spleen

Site: Usual site is inner surface (because of thinnest capsule)

Rupture: Spontaneous—accidental

Death: Usually from shock, hemorrhage or peritonitis.

**Kidneys**    MOI:
- Nonperforating: RSA, fall from a height, blow with a fist or a stick
- Perforating: Stab or gunshot wounds, fall from a height over a sharp object, fractured rib

Site: Usual site is blows upon the loin or blows from in front or crush injuries

Rupture: Usually complete tear of kidney, partial or complete avulsion from its pedicle. Tears of renal parenchyma follow the lines of the uriniferous tubules

Death: Usually from shock, hemorrhage, peritonitis or suppuration due to extravasation of urine.

**Spleen**      MOI:
- Nonperforating: RSA, fall from a height, blow with a fist or a stick
- Perforating: Stab or gunshot wounds, fall from a height over a sharp object; fracture pelvis

Site: Usual intraperitoneal

Rupture: Usually extraperitoneal (80%) while intraperitoneal (20%)

Death: Usually from shock, hemorrhage or peritonitis from the extravasation of urine in the peritoneal cavity.

**Uterus**      MOI:
- Nonperforating: RSA, fall from a height, blow with a fist or a stick
- Perforating: Stab or gunshot wounds, fall from a height over a sharp object, corrosive poisons—strong acids/alkalies.

Site: Usual sites are cesarean or operational scars

Rupture: Spontaneous during delivery

Death: Usually from shock, hemorrhage, peritonitis or septicemia.

**Vagina**      MOI:
- Fall on a projectile object
- Sexual violence (forcible rape - esp. on minor girls)
- Criminal abortion—introducing of stick, a sharp object, corrosive agent
- Obstructed labor

Site: Usual sites are walls

Rupture: Spontaneous

Death: Usually from shock, hemorrhage septic cellulitis.

**Vulva**      MOI:
- Fall on a projectile object
- Sexual violence (forcible rape - esp. on minor girls, by penetration of a large sized penis)
- Criminal abortion—introducing of stick, a sharp object, corrosive agent (inflicted as a punishment/management for adultery and the infidelity).
- Obstructed labor

Site: Anywhere

Rupture: Spontaneous

Death: Usually from shock, hemorrhage or septic cellulitis.

**Urethra**      MOI:
- Fall on a projectile object
- Fracture pelvis

- Sexual violence (forcible rape - esp. on minor girls, by penetration of a large sized penis)
- Criminal abortion—introducing of stick, a sharp object, corrosive agent
- Obstructed labor

Rupture: Spontaneous

Death: Usually from shock, hemorrhage or septic cellulitis.

**Penis**

MOI:
- Accidental: Fall astride a projecting object, cycling accidents
- Direct violence—kicking, hitting with a stick/baseball, sexual violence
- Perforating: Stab or gunshot wounds, fall from a height over a sharp object

Site: Usual sites are bulbous urethra and membranous (intrapelvic)

Rupture: Spontaneous

Death: Usually from shock, hemorrhage or peritonitis due to extravasation of urine.

**Medicolegal aspect**

- That whether the injuries are complete or incomplete, penetrating or perforating, lacerated, fracture of spine or pelvis?
- That whether the injuries are accidental, suicidal or homicidal?
- That whether injuries are the cause of death?

**Testes**

MOI:
- Accidental: Fall astride a projecting object, cycling accidents, straining at stool, lifting a heavy weight and coitus
- Direct violence—kicking, hitting with a stick/baseball, sexual violence
- Perforating: Stab or gunshot wounds, fall from a height over a sharp object

Predisposing factors: Usually inversion of the testis and rarely torsion of the testis.

Rupture: Usually the testis may be found protruding through the injured scrotum. Rarely the closed rupture of the testis from blows.

Death: Usually from shock, hemorrhage or peritonitis due to the extravasation of urine.

## Bibliography

1. Advanced Paediatric Life Support Group: Advanced Life Support: the practical approach, 3rd Ed., BMJ Books, London, 2001.
2. Bailey and Love's. Short Practice of Surgery : Cranio-Cerebral Injuries. 369–91, 13th Ed., H.K.Lewis and Co. Ltd., London, 1965.
3. Baxter CR. Emergency treatment of burn injury. Ann Emerg Med 17:1305, 1988.
4. Bohler L. The treatment of Fractures. 4th ed. Bristol; Wright, 1935.
5. British Orthopaedic Association. Memorandum on Accident Services, 1959.
6. Brown GJ, et al. Principles and Practice of Children's Emergency Care. MacLennan and Petty, Sydney, 1997.
7. Clark R. Resuscitation and Transfusion in Severe Injuries. In Modern Trends in Accident Surgery and Medicine. Ed. by R Clarke, FG Badger and S Sevitt London; Butterworths, 1959.

8. Clarke J. Late Management of Burns, Surgery Internationa 13:137, The Medicine Publishing Co. Ltd., Abingdon, OXON, 1997.

9. Colquhuon MC. Handley AJ, and Evans TR. ABC of resuscitation, ed. 4th. BMJ Books, London, 1999.

10. Coupland RM. Missile and Explosive Wounds, Surgery International 13:140–4, The Medicine Publishing Co. Ltd., Abingdon, OXON, 1997.

11. Cunningham's Manual Of Practical Anatomy, vol. I-III, 12th Ed., Oxford University Press, London, 1961.

12. Das K. Clinical Methods In Surgery, 6th Ed., Lakshman Chandra Sil, Calcutta, 1962.

13. Driscoll P, Skinner D, Earlham R. ABC of Major trauma, ed. 3rd, BMJ Books, London, 2000.

14. Edhouse J, Wardrope J. Assessment of Injured Patients. Surgery International. 13, 121–6, Medicine Publishing Co. Ltd., Oxon, 1997.

15. Evans DK. Reduction of Cervical Dislocations. J Bone Jt Surg. 43B, 552, 1961.

16. Evans R, Burke D. Key topics in Accident and Emergency Medicine, ed. 2nd, Bios Scientific Publishers, Oxford, 2001.

17. Experienced Teacher: Notes on Medical Jurisprudence and Toxicology, Current Publishers, Calcutta, 1965.

18. Eye Emergencies. Diagnosis and Management, Webb L.A., Butterworth-Heinemann, Oxford, 1995.

19. Freedlander E. Early Management of Burns, Surgery International 13:133–6. The Medicine Publishing Co. Ltd., Abingdon, OXON, 1997.

20. Gentleman D, Dearden M, Midgley S, Maclean D. Guidelines for resuscitation and transfer of patients with serious head injury. BMJ ; 307:547–52, 1993.

21. Guly HR. History Taking, Examination, and Record Keeping in Emergency Medicine, Oxford University Press, Oxford, 1996.

22. Haljamee H. The Pathophysiology of Shock. Acta Anaesthesia Scand Suppl 3–6, 1993.

23. Hill G. A&E risk management. Medical Defence Union, London, 1991.

24. Huckstep RL. A Simple Guide to Trauma, ed. 5th, Churchill Livingstone, Edinburgh, 1995.

25. Hunt J et al: Acute electrical burns: Current diagnostic and therapeutic approaches to management. Arch Surg 115:434, 1980.

26. Isacsson G, Rich CL. Management of patients who deliberately harm themselves. BJ. ; 322:213–5, 1962.

27. Kapoor PS. Accident and Emergency: Etiology, Diagnosis, and Management, 2nd Ed., CBS, New Delhi, 2016.

28. Kapoor PS. Management of multiple injuries. Accident And Emergency. 2nd Ed., CBS, New Delhi, 2016.

29. Keele CA, Neil E. Samson Wright's Applied Physiology, 10th Ed., Oxford University Press, London, 1963.

30. Krupp MA, Chatton MJ. Current Medical Diagnosis and Treatmernt, Maruzen Asian Edition, Bombay, 1975.

31. London PS. The Anatomy of Injury and its Surgical implications. Butterworth-Heinemann, Oxford, 1991.

32. Luicartti ME, Rigby H. Wound Healing—Bone Fracture, Surgery International 13:127–8, The Medicine Publishing Co. Ltd., Abingdon, OXON, 1997.

33. Management of Head Injuries, CD.G., Oxford University Press, Oxford, 1996.

34. Mattox KL. Complications of Trauma. Churchill Livingstone, Edinburgh, 1993.

35. McGREGOR AL. Layers of the Scalp. A Synopsis of Surgical Anatomy. 9th Ed., John Wright and Sons Ltd., Bristol, 1963.

36. McLatchie GR. Essentials of Sports Medicine, 2nd Ed., Churchill Livingstone, Edinburgh, 1993.

37. Medical Defence Union (MDU). Medical records. Medical Defence Union, London,. 1992.

38. Miller A. Closed Injuries of the Kidney, Bladder, and Posterior Urethra. Proc. R. Soc. Med. 54, 563, 1961.

39. Mirvis SE, Young JWR. Imaging in Trauma and Critical care, Williams and Wilkins, Baltimore, 1992.

40. Mirvis SE, Young JWR. Imaging in Trauma and Critical Care. Williams and Wilkins, Baltimore, 1992.
41. Murat JE, Huten N, Mesny J. The use of Standardised assessment procedures in the evaluation of patients with Multiple Injuries. Archives of Emergency Medicine, 2, 11–5, 1986.
42. Murat JE, Huten N, Mesny J. The use of Standardised assessment procedures in the evaluation of patients with Multiple Injuries. Archives of Emergency Medicine, 2, 11–5, 1986.
43. Raby N, Berman L, de Lacy G. Accident and Emergency Radiology, WB Saunders Co., Philadelphia, 1995.
44. Robertson C, Redmond AD. Management of Major Trauma, 2nd Ed., Oxford University Press, Oxford, 1996.
45. Robertson MA, Molyneux EM. Triage in the developing world. Can it be done? Arch Dis Child: 85:208–13, 2001.
46. Settle JAD editor: Principles and Pracice of Burns Management. Churchill Livingstone, Edinburgh, 1996.
47. Shaw's. Textbook of Gynaecology, 8th Ed., Howkins J, J & A. Churchill Ltd., London, 1962.
48. Stevenson HM, Richards D. Discussion on Non-penetrating injuries of the Chest and Abdomen. Proc. R. Soc. Med. 54, 565–6, 1961.
49. Trunkey DD, Lewis FR. Current Therapy of Trauma, 4th Ed., Mosby Year Book, St Louis, 1998.
50. United Kingdom Central Council (UKCC). Standards for Records and Records Keeping. Pp. 15–16 April, 1993.
51. Walder DN. The Shocked Patient Practitioner 187, 34 (1961).
52. Watson-Jones R. Fractures and other Bone and Joint Injuries. Livingstone, Edinburgh, 1952.
53. Wyatt JP, Illingworth RN, Robertson CE, Clancy MJ, Munro PT. Oxford Handbook of Accident and Emergency Medicine. 2nd ed. Oxford University Press Oxford, 2005.

# ORTHOPEDIC TRAUMA

## INTRODUCTION

**Orthopedic Trauma** includes fractures and dislocations as well as musculoskeletal injuries to soft tissues includs muscles, ligaments, tendons and nerves. Orthopedic trauma particularlly includes injuries to the upper limb (shoulder to hand), lower limb (hip to foot) and the spine. Orthopedic surgeons generally do not deal with injuries to the head, chest, abdomen and blood vessels. In case of a polytrauma patient, mostly caused by high velocity injuries like motor vehicle collisions or fall from a height, the orthopedic part of the patient's care is coordinated with other surgical specialties as appropriate usually in the department of A&E. Orthopedic trauma patients usually admitted via the department of A&E (emergency) or examined as an outpatient in a fracture clinic.

The management of orthopedic trauma may involve either surgery or nonsurgical treatment. Surgical management: may include: Reduction (manipulation): Closed or open reduction (relocation or realignment) of a fracture or dislocation to its original correct position, mostly followed by application of a plaster cast, brace, splint or sling.

**Fixation:** External fixation: application of a frame fixed to the bone with pins or wires (Ilizarov fixator).

**Internal fixation:** Insertion of a metal implant to fix the fracture

**Implants:** K-wires, screws, plates and intramedullary nails, etc.

**Nonsurgical management:** May include:

Plaster casts, braces, splints, crutches, slings, etc.

## References

1. Kapoor PS. Accident and Emergency: Etiology, Diagnosis, and Management, 2nd Ed., CBS, New Delhi, 2016.
2. Driscoll P, Skinner D, Earlham R. ABC of Major Trauma, 3rd Ed., BMJ Books, London, 2000.
3. Huckstep RL. A Simple Guide to Trauma, 5th Ed., Churchill Livingstone, Edinburgh, 1995.
4. Trunkey DD, Lewis FR. Current Therapy of Trauma, 4th Ed., Mosby Year Book, St Louis, 1998.
5. Robertson C, Redmond AD. Management of Major Trauma, 2nd Ed., Oxford University Press, Oxford, 1996.

# 3

# Dislocations

**Dislocation of:**
- Temporomandibular joint
- Sternoclavicular joint
- Acromioclavicular joint
- Shoulder joint
- Fracture-dislocation shoulder:
  - Dislocation shoulder with fracture neck humerus
  - Dislocation shoulder with fracture greater tuberosity
- Elbow joint:
  - Posterior
  - Anterior
- Monteggia fracture-dislocation
  - Galeazzi fracture-dislocation
- Lunate bone
- Bennett's fracture-dislocation
- Spine:
  - Atlas (C1) and Axis (C2)
  - Lumbar spine: dislocation/fracture-dislocation
- Hip joint
- Knee joint
- Patella bone
- Ankle joint: fracture-dislocation
- Peri-talar
- Talus bone

**Old unreduced dislocations:**
- Sternoclavicular joint
- Acromioclavicular joint
- Shoulder joint:
  - Anterior
  - Posterior
- Elbow joint
- Wrist joint
- Lunate bone
- Hip joint
- Knee joint
- Patella bone

- Ankle joint
- Tibiofibular joint: Proximal

**Recurrent dislocations:**
- Shoulder joint
- Elbow joint
- Knee joint
  - Patella bone
  - Ankle joint

**Pathological dislocations**

## DISLOCATION

Preface
Dislocation is defined as complete loss of contact between the articular surfaces of a joint, wherein the articulating bones displaced relatively to one another, e.g.
- Dislocation of shoulder: Complete loss of contact between humerus head and glenoid cavity.
- Dislocation of hip: Complete loss of contact between femoral head and acetabulum.

Subluxation is defined as an incomplete loss of contact between the articular surfaces of a joint, wherein the articulating bones partially displaced relatively to one another, e.g.
- Subluxation of shoulder: Partial tear of ligaments (coracoclavicular–conoid and trapezoid), may lead to complete dislocation (suppurative arthritis or RA)

  Sprain is defined as an incomplete tear of ligament/s, unrelated to stability of the joint, e.g. sprain of ankle: Partial tear of the lateral ligament/s (anterior talofibular, posterior talofibular, calcaneofibular), frequently injured in sprains.

Types
Acute dislocations
Recurrent dislocations
Old unreduced dislocations
Pathological dislocations.

Etiology
Congenital, traumatic, and pathological
Congenital dislocation:
- Congenital dislocation of hip (CDH), described in chapter on the deformities.

Traumatic dislocation: (Common in adults, separation of the epiphysis common in children, while fracture of atrophic bone in older persons)

MOI
- Direct violence
- RSA
- Sports injury
- Fall from a height
Obstetric: Difficult labor

Pathological dislocation: Occurs because of:

- Inflammation (arthritis): Tuberculous, RA, rheumatic, infective
- Deformity: Subluxation of knee in triple deformity
- Paralytic: Infantile paralysis (shoulder girdle, hip), and Little's disease (spastic paralysis of hips)
- Neuropathic: Softened ligaments cause stretching, dislocation hips.

**Pathogenesis**  Stretching, rupture of capsule, muscles, ligaments; and occasionally neurovascular rupture, e.g.

- Circumflex (auxillary) nerve injury: In dislocation of shoulder
- Sciatic nerve injury: In dislocation of hip
- Ulnar nerve and median nerve: In dislocation of elbow.

**Diagnosis**  Pain: Because of local trauma, or pressure over neurovascular structures

Deformity: Flatness (shoulder dislocation), fullness (elbow dislocation) limb shortened or legthened (hip dislocation)

Local tenderness

Unnatural rigidity of joint with elastic recoil

Movements: Painful and restricted.

**Investigation**  X-ray: Confirms diagnosis

**Management**  Conservative treatment:

First aid: Splints, arm slins, traction

Analgesics, NSAIDs

Reduction: Closed reduction by manipulation, or traction ASAP.

Anesthesia: General preferred (for muscle relaxation) to overcome muscle spasm.

### Surgical treatment

Indications:

- Failure of closed reduction/irreducible dislocation
- Old unreduced dislocation
- Recurrent dislocation.

### Procedures

- Open reduction
- Arthroplasty
- Arthrodesis.

## REGIONAL DISLOCATIONS

### Dislocation of Temporomandibular joint

**MOI**  Traumatic: Direct violence (blow on the chin of partly open mouth)

Operative: Dental procedures under general anesthesia.

**Diagnosis**  Deformity:

- Unilateral dislocation: Jaw deviated towards the opposite side, with saliva dribbling from partially open mouth, a hollow palpable in front of tragus, while mandibular condyle found little anteriorly bilateral dislocation: Locking of jaw in a partly open mouth, both condyles of mandible displaced anteriorly to their normal positions.

**Investigation**  X-ray face

| Management | Conservative treatment: |
|---|---|
| | Analgesics, NSAIDs |

Reduction: Closed reduction by manipulation.

Anesthesia: General preferred (for muscle relaxation) to overcome muscle spasm.

Method: Pressing the padded thumbs on the lower molar teeth, while rotating the body of the jaw upwards with the fingers.

Postreduction: Four tailed bandage to be worn for 4/52.

**Refer:** The patient to the next fracture clinic.

## Dislocation of Sternoclavicular Joint

| Anatomy | It is a synovial joint, wherin the medial end of clavicle fits into shallow clavicular notch of the manubrium sterni and first costal cartilage; the only point of articulation of upper limb with the axial skeleton; The bone ends connected by a fibrous capsule attached to the margins of the articular surfaces; and its anterior and posterior parts thickened to form the sternoclavicular ligaments (anterior and posterior); joint associated with a circular articular disk and (interclavicular and costo-clavicular) ligaments. |
|---|---|
| MOI | Fall on the outstretched hand |
| | Direct violence. |
| Diagnosis | Sternal end of clavicle—prominent |
| | Local tenderness |
| | Movements of shoulder—painful and restricted. |
| Investigation | X-ray clavicle (focusing sternoclavicular joint)—AP view. |
| Management | Subluxation: |

- Arm pouch for 2–3/52
- Active exercises of fingers, wrist, and elbow.

**Dislocation:**

Conservative treatment:

- Closed reduction and applying a figure of 8 bandage.

**Surgical treatment**

Surgery:

- Open reduction and fixation (ORIF) with fascia lata, Alt:
- Plating (Hook plate)

After care: Arm pouch or a sling for 2/52

Active exercises of fingers and elbow.

**Refer:** The patient to the next fracture clinic.

## Dislocation of Acromioclavicular Joint

| Anatomy | It is a synovial joint. The bone ends connected by a fibrous capsule attached to the margins of the articular surfaces; and its upper part thickened to form the acromioclavicular ligament; the joint cavity is partially divided by a wedge shaped disk with base attached to the capsule; joint surfaces slope medially and downwards (clavicle tends |
|---|---|

to glide over acromion, countered by the acromioclavicular and the coracoclavicular (conoid and trapezoid) ligaments—usually torn in subluxation/dislocation.

Movements: Little gliding and rotator, associated with the pivotal movements of shoulder girdle at the sternoclavicular joint.

| | |
|---|---|
| MOI | Fall on the outstretched hand. |
| Pathogenesis | Dislocation occurs due to tearing of acromioclavicular ligament, coracoclavicular (conoid and trapezoid) ligaments, while subluxation occurs due to tearing of acromioclavicular ligament only. |
| Diagnosis | Prominence of acromial end of clavicle |
| | Local tenderness |
| | Movements of the joint—painful and restricted. |
| Investigation | X-ray clavicle (focusing acromioclavicular joint)—AP view. |
| Management | Subluxation: |

- Arm supported in an arm pouch for 4/52
- Active exercises of fingers, and elbow.

Dislocation:

- Surgical treatment

Surgery:

- ORIF: Coracoclavicular screwing and repair of conoid and trapezoid ligaments
- Acromionectomy.

Postoperative:

- Arm supported in an arm pouch for 6/52
- Active exercises of fingers, wrist, and elbow.

**Refer:** The patient to the next fracture clinic.

## Dislocation of Shoulder Joint

| | |
|---|---|
| Preface | Dislocations of shoulder are of common occurrence, because of wide range of movement, shallow glenoid cavity, and inadequate support of rotator cuff (ligaments and muscles), and are caused by acute trauma to the joint, with the arm in abduction. In majority of cases a subcoracoid dislocation occurs. |
| Types | Anterior and posterior dislocations |
| | Anterior dislocation: Common type—head lies in front of glenoid. |
| Pathogenesis | Varieties: Subglenoid, subcoracoid, subclavicular, and posterior |
| MOI | Fal on the outstretched hand, RSA, sports injury |
| | Direct violence |
| Diagnosis | Pain |
| | Deformity: |

- Flattening of the shoulder: Rounded appearance lost due to medial displacement of humeral head
- Prominent acromion, fullness in the delto-pectoral groove

Loss of resistance beneath the acromion

Movements: Painful and restricted.

| | |
|---|---|
| Investigation | X-ray shoulder joint—AP and LAT views. |

- Hamilton's ruller test: Acromion and humeral lateral epicondyle can be touched by a ruller (humeral head displaced medially), and also possible in case of fracture scapular neck
- Dugas test: Unable to touch the opposite shoulder by the affected side's hand (due to abduction of the lower end of humerus).

| | |
|---|---|
| Management | Closed reduction under anesthesia. |
| Methods | Kocher's and Hippocratic methods. |

**Kocher's method:**
- Position: Patient either sitting or lying
- Reduction: Surgeon holds the forearm near wrist, flexes and adducts elbow, applies traction, continuing traction gradually rotates the arm externally, and once the dislocation is reduced, brings the arm across the chest, and finally rotates the arm internally. The dislocation is reduced now.
- Immobilization: Strapping arm to the front of chest.

Arm sling for 4/52 and active exercises of fingers, wrist, and elbow.

**Hippocratic's method:**
- Reduction: Surgeon places his heel of foot into the axilla of patient, with utmost care not to injure the side of chest wall, the head of the humerus is levered back into its position. Immobilization: same as for Kocher's method.

## Fracture-dislocation of Shoulder

| | |
|---|---|
| Types | Dislocation of shoulder plus fracture neck of humerus |
| | Dislocation of shoulder plus fracture greater tuberosity. |

## Dislocation of Shoulder Plus Fracture Neck of Humerus

| | |
|---|---|
| MOI | Fall on the outstretched hand |
| | Direct violence. |
| Diagnosis | Swelling, local tenderness, crepitus |
| | Passive movement of arm minus that of head of humerus. |
| | Shortening (overlapping) |
| Investigation | X-ray shoulder—AP and LAT views. |
| Management | • Elderly patient: Only arm sling and active exercises advisable. |
| | • Younger patient: Open reduction is usually indicated, as closed reduction fails due to difficulty in controlling small sized upper fragment. |

Post care: Arm sling and active exercises of fingers, wrist, and elbow.

## Dislocation of Shoulder Plus Fracture Greater Tuberosity

| | |
|---|---|
| MOI | Fall on the outstretched hand, or direct violence. |
| Diagnosis | Swelling, local tenderness, crepitus, |
| | Movements (esp. abduction): Painful and restricted. |
| Investigation | X-ray shoulder—AP and LAT views. |
| Management | Same treatment as for dislocation of shoulder. |

Apposition occurs when dislocation is reduced.

Surgery: ORIF—of fracture greater tuberosity with a screw

Indication: Marked displacement of fracture.

## Dislocation of Elbow

| | |
|---|---|
| Preface | In dislocation of the elbow the forearm is frequently displaced posterolaterally. Anterior dislocation is usually accompanied by olecranon fracture. May occur in any age, usually common in adults |
| Types | • Posterolateral: Commonest type |
| | • Anterior: Rare type. |

## Posterior Dislocation

| | |
|---|---|
| MOI | Fall on the outstretched hand. |
| Diagnosis | Age: Common in adults |
| | Deformity: |
| | • Olecranon displaced up above level of epicondyles |
| | • Relationship of olecranon, medial and lateral epicondyles disturbed, i.e. almost at same level |
| | • Shortning of forearm |
| | • Movements at elbow—painful and restricted. |
| D/d | Supracondylar fracture of lower end of humerus. |
| Investigation | X-ray elbow—AP and LAT views. |
| Management | Conservative treatment: |
| | Method: Closed reduction under general anesthesia |
| | After care: Cuff and collar sling for 3/52 |

## Anterior Dislocation: Associated with Olecranon Fracture

| | |
|---|---|
| MOI | Fall on the elbow. |
| Management | Conservative treatment: |
| | Indication: Dislocation of elbow |
| | Method: Closed reduction. |
| | Surgical treatment: |
| | Surgery: ORIF |
| | Indication: Fracture of olecranon |
| | Method: Fixation with: |
| | • Screw |
| | • Tension wire |
| | • Crooked plate and screws. |
| | Postoperative: Plaster in extension of elbow for 4/52. |
| | After care: Physiotherapy. |
| Refer: | The patient to the next fracture clinic. |

## Monteggia Fracture Dislocation

| | |
|---|---|
| Pattern | Fracture of ulna with dislocation of radial head. |
| | Types: Anterior: Common type, and Posterior: Rare type |

Anterior type: Dislocation of radial head forwards along with anterior angulation of fractured ulna

Posterior type: Dislocation of radial head backwards along with posterior angulation of fractured ulna.

| | |
|---|---|
| MOI | Fall on the outstretched hand or direct violence. |
| Diagnosis | Deformity |
| | Local tenderness |
| | Movements: Painful and restricted esp. pronation and supination. |
| Investigation | X-ray forearm includes elbow and wrist: AP and LAT views. |
| Management | Surgical treatment of choice. |
| | Surgery: ORIF of fractured ulna (plating or rush pin). |

Anterior Monteggia:
- ORIF of fractured ulna (plating or rush pin)
- Reduction of radial head is achieved by pressing backwards overhead of radius.
- For unstable radial head: Fixation with percutaneous K-wire.

Postoperative: Forearm and elbow immobilized in supination and flexion, by plaster for 6/52.

Posterior Monteggia:
- ORIF of fractured ulna (plating or rush pin)
- Reduction of radial head is achieved by pressing forwards overhead of radius, with elbow in extension position.

Postoperative: Forearm and elbow immobilized in supination and extension, by plaster for 6/52, followed by physiotherapy.

## Galeazzi Fracture Dislocation

| | |
|---|---|
| Preface | Fracture of radius with dislocation of inferior radioulnar joint. |
| MOI | Fall on the outstretched hand or direct violence. |
| Diagnosis | • Swelling |
| | • Local tenderness |
| | • Movements at wrist: painful and restricted. |
| Investigation | X-ray forearm includes elbow and wrist—AP and LAT views |
| Management | Surgical treatment: |
| | Surgery: ORIF of fractured radius (plating of radius) |

Method:
- Reduction of radius is followed by spontaneous reduction of the ulna while inferior radioulnar joint does not require any opening.

Note: All fracture-dislocations of radial shaft, best treated by ORIF.

Postoperative: Plaster slab for 6–8/52.

After care: Physiotherapy.

## Dislocation of Lunate

| | |
|---|---|
| MOI | Fall on the outstretched hand. |
| Diagnosis | Pain, swelling, local tenderness. |

| Investigation | X-ray hand includes wrist—AP and LAT views. |
| Management | Closed reduction under general anesthesia. |
| Method | Apply traction to the supinated wrist |
| | Extend the wrist, maintaining traction |
| | Apply pressure over the lunate—bone reduces (click sound) |
| | Flex the wrist |
| | Apply plaster cast with wrist in flexion for 2/52, followed by plaster cast with wrist in neutral position for another 2/52. |
| | After care: Physiotherapy—active exercises. |

## Bennett's Fracture-dislocation

| Preface | It is an intra-articular fracture through the base of first metacarpal. The shaft is dislocated laterally by the unopposed action of the abductor pollicis longus. |
| MOI | Fall on the outstretched hand |
| | Direct violence |
| | Forced abduction of thumb. |
| Diagnosis | Pain |
| | Swelling |
| | Local tenderness |
| | Movements of the thumb painful and restricted. |
| Investigation | X-ray thumb—AP, LAT, and Oblique views. |
| Management | Conservative treatment: |
| | Closed reuction under anesthesia. Reduction is easy but is difficult to maintain. |
| | Method: Apply traction to the thumb, followed by abduction of thumb and then apply pressure over the outer aspect of base of thumb. |
| | Immobilization: Plaster fixation including MP joint of the thumb, for 5–6/52. |
| | Post care: Physiotherapy. |
| | Surgical treatment: |
| | • Indication: Closed reduction is easy but is difficult to maintain |
| | Surgery: ORIF—intramedullary or percutaneous Kirschner wires |
| | Immobilization: Plaster cast (Colles type slab). |
| | Post care: Physiotherapy. |

## Dislocations Spine

| Preface | Dislocation alone can occur only in the cervical region, whereas in the dorsal and lumbar regions, always fracture-dislocations occur due to vertical or oblique directions of articular processes. |

## Dislocation between Atlas (C1) and Axis (C2)

| MOI | Hanging by neck |
| Mechanism of injury | Forward displacement of atlas following rupture of transeverse ligament or fracture of odontoid process, death usually occurs due to injury to the brainstem and respiratory failure. |

| Management | If the patient survives, then under general anesthesia: |
|---|---|
| | Closed reduction: Flexion towards opposite side |
| | Post care: Skull traction, for one week, followed by plaster cast |
| | Surgical treatment: ORIF (Open reduction and internal fixation with plate and screws) if the conservative treatment fails |
| | Post care: Head and neck in plaster cast (Minerva jacket). |

## Dislocation/Fracture-dislocation of Lumbar Spine

| Preface | With minor flexion forces applied to the lumbar/or lower dorsal spine, cord and nerve root injury is the exception rther than the rule. |
|---|---|
| MOI | Direct violence |
| | Hanging: by neck: suicidal or capital punishment |
| | RSA |
| | Fall from a height |

## Mechanism of Injury

| Management | Conservative treatment: |
|---|---|
| | Indication: If the patient survives, then under general anesthesia. |
| | Method: Closed reduction. |
| | Post care: Physiotherapy. |
| | Surgical treatment: |
| | Indication: Failure of conservative treatment. |
| | Surgery: ORIF (Open reduction and internal fixation with plate and screws). |
| | Post care: Physiotherapy. |

## Dislocation of Hip

| Preface | Dislocation or fracture-dislocation of the hip is an acute emergency and to be reduced on priority basis, as longer it remains unreduced, more chances of development of avascular necrosis and osteoarthritis. Postreduction of the dislocation, open reduction of associated femoral head or acetabular fracture may be delayed for days. |
|---|---|
| Types | • Posterior type: Commonest type, the femoral head is displaced onto the dorsum ilii. |
| | • Anterior type: Rare type, the femoral head is displaced onto the side of the symphysis pubis (pubic type) or under the adductor muscles (obturator type) |
| | • Central type is a rare type, the femoral head is pushed through the broken acetabulum. |
| MOI | • RSA (car accident, i.e. dashboard dislocation: Force transmitted up the femoral shaft) |
| | • Fall of heavy weight over the back of a stooping person, e.g. mines accidents |
| | • Fall from a height. |
| Diagnosis | Posterior dislocation: |
| | • Attitude: Flexion, adduction, and internal rotation |
| | • Shortening of limb |

- Loss of resistance in Scarpa's triangle
- Absence of femoral pulse
- Hip rigidity
- Movements of hip. Painful and restricted

Anterior dislocation:
- Attitude: Flexion, abduction, and external rotation
- Lenghtning of limb
- Loss of resistance in Scarpa's triangle
- Absence of femoral pulse
- Hip rigidity
- Movements of hip: Painful and restricted

Central dislocation:
- Greater trochanter: Moves towards pelvis
- Hip rigidity
- Movements: Painful and restricted
- Rectal examination: Head movement felt, on moving thigh

| | |
|---|---|
| Investigation | X-ray Pelvis focusing the dislocated hip—AP view confirms the clinical diagnosis and type of dislocation |
| Management | Conservative treatment: Closed reduction is treatment of choice: Anesthesia: General. |

Reduction:
- Place the patient flat on a mattress on the floor
- An assistant steadies the iliac crest
- The surgeon flexes the knee and hip at right angles, the femur is lifted vertically up with great force, maintaining the upward pull the limb is rotated internally and externally, the femoral head snaps into its socket
- Check X-ray Hip: AP view (if reduction without C-arm use).

Post care: Fixed traction in a Thomas splint for 4/52, followed by physiotherapy for 2/52, followed by weight bearing. In case of fracture of acetabular rim, weight bearing allowed after 8/52 of injury.

Alternative method: Bigelow's method:
Hip is flexed, abducted, externally rotated, extended, and finally kept in neutral position

Surgical treatment:
Indication: ORIF is indicated for a large fragment of acetabulum.

## Complications of Dislocation of Hip

**A. Irreducible dislocation:** Due to interposition of soft tissue (labrum) or bony fragment into the acetabulum

Management: Closed reduction under general anesthesia with full muscle relaxation. If closed reduction fails, then open reduction is indicated.

**B. Fracture acetabular rim:** Fracture of posterior lip of acetabulum
Management: Closed reduction followed by fixed traction in a Thomas splint for 4/52, followed by physiotherapy for 2/52, and weight bearing after 8–10/52 of injury.

Surgical treatment: ORIF.
Indication: ORIF is indicated for a large fragment of acetabulum.

### C. Fracture neck femur:
Management: Surgery is treatment of choice:
- Elderly patient: Prosthesis (Thompson or Austin Moore)
- Middle aged: Total Hip Replacement (THR)
- Younger patient: ORIF.

### D. Slipped upper Femoral epiphysis:
Management: ORIF is treatment of choice.

### E. Trochanteric (extracapsular) fracture hip:
Management: ORIF (DHS or PFN) + reduction

### F. Fracture of femoral shaft:
Management:
Conservative treatment: Reduction + fixation (traction):
Reduction of dislocation: Closed reduction of hip (Stimson's method)
Fixation: Traction (Thomas splint method).

Surgical treatment: Reduction + ORIF:
Reduction of dislocation: Open reduction of hip
Fixation: ORIF of fractured femoral shaft.

### G. Fracture of patella:
Management:
Surgical treatment of choice:
Reduction of dislocation: Open reduction of hip
Fixation: ORIF of fractured patella
Reduction of dislocated: Open reduction of hip
Fixation: Tension wiring or excision, depending upon type of fracture patella.

### H. Sciatic nerve palsy:
Management:
Conservative treatment: Majority of patients with sciatic nerve palsy are best treated by conservative measures, i.e. use of foot drop splint, and physiotherapy.

Surgical treatment:
Surgery: Exploration of nerve, indicated rarely

### I. Avascular necrosis of femoral head:
Management:
Surgical treatment of choice
Surgery: Total Hip Replacement (THR).

### J. Osteoarthritis hip:
Etiology:
- Avascular necrosis of femoral head
- Intracapsular fracture neck of femur
Management:
Surgical treatment:
Surgery: Total Hip Replacement (THR).

### K. Old unreduced dislocation of hip:

| | |
|---|---|
| Management | Conservative: Closed reduction (manipulation) within a week or skeletal traction for 3–4 weeks |

Surgical treatment:
Surgery:
- Open reduction—if conservative treatment fails
- Osteotomy—post 1 year.

## Dislocation of Knee

| | |
|---|---|
| Preface | Complete dislocation of knee is rare, while subluxation of knee joint is common, because of rupture of cruciate (anterior or posterior or both) ligaments. Dislocation of knee is a serious injury, because of injury of capsule, ligaments, and neurovascular (popliteal vessels, tibial or common peroneal nerves) damage. |
| Types | Anterior (common), posterior, medial, lateral, or rotary |
| MOI | Direct violence: RSA, sports injury, fall from a height. |
| Pathogenesis | Ruptured cruciate ligament/s, hemarthrisis, femur passed forwards over the tibia, compressed popliteal vessels |
| Diagnosis | Pain, swelling, local tenderness. |
| Investigation | X-ray knee—AP and LAT views. |
| Management | Closed reduction under general anesthesia ASAP. |

Method:
Aspiration: Aspirate the knee
Reduction: Apply traction to the flexed knee
Postreduction: Apply a posterior plaster slab/splint with knee in flexion (10–15 degree) for 1/52, followed by a long leg plaster cast applied for 7/52.

Rehabilitation:
- Active exercises (quadriceps and hamstrings)
- Postremoval of plaster cast, weight bearing with help of a long leg brace with joint at knee, to be permitted.

Open reduction:
Indication: Failure of closed reduction because of interposition of soft tissues (capsule or femoral condyle caught in a bucket handle tear of capsule)

| | |
|---|---|
| Complication | Instability due to IDK (torn ligament/s)<br>Management: Surgery: repair/replacement of torn ligament/s. |

## Dislocation of Patella

| | |
|---|---|
| MOI | Direct violence: RSA, sports injury, hit by a stick. |
| Pathogenesis | Torn quadriceps expansion, hemarthrosis, dislocated patella. |
| Diagnosis | Pain<br>Swelling<br>Local tenderness<br>Movements: Painful and restricted |

| | |
|---|---|
| Investigation | X-ray knee—AP and LAT views. |
| Management | Closed reduction under general anesthesia ASAP. |

Method:
- Apply pressure over patella (extended leg and thigh)—bone reduces
- Apply posterior plaster slab for 2/52, followed by removal of plaster cast and active and passive exercises (physiotherapy).

## Fracture Dislocation of Ankle

| | |
|---|---|
| Definition | Dislocation of ankle without fracture of either the medial or loateral malleolus or of distal articular surface (anterior or posterior lip) of the tibia is very rare, because of the deep mortice formed by the tibia and fibula, and rather dislocations of talus are more common than ankle dislocation in violent trauma, i.e. RSA, fall from height. |
| MOI | Direct trauma: RSA, sports injuries, fall from a height, hit by a stick. |
| Pathogenesis | Forced inversion stresses all ligaments attached to talus, talus dislocates, shifts in front of ankle, and ovelies on lateral side of the foot, head of talus points medially with its calcaneal surface pointed backwards. |
| Diagnosis | Pain |
| | Swelling |
| | Deformity: Talus plantar-flexed local tenderness. |
| Investigation | X-ray ankle—AP and LAT views: Confirms diagnosis. |
| Management | Closed reduction under general anesthesia. |

Method:
Plantar flex the foot
Grasp the heel and the forefoot, apply traction, evert the foot
Apply B/K plaster cast with ankle at right angle, and the foot in little eversion. For 1/52, followed by a walking plaster boot for 5/52.
Post care: Physiotherapy: active exercises.

Open reduction:
Indication: Failed closed reduction.
Surgery: ORIF.

## Peri-talar Dslocation

| | |
|---|---|
| Definition | It is defined as on injury in which the talus remins in position with the calcaneus, while the talonavicular joint dislocates, and may be followed by fractures of malleoli |
| MOI | Direct violence: Forced inversion of the plantar flexed foot |
| Pathogenesis | Forced inversion stresses lateral ligament of talus, ruptures the talo-calcaneal ligament, talus remains *in situ* (ankle mortice), yields to subtalar dislocation, forefoot remains with calcaneus, talonavicular joint dislocates; talus plantar flexed. |
| | Backwards. |
| Diagnosis | Pain |
| | Swelling |

Deformity: Talus plantar-flexed local tenderness.

Investigation          X-ray ankle—AP and LAT views: Confirms diagnosis.

Management             Closed reduction under general anesthesia.

Method:

Plantar flex the foot

Grasp the heel and the forefoot, apply traction, evert the foot

Apply B/K plaster cast with ankle at right angle, and the foot in little eversion. For 1/52, followed by a walking plaster boot for 5/52.

Post care: Physiotherapy: active exercises.

Open reduction:

Indication: Failed closed reduction.

Surgery: ORIF (Kirschner wires) of talonavicular joint.

## Dislocation of Talus

Definition             Dislocations of talus are more common than ankle dislocation in violent trauma, i.e. RSA, fall from height.

MOI                    Direct trauma: RSA, sports injuries, fall from a height, hit by a stick.

Pathogenesis           Forced inversion stresses all ligaments attached to talus, talus dislocates, shifts in front of ankle, and ovelies on lateral side of the foot, head of talus points medially with its calcaneal surface pointed backwards.

Diagnosis              Pain

Swelling

Deformity: Talus plantar-flexed local tenderness.

Investigation          X-ray ankle—AP and LAT views: confirms diagnosis.

Management             Closed reduction under general anesthesia.

Method:

Plantar flex the foot

Grasp the heel and the forefoot, apply traction, evert the foot

Apply B/K plaster cast with ankle at right angle, and the foot in little eversion. for 1/52, followed by a walking plaster boot for 5/52.

Post care: Physiotherapy: active exercises.

Open reduction:

Indication: Failed closed reduction.

Surgery: ORIF.

## Old Unreduced Dislocations

Definition             It is defined as a dislocation that remain unreduced for 3–4/52

Pathogenesis           Old unreduced dislocation; unbathed articular cartilage by the synovial fluid results in degeneration, severely damaged, and gets detached.

S/S                    Pain

Deformity

Muscular: Weakness, wasting

Movements: Painful and restricted

Neurovascular: May be impaired.

| | |
|---|---|
| Investigation | X-ray of affected joint. |
| Management | Reduction: Under general anesthesia. |

Methods:

- Closed reduction: Indicated in early cases (within 3–4/52 of trauma): By manipulation, traction (under C-arm scanner).
  Caution: An osteoporotic bone may fracture, e.g. # neck humerus and # neck femur.
- Open reduction of choice in majority of old unreduced dislocations. Indications: Irreducible dislocations, failed closed reduction, elder patients (osteoporotic bones), fracture dislocations.
- Reduction + arthroplasty
- Reduction + arthrodesis.

## OLD UNREDUCED DISLOCATIONS REGIONAL

### Old Unreduced Dislocation of Sternoclavicular Joint

| | |
|---|---|
| Definition | An old unreduced dislocation of the sternoclavicular joint usually causes little disability except cosmetic factor. |
| Etiology | Irreducible dislocation, failed closed reduction |
| Diagnosis | Sternal end of clavicle—prominent |
| | Movements of shoulder: Painful and restricted. |
| Investigation | X-ray clavicle (focusing sternoclavicular joint)—AP view. |
| Management | Surgical treatment of choice. |
| | Surgery: Excision of medial end of clavicle: |

Method:

- Incision: 5 cm long parallel to clavicle
- Exposure: Medial end of clavicle exposed subperiosteally, hold it by a forceps, lift it anterosuperior direction, strip off the attached soft tissues
- Divide: Resect 2.5 cm of the bone
- Reef and suture the periosteum
- Close skin with interrupted sutures
- ASD.

Postoperative care: Immobilize shoulder girdle in an arm pouch for 3/52, with active exercises of fingers and elbow.

- Active exercises of fingers and elbow.

### Old unreduced Dislocation of Acromioclavicular Joint

| | |
|---|---|
| Definition | An old unreduced dislocation of the acromioclavicular joint usually causes little disability except cosmetic factor, for that resection of lateral end of clavicle indicated. |
| Etiology | Irreducible dislocation, failed closed reduction |
| Pathogenesis | In complete dislocation tearing of acromioclavicular ligament, coronoid and trapezoid ligaments, while in subluxation tearing of acromioclavicular ligament only. |
| Diagnosis | Prominence of acromial end of clavicle |
| | Movements of the joint—painful and restricted. |

| | |
|---|---|
| Investigation | X-ray clavicle (focusing acromioclavicular joint)—AP view. |
| Management | Surgical treatment of choice |

### Surgery
Subluxation:

Indication: Partial tear of ligaments

Surgery: Excision of lateral end of clavicle, lateral to ligaments

Dislocation:

Indication: Complete rupture of ligaments

Surgery: Excision of lateral end of clavicle + repair of ligaments.

Technique:

- Incision: 5 cm curved incision over lateral end of clavicle
- Exposure: Lateral end of clavicle exposed subperiosteally, hold it by a forceps, lift it anterosuperior direction, strip off attached soft tissue
- Divide: Resect 2.5 cm of the bone
- Reef and suture the periosteum
- Close skin with interrupted sutures
- ASD.

Postoperative care: Immobilize shoulder girdle in an arm pouch for 2/52, with active exercises of fingers and elbow.

After care: Active exercises of fingers and elbow.

## Old Unreduced Dislocation of Shoulder

| | |
|---|---|
| Definition | It is defined as an old unreduced dislocation of shoulder, because of closed reduction failure (repeated manipulations). |
| Types | Anterior and posterior dislocations |
| | Anterior dislocation: Common type—head lies in front of glenoid. |
| Etiology | Irreducible dislocation, failed closed reduction |
| Diagnosis | Flattening of the shoulder |
| | Prominent acromion, fullness in the deltopectoral groove |
| | Loss of resistance beneath the acromion. |
| Investigation | X-ray shoulder joint—AP and LAT views. |
| Management | Conservative treatment: |
| | Closed reduction under anesthesia. |
| | Indication: in fresh cases (< 4/52). |
| | Methods: Kocher's and Hippocratic methods. |

**Kocher's method:** Apply traction, continuing traction gradually rotate the arm externally, once the dislocation is reduced, then bring the arm across the chest, and finally rotate the arm internally. The dislocation is reduced now.

Postreduction:

- Strapping arm the front of chest.
- Arm sling for 4/52 and active exercises of fingers, wrist, and elbow

**Hippocratric method:** Surgeon places his heel of foot into the axilla of patient, keeping full care not to injure the side of chest wall, the head of humerus is levered back into its position.

Postreduction: Same as for Kocher's method:

- Strapping arm the front of chest.
- Arm sling for 4/52 and active exercises of fingers, wrist, and elbow

Surgical treatment: ORIF

Indications:

- Failure of closed reduction
- Old dislocation (> 4–6/52)
- Osteoporotic bone

Technique:

- Incision: Skin incision on the anterior aspect of shoulder, from lateral third of clavicle, downwards.
- Exposure: Humeral head by separating deltoid and pectoralis major muscles, then retract biceps short head and coracobrachialis
- Open: The capsule, divide the coracohumeral ligament, clear the glenoid cavity of fibrous tissue
- Reduction of humeral head with little force, to avoid fractures of the osteoporotic bones
- Repair: The torn rotator cuff (ruptured at time of dislocation).
- Transfix: The humeal head to the glenoid with 2–3 Kirschner wires to prevent recurrence of dislocation
- Cut-off: Wires and embed under the skin.
- Closure: Wound with interrupted sutures
- ASD.

Postoperative care: Immobilize the arm on an abduction humeral splint for 2/52, followed by removal of Kirschner wires.

After care: Exercises active.

## Old Unreduced Dislocation of Shoulder (Anterior)

| | |
|---|---|
| Definition | Closed reduction may be achieved even after 4–6/52, while risking danger of fracture neck of humerus (because of osteoporotic bone) or damaging the joint surfaces. |
| Etiology | Irreducible dislocation, failed closed reduction |
| Management | Surgical treatment of choice. |

Surgery: Open reduction.

Indication:

- Closed reduction failure > twice
- Unreduced dislocations > 6/52 old, in middle aged and elderly

Technique:

- Incision: Modified anterolateral approach (Cubbins): 3 cm long curved incision extended laterally around the acromion and medially along lateral half of scapular spine

- Detach: Deltoid's origin from acromion and scapular spine
- Exposure of joint capsule by reflecting the deltoid
- Exposure of joint by incising the joint capsule along biceps tendon
- Reduction of head into glenoid cavity
- Reattach the capsule and tendons to the toberosity with interrupted chromic catgut sutures; or
- Fixation of humeral head: By the Nicola procedure (tendon of long head of biceps and portion of coracohumeral ligament, passed through tunnel in humeral head; removed bone plug impacted into distal end of tunnel so as to anchor log head of biceps)
- Reef and closure of periosteum.

Postoperatively: Immobilization of arm: An abduction humeral splint (shoulder in abduction, flexion, and externally rotation) applied for 4–6/52;

After care: Exercises.

## Old Unreduced Dislocation of Shoulder (Posterior)

Definition      Posterior dislocation is rare as compared to anterior dislocation; may remain undiagnosed for weeks or months, and to be suspected by the observing signs: humeral head more prominent posteriorly, prominent coracoid, abduction restricted, and external rotation absent, confirmed radiologically (AP & LAT views).

Etiology      Irreducible dislocation, failed closed reduction

Management      Conservative treatment:

Indication: Diagnosed early

Method: Closed reduction

Surgical treatment:

Surgery: Open reduction.

Indication:
- Closed reduction failure > twice
- Unreduced dislocations > 2/52 old, in middle aged and elderly

Technique:
- Incision: Anteromedial approach
- Exposure of joint capsule by reflecting the deltoid
- Exposure of joint by incising the joint capsule
- Reduction of head into glenoid cavity
- Fixation: Fixation with two Kirschner wires through acromion into the proximal humerus
- Reef and closure of periosteum.

Postoperatively: Immobilization of arm: an abduction humeral splint (shoulder in abduction, flexion, and externally rotation) applied for 4/52.

After care: Exercises.

## Old Unreduced Dislocation of Elbow

Definition      Dislocation of an elbow may be considered as irreducible post 3/52 of an injury; an old unreduced dislocation of the elbow (> 3/52) may become difficult to reduce because of adhesions formation that restrict mobility; elbow may be deformed (held in flexion or extension)

| | |
|---|---|
| Etiology | Irreducible dislocation, failed closed reduction |
| Pathogenesis | Fibrous tissues formed to fill up trochlear notch of ulna and olecranon fossa of humerus; capsule adherence to articular surfaces; atrophic muscles; osteoporotic bones; exorbitant callus formation; ankylosed elbow joint. |
| Diagnosis | Age: Common in adults |

Deformity:
- Olecranon displaced up above level of epicondyles
- Relationship of olecranon, medial and lateral epicondyles disturbed, i.e. almost at same level
- Shortning of forearm
- Movements at elbow—restricted.

| | |
|---|---|
| Investigation | X-ray elbow—AP and LAT views. |
| Management | Surgical treatment of choice |

Surgery: ORIF

Technique:
- Incision: 10 cm longitudinal centered over olecranon
- Exposure: Triceps aponeurosis, then reflect aponeurosis by forming a flap attached distally to the olecranon
- Release: Subperiosteally muscles from distal humerus
- Isolate: Ulnar nerve from groove on the posterior aspect of medial epicondyle; then free capsule from the humeral condyles
- Excise: Massive callus formed on the posterior aspect of distal humerus and in the olecranon fossa
- Exposure: Radial head and clear the ulnar trochlear notch free of callus and fibrous tissue
- Reduction: Reduce the radial head, by rotating the forearm, and pressing gently the capitulum posteriorly, while pushing the radial head anteriorly into its bed, then push the coronoid distally and forward over the trochlea.
- Suture: The periosteum and triceps over posterior humeral surface, and fascia over radial head, then suture the tongue flap of the triceps aponeurosis.
- Transfix: The olecranon to the humerus with two Kirschner wires to avoid recurrence of dislocation, the cut off wires underneath the skin.

Postoperatively:
- Immobilization: With elbow at right angle, the arm immobilized in a posterior splint for 3–4/52.
- Kirschner wires to be removed after 2/52.
- Active exercises of fingers and shoulder.

After care: Physiotherapy.

## Old Unreduced Dislocation of Wrist

Etiology         Irreducible dislocation, failed closed reduction

Management       Surgical treatment:

Surgery:
- 3–4/52 old: Open reduction
- >16/52 old: Open reduction + excision of proximal row of carpal bones

Method:
- Incision: Curved longitudinal or transverse dorsal incision, then deepen the incision between tendons of extensor indicis proprius and extensor pollicis longus, then excise scar tissue, and expose the carpus and the distal ends of radius and ulna
- Reduction: Insert a periosteal elevator or bone skid, between the carpus and radius, and gently place the bones into normal position.
- Immobilization: With wrist in dorsiflexion, immobilize in a plaster posterior splint for 2/52.

Postoperative care:
- Active exercises of fingers and shoulder.

After care: Physiotherapy

## Old Unreduced Dislocation of Lunate

Etiology         Irreducible dislocation, failed closed reduction

Diagnosis        Pain

Deformity

Movements: Painful and restricted.

Investigation    X-ray hand includes wrist—AP and LAT views.

Management       Surgical treatment of choice.

Surgery:
- Open reduction: Indicated for several weeks old dislocation
- Bone excision of choice in Kienbock's disease (vascular changes)

Method:
- Incision: A transverse incision over the volar aspect of the wrist in the distal flexor crease, retract the fasciae, locate the Palmaris longus tendon, and isolate the median nerve under the tendon, then retract the flexor tendons to expose the capsule, then incise the capsule to expose lunate and distal end of radius, excise the fibrous tissue and free adhesions.
- Reduction: Slip the lunate with aid of a bone skid into its space, while flexing the hyperextended hand
- Excision: Excise the lunate after freeing it from all the soft tissue attachments.

Postreduction: Apply plaster cast with wrist in flexion for 2/52, followed by plaster cast with wrist

## Old Unreduced Dislocation of Hip

| | |
|---|---|
| Definition | Postoperative restoration of function is better in anterior dislocation than in posterior dislocation (more common). |
| Etiology | Irreducible dislocation; failed closed reduction |
| Diagnosis | Pain |
| | Disability |
| Investigation | X-ray pelvis focusing affected hip. |
| Management | Conservative: Closed reduction (manipulation) within a week or skeletal traction for 3–4 weeks |

Surgical treatment:

Surgery:
- Open reduction—if conservative treatment fails
- Osteotomy—after 1 year

## Old Unreduced Dislocation of Knee

| | |
|---|---|
| Definition | A satisfactory range of motion is hardly achieved post open reduction in an old dislocation of the knee, although the articular cartilage may appear normal at surgery. |
| Etiology | Irreducible dislocation; failed closed reduction. |
| Diagnosis | Pain |
| | Disability |
| | Movements: Painful and restricted. |
| Investigation | X-ray hand includes wrist—AP and LAT views. |
| Management | Surgical treatment of choice. |

Surgery:
- Open reduction: Indicated for several weeks old dislocation
- Bone excision of choice in Kienbock's disease (vascular changes)

Method:
- Incision: A transverse incision over the volar aspect of the wrist in the distal flexor crease, retract the fasciae, locate the palmaris longus tendon, and isolate the median nerve under the tendon, then retract the flexor tendons to expose the capsule, then incise the capsule to expose lunate and distal end of radius, excise the fibrous tissue and free adhesions.
- Reduction: Slip the lunate with aid of a bone skid into its space, while flexing the hyperextended hand
- Excision: Excise the lunate after freeing it from all the soft tissue attachments

Postreduction: Apply plaster cast with wrist in flexion for 2/52, followed by plaster cast with wrist.

## Old Unreduced Dislocation of Patella

| | |
|---|---|
| Definition | Frequently, the knee functions normally inspite of an old unreduced dislocation of the patella, that is mostly diplaced laterally, and in dislocation of long duration, there may be knee in valgus, and tibia rotated externally on the femur. |

| | |
|---|---|
| Etiology | Irreducible dislocation, failed closed reduction |
| Diagnosis | Pain |
| | Disability |
| | Deformity: Knee in valgus position and leg externally rotated. |
| Investigation | X-ray knee—AP and LAT views. |
| Management | Surgical treatment of choice. |

Surgery:
- Open reduction: Indicated for several weeks old dislocation, with normal contour and alignment of tibiofemoral joint.
- Arthroplasty: For young adults (to restore contours of the joint).
- Arthrodesis: For those > 40 years of age; factory and mine workers
- Patellectomy: Degenerated articular surface of patella.

Method:
- Incision:
- Reduction:

Postreduction: Apply plaster cast with wrist in flexion for 2/52, followed by plaster cast with wrist.

## Old Unreduced Dislocation of Ankle

| | |
|---|---|
| Definition | An old unreduced dislocation of the ankle without any associated fracture/s is very rare, and usually the type and severity of the dislocation depend upon the type and severity of an associated fracture/s, e.g. an anterior dislocation is usually associated with fractured anterior margin of the distal articular surface of tibia, while a posterior dislocation is usually associated either with a fractured distal tibia or a trimollar (Pott's) fracture. |
| Etiology | Irreducible dislocation, failed closed reduction |
| Diagnosis | Pain |
| | Deformity |
| | Movements: Painful and restricted. |
| Investigation | X-ray ankle—AP and LAT views. |
| Management | Surgical treatment of choice. |
| | Surgery: ORIF. |

- Open reduction: Indicated for several weeks old dislocation
- Internal fixation of fracture/s.

Postreduction: Apply plaster cast for 4/52, followed by weight bearing in a walking plaster boot, or a long leg brace with a knee joint, for the period till firm fusion.

## Old Unreduced Dislocation of Proximal Tibiofibular Joint

| | |
|---|---|
| Definition | An old unreduced dislocation of the proximal tibiofibular joint may not disturb the normal function, thereby not to require treatment, until and unless the trauma exerts any strain upon the knee joint, causing pain, disability, and pressure upon peroneal nerve. |

Etiology             Irreducible dislocation, failed closed reduction.

Diagnosis            Pain

Nerve pressure (peroneal): May cause foot drop, talipes equinovarus, sensory loss.

Investigation        X-ray knee—AP and LAT views.

Management           Surgical treatment of choice.

Surgery:
- Open reduction + arthrodesis of proximal tibiofibular joint:

Indications:
- Strain upon the knee joint causing pain and disabilty
- Fibular head pressing upon peroneal nerve: May cause foot drop
- Excision of proximal fibula.

Indication: Fibular head pressing upon peroneal nerve: may cause foot drop.

Method (ORIF + Arthrodesis):
- Incision: An 8 cm longitudinal incision anteromedial to fibular head to expose the proximal tibiofibular joint
- Isolate the peroneal nerve
- Denude the articular surfaces of fibular head and fibular articular facet of tibia
- Reduction: Gently push the fibula into its normal position, and oppose the denuded surfaces
- Fixation (optional): Insert a screw through fibular head or neck, into the tibia.

Postreduction: Apply a long leg plaster cast for 4/52, followed by the weight bearing in a plaster boot or a long leg brace with a knee joint

Immobilization: Until solid fusion.

## Recurrent Dislocations

Definition           Recurrent dislocation of a joint following traumatic dislocation/s may occur because of an inadequate healing of its supporting soft tissues

Etiology             Congenital: Inadequate development of supporting soft tissues, or joint (weak capsule)

Traumatic: Repeated trauma (epileptics), or inadequate healing of supporting soft tissues (post-traumatic).

Pathogenesis         Relaxed supporting soft tissues (weak capsule); muscular imbalance; a prominent fibular head, or malaligned joint

Diagnosis            Pain
Disability
Movements: Impaired.

Investigation        X-ray of affected joint.

Management           Conservative treatment:
Closed reduction under anesthesia
Surgical treatment of choice in majority of cases.
Indication: Failure of conservative treatments.

Surgery:
- Open reduction

Regional:

## Recurrent Dislocation of Shoulder

Definition : Recurrent dislocation of shoulder following traumatic dislocation/s may occur because of an inadequate healing of its supporting soft tissues, and the shoulder more than any other joint is subject to recurrent dislocation, and usually the dislocation is anterior.

Etiology : Traumatic: Recurrent dislocation of shoulder occurring, due to little trauma (epileptics), and many a times the patient may be able to reduce dislocation, himself or herself.

Pathogenesis : There may be following pathological lesions:
- Bankart lesion: Separated anterior part of glenod fibrocartilage
- Flattening of posterolateral aspect of head (Hill-Sachs lesion)
- Rounding/erosion of glenoid margin
- Defective shoulder cuff includes stretched anterior part of capsule.

Investigation : X-ray shoulder—Axial view.

Management : Surgical treatment of choice

Surgery: Surgical repair: Types of repair:

Bankart repair: Anchoring the glenoid labrum and anterior capsule to the rim of the glenoid cavity by mattress sutures passed through holes in the rim.

Technique:
- Incision: A curved incision from the lateral end of clavicle, extending medially along the lateral third of clavicle to the level of coracoid process, then distally along medial border of deltoid
- Isolate and retract: The cephalic vein in the space between deltoid and pectoralis major
- Detach: Clavicular head of deltoid from clavicle and retract laterally to expose coracoid, and drill a 2.5 cm hole into it
- Divide: The coracoids and retract along with attached muscles (short head of biceps, pectoralis minor, coracobrachialis)
- Exposure: Capsule by isolate and retracting subscapularis tendon
- Incise: The capsule lateral to glenoid rim
- Drill: Holes (3–4) into the glenoid rim
- Suture: The lateral part of capsule to the glenoid rim, then lap the medial part of capsule over its lateral part and suture it.
- Suture the subscapularis tendon to its normal position, and reattach the coracoids with a screw and soft tissues with silk sutures.

Putti-plat repair: Restricting the external rotation by overlapping and shortening the subscapularis tendon, and overlapping and tightening the capsule.

Technique:

- Incision: A curved incision from the lateral end of clavicle, extending medially along the lateral third of clavicle to the level of the coracoid process, then distally along medial border of deltoid
- Isolate and retract the cephalic vein in the space between deltoid and pectoralis major
- Exposure: Coracoid process by detaching clavicular head of deltoid from clavicle and retract laterally
- Drill: Hole (2.5 cm) into it
- Divide: The coracoids and retract along with attached muscles (short head of biceps, pectoralis minor, coracobrachialis)
- Isolate and divide: Subscapularis tendon 2.5 cm from its insertion
- Exposure: And incise the capsule lateral to glenoid rim
- Drill: Holes (3–4) into the glenoid rim
- Suture: The lateral part of capsule to the glenoid rim, then lap the medial part of capsule over its lateral part and suture it.
- Suture: The free edge of lateral part of subscapularis tendon to the soft structures includes labrum (labrum and capsule not detached) along the anterior rim of glenoid cavity, or to medial part of subscapularis and capsule (detached labrum and capsule) with silk sutures (shoulder held in internal rotation)
- Suture: The lateral part of capsule to the glenoid rim, then lap the medial part of capsule over its lateral part and suture it.
- Suture: The medial part of subscapularis to the rotator cuff at the greater tuberosity or at the bicipital groove (overlapping all layers)
- Reattach: Tendons of short head of biceps brachioradialis to coracoid process, and deltoid to clavicle and pectoralis major.

Bone-block repair: Buttress the joint by fixing a bone graft to the glenoid (placed level with it), to block anterior displacement of humeral head.

Technique:

- Incision: 8 cm along deltopectoral groove, retract coracobrachialis medially to expose lesser tuberosity of the humerus by externally rotating shoulder
- Isolate and retract the cephalic vein in the space between deltoid and pectoralis major
- Exposure: Capsule by isolate and dividing subscapularis tendon
- Divide the capsule and subscapularis (1 cm. medial to its insertion)
- Prepare: A subperiosteal pocket at the inferior part of anterior lip of glenoid cavity
- Grafting: Remove an iliac crest graft (2.5 × 1 cm.) and place that into the subperiosteal pocket to form an anterior wall or buttress of bone, and to be held in position by the periosteum and labrum's remnants.
- Suturing: The subscapularis tendon to its normal position with the interrupted mattress sutures, and close the wound.

Postoperatively: Immobilization: arm kept in internal rotation for 4/52
After care: Exercises.

## Recurrent Dislocation of Elbow

| | |
|---|---|
| Definition | Recurrent dislocation of elbow is rare, and is usually posterior |
| Etiology | Congenital: Inadequate development of supporting soft tissues, or joint (weak capsule) |
| | Traumatic: Repeated trauma (epileptics), or inadequate healing of supporting soft tissues (post-traumatic). |
| Pathogenesis | Laxed collateral (ulnar and radial) ligaments; misshaped trochlear notch of the ulna (too shallow); fractured coronoid process; fractured humeral lateral epicondyle causing unstable joint. |
| Diagnosis | Pain |
| | Disability |
| | Joint: Unstable |
| Investigation | X-ray elbow—AP and Lateral views. |
| Management | Surgical treatment of choice. |

Surgery:

Tenodesis: Biceps tendon transferred to the coronoid process of ulna so as to reinforce the joint anteriorly

Technique:
- Incision: Curved anterior incision
- Excision: Devitalized and severely damaged muscle
- Drill: A transverse hole through ulna (from anterior aspect of coronoid)
- Implant: Freed biceps tendon into the hole
- Suture: End of tendon to the soft tissues over ulnar's subcutaneous border, and then insert a Bunnel pullout suture, to reinforce fixation until full healing.

Postoperative:
- Immobilization: An above elbow arm POP (elbow flexed at right angle) applied for 6/52.

After care: Active exercises of elbow.

Reinforcing/repairing of the relaxed soft tissues (capsule, collateral ligaments) by threading a part of triceps aponeurosis and a part of the biceps tendon through a hole in the distal humerus.

Technique:
- Incision: Curved anterior and posterior incisions
- Excision: Devitalized and severely damaged muscles
- Exposure: Biceps tendon and triceps aponeurosis
- Split biceps tendon and muscle up to 10 cm, free half of tendon proximally at split level while maintain its attachment to bone distally (to form a strip)
- Strip making: Similarly make a strip from middle of triceps aponeurosis

- Drill: A transverse hole through humerus at the olecranon fossa
- Implant: Freed biceps tendon into the hole
- Suture: End of tendon to the olecranon's tip and to the insertion of triceps (elbow flexed to right angle)
- Suture: Strip of triceps aponeurosis to the coronoid process or to the brachialis muscle fibers
- Suture: Defect in the triceps aponeurosis with interrupted sutures.

Bone grafting: To deepen the trochlear notch anteriorly

Technique:
- Incision: Curved 10 cm long on the anteromedial aspect of elbow
- Ligate, and divide: Median cubital vein; then expose biceps tendon; isolate and retract brachial vessels laterally, and the median nerve medially
- Exposure: Tip of coronoid process by dividing brachialis and incising the capsule
- Drill: An oblique hole through ulna
- Remove: A 3 cm long bone graft from tibia, and place it into an ulnar hole, to extend the contour of the trochlear notch

Postoperative:
- Immobilization: An above elbow arm plaster cast (elbow flexed at right angle) applied for 2/52.

After care: Exercises of elbow.

## Recurrent Dislocation of Knee

| | |
|---|---|
| Definition | Complete dislocation of knee is rare, while subluxation of knee joint is common, because of rupture of cruciate (anterior or posterior or both) ligaments. Dislocation of knee is a serious injury, because of injury of capsule, ligaments, and neurovascular (popliteal vessels, tibial or the common peroneal nerves) damage. |
| Types | Anterior (common), posterior, medial, lateral, or rotary. |
| MOI | Direct violence |
| | RSA |
| | Sports injury |
| | Fall from a height. |
| Pathogenesis | Ruptured cruciate ligament/s, hemarthrisis, femur passed forwards over the tibia, compressed popliteal vessels |
| Diagnosis | Pain |
| | Swelling |
| | Local tenderness. |
| Investigation | X-ray knee—AP and LAT views. |
| Management | Conservative treatment: |
| | Closed reduction: Under general anesthesia ASAP. |

Technique:
- Aspiration of the knee.
- Reduction: Apply traction to the flexed knee

Postreduction:
- Apply a posterior plaster slab/splint with the knee in flexion (10–15 degree) for 1/52, followed by a long leg plaster cast applied for 7/52.

After care: Rehabilitation:
- Active exercises (quadriceps and hamstrings)
- Postremoval of plaster cast, weight bearing with help of a long leg brace with joint at knee, to be permitted.

### Surgical treatment:

Indication:
- Failure of closed reduction because of interposition of soft tissues (capsule or femoral condyle caught in a bucket handle tear of the capsule).

Surgery: Open reduction.
- Instability due to IDK (torn ligament/s)

Surgery: Repair/replacement of torn ligament/s.

## Recurrent Dislocation of Patella

| | |
|---|---|
| Definition | Dislocation usually occurs towards lateral side. |
| MOI | Direct violence: RSA, sports injury, hit by a stick. |
| | Congenital: Relaxed medial part of capsule, genu valgum, or may be flattened articular surfaces of patella and lateral femoral condyle, or patellar tendon inserted too far laterally. |
| Pathogenesis | Flattened articular sufaces of patella and lateral femoral condy, degenerated articular surfaces; the patellar tendon inserted too far laterally. |
| Diagnosis | Pain |
| | Swelling |
| | Disability: Discomfort by using the affected limb |
| | Movements: Painful and restricted. |
| Investigation | X-ray knee—AP and LAT views. |
| Management | Surgical treatment of choice |
| | Procedures: Based upon age of the patient: |

Child or adolescent:
Surgery: Osteotomy to align the limb in genu valgum

Young adults:
Surgery: Hauser operation to change the direction of the quadriceps pull, by transplanting tibial tuberosity distal and medial to original attachment.

Adults:
Surgery:
- Roux-Goldthwait operaion: To create a check rein medially (patellar tendon split, lateral half transplanted medially;
- West and Soto-Hall operation: To excise the patella (patellectomy) + to change the direction of the quadriceps pull.

Postoperative:
* Immobilization: By a posterior POP slab or splint for 2/52

After care:
* Active and passive exercises and physiotherapy.
* Weight bearing with the help of crutches after 3/52.

## Recurrent Dislocation of Ankle

| | |
|---|---|
| Definition | Recurrent dislocation of the ankle usually occurs due to inadequate treatment of injured supporting soft tissues post an ankle trauma, many a times being treated as simply sprain cases, thereby causing weakness of the joint. |
| Etiology | Traumatic |
| Diagnosis | Pain |
| | Deformity |
| | Movements: Painful and restricted. |
| Investigation | X-ray ankle—AP and LAT views. |
| Management | Surgical treatment of choice. |

Surgery: ORIF.
* Open reduction: Indicated for several weeks old dislocation
* Internal fixation of fracture/s.

Postoperatively: Apply POP cast for 4/52.

After care: Weight bearing in a walking plaster boot, or a long leg brace with a knee joint, for the period till firm fusion.

## Recurrent Pathological Dislocation

| | |
|---|---|
| Definition | It is defined as a dislocation that may result from stretching of capsule and ligaments of a joint by an exudates (acute suppurative arthritis) or by destroyed articular surfaces (osteomyelitis, tuberculosis, and the neoplasms). |
| Etiology | Inflammatory: Joint destruction by the disease, e.g. |

* Travelling acetabulum: In advanced tuberculous arthritis of hip
* Triple deformity: In subluxation of knee

Paralytic: Muscles supporting a joint, e.g.
* Infantile paralysis of muscles of hip, or of shoulder girdle
* Spastic paralysis of muscles of hip (persistent adductor spasm)

Neuropathic: Stretching and dislocation by softening of ligaments, e.g.
* Charcot's joint

Congenital: CDH, congenital dislocation of patella, congenital and dislocation of radial head

Neoplastic: Joint destruction by the growth

| | |
|---|---|
| Reference | Described in the appropriate chapters for description of the pathological dislocations. |

## Bibliography

1. Adams JC. Recurrent dislocation of the shoulder. J. Bone and Joint Surg. 30-B:26, 1948
2. Bankart ASB. The pathology and treatment of recurrent dislocation of the shoulder joint, Brit. J. Surg. 26:23, 1938.

3. Barnes R. Paraplegia in Cervical Spine Injuries. J Bone Jt Surg. 30-B, 234, 1948.

4. Bennett GE. Old dislocations of the shoulder J. Bone and Joint Surg. 18:594, 1936.

5. Blount WP. Unequal leg length, American Academy of Orthopedic Surgeons Instructional Course.

6. Canale ST. Daugherty K, Jones L. Dislocations. Campbell's Operative Orthopaedics, 9th Ed. Vol I-IV, 1998.

7. Chrnley J. Dislocations. 275, 13th Ed. Bailey and Love's Short Practice of Surgery. Love M, Rains A.J. H., Capper W.M.; H.K. Lewis and Co., London, 1965.

8. Crooks F, and Birkett AN: Fractures and Fracture-dislocations of the Cervical Spine. Brit. J. Surg. 31: 252, 1944.

9. DePalma AF. Surgery of the shoulder. J.B. Lippincott Co., Philadelphia, 1950.

10. Dickson JW, Devas MB. Bankart's operation for recurrent dislocation of the shoulder, J. Bone and Joint Surg 39-B:114, 1957.

11. Evans DK. Reduction of Cervical Dislocations. J Bone Jt Surg. 43B, 552, 1961.

12. Holdsworth FW. Monteggia Fracture Dislocation. Modern Trends in Orthopedics Fracture Treatment, Clark J.M.P.; Butterworths, London, 1962.

13. Kapoor PS. Dislocations. Kapoor's Accident and Emergency: 2nd Ed. CBS, New Delhi, 2016.

14. King T. Recurrent dislocation of the elbow. J Bone and Joint Surg. 35-B: 50, 1953.

15. Knight G. Cranio; Cerebral Injuries. 369, 13th Ed. Bailey and Love's Short Practice of Surgery. Love M, Rains A.J. H., Capper W.M.; H.K. Lewis and Co., London, 1965.

16. London PS. The anatomy of injury and its Surgical Implications. Butterworth-Heinemann, Oxford, 1991.

17. Macnab I. Recurrent dislocation of the patella. J. Bone and Joint Surg 34-A: 957, 1952.

18. McLatchie GR. Essentials of Sports Medicine, 2nd Ed. Churchill Livingstone, Edinburgh, 1993.

19. McLaughlin HL. Recurrent anterior dislocation of the shoulder I. Morbid anatomy, Am. J. Surg. 99:628, 1960.

20. McRae R. Dislocation of the elbow: 117, 1st Ed. Practical Fracture Treatment, Mc Rae R, Churchill Livingstone, 1984.

21. Nicola T. Recurrent dislocation of the shoulder Am. J. Surg. 86:85, 1954.

22. Nicoll EA. Fractures and Dislocations of the Spine: 100–129:3. Modern Trends in Orthopedics Fracture Treatment Clark J.M.P.; Butterworths, London, 1962.

23. Watson-Jones R. Fractures and Joint Injuries, 4th Ed. Livingstone, Edinburgh.

# 4

# Fractures

| SECTION A: GENERAL PRINCIPLES |
|---|

- Definition of fracture
- Cause/Mode of Injury (MOI)
- Types of fracture
- Pattern of fracture
- Diagnosis of fracture
- Investigations
- Treatment of fracture
- Treatment of life-threatning situations
- Treatment of fracture
- First aid treatment
- Local treatment
- Reduction of fracture
- Fixation (immobilization) of fracture
- External fixation
- Internal fixation
- Implants
- Factors affecting healing of fracture
- Complications of fracture
- Fractures in children
- References

## FRACTURE

**Definition**   It is defined as break in the continuity of alignment of a bone, that includes all types of disruptions, i.e. hairline/or microscopic to grossly comminuted fractures.

**MOI**   Direct violence: Fracture occurring at the site of impact, i.e. Being hit by a falling or moving object.

Example:
- Fracture skull vault due to fall of heavy weight
- Fracture of hand-being struck by a stick, etc.

Indirect violence: Fracture occurring away from the site of impact, i.e. Twisting or bending force.

Example:
- Fall on outstretched hand, causing fracture of clavicle, fracture neck of humerus, dislocation shoulder, fracture shaft of the humerus, fracture supracondylar humerus.
- Rotational trauma of foot may cause spiral fracture of tibia

Muscular violence fracture: Occurring due to sudden, violent muscular contraction.

Example: Fracture patella due to sudden violent contraction of the quadriceps.

Stress (fatigue) fracture: also known as march fracture.

Example: Common in Army and Police personnel, participating in long marches and prolonged standings.

Site: Usually fracture of 2nd or 3rd metatarsals.

Pathological fracture: Fracture occurring in an abnormal or diseased bone, and a little force may be sufficient to break the affected eroded (osteoporotic), brittle (Paget's), cystic bone.

Example: Subtrochanteric fracture of femur due to secondary deposits

| | |
|---|---|
| Types of fracture | Simple fracture: Also known as closed fracture. Skin is intact. The wound, if present, does not communicate with the fracture. Hence, chances of infection, are rare. |

Compound fracture: Also known as open fracture. Skin is broken. The wound communicates with the fracture. Hence chances of infection are common.

Types:
- From without in—due to direct violence, contaminating wound, thereby entry of microorganisms from outside.
- From within out-fractured bone pierces the skin. Chances of infection are comparatively less in this type.

| | |
|---|---|
| Pattern of fracture | Transverse fracture: Descriptive of the line of fracture that is at right angle to long axis of a bone. It is a stable fracture; no shortning; angulation may occur; displacement uncommon; union favorable; and chances of early mobilization. Firm support required due to smaller area of bony contact. |
| MOI | Mostly direct violence, e.g. transverse fracture of ulna sustained by warding off a blow; transverse fracture of femoral shaft sustained by RSA, sports injury, or direct hit by a stick. |
| Oblique fracture | Descriptive of the line of fracture that is at an angle, less than right angle to the long-axis of a bone; usually an unstable fracture; sustained by indirect violence, chances of displacement and shortening are common. Union may be earlier, due to larger area of bony contact. Proper reduction and firm support required, as chances of shortening, displacement, and loss of bony contact are frequent. |
| MOI | Mostly indirect violence. |
| | Spiral fracture: Fracture occurs in a spiral form, across the bone; may be sustained by indirect violence (torsional forces); usually an unstable fracture; chances of displacement, loss of bony contact and shortening (due to unopposed muscle contraction, or premature weight bearing) are common; union may be fast, due to larger area of bony contact. Proper reduction and firm support required. |
| MOI | Mostly indirect violence. |
| | Greenstick fracture: Occurs in children. The bone bends and stays bent, one cortex (convex side) breaks, while the other cortex (concave side) remains intact (periosteum and adjoining soft tissues usually normal); mostly no displacement; healing is rapid; resulting in early obilization. |
| MOI | Direct or indirect violence. |
| | Hairline fracture: Fracture may be complete or incomplete, no displacement, difficult to detect radiologically, repeated weekly X-rays |

and oblique view may reveal the fracture clearly, healing is rapid, and require mostly conservative treatment except fracture of scaphoid and fracture neck of femur.

MOI      Mostly minimal violence.

Single fracture: The bone is fractured at one level.

MOI      Mostly direct violence.

Double fracture: The affected bone is fractured at two different levels, difficult to reduce and fix the fragments, ORIF may further impair doubtful blood supply to central segment, and delayed/non union common.

MOI      Direct violence and fall from height.

Comminuted fracture: The bone is broken into more than two fragments. Greater comminution indicates severe violence, marked damage to the adjoining muscles, tendons, nerves, vessels and skin. Comminuted fractures are mostly unstable and usually complicated ones.

Types: Minor comminution at fracture site without any displacement; major comminution at the fracture site with a large "butterfly" type fragment.

Impacted fracture: In this type of fracture, one fragment is driven into the other fagment. Usually seen at junction of cortical and cancellous bones, i.e. end of the shaft or impaction of one cancellous fragment.

Example: Fractures of vertebral bodies (flexion injuries); fractures of calcaneus (fall from height) complicated fracture (syn. complex fracture): fracture associated with neighboring structures, i.e. neurovascular, visceral injuries.

Example: Fracture shaft of humerus with radial nerve injury.

Pathological fracture: Fracture occurs in an abnormal or diseased bone.

A little force may be sufficient to break the affected brittle, eroded, osteoporotic, and cystic bone.

Avulsion fracture: Fracture occurs due to sudden, violent muscular contraction.

Example:
- Fracture patella (upper pole) due to violent contraction of quadriceps.
- Fracture tibial tuberosity, due to contraction of patellar tendon.
- Fracture base of fifth metatarsal, due to contraction of peroneus bravis.
- Fracture lesser trochanter, due to contraction of iliopsoas.

Intra-articular fracture: Fracture involving a joint, causing irregularity of joint surface, leading to complication of stiffness of joint and finally to development of secondary osteoarthritis.

Fracture-dislocation: Joint dislocation, along with fracture of one of the bony components of the joint.

Example:
- Fracture dislocation of shoulder joint.
- Monteggia fracture-dislocation.

## Diagnosis of Fracture

| | | |
|---|---|---|
| Symptoms | 1. Pain | 2. Swelling |
| | 3. Difficulty/inability to move part | 4. Bruising |
| Signs | 1. Deformity | 2. Shortening |
| | 3. Local tenderness | 4. Bone surface Irregularity |
| | 5. Crepitus | 6. Unnatural mobility |
| | 7. Loss of function | 8. Wound |
| | 9. Shock | |

Deformity: Usually characteristic of a fracture, but a bone may be broken without any deformity; the deformity means separation of bony fragments from each other due to extensive tearing of the soft tissues, fascia, intermuscular septa, etc.

Types: Displacement, angulation, and axial rotation

- Displacement: It is defined as shifting of distal fragment relative to proximal fragment. Displacement may be anterior/posterior/medial/or lateral. It may be partial or complete (no bony contact of fragments) and may lead to shortening, malunion, or nonunion due to interposition of soft tissues between fractured fragments.

- Angulation: It may be anterior/posterior/medial/or lateral, depending upon point of angle or position (tilt) of distal fragment. Angulation should never be neglected, as deformity is regarded as sign of poor treatment. It may also interfere with normal functioning esp. in upper limb, affecting pronation/supination.

- Axial rotation: In this deformity, one fragment rotates on its long axis, relative to other fragment. It may or may not be associated with displacement or angulation. It may be detected radiologically, from the position of interlocking fragments, and from the differences in the relative diameters of the fragments.

Shortening: If present, is an important sign of fracture. Occurs due to overriding of fragments.

Local tenderness: In impacted fractures, local bony tenderness is the most important clinical sign while loss of function is the most important symptom.

Bone surface irregularity: In form of a gap, elevation, or a bend, if present, is a definite sign of a fracture.

Crepitus: While palpating or testing unnatural mobility, a crepitus or grating sensation may be felt or heard. Is also a definite sign of a fracture. It may also be positive in a hematoma, gas gangrene, surgical emphysema, and osteoarthritis.

Unnatural mobility: It is elicited by moving one fragment against the other. If present is a definite sign of a fracture, but to be elicited with great care to avoid occurrence of complications. It is absent in impacted fracture and greenstick fracture loss of function: there may be complete loss of function in a fracture case. Impacted fracture may present great difficulty in clinical diagnosis. X-ray is of great helpfull in such cases.

Wound: If present may contain broken fragments, foreign body, blood clots, etc. There may be oozing of blood from the wound.

Shock: If present, is a life-threatening emergency, and to be managed on priority basis. It is oligemic due to hemorrhage and vasoconstriction (to maintain peripheral vascular resistance).

Signs of shock:
- Unconscious
- Air gasping or breathless
- Pale, cyanotic
- Hypotension.

**Investigations**
- X-Ray examination: It is the main investigation for confirming the clinical diagnosis of a fracture. X-ray of the affected bone taken, mostly in two planes (views), i.e. Anteroposterior (AP) and Lateral. views reveal upward or downward displacement

Axial view: Required esp. in fracture of calcaneum.

AP view: Reveals lateral or medial displacement, whereas lateral view reveals anterior or posterior displacement of distal fragment. Both views reveal upward or downward displacement.

Axial view: Required esp. in fracture of calcaneus.

Oblique view: Required esp. in fracture of scaphoid.

X-ray findings in a fracture, reveal:
- Site and type of fracture.
- Displacement, angulation, rotation of fragments.
- Callus formation-sign of union.
- Sclerosis, rounding of fractured ends-sign of nonunion.
- Avascular necrosis (AVN) of bone-decalcification of adjoining bones, while avascular necrotic bone preserves its density due to nonvascularization.

**Examples**
- AVN of femoral head following fracture neck of femur.
- AVN of proximal fragment following fracture of scaphoid.
- Myositis ossificans is subperiosteal ossification, following fracture.
- Elbow fractures.
- Pathological fractures: X-ray may reveal the underlying pathological condition, responsible for erosion of bone, lowering the strength of bone, lowering the strength of bone-vulnerable to fracture even from trivial trauma.

MRI of affected bone and joint
CT scan of affected bone and joint.

## Management of Polytrauma

**Preface**
Trauma is the commonest cause of death in the developed countries; usually under the age of 40 years; deaths from trauma exceed the

combined deaths from CVS disorders and cancer; about 30% of these traumatic deaths occur as RSA.

Trimodal death pattern: Post-trauma death shows a trimodial pattern:

- First peak: Mortality occurs immediately or shortly post-trauma: Etiology: Major head (brain) or vascular (hemorrhagic shock) injury; mostly unsalvageable.

- Second peak: Mortality occurs within hours. post-trauma; period spanning 1st and 2nd peaks called 'golden hr,/s' Etiology: ABC (airway, breathing, or circulatory) disorders; most of that could be treated ASAP.

- Third peak: Mortality occurs days or weeks post-trauma Etiology: Infection (sepsis) or organ/s failure.

Principles

## I. Management of Life-Threatening Situations

Airway obstruction

Breathing distress—Tension pneumothorax, hemothorax, cardiac tamponade.

Bleeding (hemorrhage)

Chest injuries—Flail chest

Head injuries and neurological disorders

Shock

Spine injuries

Abdominal injuries

Pelvis injuries

## II. Management of Fracture

Reduction of fracture

Fixation (immobilization) of fracture

External fixation and internal fixation

Rehabilitation

## MANAGEMENT OF LIFE-THREATENING SITUATIONS

### Advanced Trauma Life Support (ATLS)

**Priority of treatment:** In the management of polytrauma (multiple injuries), priority of treatment is directed to life-threatening conditions such as airway obstruction, shock, or external hemorrhage, even before a detailed examination begins. The doctor incharge should plan the line of treatment in consultation with other specialists involved in the management of various lesions. It may be possible to manage all the injuries simultaneously but at times, these lesions to be dealt with, on priority basis, e.g. in a definite sequence. Compound fractures should preferably be treated along with head, neck, or chest injuries. Operative treatment for simple fractures may better be postponed to a later stage. But it is better not to postpone the corrective orthopedic measures for more than a day or so, in the patients who appeared unlikely to recover from their associated injuries.

**Management:** Described in the section—Management of multiple injuries:

## MANAGEMENT OF FRACTURE

### First Aid Treatment

Principle
- Immobilization: To immobilize the joint above and below the fracture: upper limb: arm to be held by the side of the body by the use of arm slings and bandages; shoulder and elbow held with a sling; forearm held with crammer wire splint or card board, wooden splint; lower limb: splinted on a Thomas splint; femur held with traction or splint; tibia and ankle splinted with a wooden splint with foot piece.
- Pain relief:

Analgesics:
- Inj. Morphine 10 mg IV. Repeat 8–12 hourly.

Side effects    Nausea, vomiting, constipation, sedation, respiratory depression.

Antidote    Inj. Nalorphine 5 mg IV + Inj. Stemetil or Inj. Perinorm
- Inj. Pethidine 50 mg IV. Repeat 8–12 hourly.

Side effects: Addiction (dependence)
- Inj. Pentazocine 30–60 mg IM or IV. Repeat 3–4 hourly

Side effects: Nausea, vomiting, dependence

Bleeding control: By bandaging of wound.

Infection control: By dressing of wound, antibiotics IM or IV.

Local treatment

### Reduction of Fracture

**Aims:** To reduce a displaced fracture, so as to unite in good functional position, and the reduction is usually easier if performed without unnecessary delay, prior to surrounding soft tissues becoming swollen and turgid. Often unreduced fractures unite rapidly, but may yield to malunion. Repeated manipulations to achieve perfect radiological reduction may lead to hazards (malunion/nonunion). Slight/little displacement esp. in children and old, weak patient may often be accepted (to outweigh undesirable risks).

Indication: Correction of deformities: displacement, angulation, and rotation (cosmetic and functional issues).

Anesthesia    General, regional, or local:
- General: Provides muscle relaxation, duration, and versatility.
- Regional: Safer for minor procedures
- Local: Safer for minor procedures.

Types of reduction    Closed or open.

Closed reduction    Majority of fractures are reduced by this method.

Advantages:
- Relatively safe method—chances of infection are less.
- Relatively much cheaper.

Disadvantages:
- Failure of reduction sometimes—due to interposition of soft tissues between fragments.

- Failure to maintain reduction.
- Prolonged immobilization.

Technique:

- Most of fractures reduced manually by using longitudinal traction, angulation, or hingeing. Ideally postreduction, the limb should look similar to its fellow in length and appearance. Frequently X-ray picture may be deceptive, thereby alarming inexperienced surgeon to resort to repeated manipulations or unnecessary open reduction, that may lead to undesirable results, as loss of alignment is of more serious consequences than lacking end to end apposition, esp. in weight bearing bones.
- By continuous traction (fractures of femur and dislocation of cervical spine). In fractures of femur shaft, overlapping does not prevent union, although some shortening may occur.

Types: Skin and skeletal tractions:

- Skin traction (by using an adhesive strapping): Mostly indicated in children and young adults for fractures femur and fractures of lower end of humerus.

Method:

- Toilet of skin with spirit/alcohol/betadine scrub, post skin- shaving;
- Apply adhesive tape (of traction kit) on both sides of leg, extending beyond foot for spreader bar
- Place foam/cotton over malleoli (protection)
- To secure adhesive tapes throughout with encircling elastic crepe-bandage
- Apply desired weights to the cord.

Skeletal traction (by using a Steinmann pin through tibial tuberosity): indicated in an older patient, that require a heavy traction, but often complications like pin track infection do occur.

**Open reduction**   Should always be undertaken by a surgeon highly skilled. In fracture management. Better to be avoided in children.

Indications:

- Failure of closed reduction (fractures of medial malleolus)
- Particular fractures-in need of perfect reduction and fixation, e.g. fracture neck of femur.
- To reduce mortality and morbidity (internal fixation of trochanteric fractures)
- To achieve acceptable reduction—not possible by closed methods (depressed comminuted fractures of tibial condyle)
- To prevent occurrence of displacement, angulation, or deformity, common after closed reduction (Monteggia fracture dislocation, fracture patella, olecranon fracture)
- Compound fractures, complicated fractures.
- Early mobilization required esp. in elderly patients.

Disadvantages:

- Relatively unsafe method, as chances of infection are more.

Sometimes disastrous one: Resulting in gangrene, requiring amputation, or even death may occur.

- To impair vascularity by stripping of soft tissues for exposure of fragments, and insert implants (risk of nonunion), being absent in closed methods
- To produce scar that may impair muscle function (fractures of femur)
- To produce foreign body reaction (metallic implants)
- Relatively much costlier method.

**Fixation (immobilization) of fracture:** External and internal fixation: attention must be given not only to the broken bone, but also to the soft parts, while considering the correct method of fixation of each type of fracture.

## External fixation

**A. Plaster fixation:** It is the most widely used form of fixation, and has superseded all other forms external fixation, e.g. splints (wooden, metallic), braces for treatment of majority of fractures.

### Aims

- To retain the limb/part in the desired comfortable position, by its adaptation, and not by traction or pressure.
- To be light in weight, but strong enough to be effective in use, and to be easily removable.

### Method

*Plaster slabs*: Available in ready-made packs, or may be prepared from desired size plaster bandages, by dry method (prepared beforehand); wet method (prepared from wet bandage); pattern method (shapes prepared from wide bandages):

- Dry method: Water to be tepid (neither cold or hot), slab gripped by hands and emersed in water till no air bubbles , then held slab vertically and slightly squeezed to drain out surplus water, then placed over a flat surface and smoothed out with the palm, then apply over the desired fractured part.
- Wet method: Commonest, unroll bandage a little, immerse in water till no bubbles, squeezed, then prepare the desired sized slab, and finally apply over the desired fractured part.
- Pattern method: Unroll plaster bandage to desired size and make 4–6 layered slab, then hold the slab, immerse in water, squeeze, and apply  over the desired fractured part, often to the proximal parts first, so that moulding be carried out more profitably against a set or nearly set cuff of plaster on the calf or forearm (B/K plaster at tibial tubercle, and forearm plaster at the elbow).
- Ridging plaster slabs: To reinforce a plaster, for providing resistance to strain and stress, by ridging (central part of wet slab raised along its length, and applied to the cast, while in girdering, an additional slab, shorter than first slab is ridged and superimposed.
- Cast-bracing: Sometimes indicated in the failed initial conservative treatment of a fracture (delayed union):

Example: Fractures of femur ant tibia in same limb: separate support for each, linked together by hinges at the side of the knee, allowing early ambulation.

Post care: Should be taken of swelling, change in the skin color, numbness, etc. following application of plaster—if present, then:

- Immediately loosen the plaster by splitting, or removing/changing the plaster.
- Elevation: To wear an arm sling in case of upper limb, while in case of lower limb, elevate the leg on pillows or RBE
- Active exercises.

**B. Traction:** Fixed traction in a thomas splint or by continuous traction for couple of weeks, holding a reduced fracture. It is often used for treating fracture femoral shaft (skin traction by adhesive strapping, or skeletal traction by using a Steinmann pin).

**C.** Braces, splints, jackets, collars, belts, knee caps, anklets

**D.** Elastic crepe bandaging, adhesive strapping

**E. External fixator and ring fixator:** Bone fragments held in alignment by skeletal pins.

Indication
- Compound fractures, wherein condition of skin and other soft tissues, disapprove use of internal fixation devices
- Pin track (skeletal traction) infections

Method
- Pins insertion: Central part of each pin in the bone, with the ends protruding from the skin
- Set of pins (1–3) inserted in each bone fragment
- Reduction: Fracture reduced with the aid of pins *in situ* (by an open reduction or by using an image intensifier)
- Pins held in position by a firm external support.

Ilizarov's method
Indication:
Congenital deformities: Correction:
- Upper limb
- Lower limb
- Pseudarthrosis of tibia

Traumatic
- Fractures (transosseous osteosynthesis)
- Upper limb
- Lower limb
- Nonunion

Infective
- Compound fractures: Wherein condition of skin and other soft tissues, disapprove use of internal fixation devices
- Pin track (skeletal traction) infections

Lengthening: Bone lengthening:
- Upper limb
- Lower limb

Achondroplastic dwarfism: Limb lengthening
- Compound fractures, wherein condition of skin and other soft tissues, disapprove use of internal fixation devices
- Pin track (skeletal traction) infections

Specific
- Angular deformities: Correction
- Contractures Joints
- Arthrodesis: Local
- Widening and recontouring of leg

Method: (Ilizarov): It is mostly a nonsurgical procedure, except for the insertion of wires/pins, performed in an operation theater

Insertion of wires/pins:

- Wires/pins (bayonet type for hard cortical bone, while trocar type for metaphyseal cancellous bone), 1.5 to 1.8 mm in diameter for insertion: central part of each pin in the bone, with the ends protruding from the skin
- Drilling through both cortices, then hammer wires/pins
- Set of wires/pins (1–3) inserted in each bone fragment, with care to protect neurovascular structures (precise anatomical insertion of wires/pins.

Reduction of fracture: Fracture reduced with the aid of pins *in situ* (by an open reduction or by using an image intensifier) Fixation of wires/pims to rings: pins held in position by a firm external support rings (made of two half rings), as per maximal diameter of the limb (space to be kept between inner part of the ring and the limb all around).

Ring assembly: To place limb centrally in the ring, so as to avoid the postoperative edema, pain, and pressure ulcers. The wires on the rings to be tensioned by a pair of dynamometers or by turning wire fixation bolt, as any movement between the wires and soft tissues may cause continuous irritation and infection. Ring attachments (cannulated bolt for a wire passing centrally through ring hole; slotted bolt used for a wire passing eccentrically to ring hole; and washers used for a wire passing above or below the ring surface).

Rods assembly to connect rings: Rods (threaded or telescopic) placed parallel to one another and to bone axis, and the rods (3–4) to be placed at equidistance from each other on the ring's circumference.

## Postoperative Care

Early:
- Bedrest
- Elevate the limb
- ASD
- Physiotherapy: Exercises

Late:
- Wires checking to remain tight

## Removal of Apparatus: Based on

Limb's condition

Diagnosis and pathology: No pain, discomfort, swelling

Healing time: Often < other methods, as basically nonsurgical and utilizes biology healing.

X-ray findings: Healthy new bone formation

Postoperative complications: Instability of bone fragments in the apparatus

Injury to nerves and vessels

Infection
- Wire infections
- Bone amd soft tissue

Rehabilitation
- Instructions towards patient's behavior: exercises, occupational therapy

- Preventive and corrective methods: To avoid teethering of muscles, while passing wires through
- Rehabilitation methods and physiotherapy: Based upon a strategy to overcome resistance of powerful muscles that create deformities due to joint contractures.

## Internal Fixation

*Principles of internal fixation of fractures:*

Anatomical and physiological factors involved in the healing of a fracture are essential to perfect management, esp. in the case of treatment by open methods, using implants like plates and screws, screws, intramedullary nailing and interlocking nailing, tension wires, percutaneous wires, etc.

Aims:

- Clinical: To achieve proper union (primary object): as function of the adjoining soft tissues and joints depends upon it
- Anatomical: To restore normal anatomical position of the bones after healing: as function of the adjoining soft tissues and joints depends upon it
- Physiological: To restore normal function of the limb, relative to early mobilization of soft tissues and adjoining joints.

Circulation: To maintain/re-establish the local circulation

Example: Fracture femoral neck, or fracture scaphoid.

## Principles:

- Freedom from foreign body reaction: Implant should be biological inert, free from toxic reactions, inflammatory response, fibrous and giant cell reactions. These usually cause pain, swelling, and loss of function
- Freedom from rust: Implant should be made of high quality stainless steel, etc. to avoid rusting of implant esp. in compound fractures
- Freedom from mechanical failure: Implant should be lighter in weight of great strength and of suitable design to match the shape and size of donor bone.

## Materials Commonly Used are

- Stainless steel
- Vitallium—alloys of chromium, cobalt, and molybdenum
- Titanium.

## Advantages of Internal Fixation

- Firm fixation
- Early weight bearing
- Early return to work.

## Disadvantages of Internal Fixation

- Infection
- Failure: Due to faulty technique or faulty (wrong) selection of implant.
- Failure: Due to faulty selection of treatment (closed or internal fixation) for needs of each and every particular case.

## Implants

### Plates and Screws

*Criterias:*

- Skin incision: To be long enough, so as to provide enough exposure, with least possible retraction (reduction and internal fixation easier)

  By extending skin incision, may not interfere healing period, as healing occurs from side to side and not from end to end, and the skin incision not to be placed directly over the bone.

- Muscles: Bone to be approached through intermuscular planes, rather than through muscle bellies, and sharp dissection preferred over blunt dissection.
- Neurovascular: To be handled with utmost care, and hemostasis is mandatory.
- Bones: To be exposed by subperiosteal stripping, without dissecting unnecessarily the soft tissues from the fractured fragments. Postexposure, reduction achieved by periosteal elevators or bone levers, maintained by the holding clamp (Lane, Rush, Ochsner, Lambotte).
- Plates: To be of high quality, and malleable enough to permit adjustment to the contour of the bone (by bending irons), and the plate should be long enough and strong enough, so as to provide firm fixation. Slotted plates (bony contact established prior to screws tightening) to be preffered over Sherman or Lane bone plates, for femur, tibia, and humerus.
- Sherman plate is a lightweight, comparatively of weaker strength plate, and requires external support.
- Eggar plate is slotted, so that the screws are not fully tightened, allowing the bone ends to remain in contact. Requires external support.
- Dynamic compression plate (DCP) is slotted and tightening of plate is achieved by pinching of plate by the heads of screws.
- Nail/blade plate is being used in a fracture closer to a long bone's end.

  Insertion: Nail or blade part is driven through the cancellous part, while the plate part is fixed with the cortical screws, to the shaft of the long bone.

- Buttress plates, Y plates, Fracture plates, LC plates, cervical spine locking plates
- Screws: Cortical and cancellous screws, available in large range of lengths but restricted in range of diameters.

*Types of screws:*

- Self tapping screws: The screw cuts its own thread in the bone.

  Example: Sherman and Lanes screws.

  The screw has an OD (outside diameter) and a slot single, cruciate, or combination. Insertion: A hole is drilled through the bone, followed by driving in the screw, cutting its thread into the bone by its flutted end.

*Screws which require bone to be tapped prior to insertion:*

- AO series screws: AO cortical screw has: An OD; a hexagonal socket; a buttress thread with pitch.

  Insertion: A hole is drilled through the bone, followed by tapping with a corresponding tap and finally the screw is driven through.

*Screws which do not require bone tapping prior insertion*:

- Single cortical screw: It is a week internal support and requires external support, e.g. plaster of paris or splint.
- Cancellous screws: Indicated in cancellous bone.
- Locking screws: Cannulated, self drilling, self tapping screws.
- Dynamic hip screw (DHS).
- Transfixation screws: Indicated in long oblique or tortional fractures (butterfly fracture with two oblique surfaces)
- Spine system (Schanz screws)—for cervical spine surgery
- Pedicle screw system—for low back surgery.
- Nails/Pins:
- Intramedullary nailing for fractures of shafts of long bones, e.g. Kuntscher nail for fracture shaft femur.
- Interlocking Nails:
  - Antegrade Femoral Nail (AFN)
  - Proximal Femoral Nail (PFN)
  - Distal Femoral Nail (DFN)
  - Universal Femoral Nail (UFN)—Titanium solid nail
  - Cannulated Femoral Nail (CFN)
  - Rush pins (nails) for fracture humerus, ulna, etc.
  - Principles of medullary fixation:
- Fracture through narrowest part of medullary canal (eliminates rotation, distraction, side-to-side movement, and shearing stress)
- To eliminate need for external fixation
- To be avoided if the bone is too much curvaceous (nail may break)
- To be strong enough to maintain alignment and position, and not to bend or break by angular forces
- To be inserted in such a way, that its removal to be easy (bend or break)
- To remove the nail prior to opt for other procedures, in case of infection or nonunion.
- That a metallic nail is not a substitute for union may break or bend

Rehabilitation: Bohler introduced the importance of rehabilitation by encouraging the patient to uitilize the splinted limb (to maintain limb's circulation, minimize muscle's atrophy, and to reduce period of joint stiffness). Bohler strongly emphasized that poor results of fracture management do not result from fracture, but results from poor splintage.

*Principle/aim of rehabilitation*:

- To restore the patient to work at the earliest possible after injury, with the minimal residual disability.
- To start rehabilitation (physical, psychological, occupational) as soon as the patient overcomes the main discomfort (pain and fear of pain) in the early days, and muscle wasting and joint stiffness in the later periods of management.
- To apply a plaster cast that allows patient to feel comfortable and allows the limb to be utilized. Pain from a poorly applied plaster cast, or a joint fixed in an uncomfortable position, discourage patient to follow sugeon's instructions, e.g. pressure sore from a faulty plaster cast, may discourage the patient to use the limb.

- To encourage patients for visiting fracture rehabilitation clinics in groups for physical, mental, and occupational therapy. The idea being the fractured limb may benefit from rehabilitation a lot while still inside the plaster cast/boot (retained until patient walks in it) so as to walk freely postremoval of plaster.
- To encourage exercises, not only of the injured limb but also of he the whole body, to take place (exercises based on postural reflexes, thereby ensuring maintenance of maximum tone). The exercise chosen should produce the required movement without disturbing the patient mentally (fatigue from exercise is due rather to mental exhaustion than to physiological fatigue of muscle); balancing and ankle motion achieved by playing darts; arms and hand movements by playing with balls of different sizes or shapes; walking achieved by playing skittles or bowls. Over all the patient must keep moving.
- To confine massage and physiotherapy (poor substitute) to early period of rehabilitation, because of local trauma, or necessity of using fixed splints, active exercise not feasible.

## Factors Affecting Healing of Fracture

Definition: Following factors may affect healing in a patient with a fracture or dislocation (Table 4.1).

## Factors

**Age:** Younger the patient, better are chances of early union of fracture. In children, union of fracture is faster, which slows down as the age advances. Also power of remodelling of fracture is stronger in epiphyseal fusion is imminent; remodeling also poor in case of axial rotation.

Example: In a child, union in a fractured femur, usually expected a little post number of weeks. Equivalent to its numerical age (4 weeks vide 3 years of age), while in adults usually takes 3–6/12.

- **Type of bone:** Cancellous (spongy) bone: Healing in the fractured cancellous bone is comparatively earlier than In the fractured cortical bone, and the weight bearing usually permitted:
  - In fractures of os calcaneus usually after 6/52
  - In fractures vertebral bodies allowed after 6–8/52

**Table 4.1:** Factors affecting healing of fracture

| Factor | Healing | |
| --- | --- | --- |
| | Early | Late (slow/delay/nonunion) |
| Age | Younger | Adult/old |
| Type of bone | Cancellous | Cortical |
| Distraction of bone ends | – | Delayed/nonunion |
| Unnatural mobility | – | Delayed/nonunion |
| Infection | – | Delayed/nonunion |
| Impaired blood supply | – | Delayed/nonunion |
| Quality of bone | Clavicle | Tibia |
| Pathological fracture | – | Malignant tumors (delayed) |
| Intra-articular fracture | – | Delayed |

(*Source*: Kapoor's Accident and Emergency)

– In fractures tibial plateau allowed after 6–8/52
– In fracture pelvis bedrest advised for 6/52
– In colles fracture plaster discarded after 6–8/52
Cortical (compact) bone: Endosteal callus may be well-established in a couple of months (appx. 10–15/52 to unite), while an abundant external bridging callus may permit an early recovery, e.g.
– In fractures humeral shaft, union occurs usually in 10/52
– In fractures tibial shaft union occurs usually in 12–16/52
– In fractures metacarpals, metatarsals, phalanges (substantial callus externally bridging) firm union occurs in 4–6/52.

- **Distraction of bone ends, due to:**
  – Interposition of soft tissues between bone ends: usually fasciae or ligaments seems to be a more effective barrier to growth of external callus across a fracture than muscle's interposition (e.g. fractures of patella, olecranon, and medial malleolus), resulting in impaired apposition of fractured surfaces, may cause delayed union, or even nonunion.
  – Excessive traction force applied during immobilization period following reduction of fracture, pulls apart the fractured bone ends thus favoring growth of fibrous tissue that insulates bone ends from each other (emphasizing use of minimum traction force to obtain desired reduction).
  – Faulty internal fixation of fractures: may cause resorption of bone ends at the fracture site, thus prevents bone fragments from meeting together.

- **Unnatural movements at the fracture site:** Faulty immobilization (fixation) of a fracture, resulting in movements at the fracture site, which in turn interupts the vascularization of hematoma, leading to the impaired formation of bridging callus, finally into delayed union, nonunion.

- **Infection:** Mild infection that clears up shortly, may not cause any side effect, while severe infection (acute osteomyelitis) may result in delayed or nonunion, due to resorption of callus. Usually common in compound fractures and fractures treated by internal fixation (implant acts as a forein body and a nidus in an established infection) advisable to retain implant until healing being achieved, otherwise its removal early may results in movements of fragments and finally nonunion. Rare in fractures being treated by conservative measures.

- **Impaired blood supply:** Interruption of blood supply to the bone following fracture, may lead to avascular necrosis of the bone, due to rupture of vessels supplying bone—becomes soft and distorted in size and shape, causing pain, stiffness, and osteoarthritis.

  *Common sites:*
  – Avascular necrosis of femoral head, following intracapsular fracture of femur neck or dislocation of hip.
  – Avascular necrosis of proximal segment of scaphoid following fracture scaphoid.
  – Avascular necrosis of talus following fractures or dislocations
  – Avascular necrosis of lunate following dislocations.

- **Quality of bone:** Certain bones heal earlier or later than others following fracture, due to unknown factors, e.g.
  – Fracture clavicle that heals earlier inspite of uncontrolled movement at the fracture site.
  – Fracture tibia—heals slowly inspite of firm fixation.

## Pathological Fractures

- Occur spontaneously or after trivial trauma, in an abnormal or diseased bone due to progressive weakness of the bone that may heal slowly esp. in case of primary and secondary malignant bone tumors, due to marked erosion of bone. On the other hand, union occurs without any delay, e.g. simple bone cyst.

- **Intra-articular fractures:** Union is delayed due to dilution of the hematoma by the sunovial fluid.

## Complications of Fracture

Complications (general or local) that may occur in a patient who has suffered a fracture or dislocation may be classified in the following manner (Table 4.2).

## General Complications

**Shock:** Oligemic shock due to hemorrhage (external or internal) that may not recover within an hour or so (due to decreased blood volume) following trauma (fracture pelvis or femur), and in such a case, giving early anesthesia without fluid replacement may yield severe hypotension due to failure of protective vasoconstrictive mechanism.

Diagnosis: Unconscious, breathless, pale, cyanotic, pupils-dilated, hypotension, pulse rapid

Management: On top priority basis, measures:

A. Airway maintenance: Position of head, removal of any foreign body, endotracheal intubation, ventilator-oxygen therapy

B. Breathing monitoring: Treatment of the cause, i.e. any chest injury, tension pneumothorax, hemothorax.

**Table 4.2:** Complications of a fracture

| General complication | Local complications | |
|---|---|---|
| | Early | Late |
| Shock | Arterial injury | Avascular necrosis |
| Hemorrhage | Nerve injury | Ischemic contracture |
| Fat embolism | Infection | Tight plasters |
| Hypostatic pneumonia | | Slow union |
| Acute renal failure | | Delayed union |
| | | Nonunion |
| | | Malunion |
| | | Shortening |
| | | Joint stiffness |
| | | Myositis ossificance |
| | | Osteoarthritis |
| | | Sudeck's dystrophy |
| | | Bedsores |
| | | Visceral |
| | | Cast syndrome |

(*Source*: Kapoor P.S.: Accident and Emergency)

C. Control of bleeding: By bandage, tourniquet, etc. for external hemorrhage; by lligating torn vessel or soft tissue—for internal hemorrhage.

Re-establishment of circulating blood volume:
- IV fluids: Normal saline, dextrose
- Blood transfusion—if loss more than 1–2 litres
- Plasma or plasma expanders—if loss less than 1 litre or if whole blood not available.
- Drugs: Inj. Morphine 10 mg IV for relief from pain. Repeat after 8–12 hourly if required. Inj. Hydrocortisone 100 mg IV to combat hypotension. Repeat 4 hourly. Inj. Ephedrine IV.
- Splintage of fractured bone, by use of splints, braces, arm slings, traction.

**Hemorrhage:** External or internal—due to rupture of vessels, soft tissues, bone fragments, etc. Bleeding may be extensive, resulting in decreased blood volume.

**Management**
- External hemorrhage: Control of bleeding by applying firm bandage, tourniquet
- Internal hemorrhage: Control of bleeding by ligating the torn vessel, soft tissue repair. Blood transfusion, and if not available, then give plasma or plasma expander and IV saline.

**Fat embolism:** Due to entry of microparticles of fat particles from broken bone marrow, into the circulation. It is a serious, life-threatening emergency. Commonly seen in fracture of femoral shaft, fracture pelvis, and fracture tibia.

S/S: Confusion, irritation, or comatose, fever, patechial hemorrhages in the skin, palate, conjunctiva, renal failure, death.

Investigation: CBC: fall in hemoglobin

Sputum: Fat droplets

Eye: Fundus examination may reveal retinal hemorrhages, exudate

CXR: May show mottling of lung fields (fat embolism)

Management: Heparin IV, oxygen, IV fluids, monitoring vital signs

**Hypostatic pneumonia:** May occur in an elderly patient, confined to bed, as commonly seen in fracture neck femur, fracture pelvis.

S/S: Fever, chest pain, cough with expectoration, dyspnea, orthopnea, pulse rapid.

Investigation: CBC, ESR, Blood culture, and CXR.

**Management:**
- Make patient comfortable in the bed with support of backrest
- Oxygen therapy
- IV fluids
- Antibiotics
- Analgesics
- Expectorants
- Steam inhalation
- Monitoring-nursing care

**Acute renal failure:** Following fracture (fall from height, RSA, blows), due to shock, excessive bleeding, fat embolism.

S/S: Confusion, irritation, coma, fever, edema face and legs, oliguria

Investigation: Serum electrolytes, creatinine, ECG-to monitor the potassium level.

**Management:**
- Bedrest
- Indwelling catheterization
- Inj. Morphine for pain and sedation
- IV Dextrose 20% slowly
- Blood transfusion
- Antibiotics
- Heparinization
- Management of fracture.

## Local Complications of Fracture

### Early Complications

**Arterial injury:** Blood vessels may be torn, or occluded by pressure of bone fragments, or spasm of vessels, leading to ischemia of muscles, necrosis, fibrosis, and contractures.

Example: Volkmann's ischemic contracture:
- Brachial artery injury in a supracondylar fracture of humerus and popliteal artery injury in a fracture of lower end of femoral shaft.

S/S: Loss of distal pulses, pallor and cold skin, severe pain in the limb, paresthesia, muscle paralysis

Management: Postreduction observation of fracture:
- If pulse is doubtful, then:
  Check the reduction, loosen/remove the external fixation, i.e. POP/splint
- Still no pulse, then: Inj. papaverine.
- Still no pulse, then: Exploration of artery

## Nerve Injury

Types of injuries:
- Neurapraxia (concussion): It is the commonest nerve injury and recovery occurs within a month or so.
- Axonotmesis (lesion in continuity): It is rupture of axons within an intact neural sheath and recovery occurs within few months.
- Neurotmesis: It is complete division of nerve.

**Examples:**
- Radial nerve injury in fracture shaft humerus
- Median and ulnar nerve injuries in supracondylar fracture of humerus
- Axillary nerve injury in shoulder dislocation
- Sciatic nerve injury in hip dislocation
- Common peroneal nerve injury in knee dislocation

Management: Majority of nerve injuries are in continuity.

**Conservative treatment**
- Postreduction of fracture or of dislocation, recovery in nerve injuries, ususally starts after about 6–8/56, then progressing satisfactrily thereafter. During recovery period, the skin should be protected against trauma, burns, etc.

- Joints to be mobilized by passive exercises. Prevent deformities, by use of splints, etc.

Example: Cock up splint in wrist drop.

## Surgical treatment:

- Exploration: Indicated in cases, where recovery is delayed or absent.
- Suturing: Primary suturing of nerves, if no infection.
- Reconstructive surgery-where nerve repair not feasible.

**Infection (osteitis):** In closed fractures is rare until infection is well established. Infection in a compound fracture, or following ORIF of a fracture, may cause:

- Osteomylitis—with discharging pus for a long period, inspite of use of antibiotics and surgical measures.

Gas gangrene: A highly serious life-threatening emergency

- Delayed or nonunion.

S/S: Fever (recurrent), pain, swelling, local tenderness, mobility painful
Investigation: CBC, ESR, Blood culture, CXR.

Management of compound fracture:

- Toilet of the wound with hydrogen peroxide and sterile fluids.
- Debridement of wound and immobilization.
- Antibiotics

Management of osteomyelitis:

- Acute: Incision drainage of pus
- Chronic: Saucerization; sequesterectomy; amputation.

Management of gas gangrene:

- Oxygen; antibiotics; gas gangrene antitoxin; amputation.

**Avascular necrosis of bone (AVN):** It is defined as death of bone due to complete interruption of bood supply (torn vessels) to one of the fragments following a fracture or dislocation, common in certain bones due to specific blood supply, e.g.

- Avascular necrosis of femoral head following intracapsular fracture neck femur.
- Avascular necrosis of proximal segment of scaphoid following fracture through waist of os scaphoid.

Management:
Firm fixation (ORIF) may help in recovery, but not always successfull. In an established case-treatment of choice is THR, in case of AVN following fracture neck femur.

**Volkmann ischemic contracture (VIC):** It is due to arterial spasm, following reduction of fractures. The arterial spasm yields to interruption of blood supply to muscles, resulting in necrosis, fibrosis, and finally to contractures.

Examples: VIC of flexor group of muscles of forearm, following reduction of supracondylar fracture of humerus and fractures of forearm. Also seen in leg and calf muscles. There may be ischemia of nerves, that may cause impaired conduction.

Etiology: Exact cause of arterial spasm is unknown.

Diagnosis:

- Hand becomes white and numb
- Radial pulse-absent
- Failure to extend wrist and straighten fingers passively.

Management:
- Relax flexion at elbow and extend it beyond 90
- Exploration of artery
- Inj. papaverine 2.5% sol.—to wash segment of artery in spasm
- Physiotherapy.

## Tight Plasters

Unfortunate incidence of loss of limbs occurs frequently, after the application of plaster, due to impaired circulation often caused by arterial spasm (medicolegal problem, and surgeon held under medical negligence act). In case a tight plaster, or a tourniquet, left in position too long, the circulation fails to return because of a secondary arterial spasm, that may resist all efforts at relaxation.

Diagnosis:
- Severe pain or numbness
- Swelling of fingers/toes.
- Skin of fingers/toes: Pale, white, or cyanotic

Management: Preventive treatment:
- Elevate the limb
- Watch circulation
- Active exercises of fingers/toes

Specific treatment:
- Split the plaster
- Check circulation
- Check reduction: Clinically and radiologically.

**Slow union:** Fracture takes comparatively longer time than usual to unite without any change from normal clinically or radiologically.

Management:
- Wait and watch for normal union, clinically and radiologically, periodically
- No interference with reduction and fixation.

**Delayed union:** Fracture fails to unite within specific time. There may be variations in the time taken by the bone for clinical union to occur (appx. 6 to 10/52), and wide differences may occur even in different bones in the same patient.

Investigation: X-ray findings: no evidence of repair: no callus visible, ends of bone fragments well defined, no sclerosis, there may be generalized osteoporosis

Management:
- As spontaneous union still possible (absent sclerosis and rounding off of bone ends): to continue with the fixation.
- Active exercises.

**Nonunion:** Fracture fails to unite, and usually being the end result of few cases of delayed union, that fail to unite spontaneously by the continued fixation.

## Etiology

General:
- Old age, poor health, vitamin deficiency
- Systemic diseases: Tuberculosis and syphilis.

Local:
- Delayed union: Fails to unite spontaneously by continued fixation
- Inadequate fixation: Continuous movement of fragments leads to impaired bridging callus, bone ends insulated from each other by the formation of fibrous tissue, the bone rounded off and sclerosed (lower third of tibia).
- Distraction: Excessive traction force pulls apart the bone ends, thus favors the growth of fibrous tissue that insulates the bone ends from each other.
- Interposition of soft tissues between fragments: Interposed fasciae, ligaments, and muscles, act as barrier to the callus growth across a fracture (fractures patella, olecranon, medial malleolus).
- Infection: Acute osteomyelitis, compound fractures, may cause the delayed union, and even nonunion.

Diagnosis: Unnatural mobility at fracture site, after expiry of normal union period (appx. 6/12).

X-ray: Sclerosis, rounding off of bony ends, fracture line clearly visible, bony ends may be flared out.

Management: Internal fixation and bone grafting.

Indication: Fracture freely mobile (non-sticky).

**Malunion:** Fracture united in an abnormal anatomical position.

Etiology: Defective reduction and fixation.

Diagnosis:
- Deformity: Angulation or rotational deformity resulting in cosmetic effect and impaired functioning of the limb.
- Shortening.
- Secondary osteoarthritis.

Management:
- Early case: If detected earlier e.g. before union, the angulation may be corrected by wedging of plaster cast, and manipulation under anesthesia
- In late cases, e.g. after union of fracture: correction by osteotomy.

## Shortening

Etiology:
- Malunited fracture—due to angular, and rotational deformities
- Transverse, oblique and spiral fractures
- Epiphyseal injuries (limb lengthens due to stimulated bone growth), e.g. fracture femoral shaft in a child.

Diagnosis:
- Bones: Fractures femoral neck, fractures femoral shaft, fractures tibial shaft
- Impaired functioning of the limb.

Management:
- Up to 2.5 cm compensated by pelvis tilt
- More than 2.5 cm corrected by alteration of the footwear, e.g. raising by a wedge incorporated within the shoe
- Corrective osteotomy for shortening due to marked angulation.

**Joint stiffness:** To be expected after a fracture, that may be temporary or permanent. Intra-articular fractures, or fractures very close to the joints, more prone to joint stiffness than fractures of shaft away from the joint.

Etiology:
*   Intra-articular, e.g.
    A. Fibrous adhesions (organized hematoma)
    B. Injury to articular cartilage
    C. Prolonged immobilization (degeneration)
*   Extra-articular, e.g.
    A. Injury to joint capsule, ligaments, tendons, muscles, etc.
    B. Fibrosis
*   Mechanical obstruction, e.g.
    A. Intra-articular fractures
    B. Myositis ossificans.

**Management**

Preventive treatment:
*   First aid splintage, before reduction
*   Perfect reduction
*   Adequate fixation
*   Elevation of limb
*   Active exercises.

Specific treatment:
*   Physiotherapy

Surgical treatment: Correction of the cause.

**Myositis ossificans:** It is a complication of orthopedic trauma, wherein a bony mass appears in the tissues near a joint, resulting in restricted movements due to mechanical obstruction.

Etiology: Repeated manipulations for reduction of fracture. Elbow is the commonest site for myositis ossification; also common in other sites like shoulder, hip, and knee, and frequently seen in patients of head and spinal injuries with paraplegia.

Pathogenesis: Hematoma formation in the muscle, leading to bone formation as a result of calcification and ossification of this hematoma.

Example: Myositis ossificans of brachialis muscle at the front of elbow joint, following reduction of supracondylar fracture.

X-ray: Confirms diagnosis.

Management:
*   Early excision: Yields poor results, with recurrence
*   Late excision: Yields good results (mechanical obstruction removal) with less chances of recurrence.

**Osteoarthritis:** Degeneration of the joint, following fracture:

**Etiology**

Traumatic:
*   Intra-articular fractures
*   Malunited fractures (stressful joints)

- Injury to articular cartilage, capsule, ligament (irregular surfaces)
- Avascular necrosis (impaired blood supply of I/A bone fragment).

Infective

Malunion

## Management:

Conservative measures:

- Treatment of the cause
- Physiotherapy—Shortwave therapy, Infrared therapy, exercises
- Intra-articular injections of hydrocortisone with xylocain (Lidocain) 2%-once or twice a week.

Surgical measures:

- Synovectomy
- Excision osteophytes
- Arthroscopy
- Reconstruction
- Total joint replacement
- Arthrodesis.

**Sudeck's dystrophy:** It is a complication of orthopedic trauma, found only after removal of plaster (4–6/52 of immobilisation), seen most frequently after Colles fractures of the wrist, also seen after scaphoid fractures, or following any wrist injury.

Etiology:

- Unknown
- May be due to sympathetic response to fracture.

Diagnosis:

- Painful, restricted movements.
- Swelling of hand and fingers
- Skin-warm and shining
- Tenderness present over wrist and metacarpals.

X-ray: Fracture united, osteoporosis, mottling of carpus

Management:

- Anti-inflammatory analgesics.
- Physiotherapy: Exercises.

**Bedsores:** Due to local pressure by ridges, produced by uneven application of a bandage, loose plaster, infection, and malnutrition.

Pathogenesis: Local pressure over unprotected bony prominences by the cast indent prior to plaster setting, resulting in edema, gangrene

Diagnosis: Pain, discomfort, edema, gangrene.

Management: Cut a window in the plaster cast, for AS dressings.

**Visceral complications:** Frequently post fracture, regional visceral complications occur:

- Rupture of urethra, bladder, or rectum in fracture pelvis
- Rupture of Kidney, spleen, liver, intestine, etc. due to local trauma, e.g. compression of abdomen in RSA, fall from height, sports injury
- Paralytic ileus: In fracture pelvis or lumbar spine.

Etiology:
- Direct violence: Blows, hits with a stick
- RSA
- Fall from height

Pathogenesis: Disturbed autonomic control of bowl due to retroperitoneal hematoma.

Diagnosis: Distension abdomen, absent bowel sounds, vomiting, constipation.

Investigation:
- Serum electrolytes
- Plain X-ray abdomen
- Abdominal paracentesis
- Laparotomy
- Laparoscopy

Management: Nasogastric suction, IV fluids.

## Cast Syndrome

Etiology: Plaster jackets, hip spicas, or plaster beds
Diagnosis: Vomiting, constipation, abdominal distension.

Management:
- Removal of plaster
- Nasogastric suction
- IV fluids.

## SECTION B: PRINCIPLES OF FRACTURE TREATMENT IN CHILDREN

Preface Childhood fractures are different from adult fractures, and also the principles of treatment are quite different. The treatment of fractures in children is simple as compared to complex one in adults. Fractures of he shaft of long bones in children hardly require open reduction, as bony growth relative to patient's age, mostly compensates for disparity in apposition, malalignment, and shortening, e.g. fractures of femur may stimulate hypergrowth of the limb. In infants, fractures shaft of the femur and humerus, relatively common, majority of these result in normal growth, irrespective of the position and alignment of the bone fragments. Spontaneous correction of an angular deformity in a child depends upon the age of the child; site of the fracture; and the degree of angulation. Major angulation near the bone's end is acceptable in young children, while fracture mid shaft and near the bone end in adolescents require perfect reduction.

Principles Delayed union: Absent in children, due to remarkable osteogenic activity of all the osseous tissues (endosteum, periosteum, and cortex) that may bind large gaps, except in case of
- Deformity: It is rare in children, due to great power of remodeling.
- Shortening of limb: Self-correctable, due to stimulation of growth.
- Joint stiffness: It is rare.

- Manipulation of greenstick fracture: It is easier, due to strong periosteum.
- Immunity of certain bones: Fracture spine rare, paraplegia unknown, fracture pelvis rare.
- Problematically childhood fractures:
- Supracondylar fracture of humerus: Associated with vascular injuries.
- Fracture of capitellum: Associated with late cubitus valgus and ulnar nerve palsy.
- Separation of lower femoral epiphysis—causing gangrene of foot, due to pressing of popliteal vessels.
- Epiphyseal fractures in children, complicated by infection, open reduction, repeated manipulations, usually result in growth disturbances.

## References

1. Bohler L. The treatment of Fractures. 4th ed. Wright, Bristol, 1935
2. **Charnley J. Fractures:** Bailey and Love's Short Practice of Surgery, ed. 13th , H.K. Lewis and Co. Ltd., London, 1965
3. Clark JMP. Fracture Treatment: Modern Trends in Orthopedics, 3, Butterworths, 1962
4. Kapoor PS. Fractures: Accident and Emergency, ed. 2nd, CBS, New Delhi, 2016
5. McRae R. Fractures General Principles: 1, Practical Fracture Treatment. Churchill Livingstone, Edinburgh, 1984.
6. Keith T Oldham, Paul M Colomham, Robert P Folgia, Michel A Skinner. Principles and Practice of Pediatric Surgery. Vol I: Trauma: 357–509.
7. Smith H. Fractures: Campbell's Oerative orthopedics, vol. 1, ed. 4, C.V. Mosby Co., 1963 Kimpton, 1956.
8. Watson JR. Fracturtes and other Bone and Joint Injuries. Livingstone, Edinburgh, 1940.

## SECTION C: REGIONAL FRACTURES

## Upper Limb Fractures

### Fractures about the Shoulder Girdle

Include        Fractures of clavicle
               Fracture of scapula
               Fracture-dislocation of shoulder joint
               Shoulder cuff injuries
               Fractures of greater tuberosity
               Fracture neck of humerus
               Fracure shaft of humerus

### Shoulder Girdle

Anatomy        Shoulder girdle is formed by the bones of the shoulder, i.e. clavicle/or collar bone, and the scapula/or shoulder blade; these articulate with each other at the top of the shoulder to form the acromioclavicular joint; and the clavicle articulates with the upper end of the sternum/or breast bone to form the sternoclavicular (large synovial) joint. The clavicle lies subcutaneously at the junction of neck and thorax; the sternum lies subcutaneously in the anterior midline and is palpable throughout its length; **in contrast to the clavicle, the scapula has no direct attachment to the axial skeleton, as it is attached to the ribs and the vertebral column by muscles only; its only connection to the axial skeleton is indirect one through the clavicle.**

Function: The clavicle serves as a brace for the shoulder, helping to keep the arm sufficiently far from the body so as to allow the free movements.

## Fractures of Clavicle

| | |
|---|---|
| Preface | The clavicle (collar bone) is the commonest long bone to fracture; being subcutaneous, it is prone to indirect violence, i.e. fall on the outstretched hand; and direct violence, and RSA. |
| Sites | Fracture occurs commonly at the junction of outer flattened third and inner pyramidal portions; and may also occur in the middle third. |
| MOI | Indirect violence: Fall on the outstretched hand—commonest cause |
| | Direct violence |
| | RSA |
| | Sports injury. |
| Pathogenesis | Patterns: |
| | In children: |

- Greenstick fracture: no deformity
- Local tenderness present
- Reluctance to move the arm.

In adults:
- Separation of bony ends
- Elevation of proximal end by the pull of sternomastoid
- Displacement of outer end-downwards, forwards, and inwards by the pull of pectoralis.

| | |
|---|---|
| Diagnosis | Pain |
| | Local tenderness |
| | Bony irregularity |
| | Crepitus |
| | Unnatural mobility at fracture site. |
| Investigation | X-ray clavicle—AP view. |
| Management | Greenstick fracture in children |
| | Cuff and collar sling |
| | Analgesics |

**Refer:** To the next fracture clinic.

| | |
|---|---|
| Fractures in adults | Conservative treatment: |
| | Apply figure of 8-bandage or a clavicle brace, Alt: |
| | Three-slings method: Simplest method of all |
| Technique | • Slings made of ordinary cotton triangular bandages; two of these rolled up enclosing cottonwool, so as to make two sausage-shaped pads, that are tied round each shoulder |

- With patient sitting on a stool, and an assistant pulling patient's shoulders backwards, with his/her knee as a fulcrum the surgeon ties the ends of the two slings together, without exerting too much pressure on the patient's back
- Third bandage used to support elbow on the affected side and to elevate the shoulder

Cuff and collar sling or arm pouch

Analgesics

**Refer:** To the next fracture clinic.

## Surgical Treatment

Surgery              ORIF—medullary fixation with 2 medullary pins, Alt:
- Plate and screws

Indications:
- Failure of conservative treatment, e.g. persistent separation of fragments
- Neurological due to pressure exerted by displaced fragment upon the brachial plexus
- Ligament injury (coracoclavicular) by distal fragment

After care: Arm supported in an arm pouch for 1–2/52.

Removal of pins after 8–12/52

**Refer:** To the next fracture clinic.

## Fractures of Scapula

Preface              Fractures of the glenoid and neck of the scapula are difficult to treat both conservatively (closed reduction by skeletal traction) and surgically (ORIF); usually, inspite of medial displacement of the lateral acromionectomy is indicated for acromion obstructing abduction.

Sites                Common sites are neck, body, and glenoid of scapula.

MOI                  Direct violence.

Diagnosis            Flattening and drooping of shoulder

                     Lengthening of arm

                     Local tenderness

                     Movements of shoulder painful and restricted.

Investigation        X-ray scapula—PA view.

Management           Conservative treatment:

                     Warm fomentation

                     Massage—with warm oil or an anti-inflammatory cream.

                     Strapping—adhesive

                     Analgesics

                     Arm pouch for 2–3/52

                     Active exercises of fingers, wrist, elbow

                     Surgical treatment:

                     Surgery: Open reduction

                     Indication: Dislocation of shoulder plus fracture neck of humerus.

**Refer:** To the next fracture clinic.

## Shoulder Cuff injuries

Described in Chapter of Affections of muscles, tendons, and tendon sheaths.

## Fracture Neck of Humerus

| | |
|---|---|
| Preface | Many classifications have been introduced, i.e. surgical or anatomical neck fractures, or as abduction or adduction fractures, but there is hardly any difference in their method of management (better all grouped as 'fracture of surgical neck'; leading factor in fractures of this area is that the fracture being nearer to a joint demands an early movement (ASAP). |
| Definition | Fracture line passes through the surgical neck, and rarely through the anatomical neck. |
| MOI | • Indirect violence: Fall on the outstretched hand; sports trauma<br>• Direct violence<br>• RSA |
| Pathogenesis | Patterns:<br>• Greenstick fracture—in children<br>• Impacted (abduction and adduction) fracture—in adults<br>• Unimpacted fracture. |
| MOI | Fall on the outstretched hand, or direct violence. |
| Diagnosis | Patient supports the arm with the other hand<br>Local tenderness<br>Deformity. |
| Investigation | X-ray shoulder—AP view. |
| Management | Conservative treatment:<br>• Impacted fracture: Arm sling or cuff and collar sling for 4/52<br>After care—Physiotherapy<br>• Unimpacted fracture: Closed reduction and arm sling<br>After care: Physiotherapy.<br><br>Surgical treatment:<br>Surgery: Internal fixation with:<br>• Rush pinning/ender nailing, Alt:<br>• Plate and screws—Locking Compression Plate (LCP)<br>After care: Physiotherapy. |

**Refer:** To the next fracture clinic.

## Fracture Shaft of Humerus

| | |
|---|---|
| Preface | Fracture shaft of the humerus usually occur close to the midpoint; easily diagnosed by the visible deformity and unnatural mobility; radial nerve injury is common |
| MOI | Fall on the outstretched hand, or direct violence. |
| Pathogenesis | Deformity:<br>• In fractures of proximal third: Proximal fragment adducted due to pull of pectoralis<br>• In fractures of middle third: Proximal fragment abducted due to pull of deltoid. |

| | |
|---|---|
| Diagnosis | Patient supports the arm with the other hand |
| | Deformity—mostly angulation |
| | Local tenderness |
| | Unnatural mobility. |
| Complication | Radial nerve palsy (wrist drop) may accompany the fracture. |
| Investigation | X-ray humerus—AP and LAT views. |
| Management | Conservative treatment: |

- U-plaster method: Apply a U-slapped plaster slab, starting from axilla, to under the elbow, to the top of shoulder, supported by elastic crepe bandage
- Hanging cast method: The weight of the limb plus that of plaster, reduce fracture and maintain reduction. It may lead to nonunion due to distraction

After care: Cuff and collar sling. Union normally occurs in about 6–8/52.

## Surgical Treatment

Surgery          Internal fixation

Indications:

- Patient bedridden
- Double/or comminuted fracture
- Radial nerve palsy
- Compound fracture.

Methods:

- Rush pinning/ender nailing—antegrade or retrograde
- Intramedullary nailing—Solid humeral nail (UHN), PHN
- Interlocking nailing under C-arm supervision
- Interlocking nailing (open) without C-arm supervision
- Plate and screws.

## Management of Complications of Internal Fixation

- Nonunion: ORIF + bone grafting.
- Radial nerve palsy: Usually the recovery begins 8/52 after the injury/palsy. Provide the patient with a wrist drop splint and the regular physiotherapy.
- Wait for 8/52.
- Exploration of radial nerve—If no evidence of recovery.

**Refer:** To the next fracture clinic.

## Fractures About the Elbow

Preface          Elbow trauma demand respect; result in a greater variety of fractures and epiphyseal injuries; usually associated with neurovascular damage than any other portion of the body; the intractable joint stiffness that occasionally occurs following the comparatively minor trauma; and the marked sensitivity of the traumatized joint to the early passive mobility aggravates the difficulties of the management and prognosis;

certain injuries require early open surgery and perfect reduction, some skilled manipulation, and knowledgeable remodeling possibilities as the growth proceeds, while in others the best results obtained by confining to the inevitable joint disturbance and encouraging early movement.

| | |
|---|---|
| Anatomy of elbow | Described in Chapter of Dislocations |
| Fractures | Classification (Table) |

**Fractures in children:**
- Supracondylar fracture
- Lateral condyle fracture
- Medial epicondyle fracture
- Lateral epicondyle fracture
- Fracture neck of radius

**Fractures in adults:**
- Fracture of lower end of Humerus (Y or T shaped)
- Fracture of capitellum
- Fracture of olecranon
- Fracture head of radius

Injuries of muscles and tendons:
- Tennis elbow (lateral epicondylitis)

## Supracondylar Fracture of Humerus

| | |
|---|---|
| Preface | The supracondylar fracture in children, when grossly displaced is one of the most difficult fractures to manage perfectly; being notorious for the neurovascular complications (partly attributed to the inadequate treatment). |
| Definition | It is one of the commonest fracture of childhood, involving distal end of humerus |
| Pathogenesis | Fracture line is proximal to trochlea and capitulum. |
| Types | Postertior—common type and Anterior—rare type. |
| MOI | Fall on the outstretched hand. |
| Etiology | Direct violence RSA Sports injury. |
| Diagnosis | Deformity—Distal fragment is displaced backwards, upwards, and outwards Swelling Pain Local tenderness Olecranon, medial and lateral epicondyles—preserve their relation Shortening of the arm Movements at the elbow painful and restricted. |
| Investigation | X-ray elbow—AP and LAT views. |

| | |
|---|---|
| Complications | • Injury to brachial vessels |
| | • Injury to ulnar, median, or radial nerves |
| | • Movements of elbow—painful and restricted |
| | • Malunion |
| | • Deformity: cubitus valgus or varus |
| | • Volkmann's ischemic contracture |
| | • Myositis ossificans. |
| Management | Conservative treatment: Closed reduction under C-arm supervision |
| | Anesthesia: General |
| | Technique: |
| | • Traction is applied to extended elbow—to disengage fragments |
| | • Correction of lateral displacement |
| | • Maintaining traction in the length of arm, flex the elbow |
| | • Forward drawing of posterior displaced lower fragment—into line with axis of humerus |
| | • Finally flex the elbow to 60–70 degree—to lock reduced fragments by taught triceps |
| | Check the radial pulse before applying plaster slab for 6–8/52 |
| | Remanipulation: In case of previous poor reduction |
| | After care: |
| | • Admit the child for overnight stay in the hospital, for observation of circulation. |
| | • Elevate the arm cuff and collar sling. |
| | Surgical treatment |

**Refer:** The child to orthopedic team for surgery

| | |
|---|---|
| Indication | • Failure of conservative treatment |
| | • Instability. |
| Surgery | Internal fixation—Rush pin/ender nails, followed by plaster fixation. |

**Refer:** The child to next fracture clinic.

## Fracture of Lateral Condyle

| | |
|---|---|
| Preface | It is the commonest epiphyseal injury around the elbow in children; It is an intra-articular fracture, therefore accurate reduction is essential. |
| Pathogenesis | The detached fragment (includes capitellum and half of trochlea) is displaced and rotated by forearm extensors and lateral ligament, resulting in deformity of cubitus valgus with late ulnar palsy. |
| MOI | Fall on the outstretched hand or fall on the point of olecranon. |
| Etiology | Direct violence |
| | RSA |
| | Sports injury. |
| Diagnosis | Pain |
| | Swelling |
| | Deformity—cubitus valgus |
| | Local tenderness |
| | Movements at elbow—painful and restricted. |

| Investigation | X-ray elbow—AP and LAT views. |
|---|---|
| Complications | • Nonunion |
| | • Deformity—cubitus valgus |
| | • Late ulnar nerve palsy |
| Management | The lesion being an intra-articular fracture, needs perfect reduction; even minor degrees of displscement may indicate periosteal or soft-tissue interposition that may cause delayed/or nonunion; thus ORIF is the treatment of choice in majority of cases. |
| | Surgical treatment: |
| | Surgery: ORIF: Kirschner wiring/or screw fixation through metaphyseal portion of the fracture, is the treatment of choice. |
| | After care: Immobilization: plaster cast from knuckles to middle of arm |

**Refer:** The child to the next fracture clinic.

## Fracture of Medial Epicondyle

| Etiology | Indirect violence: Fall on the outstretched hand |
|---|---|
| | Direct violence |
| | RSA |
| | Sports injury |
| Pathogenesis | Valgus strain with or without lateral dislocation of the elbow; probably an associated subluxation of the joint that has reduced spontaneously; the epicondyle may be retained postreduction of a dislocation—causing blockage of the joint in flexion. |
| Diagnosis | Pain |
| | Swelling |
| | Deformity—cubitus valgus |
| | Local tenderness |
| | Movements at elbow—painful and restricted. |
| Investigation | X-ray elbow—AP and LAT views |
| | Absence of medial epicondyle from its normal position |
| | Inclusion of fragment inside the joint. |
| Management | Conservative treatment: Closed reduction under general anesthesia |
| | Technique: |
| | • Reduction: Forced valgus, supination, extension, dorsiflexion of wrist |
| | • Immobilization: Plaster cast for 4/52; Alt: |
| | • Cuff and collar sling for 2–3/52, with the elbow at a right angle |
| | • Exercises |

**Refer:** The child to next fracture clinic.

Surgical treatment:

Surgery: Internal fixation—Kirschner wire fixation followed by plaster fixation.

Indication: Failure of conservative treatment.

**Refer:** The child to the next fracture clinic.

## Fracture of Lateral Epicondyle

| | |
|---|---|
| Etiology | Indirect violence: Fall on the outstretched hand |
| | Direct violence |
| | RSA |
| | Sports injury |
| MOI | Fall on ther outstretched hand or direct violence. |
| Diagnosis | Pain |
| | Swelling |
| | Local tenderness |
| | Movements at elbow—painfull and restricted. |
| Investigation | X-ray elbow—AP and LAT views. |
| Management | Conservative treatment: |
| | Reduction: Closed reduction |
| | Immobilization: In a plaster cast for 3–4/52. |

**Refer:** The child to next fracture clinic.

## Fracture Neck of Radius

| | |
|---|---|
| Preface | Usually a greenstick fracture |
| Etiology | Indirect violence: Fall on the outstretched hand |
| | Direct violence |
| | RSA |
| | Sports injury |
| Pathogenesis | Fall on the outstretched hand causes a valgus strain on the elbow joint that drives the capitellum against the outer side of radial head, resulting in tilting and outward displacement; associated with a traction lesion of the inner side of the joint that may assume the form of a strain or rupture of the medial collateral ligament, avulsion of the medial condyle, or an associated fracture of the upper end of the ulna. |
| Diagnosis | Pain |
| | Deformity: Angulation |
| | Swelling |
| | Local tenderness |
| | Movements at elbow—painful and restricted. |
| Investigation | X-ray elbow—AP and LAT views. |
| Complications | • Nonunion |
| | • Cross-union. |
| Management | Conservative trteatment: |
| | Indication: |
| | • For little/or no tilt: Cuff and collar sling and analgesics |
| | • For marked tilt: Manipulation (traction, pronation, supination) under anesthesia. |

**Surgical treatment:**
Surgery:
• Open reduction

Indication:
- Failure of conservative treatment
- Marked displacement
- Excision of radial head

Indication: Danger of cubitus valgus development.

**Refer:** To the next fracture clinic.

## Fracture of Lower end of Humerus (Intercondylar)

Preface
: T or Y shaped fractures of lower end of humerus, usually occur as a result of fall on the point of the elbow; are very difficult fractures to treat; both occur in the adult; being intra-articular fractures, the fundamental principle is early movement (ASAP), current tendency is to favor this at the expense of the anatomical position of the fragments

Etiology
: Indirect violence: Fall on the point of the elbow
Direct violence
RSA
Sports injury

Pathogenesis
: Fall on the point of elbow, the olecranon wedges into the lower end of humerus, causing separation and comminution of the articular surface

Diagnosis
: Deformity
Swelling
Local tenderness
Crepitus
Unnatural mobility
Movements at elbow—painful and restricted.

Investigation
: X-ray elbow—AP and LAT views.

Management
: Conservative treatment:
Indication: Comminuted fracture
Technique:
- Closed reduction
- Immobilization: Plaster (POP) cast for 2–3/52; Alt:
Cuff and collar sling for 2–3/52
After care: Exercises.

**Refer:** The patient to next fracture clinic

**Surgical treatment:**
Indication: Noncomminuted fracture
Surgery: ORIF: Plate and screws (LCP), rush pin/ender nail, or screws.
Immobilization: POP cast—knuckles to above elbow.
After care: Physiotherapy.

**Refer:** To the next fracture clinic.

## Fracture of Capitellum

Preface
: An isolated fracture of the capitellum is a common injury of childhood; one of considerable importance; in case of slight displacement, the elbow may be managed in a cuff and collar sling, with active movements

starting post 3/52; while in cases of gross displacement (capitellum often rotated through 180 degrees with articular surface of the capitellum facing fractured surface of the humerus.

| | |
|---|---|
| Etiology | Indirect violence: Fall on the outstretched hand |
| | Direct violence: Hit by a stick/rod |
| | RSA |
| | Sports injury. |
| MOI | Fall on the outstretched hand, causing fracture of the capitellum by an upward thrust transmitted by the radial head. |
| Diagnosis | Pain |
| | Swelling |
| | Local tenderness |
| | Movements at elbow painful and restricted. |
| Investigation | X-ray elbow—AP and LAT views. |
| Management | Conservative treatment: |
| | Technique: |

- Reduction: Closed reduction
- Immobilization: In a plaster cast applied to the extended elbow.

**Refer:** The patient to next fracture clinic

**Surgical treatment:**
Surgery: ORIF (Smiley pins)
Immobilization: In a plaster cast for 4–6/52
After care: Physiotherapy.

**Refer:** To the next fracture clinic.

## Fracture of Olecranon

| | |
|---|---|
| Preface | Majority of olecranon fractures usually occur in middle age; fractures frequently comminuted; often associated with abrasions; may be open fractures; an early movement is desirable of any type of management; attempts to replace and hold the displaced fragment in good position by closed reduction (manipulation) and plaster cast immobilization are to be avoided. |
| Etiology | Indirect violence: Fall on the outstretched hand |
| | Direct violence |
| | RSA |
| | Sports injury |
| MOI | Avulsion injury caused by the opposing strains of sudden flexion of the elbow joint against the violent contraction of the triceps muscle. |
| Diagnosis | Pain |
| | Swelling |
| | Local tenderness |
| | Bone irregularity |
| | Movements at elbow: Painful and restricted. |
| Investigation | X-ray elbow—AP and LAT views. |

Management     Conservative treatment:
               Technique: Plaster cast above elbow for 6–8/52
               Indication: Hairline and undisplaced fracture.
**Refer:** The patient to next fracture clinic.

### Surgical treatment:
Surgery: ORIF
Indications:
- Displaced closed fractures (transverse, oblique, comminuted)
- Open fractures

### Methods:
Displaced closed fractures:
- Zuelzer hooked plate and screws
- Croll olecranon screw
- Lag screw
- Tension band wiring (Kirschner wires, Rush pin)

Open fractures:
- Clamp cum compressor device

After care: Physiotherapy.

**Refer:** To the next fracture clinic.

## Fracture Head of Radius

Preface          Usually the extent of bone damage cannot be asessed radiologically and that relatively trivial fissure or marginal fractures may be associated with severe articular damage, often with disturbed capitellum; elderly patients unlikely to subject the joint to any vigorous use, to be managed with the arm in a sling until the acute symptoms subside, only then to utilize the elbow gradually; younger patients with comminuted fractures (esp. damaged capitellum), are to be managed by excision of the whole of radial head better within 3–4/7 of initial injury, to rlieve pain/stiffness and for increased range of movement.

Etiology         Indirect violence: Fall on the outstretched hand
                 Direct violence
                 RSA
                 Sports injury

MOI              Fall on the outstretched hand, with the elbow extended, besides a valgus strain causing a compression injury of the radial head

Types            Chip fracture involving less than a third of periphery
                 Comminuted fracture of whole head.

Diagnosis        Pain
                 Swelling
                 Local tenderness
                 Movements at elbow—painful and restricted.

Investigation    X-ray elbow—AP and LAT views.

Management       Conservative treatment:
                 Indication: Chip fractures
                 Method: Plaster cast above elbow

**Refer:** The patient to next fracture clinic.

> **Surgical treatment:**
> Indication: Comminuted fractures
> Surgery: Excision of radial head.
> After care: Physiotherapy.

**Refer:** To the next fracture clinic.

## Tennis Elbow (Lateral Epicondylitis)

Described in Chapter of Traumatic affections of Ligaments, tendons, and muscles.

## Forearm Bones Injuries

Types
- Fracture both bones forearm
- Isolated fracture radius
- Isolated fracture ulna

## Fracture Both Bones Forearm In Adults

Preface
Complete functional recovery of forearm post fractured shafts of radius and ulna depends upon the restoration, not only of full flexion and extension of wrist and elbow, but also of full pronation and supination (urgency to restore full pronation and supination make these fractures more difficult to manage.

Etiology
Direct violence: Hit by a stick/or rod
Indirect violence: Fall on the outstretched hand
RSA
Sports injury

Pathogenesis
Post fractured bones, if the radial fragments unite with one rotated corresponding to the other one, then loss of corresponding degree of rotation inevitable; scarring with resultant shortening of interosseous membrane may bind radius to the ulna tightly causing restricted rotation (pronation and supination); massive scarring and shortening in case of bones uniting with deformity and the radius angulated towards ulna.

Diagnosis
Pain
Deformity: Angulation, rotation
Shortening
Local tenderness
Unnatural mobility
Loss of function
Movements: Painful and restricted

Investigation
X-ray of forearm including elbow and wrist—AP and LAT views.

Management
Conservative treatment:
Reduction: Closed reduction under C-arm supervision.
Indications:
- Elderly patient
- Undisplaced fractures
- Multiple injuries.

Disadvantages:
- Difficulty in reduction
- Failure to maintain reduction
- Displacement—marked
- Rotational deformities—common
- Volkmann ischemic contracture

Immobilization: In a cast for 6–8/52.

After care: physiotherapy—exercises.

### Surgical treatment:

Surgery: ORIF is treatment of choice in adults.
- Plating of both fractured bones, or
- Plating of radius and nailing of ulna

Technique:
- Apply a tourniquet
- Exposure (Henry):
- Radius: Anterior incision
- Ulna: Posterior incision

Postoperative: Plaster cast for 6–8/52.

After care: Physiotherapy.

**Refer:** To the next fracture clinic.

## Fracture Both Bones Forearm in Children

| | |
|---|---|
| Preface | Mostly greenstick fractures (undisplaced). |
| Etiology | Direct violence |
| | Indirect violence; fall on the outstretched hand |
| | RSA |
| | Sports injury. |
| MOI | Fall on the outstretched hand or direct violence. |
| Pathogenesis | Patterns: Mostly undisplaced greenstick fractures of radius and ulna in middle thirds; distal fragments tilted anteriorly (posterior angulation) without any displacement; an intact posterior hinge (beneficial in the reduction); displaced fractures: off ending of one or both bones; with potential instability; deformities: shortening, angulation, and axial rotation may occur. |
| Diagnosis | Deformity—angulation, rotation |
| | Shortning |
| | Unnatural mobility |
| | Loss of function. |
| Investigation | X-ray of forearm including elbow and wrist—AP and LAT views. |
| Management | Conservative treatment: |
| | Indication: |
| | • Undisplaced greenstick fractures |

Technique:

Reduction: Closed eduction of angulation deformity; usually the deformity is overcorrected, so as to prevent recurrence of angulation due to sagging.

Immobilization: POP cast for 4–6/52

After care: Physiotherapy.

- Displaced fractures:

Reduction: Closed reduction of angulation, and rotation, deformities, and correction of displacement, under C-arm control.

Immobilization: Pop cast for 4–6/52.

After carte: Physiotherapy.

Surgical trteatment:

Indication: Failure of closed reduction.

Surgery: ORIF.

Postoperative: POP slab with flexed (90 degree) elbow, for 4–6/52.

After care: Physiotherapy.

**Refer:** To the next fracture clinic.

## Isolated Fracture of Radius

| | |
|---|---|
| Preface | Isolated fracture of the shaft of radius or ulna with deformities, i.e. of angulation or shortening, without involvement of inferior radioulnar joint, is a rare entity; failure to consider this primary fact results in permanent disability—not only from unreduced dislocation, but usually from difficulty in reducing fracture in presence of dislocation; thereby for isolated fractures of shafts of radius or ulna, superior and inferior radioulnar joints must be included radiologically. |
| Etiology | Direct violence |
| | Indirect violence |
| | RSA |
| | Sports injury. |
| Pathogenesis | Oblique or comminuted fracture; radius shortened with rotated lower fragment; radial fragments angulated towards ulna; dislocated inferior radioulnar joint. |
| Diagnosis | Pain |
| | Swelling |
| | Deformity: Angulation, rotation, shortening |
| | Local tenderness |
| | Movements at wrist: Painful and restricted. |
| Investigation | X-ray forearm including wrist and elbow—AP and LAT views. |
| Management | Conservative treatment: |
| | Reduction: Closed reduction |
| | Immobilization: In a POP cast |

Disadvantage:

- Difficulty in maintaining reduction by external splinting, due to muscle pull that invariably angulates the lower fragment towards ulna and the inferior radioulnar joint redislocates

Surgical treatment of choice.

Surgery: ORIF of fractured radius (plating).

Indication: Failure of conservative measures.

Postoperative: POP for 6–8/52.

After care: Physiotherapy.

**Refer:** To the next fracture clinic.

## Isolated Fracture of Ulna

| | |
|---|---|
| Pattern | Mostly greenstick fractures. |
| MOI | Fall on the outsretched hand or direct violence. |
| Diagnosis | Swelling, tenderness, bone irregularity, ulnar angulation. |
| Investigation | X-ray forearm includes elbow and wrist—AP and LAT views |
| Management | Conservative treatment: |

Indication: Displacement slight: Plater in mid-pronation for 8–10/52.

Surgical treatment:

Indication: Displacement/angulation marked

Surgery: ORIF

Postoperative: POP for 6–8/52.

After care: Physiotherapy.

## INJURIES ABOUT THE WRIST AND HAND

### A. Closed Hand Injuries

   i. Colles fracture

  ii. Smith's fracture  (Syn. reversed Colles fracture)

 iii. Barton's fracture

 iv. Slipped radial epiphysis

  v. Fracture of the radial styloid

 vi. Scaphoid fracture

 vii. Metacarpal fractures

viii. Rupture of ulnar collateral ligament (Gamekeeper's thumb)

 ix. Fractures of phlanges

  x. Mallet finger

### B. Open Hand Injuries

**Colles fracture**

| | |
|---|---|
| Preface | It is defined as a fracture of radius within 2.5 cm of the wrist and usually occurs in old ladies; associated with either avulsion of the styloid process of the ulna or ruptured triangular fibrocartilage of the wrist joint; shortening of radius causes subluxation of the inferior radioulnar joint and a prominent ulnar styloid; lower fragment of radius displaced backwards and radially, and rotated so that the articular surface points backwards, i.e. displaced and rotated in the direction of violence; all these deformities results in 'dinner fork' deformity; radial styloid process is at par with ulnar styloid process (instead of 1.25 cm below that of ulna). |
| Etiology | Indirect violence: Fall on the outstretched hand |
| | Direct violence: Fighting |
| | RSA |
| | Sports injury. |

| MOI | Fall on the outstretched hand. |
| Pathogenesis | Avulsed ulnar styloid process; ruptured triangular fibrocartilage of the wrist joint; shortened radius; subluxated inferior radioulnar joint; prominent ulnar styloid; dinner fork deformity; radial styloid at par with ulnar styloid process. |
| Diagnosis | Deformity: Dinner fork, i.e. lower end of radius is displaced backwards, radially and rotated; radial and ulnar styloid processes are on same level<br>Pain<br>Swelling<br>Local tenderness<br>Movements painful and restricted |
| Investigation | X-ray forearm including wrist—AP LAT views. |
| Management | Closed reduction under general anesthesia. |

Technique:

- Position: The assistant holds the arm above the flexed elbow. The surgeon grips the patient's wrist with one hand above and the other below the level of fracture, changing hands accordingly to suit patient's left or right wrist. For patient's left wrist, surgeon places palm of his left hand on the palmar surface of patient's wrist above level of proximal fragment, the palm of his right hand is then applied to the dorsal surface of patient's wrist distal to level of fracture.

Reduction:

- Disimpaction of distal fragment: Surgeon applies traction with the right hand, in line of forearm, and increases the deformity a little by extending the wrist.
- Palmar flexion: Maintaining traction to disengage the fractured fragments, the distal fragment is flexed gently, followed by direct pressure exerted by right hand on the dorsal surface of distal fragment, while in the opposition direction, by left hand on the ventral surface of the proximal fragment.
- Maintaining traction, the patient's wrist is pronated by surgeon by pronating his own right hand, while maintaining his left hand stationary, to prevent proximal fragment from following the distal fragment.
- Ulnar deviation of patient's wrist is the final movement.

Postreduction position: Palmar flexion, ulnar deviation, and the pronation

Immobilization: The reduction is maintained by applying plaster slab to the dorsal and radial surfaces of the wrist, and the plaster extends from the level of metacarpal heads to the elbow—below its crease in front while up to olecranon level posteriorly.

After care:

- Elevate the hand in a cuff and collar sling; watch the circulation for any impairment, i.e. any swelling of the fingers, and numbness or severe pain in the fingers
- Active exercises of fingers, thumb, elbow, and shoulder

- Anti-inflammatory analgesics.
- Removal of cast: After 6–8/52, followed by physiotherapy.

Complications   • Malunion

Management: Physiotherapy. Surgery—rarely indicated

- Rupture of extensor pollicis longus

Management: In elderly—Physiotherapy

- Sudeck's atrophy:

S/S: Swelling of fingers, skin of hands—warm and tendered, movements—painful and restricted.

X-ray—shows osteoporosis.

Management: Physiotherapy.

**Refer:** The patient to next fracture clinic.

## Smith's Fracture (Syn. Reversed Colles Fracture)

| | |
|---|---|
| Definition | It is defined as the deformity characterized by the reverse of that which occurs in Colles fracture; the distal fragment being displaced in front of the lower end of the radius. |
| Etiology | Indirect violence: Fall on the back of hand |
| | Direct violence |
| | RSA |
| | Sports injury. |
| Pathogenesis | Fall on the back of hand; distal fragment displaced in front of lower end of radius; articular surface looks forwards, i.e. displaced and angulated in the direction of violence. |
| Diagnosis | Deformity: In the opposite direction to that of Colles' fracture, i.e. lower end of radius is displaced forwards in front of lower end of radius, and tilted anteriorly (posterior angulation). |
| | Fracture: Usually impacted. |
| | Pain |
| | Swelling |
| | Local tenderness |
| | Movements: Painful and restricted. |
| Investigation | X-ray forearm including wrist—AP and LAT views |
| Management | Closed reduction under general anesthesia |

Method:

- Position: The assistant holds the arm above the flexed elbow. The surgeon grips the patient's wrist with one hand above and the other below the level of fracture, changing hands accordingly to suit patient's left or right wrist. For patient's left wrist, surgeon places palm of his left hand on the palmar surface of patient's wrist above level of proximal fragment, the palm of his right hand is then applied to the dorsal surface of patient's wrist distal to level of fracture.

Steps:

- Disimpaction of fragments: Apply traction to the supinated arm
- Dorsiflexion: Maintaining traction to disengage the fractured fragments, fragments, the distal fragment is extended gently,

followed by direct pressure exerted by the right hand on the ventral surface of the distal fragment, while in the opposition direction, by left hand on the dorsal surface of the proximal fragment.

Immobilization: The reduction is maintained by applying plaster slab to the dorsal and radial surfaces of the wrist, and the plaster extends from the level of metacarpal heads to above elbow.

After care:
- Elevate the hand in a cuff and collar sling, watch the circulation for any impairment, i.e. any swelling of fingers, numbness or severe pain in the fingers.
- Active exercises of fingers, thumb, elbow, and shoulder
- Anti-inflammatory analgesics.
- Removal of cast post 6–8/52, followed by physiotherapy.

**Refer:** The patient to next fracture clinic.

## Barton's Fracture

| | |
|---|---|
| Definition | It is defined as a form of Smith's fracture, characterized by involving only the anterior part of the radius. |
| Etiology | Indirect violence: Fall on the outstretched hand |
| | Direct violence |
| | RSA |
| | Sports injury. |
| Pathogenesis | Fall on the outstretched hand resulting in fractured anterior portion of the radius. |
| Diagnosis | Deformity |
| | Pain |
| | Swelling |
| | Local tenderness |
| | Movements of wrist: Painful and restricted. |
| Investigation | X-ray forearm including wrist—AP and LAT views |
| Management | Conservative treatment: |
| | Reduction: Closed reduction as for Smith's fracture. |
| | Immobilization: As for Smith's fracture. |
| | Surgical treatment: |
| | Indication: Failure of closed reduction. |
| | Surgery: ORIF (Screw—cancellous, or buttress plate). |

**Refer:** The patient to next fracture clinic.

## Slipped Radial Epiphysis

| | |
|---|---|
| Definition | Common in adolescence and in childhood, is the counterpart of colles fracture; displaced distal radial epiphysis is usually associated with a small fracture of the metaphysis (Salter Harris type II injury); deformity of the wrist occurs due to unequal growth of the radius and ulna. |
| Etiology | Direct violence |
| | Indirect violence: Fall on the outstretched hand |

RSA

Sports injury.

**Pathogenesis**      Fall on the outstretched hand; displaced distal radial epiphysis; mataphyseal fracture.

**Diagnosis**         Deformity: Displacement of distal radial epiphysis along with a small piece of metaphysis (Salter Harris injury)

Pain

Swelling

Local tenderness

Movements: Painful and restricted

**Investigation**     X-ray wrist—AP and LAT views.

**Management**        Conservative treatment:

Closed reduction and plaster fixation (same as for Colles fracture).

**Refer:** The child to the next fracture clinic.

## Fracture of the Radial Styloid (Chauffer's Fracture)

**Definition**        It is defined as a fracture of radial styloid; fracture line that involves the radiocarpal joint surface, is mostly without any gross displacement; that often involves a much larger piece of radius; so-called ~Chauffer's fracture' sustained by 'back fires' while starting internal combustion engines (generators).

**Etiology**

**MOI**               Fall on the outstretched hand

Engine (generator, pump, auto) starting handle–back-fires.

**Diagnosis**         Deformity—slight displacement

Pain

Swelling

Local tenderness

Movements at wrist: Painful and restricted.

**Investigation**     X-ray wrist—AP and LAT views.

**Management**        Conservative treatment:

• Closed reduction and plaster fixation (same as for colles fracture).

Surgical treatment:

Indication: Failure of conservative measures.

Surgery: ORIF (Screw—cancellous, or buttress plate).

After care: Physiotherapy.

## Scaphoid Fracture

**Definition**        It is defined as the commonest bone to be fractured in the wrist; a sprained wrist following fall on a stretched hand, should arouse suspicion; with thumb and fingers fully extended, fullness of the anatomical snuff-box with local tenderness may happen due to fracture scaphoid.

**Etiology**          Indirect violence: Fall on the outstretched hand

Direct violence

RSA

Sports injury.

| | |
|---|---|
| Pathogenesis | Fall on the outstretched hand in men aged 20–40 years. |
| | Engine (generator, pump, auto) starting handle—back-fires. |
| Diagnosis | Pain—outer aspect of wrist |
| | Fullness of snuffbox |
| | Local tenderness |
| | Movements at wrist: Painful and restricted. |
| Investigation | X-ray wrist—AP, LAT, and oblique—views |
| | Certain cases—Fractures become visible only after 2–3/52. |
| Management | Conservative treatment: |

Indication: Every case of sprained wrist, to be suspected as case of fracture scaphoid, even if the X-ray being negative, and should be treated with the wrist in plaster cast (scaphoid cast) and X-ray repeated after 3/52, to confirm diagnosis of scaphoid fracture.

Method: Cock-up plaster cast for 8–10/52:

Position: Patient keeps the hand—as if holding a glass

Cast: Plaster cost includes metacarpal bone of thumb

- Embraces sides of forearm and wrist—to prevent lateral displacement
- Not to interfere with free movements of fingers.

Post care: Physiotherapy.

Surgical treatment:

Surgery: ORIF (cancellous screw fixation).

Indication:

- Displaced unstable fracture of scaphoid
- Failure of conservative treatment.

| | |
|---|---|
| Complications | Nonunion: Symptomless or wrist pain, difficulty in performing work. |
| | Management: Symptomless—active exercises |

Symptoms (marked):

- Early case: Screw fixation plus bone grafting
- Late case: Excision radial styloid

Sudeck's atrophy: Pain, swelling, local tenderness, painful and restricted movements of fingers and wrist

Management: Analgesics; immobilization of wrist—for 2–3/52.

Post care: Physiotherapy—active exercises.

Osteoarthritis: Pain, swelling, painful and restricted movements of fingers and wrist.

Management: Analgesics and physiotherapy.

## Fractures of Metacarpals

| | |
|---|---|
| Definition | It is defined as fractures involving the shaft of one or more of the inner four metacarpals as a result of knuckles striking objects, e.g. in boxing, or by objects striking the dorsum of the hand, as in industrial injuries. |
| Etiology | Direct violence |
| | Indirect injury |

| | |
|---|---|
| | RSA |
| | Sports injury: Knuckles striking face (boxing). |
| Pathogenesis | In sports injury, e.g. boxing—knuckles striking face, etc. in industrial injuries, e.g. objects striking the dorsum of the hand. |
| | Types: Transverse, oblique, or spiral. |
| Diagnosis | Pain |
| | Swelling |
| | Local tenderness |
| | Bone irregularity |
| | Movements of hand painful and restricted. |
| Investigation | X-ray hand—AP and LAT views. |
| Management | Conservative treatment: |
| | Indication: Undisplaced fractures |
| | Technique: Plaster fixation (Colles type slab) for 3–4/52. |
| | After care: Physiotherapy—active exercises. |
| | Surgical treatment: |
| | Indication: Displaced fractures |
| | Surgery: ORIF: |

- Intramedullary (single/multiple) Kirschner wires, Alt:
- Percutaneous Kirschner wires

Postoperative: Plaster cast (Colles type slab).

After care: Physiotherapy

**Refer:** The patient to next fracture clinic.

## Fracture neck of Fifth Metacarpal

| | |
|---|---|
| Definition | Defined as fractures usually caused by clenched fist facing resistance, e.g. as a result of a fight; angulation and impaction are common. |
| Etiology | Direct violence: Fighting—clentched fist facing resistance |
| | Indirect violence: Fall on a outstretched hand |
| | RSA |
| | Sports injury: Boxing. |
| Pathogenesis | Fractured neck 5th metacarpal; angulated; impacted fragment. |
| Diagnosis | Deformity—angulation |
| | Pain |
| | Swelling |
| | Local tenderness |
| | Movements: Painful and restricted. |
| Investigation | X-ray hand—AP and LAT views. |
| Management | Conservative treatment: |
| | Indication: Angulation—slight/or moderate. |
| | Method: Closed reduction and plaster slab for 4/52. |
| | Surgical treatment: |
| | Indication: Angulation—marked |
| | Surgery: ORIF (percutaneous/or intramedullary Kirschner wiring). |

**Refer:** The patient to next fracture clinic.

## Rupture of Ulnar Collateral Ligament (Gamekeeper's Thumb)

Described in Chapter of Traumatic Affections of Ligaments, Tendons, and Muscles.

## Fracture of Phalanges

| | |
|---|---|
| Principles | 1. Post-traumatic swelling: |

- Every effort to be made to limit the swelling that may lead to chronic edema and irreparable fibrosis
- Elevation of the arm in a sling may be beneficial, provided the hand not to be made dependent
- Pressure dressing (if reqd.) to be applied with utmost care—to avoid local constriction

2. Splintage:

- For splintage only few joints as possible to be immobilized, for minimum possible time; MP joints of fingers—never to be splinted in extension
- Exercises: Active exercises of free fingers vigorously
- Garter strapping: An undisplaced fracture of a phalanx strapped to an adjoining normal finger provides an ideal combination of stability while retaining movement.

3. Rotational (tortional) deformity:

- Of phalanx or metacarpal may not be observed in extension, while causing deformity and impaired function in flexion (by checking the power of injured finger by flexing it prior to fixation, the rotational deformity can be avoided).

| | |
|---|---|
| Definition | It is defined as fractures sustained by direct violence (blow) or as a crush injury sustained by pressing in a door or window sash; fractures of the proximal phalanges are more difficult to manage than metacarpal injuries as the flexor tendon sheath may be involved in a displaced fracture. |
| MOI | Direct violence, e.g. by a Hammer's blow, or <br> Crush injury: Pressed by a door/or window sash. |
| Diagnosis | Deformity: Angulation <br> Pain <br> Swelling of finger <br> Local tenderness <br> Bone irregularity <br> Movements: Painful and restricted. |
| Investigation | X-ray hand (focusing affected finger)—AP and LAT views. |
| Management | Fractures of phalanges are difficult to treat, due to involvement of flexor tendon sheath. |

Conservative treatment:

**A.  Fracture of proximal and middle phalanges:**

Methods: Closed reduction and fixation with:

- Splintage: Aluminium splints covered with foam-plastic or rolled bandage held in the palm
- Plaster slab (volar) for 3/52.

Surgical treatment:
Surgery: Intramedullary Kirschner wires.
After care: Physiotherapy—active exercises.

### B. Fracture of terminal phalanx:
Surgery: Toilet of wound, debridement and suturing, followed by:
- Strapping of finger to adjacent normal finger
- Splintage—aluminium splints covered with foam-plastic.

**Refer:** The patient to next fracture clinic.

## Mallet Finger
Described in Chapter of Traumatic affections of Ligaments, tendons, and muscles.

## Trigger Finger
Described in Chapter of Traumatic affections of Ligaments, tendons, and muscles.

## Open Hand Injuries

| | |
|---|---|
| Principles | Post-traumatic: |
| | • To restore its function |
| | • To prevent infection |
| | • To salvage injured parts |
| | • To promote primary healing |
| | • To realign fractures and suturing nerves and tendons as secondary repairs to primary toilet (cleansing) of the wound of foreign bodies and debridement of devitalized tissue/s |
| | • To provide skin coverage even with skin grafing if required. |
| Types | Cuts, lacerations, injection injuries |
| | Crush injuries |
| | Compound injuries |
| | Burns injuries. |
| Etiology | Direct violence, e.g. by a hammer's blow |
| | Crush injury: Pressed by a door/or window sash |
| | RSA |
| | Sports injury. |
| Pathogenesis | Wound may be lacerated, clean or dirty; foreign body/clots may be visible; skin may be denuded or lacerated; tendons may be torn; nerves may be torn; bones may be fractured. |
| Diagnosis | History of injury |
| | • Mode of injury |
| | • Time of injury |
| | • Any first aid treatment received |
| | • Any food taken and when it was taken |
| | • Any history of allergy |
| | Examination. |
| Investigation | X-ray examination. |
| | Pus/wound secretion: For culture sensitivity test |
| | CBC, ESR |

Management:          Aims:
- To prevent infection
- To promote primary healing
- To salvage injured parts.

Conservative treatment:
- Antibiotics, Inj. Tetanus toxoid
- Analgesics and NSAIDs.

Surgical treatment:
Surgery: Debridement of wound and repair of tissues.
- Anesthesia: General or regional block.
- Tourniquet: Required during procedure
- Toilet of wound
- Examination of wound's depth
- Repair of deep structures

Caution: Tourniquet to be used as briefly, when the viability of skin is questionable.

Technique:
- Shave and prepare: Shave the surrounding uninvolved skin
- Toilet of wound: With antiseptic (betadine) solution, followed by saline irrigation

Debridement: Excision of dead skin, removal of foreign material
- Bleeders: Clamped

Repair:
- Tendons: Flexor tendons—primary suturing
           Extensor tendons—primary suturing
- Nerves:  Clean wounds—primary suturing
           Crush injury—secondary suturing
- Skin:    Clean wounds—primary suturing
           Infected wounds—secondary suturing
- Fractures: Clean wounds—primary procedure
             Infected wounds—late reconstructive surgery

After care: Physiotherapy after 3/52.

**Refer:** The patient to next fracture clinic.

## Lower Limb Fractures and injuries

### Fractures pelvis and hip

- Fractures iliac crest
- Fractures true pelvis
- Fractures sacrum
- Fractures coccyx
- Fracture neck femur
- Intracapsular fractures
- Extracapsular fractures (Trochanteric fractures)

## Fractures Pelvis

Principles
- Pelvic ring: The pelvic ring is formed by union of two halves of pelvis to the sacrum by sacroiliac ligaments posteriorly, and by symphysis pubis anteriorly. This pelvic ring protects the pelvic organs
- Fracture of hip bone may result from a blow or compression of pelvic ring by a crushing force, i.e. in RSA or fall of heavy weight, i.e. in mine industries
- Fracture usually occurs across a weaker part of the bone, i.e. wing of the ileum or the obturator foramen

- Displacement: Little in case of isolated/single fracture; while fractures across both the iliac wings and the obturator foramen, or across both obturator foramina, permits displacement of a part of the pelvis.
- Fractures of pelvic ring at two different levels, lead to marked separation of the ring, while isolated fractures are mostly stable injuries.
- Internal hemorrhage: Pelvis is richly supplied with blood vessels, which are damaged by fractures. Internal hemorrhage is mostly severe, leading to oligemic shock.
- Visceral injury: Pelvic fractures with displacement esp. of anterior parts, are often associated with damage to the viscera within the pelvis, the male urethra and urinary bladder being particularly vulnerable, and rarely the rectum.

## Types of Pelvic Fractures

- Fractures of iliac crest
- Fractures of true pelvis

## Fractures of Iliac Crest

| | |
|---|---|
| Preface | Fractures of the iliac crest are not of significance as these are stable fractures, due to support from muscles on the inner side (iliacus) and outer side (glutei) of pelvic bone; displacement is slight. |
| MOI | Direct violence |
| | Fall from height |
| | RSA |
| | Sports injury. |
| Pathogenesis | Crush injury causing isolated fractures of the ileum or obturator foramina; little displacement. |
| Diagnosis | Pain |
| | Swelling |
| | Local tenderness |
| | Movements: Painful and restricted |
| Investigation | X-ray pelvis—AP view |
| Management | Conservative treatment: |
| | Bedrest |
| | Analgesics and NSAIDs |
| | Support: A wide cloth support is sufficient for 2–3/52. |

**Refer:** The patient to next fracture clinic.

## Fractures of True Pelvis

| | |
|---|---|
| Principles | • Fractures of the true pelvis can occur either in the oblique diameter, i.e. through obturator foramen on one side and the sacral ala on the opposite side, or the pelvic ring may be fractured at two places on the same side |
| | • Fractures can occur at two levels on the same side or on the opposite side |

- Fractures of pelvis in trauma patients are reported to be 3–8.2%, with approximately half of these fractures being caused by high energy injuries with a potential for catastrophic hemorrhage and death
- Fractures of anterior pelvic ring are important from treatment point of view (ORIF controversial because of fears of disturbing pelvic hematoma and causing additional hemorrhage).

| | |
|---|---|
| MOI | Direct violence |
| | Fall from height or fall down stairs |
| | RSA |
| | Sports injury. |
| Diagnosis | Local signs: Bruising over the ileum, groin, or perineum |
| | Local tenderness |
| | Bone irregularity |

Signs of visceral complications:
- Urethral injury: Blood per urethra, perineal hematoma, distended bladder
- Bladder injury: Suprapubic tumor like mass, strangury, local tenderness
- Rectal and vaginal examinations—helpful in diagnosis

| | |
|---|---|
| Investigation | X-ray pelvis—AP view |
| | Hemogram, PCV, blood electrolytes |
| | Blood urea, blood sugar, serum proteins |
| | Blood grouping and cross matching |
| Management | Conservative treatment: |
| | General or first aid treatment: |

Treatment of shock (if present):
- Airways maintenance, oxygen therapy
- IV fluids, blood transfusion, plasma or plasma expander
- Inj Hydrocortisone IV, Inj Ephedrine—if reqd. urgently
- Inj Morphine or Pethidine or Pentazocine (Fortwin)

Bedrest
Traction.
Local treatment:

Reduction and immobilization:
- Closed reduction and traction, Alt:
- Closed reduction and plaster hip spica

**Surgical treatment:**
Surgery:
Indication: Associated bladder injury; early mobilization desirable.
- ORIF (plating and screws), Alt:
- Fixation of the anterior pelvic ring fractures with percutaneous cannulated screw under fluoronavigation

Advantage: Minimally invasive surgery under fluoronavigation.
After care: Walking prohibited for 2–3/12.

**Refer:** The patient to next fracture clinic.

## Fracture of Sacrum

| | |
|---|---|
| MOI | Direct violence: kicks |
| | Fall from height |
| | RSA |
| | Sports injury. |
| Diagnosis | Pain |
| | Swelling |
| | Local tenderness |
| | Bone irregularity. |
| Investigation | X-ray sacrum—AP and LAT views |
| Management | Conservative treatment: symptomatic: |
| | Bedrest for 2–3/52 |
| | Analgesics: Paracetamol, NSAIDs, PO or IM |
| | Local block (puncture): inj. Lignocaine 2% infiltration |

**Refer:** The patient to next fracture clinic.

## Fracture of Coccyx

| | |
|---|---|
| MOI | Direct violence —fight, or kicks |
| | Fall from height |
| | RSA |
| | Sports injury. |
| Diagnosis | Pain: Often severe, occurs on walking, sitting, and aggravates on coughing or defecation |
| | Swelling |
| | Local tenderness |
| | Bone irregularity. |

**Refer:** The patient to next fracture clinic.

## Traumatic Coccydinea

| | |
|---|---|
| MOI | Direct violence |
| | Fall from height |
| | RSA |
| | Sports injury. |
| Diagnosis | No fracture |
| | Pain: Mostly severe |
| | Local tenderness |
| Investigation | X-ray pelvis—AP view |
| Management | Conservative treatment: symptomatic treatment, e.g. |
| | Bedrest |
| | Warm fomentation, SWD, or IR therapy |
| | Seitz baths |
| | Analgesics and NSAIDs |

Local block—inj lignocaine 2% infiltration

Preventive: To sit on an inflated tube; avoid sitting on hard surface.

**Surgical treatment:**

Indication: Failure of conservative treatment.

Surgery: Excision in extreme cases.

**Refer:** The patient to next fracture clinic.

## Fracture Neck of Femur

Preface      Fracture neck femur is one of the most common injuries amongst the geriatric population; prevalence of these fractures has further increased with improved life expectancy; aim of management of these fractures is restoration of pre-fracture function without associated morbidity; management of displaced femoral neck fractures in elderly has been controversial; in elderly ORIF of these fractures has poor outcome includes high rate of nonunion and avascular necrosis; problems encountered are acetabular erosion and loosening of stem causing pain; inspite of these, superiority of prosthetic replacement over internal fixation well established.

Types      Intracapsular and Extracapsular (Sir Astley Cooper division).

## Intracapsular Fractures

Preface      Intracapsular fractures are prone to complications (nonunion and avascular necrosis of femoral head) because of impaired blood supply to femoral head due to intracapsular fracture, leading to avascular necrosis; joint reconstruction (total hip replacement) revolutionized management of patients with advanced hip disorders; arthroplasty is a reconstructive procedure that alters the structure or function of a joint; many different types of hip arthroplasties have been introduced over the years.

Anatomy      Blood supply of head and neck of femur (Trueta): The medial femoral; circumflex artery is the main vessel supplying the upper end of femur; its branches pierce the capsule of the hip joint at its femoral attachment and are disposed as two main groups on the superior and inferior aspects of femoral neck; posterosuperior group of arteries are the main source of blood supply to the femoral head and neck; terminal branches of this group (lateral epiphyseal arteries of Trueta) supply that part of the femoral head (developed from epiphysis) are damaged in most of displaced intracapsular fractures; role of arteries of ligamentum teres (medial epiphyseal arteries of Trueta) supplying femoral head is doubtful regarding its viability.

Types      Subcapital and transcervical.

Femoral head ischemia: More common in the subcapital than in the transcervical type.

MOI      Direct trauma in young adults

Fall from height

RSA

Sports injury

Indirect trauma (missing a step) in elderly.

**Pathogenesis**      Osteoporotic bone (in elderly); healthy bone (in young adults); avascular necrosis of femoral head (increased density of femoral head).

**Diagnosis**         Age: Common in elderly persons (> 80%), while uncommon in young adults.

Sex: Common in females (> 80%)

Deformity:

- Externally rotated lower limb (like paralysed)
- Coxa vara (syn. adduction fracture) is more serious (tendency to nonunion) as the fracture line exposed to the shearing strain while weight bearing attempt by the patient.
- Coxa valga (syn. abduction fracture)—the strain of weight bearing further imacts the fracture (unfortunately less common) shortening of limb (due to coxa vara)

Elevated greater trochanter: As confirmed by measurements:

Measurements:

- Bryant's triangle: Patient lies supine, three lines drawn on both sides; first line from anterosuperior iliac spine, vertically down to the bed, second line horizontally from top of greater trochanter to join the first line at right angle, and third line from anterosuperior iliac spine to the top of greater trochanter.

  Interpretation: Comparative second line decrease indicates upward elevation of greater trochanter.

- Nelaton's line: Patient turned to healthy side. A measuring tape is placed from anterosuperior iliac spine to the ischial tuberosity.

  Interpretation: Normally the tape (vide this line) touches the top of the greater trochanter, and any upward displacement is demonstrated.

- Schoemaker's line: A line from the tip of greater trochanter to the anterosuperior iliac spine is extended over the anterior abdominal wall, it should normally coss the midline at or above the umbilicus, while crossing below the umbilicus shows elevation of trochanter.

- Chiene's test: Normally a measuring tape joining the tips of the greater trochanters is parallel to another between the anterosuperior iliac spines; these two lines converge towards the affected side when the trochanter is elevated (+ve test).

- Morris's bitrochanteric test: Distance from the outer border of the greater trochanter to the symphysis pubis measured on both sides by a pair of calipers or a graduated ruler, and compared; denotes medial or lateral displacement of the trochanter, i.e. reduced distance on the affected side in cases of posterior and central dislocations/fracture dislocations.

  Loss of function: Movements painful and restricted esp. in case of the recent trauma.

| | |
|---|---|
| Grading | Garden: Grade I and II: Undisplaced fractures |
| | 　　　　Grade III and IV: Displaced fractures |

Pauwels': Based on Pauwels' angle formed by the fracture line with the horizontal plane, i.e.
- Type I (< 30 degree)
- Type II (30–50 degree)
- Type III (> 50 degree)

| | |
|---|---|
| Complications: | • Nonunion of fracture neck femur |
| | • Avascular necrosis (AVN) of femoral head. |
| Investigation | CBC, ESR, serum electrolytes, serum proteins, BUN |

Blood grouping and cross matching

Urine analysis

ECG

X-ray pelvis—AP view, to study type of fracture and the distorted Shenton's line.

X-ray of affected hip—LAT view, to study angulation of femoral head over neck, and fragmentation

CXR—PA view to rule out any pathology.

| | |
|---|---|
| Management | Has evolved significantly. |

### Principles of treatment:
- Problem of union of fracture (due to interruption of blood supply) and not of survival of patient
- Surgical treatment—Internal fixation is treatment of choice
- Surgery may preferably be delayed for few days if the patient is very old and whether in shock.

Conservative treatment: Satisfactory as far as the union of fracture is the aim, but the mortality rate is relatively high, and also because of prolonged immobilization, restoration of function of the limb esp. of knee may be slow or even restricted permanently, besides cardiorespiratory complications.

Method:
- Closed reduction
- Immobilization: In POP hip spica in abduction and internal rotation (Whitman abduction plaster)

Complications of conservative treatment:
- Nonunion
- Avascular necrosis of femoral head
- Bedsores: Prolonged immobilization in the bed
- Osteoporosis: Disuse
- Respiratory
- Cardiovascular.

Surgical treatment of choice:

Surgery: Methods:
- Reduction and internal fixation
- Prosthesis
- Total Hip Replacement (THR)

Reduction and internal fixation

Preoperative treatment (first aid):
- Analgesics
- Antibiotics
- IV fluids
- Blood transfusion—to combat loss of blood due to fracture and to treat anemia
- Skin traction—to relieve muscle spasm and to prevent further displacement of fragments to combat shortening.

Reduction:
- Position: Patients fixed on a fracture table, in supine position, with normal limb tied to the foot stirrup
- An assistant steadies the pelvis, while the surgeon holding the affected limb, flexes the hip and knee to right angle, then rotates the hip to disengage any impaction, then exerts traction longitudinally to restore normal length and the neck engages the head; abduct, extend, and internally rotate the limb, thus locking the head in position with the neck. Thereafter tie the foot to the foot stirrup, with the limb in 20 degree abduction, internally rotated.

Check rays AP and LAT views (or under C-arm vision) to confirm the reduction: Interpretation:
- AP view: Neutral position or slight valgus of head v/s neck reqd.
- LAT view: Slightest variation permissible.

Failed reduction: Remanipulation.

## Methods of Internal fixation:

Hip screws:
- Cannulated hip screws/cancellous partially threaded screws
- Cannulated screws/cancellous partially threaded screws with fibular strut graft
- Sliding hip screw (SHS)

DHS (nail plate)—to prevent extrusion and rotation of the nail

Antegrade Femoral Nailing (AFN)

Moore/Knowles pins—to prevent avascular of head; of choice for children

Procedure:

Draping: Lateral aspect of the hip, by squaring off the operative field

Anesthesia: General
- Incision: A lateral incision centered over the greater trochanter.
- Exposure: Expose the trochanteric ridge
- A guide wire is inserted at 45 degree to horizontal plane, through neck into head (preferably into posteroinferior part of neck and center of head)
- Length of nail, measured by substracting the length of protruding part of guide wire from its total length
- Cortical opening widened by nail starter driven over guide wire

- Selected nail is driven along the guide wire and hammered home
- Check the position
- If plate is to be used, then the plate is attached to the nail and bone with cortical screws.

Post care: Patient allowed out of bed within a few days; weight bearing allowed after 2–3/12, depending upon union of fracture, and general condition of the patient.

Complications:
- Nonunion of fracture neck of femur
- Avascular necrosis of femoral head
- Traumatic arthritis hip.

## Nonunion

| | |
|---|---|
| Etiology | • Inadequate immobilization (failure of internal fixation)<br>• Ischemia of femoral head. |
| Management | Head viable: Treatment of choice is:<br>• Subtrachanteric displacement osteotomy:<br>• McMurray—no longer in vogue<br>• Pauwel's valgization osteotomy<br>• Nailing and bone grafting (Peg graft) in younger patient.<br><br>Head nonviable: Either treatment is:<br>• Prosthesis<br>• Total Hip Replacement (THR). |

## Subtrochanteric Displacement Osteotomy

| | |
|---|---|
| Definition | It is defined as a displacement or high osteotomy, wherein bony support may be restored, either by the healing of the nonunion or by changing the line of weight bearing, thus inspite of persisting nonunion, weight bearing borne directly beneath the femoral head. |
| McMurray | Modifications: two:<br>A. Nonunion fixed with two Knowles pins and the osteotomy fixed with a reversed Neufeld or Blount nail (for well preserved neck and reducible fragments)<br>B. Nonunion fixed with a reversed Neufeld nail (for a short neck), while Knowles pins omitted |

Caution: Osteotomy not to be too oblique, nor to include any part of the base of the neck (medial projecting bone may prevent shaft to displace beneath the head).

Method:
- Patients fixed on a fracture table, in supine position, with normal limb tied to the foot stirrup
- Check the position of head vs neck by X-ray or C-arm vision
- Incision: 15 cm long along to femoral shaft, from greater trochanter
- Incise vastus lateralis and strip from anterior surface of femur at the site of desirable osteotomy insert one guide wire into femur, at surface

level with lesser trochanter; advance obliquely—medially and proximally, to emerge medially just proximally to lesser trochanter

- Insert second guide wire proximal to the first one, through greater trochanter, neck, into the head
- Insert two Knowles pins through greater trochanter, neck, into head
- Divide the femur (by an osteotome or Gigli saw) next to distal guide wire
- Displace medially the distal fragment beneath the femoral head
  Fixation of osteotomy blade plate: Insert the blade through greater trochanter, then fix the osteotomy plate (Neufeld or Blount) to the abducted femoral shaft by 3 screws
- Confirm position by X-ray or C-arm vision.

Postoperative: No immobilization reqd.

After care: Exercises, and after 8/52 partial weight bearing allowed on crutches, till firm union (appx. 6/12).

## Pauwels Y Osteotomy

| | |
|---|---|
| Indication | Unusual pseudarthrosis of femoral neck (neck absorption + proximal displacement of distal fragment). It is indicated only in case of viable head and in the healthy patient that allows prolonged plaster immobilization to achieve union. |

Aims:
- To enlarge femoral neck, so as to increase apposition between neck and the head
- To improve the function of hip abductors, by distal displacement of the greater trochanter.

Method: Pauwels advocates nailing + osteotomy:
- Osteotomy made at the intertrochanteric level
- Lateral wedge—removed
- Fixation of osteotomy—with a plate and screws.

## Nailing and Bone Grafting (Peg Graft)

| | |
|---|---|
| Indication | Younger patient |
| Method | Fixation with screw + fibular strut graft: |

- Cannulated screws/cancellous partially threaded screws + fibular strut graft.

## Prosthesis Replacement (Medullary/Stem syn. Femoral Endoprosthesis)

| | |
|---|---|
| Indication | Suitable for a frail/elderly patient who is unlikely to have a long/or active life subsequently. The morbidity is appreciable esp. when a posterior approach is used |
| Method | Excision of the femoral head, and replacement with a Thompson or Austin moore prosthesis: |
| Thompson | Head dimension: 39; 41; 43; 45; 47; 49; 51; 53 mm |
| | Stem:                    105 mm |

| Austin moore | Head dimension: 39; 41; 43; 45; 47; 49; 51; 53; 55; 57 mm |
|---|---|
| | Stem: 127.................; 140 .............; 152 ......... mm |

Technique: Preoperative planning:
- Exposure: Lateral, anterolateral, or posterior approach
- Femoral neck resection
- Femoral preparation
- Removal of femoral head
- Measuring of femoral head size
- Acetabular cleaning
- Trial reduction of head into acetabulum
- Femoral cementing
- Stem implantation
- Reduction—by gentle delivery of head into the acetabulum
- Check X-ray
- Closure of wound after putting in a drain.

Post care: Exercises:
- Breathing exercises, starting on the same day of operation
- Quadriceps, toes, ankle exercises—first day onwards.

**Refer:** The patient to fracture clinic after 2–3/12. If satisfactory, then next visit after one year and so on for five years, with periodical check X-rays.

## Total Hip Replacement (THR)

| Definition | Affords an early immobilization and returning to initial, prefracture state is fully justified, provided the patient's condition is satisfactory, for this major surgery |
|---|---|
| Technique | Preoperative planning: |

- Exposure: Lateral, anterolateral, or posterior approach
- Femoral neck resection
- Femoral preparation
- Acetabular preparation
- Acetabular cementing and pressurization
- Acetabular implantation
- Trial reduction
- Further femoral preparation
- Femoral cementing
- Stem implantation
- Reduction by gentle delivery of head into the acetabulum
- Check X-ray

Post care: Exercises:
- Breathing exercises: Starting on the same day of operation
- Quadriceps, toes, ankle exercises: First day onwards.

**Refer:** The patient to fracture clinic after 2–3/12. If satisfactory, then next visit after one year and so on for five years, with periodical check X-rays.

## Avascular Necrosis (AVN)

| | |
|---|---|
| Etiology | In majority of patients, the cause is interruption of blood supply due to rupture of blood vessels by the fracture. Although AVN of the femoral head is usually a deciding factor for nonunion, it may not prevent union (neck absorption may not prevent union when fixation used permits nail extrusion, maintaining contact of fractured surfaces). |
| Diagnosis | Pain: Increasing type |
| | Disability: Limp |
| | Movements: Painful and restricted |
| Investigation | X-ray: Changes (sclerosed head, narrowed joint space, irregular articular surfaces, lipping of acetabulum) usually appear within a year or so of trauma. |
| Management | • Total Hip Replacement (THR): It is the treatment of choice in elderly |
| | • Prosthetic replacement: In frail, elderly |
| | • Prompt reduction + stable fixation, or osteotomy: In younger |
| | • Arthrodesis hip: In difficult and unusual cases. |

## Traumatic Arthritis (Osteoarthritis) Hip

| | |
|---|---|
| Definition | Incidence and severity of traumatic arthritis post fracture-dislocation or dislocation of hip is as per severity of trauma to osseous tissue and soft structures. |
| Management | Osteotomy: Valgus (abduction) |

## Extracapsular Fractures or Trochanteric Fractures

| | |
|---|---|
| Definition | It is defined as any fracture from the extracapsular part of the femoral neck, to a point 5 cm distal to the lesser trochanter. These fractures are becoming more common than the intracapsular fractures, as they usually occur in the oldest age (average age steadily increasing). Mostly the type of management (internal fixation and other treatment) remain the same for entire group. |
| Types | Based on anatomy: |

• Intertrochanteric: Fracture line extending from greater trochanter to lesser trochanter, along the intertrochanteric line.
Reduction: Simple and easily maintained.
• Pretrochanteric (comminuted fractures): Main fracture along the intertrochanteric line, along with multiple fractures in the cortex.
Reduction: Difficult to achieve.
• Subtrochanteric: Fracture of the trochanter extending from lesser trochanter to 5 cm distally, into the femoral shaft.
Reduction: Difficult to achieve and maintained.

Based on stability:
• Stable: Undisplaced, noncomminuted, intertrochanteric fractures
• Unstable fractures:
    – Displaced, comminuted, pertrochanteric
    – Subtrochanteric fracture extending into femoral neck
    – Reverse oblique fracture

– Trochanteric fracture (comminuted) extending into femoral neck
– Trochanteric wall (lateral) fracture.

| | |
|---|---|
| Principles | • Problem is of survival: As these fractures occur in comparatively older age, and longer period of immobilization.<br>• Fractures occur in the cancellous bone, thereby chances of an early union are comparatively better due to:<br>  – Safe blood vessels: hence no chances of avascular necrosis<br>  – Adequate size of neck and head fragments: good fixation achieved<br>• Nonunion: Extremely rare<br>• Early weight bearing possible: postinternal fixation<br>• Early mobilization: postinternal fixation |
| MOI | Indirect violence, i.e. missing a step by an elderly patient<br>Direct violence |
| Diagnosis | An elderly lady<br>Lower limb externally rotated<br>Shortening of limb<br>Local tenderness<br>Loss of function |
| Investigation | X-ray Hip – AP view to confirm type of fracture |
| Management | Conservative treatment: For patient unwilling, or unfit for surgery.<br>Bedrest<br>Traction: Fixed in Thomas splint.<br>Analgesics, NSAIDs |

Surgical treatment:

Surgery: Internal fixation is treatment of choice

Methods of internal fixation:

- SP nail plate
- McLaughlin nail-plate
- Sliding compression screws:
  – Dynamic hip screw (DHS)
  – Dynamic condylar screw (DCS): Blade plate (95 degree)
- Intramedullary nailing (IMN) with sliding hip screws (SHS)
  – Proximal femoral nail (PFN)
  – Gamma nail
  – Ender nails
- Arthroplasty (bipolar or total hip replacement)
- External fixator (Ilizarov).

| | |
|---|---|
| Indications | Stable fracture:<br>• DHS is the gold standard<br><br>Unstable fracture:<br>• DHS—yields poor results<br>• DHS with modification, or IMN with SHS<br>• IMN (intramedullary nailing)<br>• DCS—sparingly used in reverse oblique fracture<br>• Used in subtrochanteric fracture. |

## Dynamic Hip Screws (DHS)

Indication:        Intertrochanteric fracture: Stable and unstable (moderate)
                   Types: Long barrel plate: For larger femoral head and neck length
                   Short barrel plate: For shorter femoral head and neck length.

## Intramedullary Nailing (IMN)

Advantages         Reduction (closed) easy, short invasive surgery, less blood loss, early
                   mobilization, and reduced mechanical (fixation) failure.
                   Disadvantage: Mechanical (fixation) failure, pain in the thigh, stiffness,
                   deformity, nail extrusion.

## Arthroplasty (Bipolar or Total Hip Replacement)

Indication         Pathological fractures, neglected fractures, fixation failure
                   Advantages: Pain relief, early mobilization, lower revision rates
                   Disadvantages: Extensive surgery and cemented implants.

                   External fixator
                   Indication: Poor risk patients
                   Disadvantage: Infection
                   Alternative: Sliding hip screw (SHS).
Technique          Of internal fixation:
                   Anesthesia: General
                   Position: Patient placed supine on the orthopedic table
                   Reduction: Indicated in displaced fracture
                   Method: By traction in neutral position
                   Exposure: Lateral approach
                   Fixation: Blade plate, nail plate, or proximal femoral nail

                   Indications:
                   • Stable fracture: Blade plate, or nail plate (DHS)
                   • Unstable fracture, or fracture extending into femoral shaft.

                   Post care: Same as for intracapsular fractures.

## Complications of Fixation of Trochanteric Fractures

                   Comparatively minimal vs of intracapsular fractures:
                   • DHS failure: Due to faulty placement in neck and head
                   Management: Revised surgery
                   • Nail breakage: Due to faulty fixation
                   Management: Replacement of broken nail
                   • Nonunion: Due to faulty implant/bony failure
                   Management:
                   • Revised surgery: Removal of implant and fixation in valgus + bone
                   Grafting
                   • THR: In elderly
                   • Malunion (varus and external rotation): Due to faulty fixation
                   Management: Valgus osteotomy.

## Slipped Upper Femoral Epiphysis

| | |
|---|---|
| Preface | Slipped upper femoral epiphysis (traumatic) usually occurs as a sudden epiphyseal separation; condition resembles fracture femoral neck; union often takes place in the deformed position leading to diminished neck-shaft angle, i.e. coxa vara; occurs in adolescence. |
| Etiology | Hormonal imbalance—Frohlich syndrome, gigantism |
| | History of trauma |
| Diagnosis | Adolescent, fatty, sexually immature, pain in groin or knee, limp |
| | Leg—externally rotated |
| | Movement (internal rotation)—painful and restricted |
| Investigation | X-ray Hip—AP and LAT views, to confirm slip esp. in LAT view |
| | X-ray normal Hip—AP view, for comparison purpose |
| Management | Conservative treatment: |
| | Rest |
| | Reduction |
| | Immobilization: Traction |
| | Analgesics and NSAIDs |
| | Surgical treatment of choice |
| | Surgery: |
| | • Reduction and pinning |
| | • Osteotomy: For deformed late cases. |
| Complications | Avascular necrosis: |
| | Management: |
| | Preventive: Avoid forced manipulation to correct deformity |
| | Surgical treatment: Osteotomy: indicated in established cases. |

## Fractures of Femur and Injuries about Knee

1. Fractures of femoral shaft
2. Fractures of upper third of femur
3. Supracondylar fracture of femur
4. Femoral condylar fractures
5. Fractures of Patella
6. Internal derangements of knee (IDK)
    i. Injury medial collateral ligament and lateral collateral ligament
    ii. Injury medial meniscus
    iii. Injury cruciate (anterior and posterior) ligaments
    iv. Injury to infrapatellar pad of fat
    v. Fracture to tibial spine
    vi. Loose bodies.
7. Fractures lateral tibial plateau (Bumper fracture).

## Fractures of Femoral Shaft

| | |
|---|---|
| Preface | Modern trend in the management of fractures of femoral shaft is towards an increasing use of ORIF; introduction of intramedullary nailing and similar methods (intralocking nailing, external fixator, etc.) |

has been a noticeable advance, while limitations associated with such methods have not yet been overcome completely; there are still occasions when it is better to be a little conservative; surgeon does not repair a fracture; he simply does his best to create the best possible circumstances for natural repair of the fracture (paraphrase Ambroise Pare: 'I splint the fracture; God heals it'.

| | |
|---|---|
| **Sites** | Fractures of proximal third |
| | Fractures of middle third |
| | Fractures of distal third |
| **MOI** | Direct trauma: hit by a stick |
| | Fall from height |
| | RSA |
| | Crush injuries |
| | Sports injury. |

**Diagnosis**    Deformity:

- In fractures of proximal third:
  Proximal fragment: Flexed by iliopsoas, abducted by glutei, everted by external rotators
  Distal fragment: Adducted by adductors, upwards by hamstrings and quadriceps, everted by weight of limb
- In fractures of middle and distal third:
  Backward angulation, shortening by quadriceps and hamstrings.
  Local tenderness
  Unnatural mobility
  Loss of function

**Investigation**    X-ray thigh including knee and hip—AP and LAT views
CBC, ESR, serum electrolytes, proteins, blood urea.
Blood grouping and cross matching

**Management**    Aims of treatment: Three main aims:

1. Restoration of alignment: It is essential as malalignment results in undue strain upon the knee joint, and later on development of osteoarthritis
2. Restoration of length: By prevention and correction of shortening due to contraction of powerful muscles of thigh
3. Prevention of knee stiffness by prevention and correction.

Conservative treatment:

- Traction, and hip spica
- Traction and counter-traction: To prevent and correct shortening.

Traction: It is applied to the distal fragment and counter-traction, is applied to the proximal fragment, to prevent the trunk and pelvis following the traction force and to prevent the recurrence of shortening.

Methods of applying traction and counter-traction:

- Fixed traction: Traction is applied by tying the cords to the foot end of the Thomas splint, which is passed over the limb, so that padded ring of splint rests against the ischial tuberosity, which provides counter-traction.

Types of traction:
- Skin traction: Indicated in children and younger patients, using adhesive plaster
- Skeletal traction: Indicated in older patients and where heavy traction is required, using a Steinmann pin
- Gallows traction: Indicated in children below the age of five years, using strapping, and the legs are hung up by overhead pulley, so that buttocks are lifted up from the bed. The child's weight acts as the counter-traction.
- Continuous traction (syn. balanced traction): More comfortable and precise method. It is attached to the limb by skin or skeletal traction which is applied to the pulleys of Bohler Brawn splint.

Hip spica: Indicated in a fretful child, and in a compound fracture

Method: Hip spica to include:
- From nipple line to the:
  - Injured leg—up to toes
  - Normal leg—above knee.

Surgical treatment:

Indications:
- Failure of closed reduction
- Multiple fractures
- Early mobilization required.

Methods:
- Intramedullary nailing
- Intertlocking nailing under C-arm
- Interlocking nailing (open) without C-arm
- Plating and screws
- External fixator.

Nails:
- Universal Femoral Nail (UFN): It is a solid nail available in diameters of 9, 10, 11, and 12 mm
- Cannulated Femoral Nail (CFN): A Kuntscher nail is commonly used, available in diameters of 10 to 15 mm

Both the nails are part of the same system UFN/CFN have two proximal locking holes (1 dynamic and 1 static) and two distal locking holes (static) and are locked with 4.9 mm locking bolts.

| Intramedullary nailing | A Kuntscher nail is commonly used |
|---|---|

Anesthesia: General or spinal

Method: Retrograde or antigrade approach

Incision: An anterolateral or lateral

Exposure: The fracture site is exposed:
- Proximal fragment reamed up
- Selected nail is driven up into the proximal fragment, till it appears in the buttock
- Nail delivered through skin incision

- Fracture reduced by traction and manipulation by using bone holding clamps
- Nail hammered and driven down into the distal fragment
- Check up the reduction and position of nail by X-ray or C-arm.

Post care: Physiotherapy: active exercises of the knee.

- Weight bearing after formation of callus, i.e. few weeks time.

## Management of Special Situations

### Fractures of femur and tibia in the same leg

Management        Conservative treatment: Closed reduction of tibial fracture and below knee plaster cast, incorporating a Steinmann pin (skeletal traction) through tibial tubercle, using Thomas splint, for reduction and immobilization of femoral fracture.

Surgical treatment:
Surgery: Intramedullary nailing of femur and plating of tibia

### Pathological fracture

Management        Surgical treatment of choice
Surgery: Intramedullary nailing and bone grafting.

### Vascular trauma

Management        Surgical treatment of choice
Surgery: Intramedullary nailing of femur followed by vessel repair.

### Nerve trauma

Management        Majority of nerve lesions are in continuity and are recoverable. In case of compound fractures, where nerve division is suspected, treatment required is nerve exploration and internal fixation of femoral fracture.

### Fractures of femoral neck and shaft

Management        Surgical treatment of choice
Surgery: Proximal femoral nailing (PFN) is the treatment of choice.

### Fracture of femoral shaft and dislocation of hip

Management        Surgical treatment of choice
Surgery: Reduction of dislocated hip, followed by internal fixation of femur.

### Fracture of upper third of femur

Management        Surgical treatment of choice
Surgery: Intramedullary nailing, followed by traction in a Thomas splint.

### Compound fractures

Management        Conservative: Easier, partly because the reduction of displacement accompalished under direct control through the wound, and partly because the difficulties of securing length and alignment are less.

Method: Toilet of wound + reduction + plaster fixation/traction
Surgical: External fixator.

## Complications of Fractures of Femur

- **Shock (oligemic):** Described in Management of Multiple Trauma.
- **Embolism (fat):** Described in Management of Multiple Trauma.
- **Delayed union:**
  Management: Prolonged immobilization.

- **Nonunion:**
  Management: Surgical treatment of choice
  Surgery: Intramedullary nailing and bone grafting.

- **Malunion:**
  Management: Surgical treatment of choice
  Surgery: Corrective osteotomy/osteoclasis.

- **Knee stiffness:**
  Etiology:
  - Quadriceps tethering: Leading to adherence to fracture site
  - Intra-articular fractures: Leading to adhesions formation or formation of a mechanical block
    - Prolonged immobilization: Esp. in delayed union.
  Management: Physiotherapy: Active exercises, SWD/IR

- **Shortening:**
  Management:
  - Up to 2.5 cm (1") corrected by shoe modification
  - > 2.5 cm (1") corrected by surgery, i.e. osteotomy.

## Supracondylar Fracture of Femur

| | |
|---|---|
| Preface | Most supracondylar fractures of the femur may be treated with the skeletal traction by Kirschner wires/Steinmann pin through the proximal tibia; perfect reduction neither necessary nor possible in comminuted fractures. |
| MOI | Direct violence<br>Fall from height<br>RSA<br>Sports injury |
| Diagnosis | Deformity: Angulation<br>Swelling<br>Local tenderness<br>Movements: Painful and restricted<br>Shortening. |
| Investigation | X-ray thigh including knee—AP and LAT views |
| Management | Conservative treatment:<br>In children: Minimal displacement in majority of cases:<br>• Closed reduction and a cylinder plaster<br>• Walking with crutches<br>• Weight bearing after formation of callus |

In adults: Distal fragment is angulated posteriorly by the pull of gastrocnemius.

- Traction to the limb with knee in flexion by bending the Thomas splint at the fracture level.

After care: Physiotherapy: Active exercises of the knee.

### Surgical treatment:

Surgery: ORIF:

Implant: Blade plate, nail plate, or distal femoral nail (DFN):

DFN: It is available in diameters of 9 mm (solid), and 10, 11 mm (cannulated) and in long and short version, with distal locking options. DFN short has 2 mL holes for proximal locking while the DFN long has 2 AP and 1 mL proximal locking holes.

## Fractures of Lateral Tibial Condyle (Bumper's fracture)

| | |
|---|---|
| Preface | Bumper fracture is the commonest of all the condylar fractures caused by an abduction strain that forces the lower leg into valgus; usually associated with a downward thrust of the bodyweight. |
| MOI | Direct violence<br>Fall from height<br>RSA<br>Sports injury. |
| Pathogenesis | An abduction strain, forces the leg into valgus; resulting fracture. |
| Pattern | • Vertical splitting of lateral tibial condyle caused by lateral femoral condyle, driven down into the tibial head<br>• Depressed lateral tibial condyle along with fracture of neck of fibula is the commonest condylar fracture<br>• Comminuted fracture of lateral tibial plateau. |
| Diagnosis | Swelling<br>Local tenderness<br>Movements of knee—painful and restricted. |
| Investigation | X-ray knee—AP and LAT views. |
| Management | Conservative treatment:<br>Closed reduction and immobilization in a plaster cylinder for 4–6/52, followed by physiotherapy<br>Surgical treatment:<br>Surgery: ORIF<br>Indication: Fracture with displacement. |

## Fracture of Medial Tibial Condyle

| | |
|---|---|
| Preface | It is a rare injury; may be associated with ruptured lateral collateral ligament or avulsed styloid process of the fibula; may be complicated by common peroneal nerve palsy (appear postimmobilization of limb in a plaster cast—due to post-traumatic edema). |
| MOI | Direct violence<br>RSA<br>Sports injury. |

| Pathogenesis | An adduction strain, forces the leg into varus; resulting fracture. |
| Diagnosis | Swelling |
| | Local tenderness |
| | Movements of knee—painful and restricted |
| Investigation | X-ray knee—AP and LAT views |
| Management | Conservative treatment: |
| | Closed reduction and immobilization in a plaster cylinder for 4–6/52, followed by physiotherapy. |

**Surgical treatment:**

Indication: Torn lateral collateral ligament

Surgery: Repair of ligament.

## Fractures of Patella

| Preface | Fracture of the patella is the commonest fracture around the knee; majority of these fractures are undisplaced; prepatellar fibres remain intact and the power and mobility of the knee remains unaffected. |
| Pattern | Of fractures: |

- Vertical fracture
- Transverse fracture
- Comminuted (Stellate) fracture
- Avulsion fracture of upper pole
- Avulsion fracture of lower pole

| MOI | Direct trauma |
| | Indirect trauma: Violent contraction of the quadriceps |
| | RSA |
| | Sports injury. |
| Diagnosis | |

- Vertical fracture: Swelling, local tenderness, movements painful and restricted
- Transverse fracture: Swelling, local tenderness, gaping between two fragments, movements painful and restricted
- Comminuted fracture: Mostly a compound fracture, articular surface of patella is damaged beyond repair, patella appears broader, and fragmented with grating on movement: swelling, local tenderness, movements of knee painful and restricted.
- Avulsion fracture of upper pole: A distinct gap between the tendon and the patella
- Avulsion fracture of lower pole: A distinct gap between the ligament and its bony attachment.

| Investigation | X-ray knee – AP and LAT views. |
| Management | |

- Vertical fracture:

  Conservative treatment: Splintage of leg in full extension

  Surgical treatment: Internal fixation (for irregular articular surface)
- Transverse fracture:

  Surgical treatment: ORIF of fracture patella + repair of torn quadriceps:

Methods of repair:
- Tension band wiring
- Figure of 8 wiring
- Vertical screw/s
- Comminuted fracture:
  Surgical treatment: Partial patellectomy and repair of torn quadriceps
- Avulsion fracture:
  Surgical treatment: Repair.
  Post care: Physiotherapy—active exercises, SWD, or IRD.

## Internal Derangements of Knee (IDK)

| Classification | IDK includes following: |
|---|---|

   i.   Injury to collateral ligaments—commonly medial
   ii.  Injury to meniscus or cartilage—commonly medial
   iii. Cysts of lateral meniscus
   iv.  Injury to cruciate ligaments
   v.   Injury to infrapatellar pad of fat
   vi.  Fracture of tibial spine
   vii. Loose bodies

## Injury of Collateral Ligaments

| | |
|---|---|
| MOI | Traumatic—forced abduction to the extended leg. |
| | RSA |
| | Sports injury—esp. common in foot ballers. |
| Mechanism of injury | Medialal one—commonly injured: Usually associated with injury to the medial meniscus, due to attachment of its deeper fibers to meniscus. With further continued strain, the cruciate ligament esp. the anterior one may rupture. |
| Diagnosis | Pain, tenderness over bony attachments of the ligament, movements of knee (esp. abduction) painful and restricted. |
| Investigation | X-ray knee—AP and LAT views, to rule out any bony lesion |
| | MRI |
| | Arthroscopy (endoscopy)—diagnostic |

## Management

| Conservative | Analgesics, |
|---|---|
| | SWD/IRD, local massage |
| | Elastic crepe bandage/knee cap/or brace, |
| | Plaster cylinder with knee flexed at 20 degree |
| | Bedrest for 2/52. |
| Surgical | Refer: The patient to the orthopedic team for surgery |
| Surgery | Repair of collateral ligament |
| | Meniscectomy |
| | Repair of anterior cruciate ligament (ACL). |

## Injury of Medial Meniscus

| | |
|---|---|
| MOI | Traumatic—RSA |
| | Sports injury—esp. common in foot ballers. |
| Mechanism of injury | The flexed knee is subjected to rotational and abduction strains. The knee momentarily opens upon the medial side, the meniscus is sucked inside and gets nipped between the condyles of femur and tibia, resulting in a tear. Repeated strains lead to a 'Bucket handle' tear. |
| Diagnosis | Common in footballers and mine workers |
| | Pain, tenderness over joint line—midway between patellar and medial collateral ligaments |
| | History of locking of knee, followed by sudden unlocking and effusion |
| | Local tenderness |
| | Mc Murray's test—positive. |
| Investigation | X-ray knee—AP and LAT views, to rule out any bony lesion |
| | MRI. |
| | Arthroscopy (Endoscopy)—diagnostic |

### Management

| | |
|---|---|
| Conservative | Analgesics |
| | Eelastic crepe bandage/knee cap/or brace |
| | SWD/IRD, local massage |
| | Plaster cylinder with knee flexed at 20 degree |
| | Bedrest for 2/52. |
| Surgical | **Refer:** The patient to the orthopedic team for surgery |
| Surgery | Meniscectomy—in confirmed cases |
| Method | Endoscopic or open surgery |

## INJURY TO LATERAL MENISCUS

### Is a Rare Injury

| | |
|---|---|
| MOI | Sports injury. |
| Management | Analgesics |
| | SWD/or IRD |
| | Knee cap. |

## Cysts of Lateral Meniscus

| | |
|---|---|
| Diagnosis | Pain on the lateral side of knee |
| | A round hard swelling over lateral side of knee. |
| Management | **Refer:** The patient to the orthopedic team for surgery |
| Surgical | Excision of cyst. |

## INJURY TO CRUCIATE LIGAMENTS

### Anterior Cruciate Ligament (ACL) Injury

| | |
|---|---|
| MOI | Direct violence. |
| | Traumatic—RSA, sports injury, fall from height. |

| Pathogenesis | Isolated tears are uncommon, and usually associated with tears of medial collateral ligament and/or medial meniscus. |
| Diagnosis | Anterior cruciate ligament (ACL)—commonly injured |
| | Pain, swelling, tenderness |
| | Movements: Abnormal forward/backward movements of tibia over femur |
| | Knee can be hyperextended. |
| Investigation | X-ray knee—AP and LAT views, for any bony lesion |
| | MRI. |
| | Arthroscopy (Endoscopy)—diagnostic |

## Management
| Conservative | Analgesics |
| | Elastic crepe bandage/or knee cap |
| | Plaster cylinder with knee flexed at 20 degree, for 6/52—If anterior tibial spine is intact. |
| | Bedrest for 2/52. |
| After care | Physiotherapy. |
| Surgical | **Refer:** The patient to the orthopedic team for surgery |
| Surgery | • ORIF (screw fixation)—if anterior tibial spine is fractured |
| | • Re-attach/or ACL replacement (tendon of semitendinosus) is the treatment of choice—if ACL is avulsed |
| | • Repair of associated tears of medial collateral ligament and media meniscus. |

## Posterior Cruciate Ligament (PCL) Injury
| MOI | Direct violence. |
| Pathogenesis | Tibia is forced backwards. |
| Diagnosis | Abnormal backward movement of tibia over femur. |
| Investigation | X-ray knee—AP and LAT views, for any bony lesion |
| | MRI |
| | Arthroscopy (endoscopy)—diagnostic |
| Management | Same as for ACL injury. |

## Injury to Infrapatellar Pad of Fat
| MOI | Traumatic—when hypertrophied, may be nipped in between the femur and tibia during extension of the knee. |
| Diagnosis | History of pain and locking of knee without being followed by sudden unlocking (cf. medial meniscus injury). |
| | Local tenderness over sides of ligamentum patellae. |
| Investigation | X-ray knee—AP and LAT views, for any bony lesion |
| | Arthroscopy (endoscopy)—diagnostic |
| Management | **Refer:** The patient to the orthopedic team for surgery |
| Surgery | Excision of hypertrophied fat—by endoscopic surgery |

## Fracture of Tibial Spine

It is a rare injury, mostly found in children

| | |
|---|---|
| MOI | Traumatic—RSA, sports injury. |
| Mechanism | Fall on the bent knee with a violent twist of tibia over the femur |
| Diagnosis | Pain, swelling, tenderness, restricted extension of knee. |
| Investigation | X-ray knee—AP and Lateral views. |

### Management

Conservative:

| | |
|---|---|
| Indication | Undisplaced fracture |
| Treatment | Aspiration of knee |
| | Elastic crepe bandage/or knee cap/or brace, or |
| | Plaster cylinder |
| | Bedrest for 2/52 |

Surgical treatment

**Refer:** The patient to the orthopedic team for surgery

| | |
|---|---|
| Indication | Displaced fracture |
| Surgery | ORIF of fragment with a screw, or |
| | Excision of fragment. |

## Loose Bodies

| | |
|---|---|
| MOI | Direct violence |
| Diagnosis | History of locking at different angles each time |
| Investigation | X-ray knee—AP and LAT views |
| | Arthroscopy (endoscopy)—diagnostic |

### Management

| | |
|---|---|
| Surgery | Surgical removal by endoscopic or by open surgery. |

**Refer:** The patient to the orthopedic team for surgery.

### References

1. Attenberg AR, Shorkey RL. Blade-plate Fixation in Non-union and in Complicated Fractures of the Supracondylar Region of the Femur. J Bone Jt Surg 31A, 312, 1949.
2. Apley AG. Fracture of the Lateral Tibial Condyle Treated by Skeletal Traction and Early Mobilisation. J Bone Jt Surg 38B, 699, 1956.
3. Bohler L, Bohler J. Kuntscher's Medullary Nailing. J Bone Jt Surg 31A, 295, 1949.
4. Bradford CH, Kilfoyle RM, Kellcher JJ. Fracture of the Lateral Tibial Condyle. J Bone Jt Surg 32A, 39, 1950.
5. S Terry Canale, Kay Daugherty, Linda Jones. Campbell Operative Orthopaedics 9th Ed. Vol I-IV. Mosby, 1998.
6. Charnley JC, Baker SL. Compression Arthrodesis of the Knee. A Clinical and Histological Study. J Bone Jt Surg 34B, 187, 1952.
7. Dehne E, Immermann EW. Dislocation of Hip Combined with Fracture of Shaft of Femur on same side. J Bone Jt Surg 33A, 731, 1951.
8. Duthie HL, Hutchinson JR. The Results of Partial and Total Excision of the Patella. J Bone Jt Surg 40B, 75, 1958.
9. Hohl M, Luck JV. Fractures of the Tibial Condyle. J Bone Jt Surg 38A, 1001, 1956
10. Jackson JP, Waugh WL. Tibial Osteotomy for Osteoarthritis of the Knee. J Bone Jt Surg 43B, 114, 1961.

11. Kapoor PS. Internal derangements of knee: Accident and Emergency, ed. 2nd, CBS, New Delhi, 2016.

12. Kapoor SK, et al. Expandable self-locking nail in the management of closed diaphyseal fractures of femur and tibia. Indian Journal of Orthopaedics. Vol. 43 No.3, 264–270, 2009.

13. Krettek C, Manss J, Konemann B, et al. Deformation of Femoral Nails with Intramedullary insertion. J Orthop. Res 16 (5) 572–5, 1998.

14. Krettek C, Konemann B, Miclau T, et al. A New Technique for the Distal Locking of Solid AO Unreamed Tibial Nails. J Orthop Trauma 11 (16) 446–51, 1997.

15. Kulkarni GS, et al. Intertrochanteric fractures. Indian Journal of Orthopaedics. Vol. 40 No.1, 16–23, 2006.

16. Meyers MH, McKeever FM. Fracture of the Intercondylar Eminence of the Tibia. J Bone Jt Surg 41A, 209, 1959.

17. O Donoghue DH. Surgical Treatment of Fresh Injuries to the Major Ligaments of the Knee. J Bone Jt Surg 32, 725, 1950. An Analysis of End-results of Surgical Treatment of Major Injuries to Ligaments of the Knee. J Bone Jt Surg 37A, 1955.

18. Palmar I. Fracture of the Upper end of the Tibia. J Bone Jt Surg 33B, 160, 1951.

19. Shekhar L, Mayanger JC. A clinical study of Ender nails fixation in femoral shaft fractures in children. Indian Journal of Orthopaedics. Vol. 40 No. 1, 16–23, 2006.

20. Shetty MS, Kumar A, Kanthi KG: Locking Compression Plate—LCP—A Boon in Traumatology

21. Shorbe HB, Dobson CH. Patellectomy (Repair of Extensor Mechanism) J Bone Jt Surg 40A, 1281, 1958.

22. Slee GC. Fractures of Tibial Condyles. J Bone Jt Surg 37B, 427, 1955.

23. Smillie IS. Injuries of the Knee Joint. Edinburgh ; Livingstone, 1951.

24. Wilson EF. Repair of Cruciate Ligaments. J Bone Jt Surg 43B, 342, 1961.

## FRACTURES OF TIBIA AND FIBULA

Principles
- It is vital to correct angulation deformity in fractures of this weight bearing bone, to prevent development of osteoarthritis in ankle and knee
- Prone to infection, as one-third of tibia is subcutaneous
- Prone to torsional forces, causing oblique and spiral fractures as commonly seen in this bone
- Prone to Volkmann ischemic contracture due to injury to the popliteal artery in fractures of upper third.

## Fractures in Children

| | |
|---|---|
| Types | Undisplaced (syn. Greenstick) fractures of Tibia |
| | Displaced fractures of tibia. |
| Pattern | Mostly greenstick fractures |
| MOI | Direct violence |
| | Fall from a height |
| | RSA |
| | Sports injury. |
| Diagnosis | Swelling |
| | Local tenderness |
| | Movements: Resents moving leg. |
| Investigation | X-ray leg including ankle and knee—AP and LAT views |
| Management | Conservative treatment |

Undisplaced fractures of tibia:

Management: Plaster cast from groin to toes, with knee slightly flexed, for 4–6/52.

After care: Apply elastic crepe bandage for 1/52 post removal of the plaster.

Displaced fractures of Tibia:

Management: Closed reduction

Method: Traction, manipulation, and plaster cast above knee for 6/52.

After care: Same as for greenstick fractures.

## Fractures of Tibial Tuberosity

| | |
|---|---|
| Definition | Individual fractures of tibial tuberosity are rare, although it is usually involved in major fractures of the tibial head. It may be injured during its development period (evidence of apophyseal osteochondrosis) |
| MOI | Direct trauma: May separate small fragments from the apophysis. |
| | Indirect trauma: Violent quadriceps contraction. |
| Pathogenesis | Small fragments, separated from tibial apophysis. |
| Diagnosis | Pain |
| | Swelling |
| | Disability |
| D/d | Pathological fracture: |
| | • Paget's disease |
| | • Osteoclastoma. |
| Investigation | X-ray leg including Knee—AP and LAT views. |
| Management | Conservative treatment: |
| | Rest |
| | Analgesics, NSAIDS |
| | SWD, IR therapy |
| | Surgical treatment of choice. |
| | Surgery: |
| | ORIF: In isolated fractures with separated tibial tuberosity. |
| | Excision of small fragments detached from tibial apophysis. |

## Fracture of Tibial Spine

| | |
|---|---|
| Definition | It is a rare injury, common in children |
| MOI | Fall on the bent knee with a violent twist of tibia over the femur |
| Diagnosis | Local tenderness underneath lgament patellae |
| | Extension knee—painful and restricted |
| Investigation | X-ray knee—AP and LAT views |
| Management | Conservative treatment: |
| | Indication: Undisplaced fracture |
| | Method: Aspiration of knee and plaster cylinder |
| | Surgical treatment: |
| | Indication: Displaced fracture |

Surgery:
- ORIF of fragment with a screw, or
- Excision of fragment.

# Fractures in Adults

## Intra-articular fractures

| | |
|---|---|
| Preface | Intra-articular fractures are usually caused by direct violence on the extended knee, e.g. pedestrian suffering from a 'Bumper' injury. |
| MOI | Direct trauma: To the extended knee (syn. Bumper/compression fractures: femoral condyle forced into the tibial condyle) |
| | RSA |
| | Fall from a height |
| | Sports injury: Athletics, cycling, jumps |
| Types | • T-shaped vertical split in the tibial head |
| | • Y-shaped involving both condyles, with the tail extending down into the upper end of tibial shaft |
| | • Inverted Y-shaped (transverse fracture of upper end of tibia, with the tail extending upward into the knee joint) |
| Pathogenesis | Ruptured opposite collateral ligament and capsule; ruptured cruciate ligaments (by rotational or anteroposterior forces); torn menisci in the crush injury; fractured bony fragments; hemarthrosis. |
| Diagnosis | Pain |
| | Swelling |
| | Local tenderness |
| | Movements: Painful and restricted |
| Investigation | X-ray knee—AP and LAT views. |
| Management | Principles of treatment are common to all types: |

- Linear fractures: Anatomical reduction possible; exception: in gross comminution due to the damaged soft tissues (< anatomical reduction acceptable)

Conservative treatment: (85% successful).
- Aspiration and compression
- Closed reduction (usually not possible because of intact fibula)
- Plaster cylinder

### Surgical treatment:
Indication:
- Failed conservative measures (15%).
- Depressed large fragment

Surgery: ORIF (screw/or bolt)

After care: Immobilization (damaged articular surface) for 6/52, followed by active exercises.

# Fractures of upper Shaft

| | |
|---|---|
| Preface | Extra-articular fractures of tibial head and upper shaft, often difficult to manage because of certain problems, e.g. grossly comminuted, and compound fractures |

| MOI | Direct trauma: Hit by a stick |
| | Fall from a height |
| | RSA |
| | Sports injury. |
| Diagnosis | Pain |
| | Swelling |
| | Wound (open fracture) |
| | Local tenderness |
| | Movement: Painful and restricted |
| Investigation | X-ray leg including Knee—AP and LAT views. |
| Management | Conservative treatment: |
| | Rest |
| | Analgesic/NSAIDs |
| | Antibiotics |
| | Toilet of wound (open fracture) |
| | Closed reduction under anesthesia |
| | Immobilization: A long plaster cast from upper thigh to toes with knee flexed to 15 degree flexion for 8/52. |

**Surgical treatment:**
Indications:
- Failed closed reduction
- Compound fractures
- Severe comminuted fractures

Surgery: ORIF.

After care: Immobilized leg in a long plaster cast above knee to toes for 8/52.

## Fractures Both Bones (Tibia and Fibula) of Leg

| Preface | Fractures of tibia and fibula usually occur either as a result of direct or indirect violence; very commonly seen as RSA; in direct violence both bones fractured at same level, while in indirect violence the tibia usually fractured at the junction of its middle and lower thirds, and the fibula at its centre; fractures of the tibial shaft, without involvement of the fibula, are usually because of indirect violence, in that case the fracture is oblique or spiral; open (compound) fractures of tibia are common because of subcutaneous bone in its entire length, and displacement likely to cause the fragment/s to puncture the skin. |
| MOI | • Direct trauma: Bones fractured at same level |
| | • Indirect trauma: Tibia usually fractured at junction of middle and lower thirds, while fibula at its centre |
| | • Torsional stresses: Fractured tibial shaft alone (# oblique or spiral) |
| | • RSA |
| | • Sports inuries (torsional stresses) |
| | • Fall from a height |
| Pathogenesis | Compound tibial fractures usually occur (subcutaneous bone). |

| | |
|---|---|
| Diagnosis | Pain |
| | Swelling |
| | Local tenderness |
| | Wound (usually contaminated—tibial fragment penetrating skin) |
| | Movements: Painful and restricted. |
| Investigation | X-ray leg including Knee and ankle—AP and LAT views. |
| Management | Conservative treatment: |

Reduction: Closed reduction

Indications:

- Transverse fractures (if fragments engaged in stable position)
- Oblique fractures (short oblique)
- Undisplaced fractures
- Greenstick fractures

Method: Closed reduction followed by immobilization in a long plaster cast for 12/52, then weight bearing allowed with help of crutches/cast brace till firm union.

**Surgical treatment:**

Methods:

- External fixator (Ilizarov):

  Indications:
  - Compound fractures
  - Delayed union
- ORIF:

  Indications:
  - Oblique fractures (long oblique)
  - Spiral fractures
  - Compound fractures (clean)

Methods:

- Nailing (medullary fixation of tibia): Interlocking nailing
- Plate and screws: Dynamic compression plate (DCP)
- Screws for long oblique or spiral fractures
- Amputation:

Indications:

- Contaminated compound fractures
- Ischemia of the part distal to the septic wound

Postoperative: Immobilization in a plaster cast or traction for 10–12/52.

After care: Active exercises, walking with crutches/cast brace till firm union.

## Fractures of Tibial Shaft Without Fracture of Fibula

| | |
|---|---|
| Definition | Are usually because of indirect trauma, and are mostly oblique or spiral. |
| MOI | Indirect trauma |
| | RSA |

|              | Sports injuries |
|--------------|-----------------|
|              | Fall from a height |
| Diagnosis    | Swelling |
|              | Local tenderness |
|              | Bone irregularity |
| Investigation | X-ray leg including ankle and knee—AP and LAT views |
| Management   | Conservative treatment: |

Reduction: Closed reduction:

Method: Traction and manipulation

Immobilization: In a plaster cast from groin to toes for 8–10/52.

After care: Check X-ray, and if fracture united, then partial weight bearing with the help of crutches for 2/52, followed by full weight bearing.

### Surgical treatment:
ORIF:

Indications:
- Displaced fractures.
- Oblique fractures (long oblique)
- Spiral fractures
- Compound fractures (clean)

Methods:
- Plating and screws—Dynamic compression plate (DCP)

  Indications:
  - Transverse and short oblique fractures
- Intramedullary nailing: Tibia is less suitable for medullary fixation than the femur, because of rotation, and requires an external support.
- Interlocking nailing

  Nails:
  - Solid Tibial Nail (STN):

  Indications:
  - Compound tibial diaphyseal fractures
  - Unstable closed fractures
  - Comminuted fractures of tibia with small medullary canals
  - Fractures of middle third of tibial shaft
  - Transverse and short oblique fractures

  Features:
  - 9 degree proximal bend for easy insertion
  - Proximal locking holes (1 Dynamic and 1 Static ML holes)
  - Distal locking holes (2 ML and 1 AP hole).
  - Titanium Elastic Nail (TEN):

  Indications:
  - Diaphyseal fractures of long bones with narrow medullary canal, i.e. lower limb in pediatric patients, lower limb in small-stature patients

Features:

- 2 to 4 mm diameters (color coded)
- Tip of nail is curved for easy insertion

- Screws for long oblique or spiral fractures
- Amputation:

Indications:

- Contaminated compound fractures
- Ischemia of the part distal to the septic wound

- External fixator (Ilizarov):

Indications:

- Compound fractures
- Delayed union
- ORIF:

Post care: Immobilization in a plaster cast or traction for 10–12/52.

After care: Active exercises, walking with crutches/cast brace till firm union.

## Double/Treble Fractures of Shaft

| | |
|---|---|
| Definition | Defined as fractures, that are mostly transverse, and angulated, resulting in delayed or nonunion of one end of the double fragment. |
| MOI | Direct trauma: Hit by a stick, iron rod, blows, kicks, torture |
| | RSA |
| | Sports injuries |
| | Fall from a height |
| Diagnosis | Swelling |
| | Local tenderness |
| | Bone irregularity |
| | Movements: Painful and restricted. |
| Investigation | X-ray leg including ankle and knee—AP and LAT views |
| Management | Conservative treatment: |

Reduction: Closed reduction under anesthesia and C-arm screening: little angulation at both fractures may be accepted without any consequence

Immobilization: In a long leg plaster cast or traction for 10–12/52.

After care: Active exercises, walking with crutches/cast brace till firm union.

Surgical treatment:

- ORIF:

Indications:

- Failed closed reduction
- Displaced fractures.
- Angulated (considerable)
- Compound fractures (clean)
- Volkmann's ischemia

Methods:
- Plating and Screws—Dynamic compression plate (DCP)
  Indications:
  - Transverse, angulated fractures
- Intramedullary nailing: Tibia is less suitable for medullary fixation than the femur, because of rotation, and requires an external support.
- Interlocking nailing of choice (done without exposing fracture/s)
  Nails:
  - Solid Tibial Nail (STN):
  Indications:
  - Compound tibial diaphyseal fractures
  - Unstable closed fractures
  - Comminuted fractures of tibia with small medullary canals
  - Fractures of middle third of tibial shaft
  - Transverse and short oblique fractures
  Features:
  - 9 degree proximal bend for easy insertion
  - Proximal locking holes (1 dynamic and 1 static ML holes)
  - Distal locking holes (2 ML and 1 AP hole).
- Titanium Elastic Nail (TEN):
  Indications:
  - Diaphyseal fractures of long bones with narrow medullary canal, i.e. lower limb in pediatric patients, lower limb in small-stature patients
  Features:
  - 2 to 4 mm diameters (color coded)
  - Tip of nail is curved for easy insertion
- Screws for long oblique or spiral fractures
- Amputation:
  Indications:
  - Contaminated compound fractures
  - Ischemia of the part distal to the septic wound
- External fixator (Ilizarov):
  Indications:
  - Compound fractures
  - Delayed union
  - ORIF:

Post care: Immobilization in a plaster cast or traction for 10–12/52.
After care: Active exercises, walking with crutches/cast brace till firm union.

## Fractures of Distal Shaft

MOI        Direct trauma: Hit by a stick, iron rod, blows, kicks, torture
RSA

|               |                                                            |
|---------------|------------------------------------------------------------|
|               | Sports injuries                                            |
|               | Fall from a height                                         |
| Diagnosis     | Swelling                                                   |
|               | Local tenderness                                           |
|               | Bone irregularity                                          |
|               | Movements: Painful and restricted.                         |
| Investigation | X-ray leg including ankle—AP and LAT views.                |
| Management    | Conservative treatment:                                    |

Closed reduction: Amenable to treatment

Immobilization in a plaster cast for 8/52, followed by weight bearing in a walking cast till firm union.

Surgical treatment:

Indication:

- Failed closed reduction

Surgery: ORIF:

Method: Plate (DCP) with cortical screws proximally and cancellous screws

Distally

Postoperative: Immobilization: in a plaster cast for 8/52, followed by weight bearing in a walking cast till firm union.

## Compound Fractures

| Preface     | Primary excision (debridement) and toilet of an open (compound) of the tibia and fibula is an urgent procedure that commands greater skill and experience (not only technically difficult, but decision to manage skin loss, muscle mass to excise, and whether bone fragments to be removed, demands expert judgment); all devitalized muscle to be excised, and bone fragments (completely detached) may not be left behind in the hope of their survival. |
|-------------|--------|
| Management  | Conservative treatment: |

Indication: Stable fracture

- Debridement of wound
- Toilet of wound (avoid undue irrigation pressure); removal of foreign body/bodies
- Reduction of fracture
- Immobilization: Apply a plaster cast above knee.

**Surgical treatment:**

Method: ORIF

Indication: Unstable fracture and clean wound.

Method: External Fixator application (allows free dressings)

Indication: Unstable fracture and wound infective.

## References

1. Kapoor PS. Fractures management: Accident and Emergency, ed. 2nd, CBS, New Delhi, 2016.
2. Krettek C, Konemann B, Miclau T, et al. A New Technique for Distal locking of Solid AO Unreamed Tibial Nails, 1997.

3. Moore JR. The Closed Fracture of the Long Bones. J Bone Jt Surg 42A, 869, 1960.
4. Nicoll EA. The Treatment of gaps in Long Bones by Cancellous Insert Grafts. J Bone Jt Surg 38B, 70, 1956-(1960) Personal communication.
5. Rahman MM, Taha WS, Shaheen MM. A Simple Technique for Distal Locking of tibial nails. Injury 29 (10) 789–90, 1998.

## Injuries About the Ankle and Foot

Anatomy  Ankle joint is a synovial joint of the hinge variety; is a joint of great strength; its stability is provided by the strong ligaments, adjoining tendons, and by the close interlocking of the articular surfaces. The ankle joint resembles a mortise e.g. tenon joint of a carpenter. The tenon is talus, whereas the mortise is formed by the inferior articular surface of tibia and medial and lateral malleoli. The lateral malleolus of fibula is firmly attached to the tibia by anterior and posterior tibiofibular ligaments. The ankle is firmly supported by the strong deltoid ligament on the medial side and lateral ligament on the lateral side. Ankle joint transmits more weight than any other body joint; thereby a very stable joint, with limited mobility.

Movements:

At ankle:

- Flexion (plantar-flexion)
- Extension (dorsiflexion

At subtalar joint:

- Inversion
- Eversion

At midtarsal joints:

- Abduction
- Adduction of forefoot.

## Ankle Trauma

Injuries about the ankle and foot

- Pott's fracture
- Isolated fracture malleolus
- Avulsion fracture of isolated malleolus
- Displaced medial malleolar fracture
- Fracture posterior malleolar
- Bimalleolar or trimalleolar fractures
- Fracture lower end of fibula
- Ankle sprain
- Epiphyseal injuries
- References.

## Pott's Fracture

Definition  It is a fracture-dislocation of the ankle joint and requires accurate reduction and fixation; many patterns of Pott's fracture recognized, and all these differ, being caused by different types of violence; common

Pott's fracture results from continuation of the same force/stress (external rotation and eversion) that causes an uncomplicated fracture of the lateral malleolus (spirally/or obliquely); followed by fractured tip of the medial malleolus; then posterolateral subluxation of talus from tibia; a bone chip avulsed from the posterior surface of tibia.

**MOI**
Direct trauma
RSA
Sports injuries
Fall from a height.

**Classification**
A. Anatomically:
- Type I: Fracture of one malleolus
- Type II: Fractures of two malleoli (bimalleolar): commonest injury
- Type III: Fractures of three malleoli (trimalleolar): displacement appreciable

B. Diastasis of ankle/or vertical compression:
1st degree potts fracture with diastasis
2nd degree potts fracture with vertical compression

C. Genetic (Lauge-Hansen):
- Supination/external rotation (SE)
- Pronation/abduction (PA)
- Pronation/external rotation (PE)
- Supination/adduction (SA)
- Pronation/dorsiflexion (PD)

D. Traumatic (mode of violence):

External Rotation and Eversion Fractures:
- Fracture of lateral malleolus (oblique or spiral)
- Fracture of medial malleolus (tip)
- Subluxation of talus—posterolaterally causing
- Fracture of posterior surface of tibia (third malleolus)

Eversion Fractures (syn. abduction fractures):
- Fracture of fibula—5–7 cm above its lower end
- Subluxation of talus—laterally, leading to avulsion fracture of medial malleolus.

**Pathogenesis**
Staging (S-1 to S-5) based upon the position of the foot at the time of trauma, and the direction—the talus rotates in the ankle mortice, as a result of the torque convertor effect (Lauge-Hansen):

A. Supination/external rotation:
- S-1: Inverted foot (talus rotated externally in ankle mortise)
- S-2: Torn tibiofibular ligament
- S-3: Fracture fibula (oblique or spiral)
- S-4: Torn medial ligament (unstable injury)
- S-5: Avulsion fracture of medial malleolus (very unstable injury).

B. Pronation/abduction:
- S-1: Everted foot (talus abducted); torn deltoid ligament, or avulsion fracture of medial malleolus; horizontal fracture line

- S-2: Torn tibiofibular ligaments (anterior and posterior)
- S-3: Fracture fibula (distal fragment angulated medially); horizontal fracture line

C. Pronation/external rotation:
- S-1: Everted/or neutral position foot (talus externally rotated); torn deltoid ligament, or fracture medial malleolus (oblique)
- S-2: Avulsed anterior tibiofibular ligament (Tillaux fracture)
- S-3: Fracture fibula (oblique or spiral)
- S-4: Fracture neck of fibula (Maisonneuve fracture)

D. Supinated/adduction:
- S-1: Inverted foot (talus externally rotated, but countered by the forces impact on the forefoot, resulting in mainly the adduction of the talus in the mortise).
- S-2: Torn lateral ligament, or avulsion fracture of lateral malleolus; horizontal fracture line
- S-3: Fracture medial malleolus (high oblique or vertical)

E. Pronation/dorsiflexion (compression trauma):
- S-1: Dorsiflexed foot (talus dorsiflexed—its wider anterior part pushed between the malleoli, shearing off the medial malleolus)
- S-2: Fracture anterior tibial margin; then fracture lateral malleolus
- S-3: Subluxated talus anteriorly, carrying along marginal fracture
- S-4: Comminuted tibial fractures; irregular lower articular surface of the tibia; fracture all maleoli (plantarflexed trauma).

| | |
|---|---|
| Diagnosis | Pain |
| | Swelling: Diffuse in front of lateral malleolus; over lateral malleolus (sprain or fracture) |
| | Deformity: Prominent distal end of tibia (laterally displaced fracture medial malleolus); posterior displaced foot (fracture posterior malleolus |
| | Disability: Difficulty in walking |
| | Movements: Painful and restricted |
| Investigation | X-ray ankle—AP and LAT views |
| | Interpretation: |

- Site and slant of fracture
- Ligament integrity for avulsion
- Talar tilt

**Management**    Conservative treatment:

Type I:
- Rest
- Heat—SWD or IRD
- Elastic crepe bandage, or adhesive plaster.
- Analgesics

Type II:
- Below knee plaster cast for 4–6/52.

Type III:
- Manipulation of ankle, followed by plaster cast for 4–6/52.

Surgical treatment:

Indication: Failure of conservative treatment.

Surgery: Cross screwing, to avoid injury to the epiphyseal plate.

Type IV: Open reduction

Type V: Osteotomy may be required as corrective measure.

## Fractures of Foot

Include

1. Fractures of talus
2. Fractures of calcaneus
3. Rupture of tendo-achilis
4. Fracture of fifth metatarsal
5. Fractures of metatarsals
6. Crush injuries of the foot

Anatomy

The foot (pes) extends from the heel (calx) to the roots of toes; its superior surface called dorsum, while inferior surface the plantar (sole); divided into the tarsus, metatarsus, and the toes.

Tarsus: Posterior half of foot; its bones called tarsal bones (7), arranged in two rows (posterior and anterior), one intervening bone (navicular—separates talus from cuneiforms).

Arrangement of tarsal bones:

• 1st row: two bones, set one (talus lies below tibia) above the other (calcaneus—the largest tarsal bone).
• 2nd row: four bones (cuboid— most lateral, and three wedge shaped cuneiforms) placed side by side.

Metatarsals: Five, set side by side, behind toes

Toes (digits): Five (greater toe or hallux—most medial, little toe or digitus minimus); bones of toes called phalanges (proximal, middle, distal; exception—greater toe having proximal and distal)

Joints of foot: All bones of the foot participate into joints formation:

• Intertarsal joints: Tarsal bones articulate with one another
• Tarsometatarsal joints
• Intermetatarsal joints
• Metatarsophalangeal joints
• Interphalangeal joints

Arches of foot: Longitudinal and transverse, formed by bones (tarsals and metatarsals) bound together by ligaments; integrity maintained by the bones, soft tissue—ligaments and plantar fascia, and muscles.

## Fractures of Talus

Abstract

Fractures of talus create many problems pertaining to this bone, due to its wide articular surface. The vascular supply of talus is analogous to that of femoral head, i.e. talus receives its main vascular supply from a branch of dorsalis pedis artery that enters the neck (prone to trauma—fracture/fracture dislocation of proximal part of talar neck impairs blood supply—causing avascular necrosis of talar body and arthritic changes).

| Anatomy | The talus (astragalus), is the 2nd largest tarsal bone, that has a unique structure designed to channel and distribute body weight as it has no muscular or tendinous attachment; the talus rests on the superior surface of the calcaneus, its body hidden below the tibia, amongst the malleoli, while its anterior part ejects from underneath the tibia in an extended foot; its head rounded appears in front of lateral malleolus in an inverted foot. |
|---|---|

Joints of Talus: Talus plays a main role in the following joints:

- Ankle joint: Formed by the talus and the distal ends of the tibia and fibula; talus articulates by its three surfaces (superior, medial and lateral)
- Talocalcanean joint: Gliding synovial, formed by bones (talus and calcaneus), supported by ankle's deltoid and calcaneofibular ligaments
- Talocalcaneonavicular joint: Ball and socket (ball is anterior talus and socket formed by anterior calcaneus, spring ligament (plantar calcaneonavicular), and navicular bone).

## Fracture Neck of Talus

| Preface | Fracture neck of talus is the commonest amongst fractures of the talus; the neck of talus may be shorn through by the sharp anterior border of the articular surface of the tibia; comminution is common, are often associated with injury to neighboring bones; usually the body of talus extruded from the ankle joint by the velocity of the injury, leaving the head and neck *in situ*; displaced body may be palpable underneath the skin; defy all attempts at closed reduction. |
|---|---|
| MOI | Direct trauma |
| | RSA |
| | Fall from a height |
| | Sports injuries. |
| Mechanism | Fracture of neck of talus occurs as a result of acute dorsiflexion and upward force resulting in shearing of talar neck by the sharp anterior border of the articular surface of the tibia: |

- Type I: Fracture talar neck without any displacement
- Type II: Continuing dorsiflexion force—resulting in fracture neck of the talus with displacement of proximal talar segment (plantar flexion) and subluxation of subtalar joint
- Type III: And further continuation of force—resulting in thrusting of the tibia between the two talar fragments
- Type IV: Rare Type: dislocation of talar head from the navicular bone along with Type III injury.

| Diagnosis | Pain |
|---|---|
| | Swelling |
| | Local tenderness |
| | Disability: Difficulty in walking |
| | Movements of ankle: Painful and restricted |

Investigation    X-ray foot including ankle—AP, LAT and oblique views:
                 AP and oblique views
Management       Conservative treatment:
                 Closed reduction
                 Immobilization: Below knee plaster cast for 6/52.
                 Surgical treatment:
                 Indication of surgery: failure of conservative treatment
                 Surgery: ORIF (K-wire)
                 Specific treatment of:
                 Type I:
                 • Below knee plaster cast for 6/52
                 • Non weight bearing with crutches.
                 After care: Physiotherapy.
                 Type II: Closed reduction under anesthesia
                 Method: Foot is plantar flexed and everted
                 Immobilization: Below knee plaster cast for 8–10/52.
                 ORIF (K-wire) in case the closed reduction fails
                 After care: Physiotherapy.
                 Type III: Closed reduction under anesthesia
                 Method: By holding heel, apply traction, then dorsiflex the foot and
                 pull the heel forward and evert it, to open up space for talus, then
                 press the talus firmly into this space, finally planter flex the foot.
                 Immobilization: Apply below knee plaster cast for 8–10/52.
                 ORIF (K-wire) in case the closed reduction fails.
                 After care: Physiotherapy.
                 Type IV: ORIF is the treatment of choice.

## Complications of Fracture Talus

- Avascular necrosis: Leading to osteoarthritis of the ankle joint
  Management: Arthrodesis of ankle joint.
- Pott's fracture: Malleolar fractures may complicate fracture neck of
  talus.0
  Management: ORIF of malleolar fracture is treatment of choice.
- Osteoarthritis: Due to avascular necrosis or malunion.
  Management: Arthrodesis of ankle joint is treatment of choice.

## Fracture Body of Talus

Preface          The superior articular surface of the talus may be fractured by the same
                 mechanisms that result in compression fractures of the ankle; vertical
                 splits without major disturbance of the ankle or subtalar joints may be
                 managed as Type 1 talar neck fractures; any displacement commands
                 perfect reduction and cross screwing; for high degree of comminution
                 (body convexity flattened; talus compressed between the tibia and the
                 calcaneus; ankle and subtalar joints damaged) surgical reconstruction
                 seldom possible.

| MOI | Direct trauma |
|---|---|
| | RSA |
| | Fall from a height |
| | Sports injuries. |

Pattern
- Fracture of superior articular surface of the talus
- Vertical fracture-splitting, without disturbing the ankle or subtalar joints

Management  Conservative treatment:

Indications:
- Impacted fractures of talar head, usually associated with compression fractures of navicular
- Incomplete fractures of talar neck without displacement.

Method: Closed reduction.

Immobilization: In a plaster cast from below knee to toes, for 8–10/52.

After care: Walking in plaster cast/brace, till firm union.

Surgical treatment:

Indications:
- Fracture with displacement: ORIF (reduction and cross screwing)
- Comminuted fractures of body with displacement: Arthrodesis.
- Avascular necrosis: Arthrodesis.

## Fracture of Calcaneus (os Calcis)

Preface  The os calcaneus is usually fractured by falls from heights or by mine explosions; usually shattered like an eggshell involves the subtalar joint; degree of displacement variable as per violence (minor displacement to whole os calcis flattened and widened); tendo-achillis pulls up the loose fragment of tuberosity and heel everted (traumatic flat-foot); injury despite various types of management tried, causes stiff foot in the subtalar area, resulting in walking difficult on irregular surface; may experience incapacitating pain; best results achieved by accepting deformity and aiming for early mobilization.

MOI  Fall from a height: Common in window cleaners, construction workers

Impact from below: Mine explosions, below deck explosion on a boat

RSA

Sports injuries

Mechanism of fracture

The degree of displacement depends upon the force of violence. Sometimes there is no displacement, i.e. if fallen height is comparatively small. With greater fallen height, there may occur flattening and widening of calcaneum, with involvement of subtalar joint.

Pathogenesis  Type I: Isolated, single fractures of the body, anterior end, or tuberosity, with minor/or no displacement, and without involvement of the articular surfaces.

Typer II: Intra-articular fractures involving subtalar joint (tongue, and joint depression fractures).

| | |
|---|---|
| Diagnosis | Pain |
| | Swelling |
| | Local tenderness |
| | Deformity: Broadening of heel |
| | Movements: Inversion and eversion at the subtalar joint—painful and restricted |
| Investigation | X-ray foot—AP and LAT views |
| Management | Conservative treatment: |

Indications:

- Type I: Isolated, single fractures (of body, anterior end, or tuberosity) without/or minor displacement: plaster cast, with early weight bearing
- Type II: Fractures without displacement, irrespective of involvement of the subtalar joint: plaster cast, with early weight bearing.

Surgical treatment:

Indications:

- Type I: Avulsion fracture of tuberosity with displacement:

Surgery: ORIF (reduction and screw fixation of fragment + tendo-calcaneus insertion into calcaneus distally)

- Type II: Fractures involving subtalar joint (tongue fractures and joint depression fractures)

Surgery: ORIF (reduction and axial pin/screw fixation) for tongue fracture

- ORIF for joint depression fractures.
  After care: Immobilization in a plaster cast for 8/52, with exercises, weight bearing after 8/52 (post radiological confirmation of union).
- Arthrodesis (tripple): For permanent disability (incapacitated for work) and for avascular necrosis of fragment/s.

## Rupture of Tendo-achillis

Described in Chapter of Traumatic affections of ligaments, tendons, and muscles.

## Fracture of Metatarsals

| | |
|---|---|
| Anatomy | The metatarsus is formed by five matatarsals; set side by side behind toes; each consists of a base (posterior end), shaft, neck, and a head (anterior end). |
| | Joints: |

- Intermetatarsal: Bases articulate with one another
- Tarsometatarsal: Bases articulate with cuboid and cuneiform bones

| | |
|---|---|
| MOI | Direct trauma: Crush injury, i.e. falling of heavy weight on the foot or |
| | RSA: Vehicle wheel running over the foot |
| | Sports injuries |
| | Professionals: March fractures in soldiers, policemen, workers on strike |
| Diagnosis | Pain |
| | Swelling |

Local tenderness

Movements—Painful and restricted

Investigation            X-ray foot—AP and LAT views

Management               Conservative treatment:

Heat—SWD/IRD

Elastic crepe bandage

Analgesics/NSAIDs

Walking plaster shoe in severe cases

Surgical treatment:

Indications:
- Failed conservative treatment
- Muptiple displaced fractures

Surgery: ORIF (open reduction and Kirschner wire fixation)

**Refer:** The patient to the next fracture clinic

## Fracture of Fifth Metatarsal

Preface                  It is the commonest, but often overlooked fracture of the lower limb; is a minor injury that causes unnecessary disability when treated in a walking plaster.

MOI                      It is an avulsion fracture of base of fifth metatarsal due to the sudden contraction of peroneus brevis muscle, as a result of inversion strain.

Diagnosis                Pain

Swelling

Local tenderness

Disability

Movements of adduction and abduction—painful and restricted.

Investigation            X-ray foot—AP and LAT views

Management               Conservative treatment:

Heat—SWD/IRD

Elastic crepe bandage

Analgesics/NSAIDs

Plaster cast below knee for 3/52 in severe cases.

**Refer:** The patient to the next fracture clinic

## March Fracture (syn. Fatigue Fracture)

Preface                  March fracture usually occur near the necks of the second or third metatarsals; fracture occurs spontaneously, predisposed to by a short metatarsal, causing undue strain upon the heads of the sceond and third metatarsals by exertion, e.g. standing on toes; encouraged by loss of muscular tone, that is predisposed to by wearing heavy leather boots.

MOI                      Repeated stress: As seen commonly in the Army and the Police recruits (long marches).

Diagnosis                Pain: sudden, localized over the dorsal aspect of the bone

Local tenderness

Disability on walking

Movements: Painful and restricted in severe cases.

| Investigation | X-ray foot—AP and LAT views |
|---|---|
| Management | Conservative treatment: |
| | Rest |
| | Elastic crepe bandage |
| | Analgesics and NSAIDs |
| | Plaster shoe in severe cases |

**Refer:** The patient to the next fracture clinic

## Phalangeal Fractures

| MOI | Direct trauma |
|---|---|
| | RSA |
| | Sports injury |
| | Fall of heavy weight on the foot |
| Diagnosis | Pain |
| | Swelling |
| | Disability: Difficulty in walking |
| | Wound |
| Investigation | X-ray foot—AP and LAT views |
| Management | Conservative treatment: |
| | Toilet of the wound |
| | Debridement of wound |
| | Reduction: Closed reduction |
| | Immobilization of toe: |

- By adhesive strapping to adjacent toe
- A walking plaster with toe platform for 4/52.

**Refer:** The patient to the next fracture clinic

Surgical treatment:

Surgery:

- ORIF (open reduction and Kirschner wire fixation) of fracture

## Crush Injury of the Foot

| MOI | Direct trauma |
|---|---|
| | RSA |
| | Fall of heavy weight on the foot |
| | Sports injuries |
| Diagnosis | Pain |
| | Swelling |
| | Local tenderness |
| | Wound |
| | Disability: difficulty in waklling |
| Management | Conservative treatment: |
| | Toilet of the wound |
| | Debridement of wound |
| | Dressing |
| | Immobilization: With POP cast or brace for 2/12 |

Antibiotics

Analgesics and NSAIDs

After care:

Physiotherapy:

- Heat: SWD/IRD
- Elastic crepe bandage
- Exercises

**Refer** the patient to the next fracture clinic

Surgical treatment:

Surgery: ORIF (open reduction and Kirschner wire fixation) of fractures

Postoperative: Immobilization with a POP cast for 2/12

After care:

Physiotherapy:

- Heat: SWD/IRD
- Elastic crepe bandage
- Exercises

**Refer:** The patient to the next fracture clinic.

## Bibliography

### *Upper limb fractures*

1. Charnley J. The Closed Treatment of Common Fractures. Churchill Livingstone, Edinburgh (Recently reprinted by the John Charnley Trust), 1968.
2. Einarsson F. Fracture of the upper end of the humerus. Discussion based on the follow up of 302 cass. Acta orthop. Scandinav. (supp. 32), 1958.
3. Gilfillan C. Replacement prosthesis in shoulder injuries, Am. J. Surg. 91:900, 1956.
4. Gille J, et al. Hook plate for medial clavicle fracture. Indian Journal of Orthopaedics, Vol 44–2, 221–223, 2010.
5. Henderson RS. Fracture-dislocation of the shoulder with interposition of long head of biceps, J. Bone and Joint Surg. 34-B:240, 1952.
6. Kapoor PS. Fractures treatment: Kapoor's Accident and Emergency, ed. 2nd, CBS, New Delhi, 2016.
7. Lee HG. Treatment of fracturte of the clavicle by internal nail fixation; report of case, New England J. Med. 234: 222, 1946.
8. McRaer, Esser M. Practical Fracture Treatment, ed. 4th , Churchill Livingstone, Edinburgh, 2002.
9. McGregor AL. A Synopsis of Surgical Anatomy, 9th Ed., John Wright and Sons Ltd., Bristol, 1963.
10. Robinson CM, Bell KM, Court Brown CM, et al. Locked Nailing of Humeral Shaft Fractures: experience in Edinburgh over a two year period. J Bone Joint Surg (Br) 74B: 558–62, 1992.
11. Rommens PM, Blum J, Runkel M. Retrograde Nailing of Humeral Shaft Fractures. Clin. Orthop. 350: 26–39, 1998.
12. Stern PJ, Mattingly DA, Pomeroy DL, et al. Intramedullary Fixation of Humeral Shaft Fractures. J Bone Joint Surg (Am) 66A: 639–46, 1984.
13. Throckmorton T, Kuhn JE. Fractures of the medial end of the clavicle. J Shoulder Elbow Surg, (2007) 16:49–54.
14. Vander Griend R, Tomasin J, Ward Ef. Open Reduction and Internal Fixation of Humeral Shaft Fractures: results using AO Plating Techniques. J Bone Joint Surg (Am) (1986) 68A: 430–3.

### Fractures elbow

1. Charnley J. The Closed Treatment of Common Fractures. Churchill Livingstone, Edinburgh (Recently reprinted by the John Charnley Trust), 1968.
2. Einarsson F. Fracture of the upper end of the humerus. Discussion based on the follow up of 302 cass. Acta orthop. Scandinav. (supp. 32), 1958.
3. Gilfillan C. Replacement prosthesis in shoulder injuries, Am. J. Surg. 91:900, 1956.
4. Gille J, et al. Hook plate for medial clavicle fracture. Indian Journal of Orthopaedics, Vol 44–2, 221–3, 2010.
5. Henderson RS. Fracture-dislocation of the shoulder with interposition of long head of biceps, J. Bone and Joint Surg. 34-B:240, 1952.
6. Kapoor PS. Fractures treatment: Kapoor's Accident and Emergency, ed. 2nd, CBS, New Delhi, 2016.
7. Lee HG. Treatment of fracturte of the clavicle by internal nail fixation; report of case, New England J. Med. 234:222, 1946.
8. McRaer, Esser M. Practical Fracture Treatment, ed. 4th, Churchill Livingstone, Edinburgh, 2002.
9. Robinson CM, Bell KM, Court Brown CM, et al. Locked Nailing of Humeral Shaft Fractures: experience in Edinburgh over a two year period. J Bone Joint Surg (Br) 74B: 558–62, 1992.
10. Rommens PM, Blum J, Runkel M. Retrograde Nailing of Humeral Shaft Fractures. Clin. Orthop. 350: 26–39, 1998.
11. Stern PJ, Mattingly DA, Pomeroy DL, et al. Intramedullary Fixation of Humeral Shaft Fractures. J Bone Joint Surg (Am) 66A: 639–46, 1984.
12. Throckmorton T, Kuhn JE. Fractures of the medial end of the clavicle. J Shoulder Elbow Surg, (2007) 16:49–54.
13. Vander Griend R, Tomasin J, Ward Ef. Open Reduction and Internal Fixation of Humeral Shaft Fractures: results using AO Plating Techniques. J Bone Joint Surg (Am) (1986) 68A: 430–3.

### Forearm bones injuries

1. Evans EM. Fractures of the Radius and Ulna. J Bone Jt Surg. 33B, 548, 1951.
2. Hodsworth F. Fractures of the Radius and Ulna. Modern Trends in orthopaedics, 3, 84, 1962.
3. Kapoor PS. Fractures treatment: Accident and Emergency, ed. 2nd, CBS, New Delhi, 2016.
4. Knight RA, Purvis GD. Fractures of Both Bones of the Forearm in Adults J Bone Jt Surg. 31A, 755, 1949.
5. Moore JR. The closed Fractures of the long bones. J Bone Jt Surg. 42A, 869, 1960.
6. Robertson RC. Intramedullary Fixation of Fractures of the Forearm. Amer J Surg. 85, 496, 1953.
7. Smith H, Sage FP. Internal Fixation of Fractures of the Radius and Ulna. J Bone Jt Surg. 41B, 172, 1959.

### Wrist and hand

1. Furlong R. Injuries of the hand. Boston, Little, Brown, and Co., 1957.
2. Holdsworth F. Fractures of the Radius and Ulna. Modern Trends in Orthopaedics. 3, 84, 1962
3. Kapoor PS. Fractures treatment: Accident and Emergency, ed. 2nd, CBS, New Delhi, 2016.
4. Milford L. Hand Surgery. Campbell's Operative Orthopaedics. IGAKU SHOIN Ltd. Tokyo, 1965.
5. Riordan, Daniel C. Emergency treatment of compound injury of the hand. Orthopedics 1:30, 1957 Lower limb Fractures and injuries.

### Fractures pelvis and hip

1. Addison J. Prosthetic Replacement in the Primary Treatment of Fracture of Femoral Neck. Proc. R. Soc. Med 52, 908, 1959.
2. Blocky NJ, Purser DW. The treatment of Displaced Fractures of the Neck of the Femur by Compression. A Preliminary report. J Bone and Joint Surg. 39-B, 45, 1957.

3. Charnley J. The treatment of Fractures of the Neck of the Femur by Compression. Acta orthop. Scand 30, 29, 1961.

4. Charnley J. Total Hip Replacement by Low Friction Arthroplasty. Clin Orthop 72, 7–21, 1970.

5. Claffey TJ. Avascular Necrosis of the Femoral Head. An Anatomical Study. J Bone and Joint Surg. 42-B, 802, 1960.

6. Coleman SS, Compere CL. Femoral Neck Fractures, pathogenesis of Avascular Necrosis, Non-union, and Late Degenerative Changes. J Bone and Joint Surg 39A, 1419, 1957.

7. Crawford HB. Conservative Treatment of Impacted Fracture of the Femoral Neck. A report of fifty cases. J Bone Jt Surg 42A, 471, 1960.

8. Eftekhar NS. Principles of Total Hip Replacement. St. Louis Mosby, 1978.

9. Garden RS. Low-angle Fixation in Fractures of the Femoral Neck. J. Bone and Joint Surg 43B, 647, 1961.

10. Kapoor PS. Fractures treatment: Accident and Emergency, ed. 2nd, CBS, New Delhi, 2016.

11. Marya SKS, Thukral R, Bawri R, Gupta R. Failed fixation: Trochanteric Fracture: Revision Hip Arthroplasty. Indian Journal of Orthopaedics Vol 38:3, 2004.

12. Oh I, Harris WH. A cement Fixation System for Total Hip Arthroplasty Clin Orthop 164, 221–9, 1982.

13. Phemister DB. The Recognition of Dead Bone based on Pathological and X-ray studies. Ann Surg 72, 466, 1920.

14. Trueta J. The Normal Vascular Anatomy of the Human Femoral Head during Growth. J Bone Jt Surg 35B, 442, 1957.

### Fractures femur and knee

1. Apley AG. Fracture of the Lateral Tibial Condyle Treated by Skeletal Traction and Early Mobilisation. J Bone Jt Surg 38B, 699, 1956.

2. Aritomi H, Yamamoto M. A method of Arthroscopic Surgery. Clinical evaluation of Synovectomy with the Electric Resectoscope and Removal of Loose bodies in the Knee Joint, Orthopedic Clinics of North America 10: 565–84, 1979.

3. Arthroscopy of the Knee: Evaluation of an out-Patient Procedure under Local.

4. ASAMI Group. Operative Principles of Ilizarov: Fracture Treatment—Nonunion, Osteomyelitis—Lengthening, Deformity correction, Williams and Wilkins, Milan, Italy, 1991.

5. Attenberg AR, Shorkey RL. Blade-plate Fixation in Non-union and in Complicated Fractures of the Supracondylar Region of the Femur. J Bone Jt Surg 31A, 312, 1949.

6. Bohler L, Bohler J. Kuntscher's Medullary Nailing. J Bone Jt Surg 31A, 295, 1949.

7. Bradford CH, Kilfoyle RM, Kellcher JJ. Fracture of the Lateral Tibial Condyle. J Bone Jt Surg 32A,39, 1950.

8. Charnley JC, Baker SL. Compression Arthrodesis of the Knee. A Clinical and Histological Study. J Bone Jt Surg 34B, 187, 1952.

9. Dehne E, Immermann EW. Dislocation of Hip Combined with Fracture of Shaft of Femur on same side. J Bone Jt Surg 33A, 731, 1951.

10. Duthie HL, Hutchinson JR. The Results of Partial and Total Excision of the Patella. J Bone Jt Surg 40B, 75, 1958.

11. Gilltes H, Seligson D. Arthrograpgy and Arthroscopy: Precision in the Diagnosis of Meniscal Lesions: A comparison of Clinical Evaluation, J Bone and Joint Surg. 61-A: 343–6, 1979.

12. Gilltes H, Seligson DJ. Arthrograpgy and Arthroscopy: Precision in the Diagnosis of Meniscal Lesions: A Comparison of Clinical Evaluation, Bone and Joint Surg. 61-A: 343–346, 1979.

13. Hargreaves DJ, Seedhom BB. On the 'bucket-handle' tear: Partial or total meniscectomy? A quantitative study. J Bone and Joint Surg. 61-B: 381, 1979.

14. Hohl M, Luck JV. Fractures of the Tibial Condyle. J Bone Jt Surg 38A, 1001, 1956.

15. Jackson JP, Waugh WL. Tibial Osteotomy for Osteoarthritis of the Knee. J Bone Jt Surg 43B, 114, 1961.

16. Kapoor PS. Internal derangements of knee: Accident and Emergency, ed. 2nd, CBS, New Delhi, 2016.

4

17. Kapoor SK, et al. Expandable self-locking nail in the management of closed diaphyseal fractures of femur and tibia. Indian Journal of Orthopaedics. Vol. 43 No.3, 264–70, 2009.

18. Krettek C, Konemann B, Miclau T, et al. A New Technique for the Distal Locking of Solid AO Unreamed Tibial Nails. J Orthop Trauma 11 (16) 446–51, 1997.

19. Krettek C, Manss J, Konemann B, et al. Deformation of Femoral Nails with Intramedullary insertion. J Orthop. Res 16 (5) 572–5, 1998.

20. Kulkarni GS, et al. Intertrochanteric fractures. Indian Journal of Orthopaedics. Vol. 40 No.1, 16–23, 2006.

21. McGinty JB, Matza RA. Arthroscopy of the Knee: Evaluation of an out-Patient Procedure under Local Anesthesia, J Bone and Joint Surg. 60-A: 787–9, 1978.

22. McGinty JB, Matza RA. Arthroscopy of the Knee: Evaluation of an out-Patient Procedure under Local Anesthesia, J Bone and Joint Surg. 60-A: 787–9, 1978.

23. McGinty JB, Matza RA. Arthroscopy of the Knee: Evaluation of an out-Patient Procedure under Local Anesthesia, J Bone and Joint Surg. 60-A: 787–9, 1978.

24. Meyers MH. McKeever FM. Fracture of the Intercondylar Eminence of the Tibia. J Bone Jt Surg 41A, 209, 1959.

25. O Donoghue DH. Surgical Treatment of Fresh Injuries to the Major Ligaments of the Knee. J Bone Jt Surg 32, 725, 1950—An Analysis of End-results of Surgical Treatment of Major Injuries to Ligaments of the Knee. J Bone Jt Surg 37A, 1955.

26. Palmar L. Fracture of the Upper end of the Tibia. J Bone Jt Surg 33B, 160, 1951.

27. S Terry Canale, Kay Daugherty, Linda Jones. Campbell Operative Orthopaedics 9th Ed. Vol I-IV. Mosby, 1998.

28. Shekhar L, Mayanger JC. A clinical study of Ender nails fixation in femoral shaft fractures in children. Indian Journal of Orthopaedics. Vol. 40 No.1, 16–23, 2006.

29. Shetty MS, Kumar A, Kanthi KG. Locking Compression Plate – LCP – A Boon in Traumatology.

30. Shorbe HB, Dobson CH. Patellectomy (Repair of Extensor Mechanism) J Bone Jt Surg 40A, 1281, 1958.

31. Slee GC. Fractures of Tibial Condyles. J Bone Jt Surg 37B, 427, 1955.

32. Smillie IS. Injuries of the Knee Joint. Edinburgh ; Livingstone, 1951.

33. Wilson EF. Repair of Cruciate Ligaments. J Bone Jt Surg 43B, 342, 1961.

## Ankle and foot

1. Allan JH. The open reduction of fractures of the os calcis. Ann. Surg 141:890, 1955.

2. Bailey and Love's. Short Practice of Surgery. Injuries to bones: 13: 184, Charnley J.: H.K. Lewis & Co., London, 1965.

3. Blair HC. Comminuted fractures and fracture dislocations of the body of the astragalaux. Am J Surg 59: 37–43, 1943.

4. Blount WP. Fractures in children. Williams and Wilkins Co., Baltimore, 1954.

5. Bohler L. The Treatment of Fractures. 4th Ed. Wright, Bristol 1935.

6. Breathnach AS. The skeleton of the foot. In: Frazer's Anatomy of the human skeleton. 2nd Ed: 141–5, Churchill Livingstone, 1965.

7. Canale ST, et al. Campbell's Operative Orthopaedics, ed. 9th, Vol I-IV. C.V. Mosby Co., Saint Louis, 1998.

8. Canale ST, Kelly FB Jr. Fractures of the neck of the talus. J Bone Joint Surg 62A: 97–102, 1980.

9. Clark JMP. Modern Trends in Orthopedics Fracture Treatment, Butterworths, London, 1962.

10. Clark JMP. Modern Trends in Orthopedics Fracture Treatment. Butterworths, London, 1962.

11. Hawkins LG. Fractures of the neck of the talus. J Bone Joint Surg. 52A: 991–1002, 1970.

12. Jones FW. The foot. In: Structure and function as seen in the foot. 2nd Ed. 68–74, Covent Garden W Co., London, 1946.

13. Kapoor PS. Accident and Emergency: Fractures Management. 2nd Ed. CBS, New Delhi, 2016.

14. Kapoor PS. Pott's fracture: Accident and Emergency, ed. 2nd, CBS, New Delhi, 2016

15. Kleiger B. Fractures of the talus. J Bone Joint Surg. 30A: 735–43, 1948.

16. McMinn RMH. Bones of the foot. In: Lasst's Anatomy—Regional and Applied. 9th Ed. 231–3, Churchill Livingstone, London 1993.

17. McRae R. Practical Fracture Treatment. p. 289–93, Churchill Livingstone, Edinburgh, 1984.

18. Stewart MJ. Twenty five years of progress in the treatment of fractures. Am. Surgeon 22: 485, 1956.

19. Watson-Jones R. Fractures and Joint Injuries. 4th Ed. Williams and Wilkins Co. Baltimore, Vol. 1, 1952 and vol. 2, 1955.

# 5

# Spinal Trauma

## ANATOMY OF VERTEBRAL COLUMN

Preface   The vertebral column usually formed by 33 vertebral (vertebrae) bones: (cervical-7; dorsal/thoracic-12; lumbar-5; sacral-5; coccyx-4); sacrum forme by fusion of 5 sacral vertebrae, while coccyx formed by fusion of 4 coccygeal vertebrae.

Curves of colum: Primary and secondary:
- Primary: Present at birth (dorsal/thoracic, and sacral)
- Secondary: Develop post birth (cervical, and lumbar):
  - Cervical: Appears post holding up of head by the child (3rd month)
  - Lumbar: Develops post sitting up of the child (5th month).

## Anatomy of Typical Vertebra

Composition:   The elements comprise the:
- Vertebral body: Kidney shaped, consisting of cancellous bone, enveloped by cortical bone.
- Neural arch: Horseshoe shaped, attached to posterior surface of vertebral body, thus forming a ring called neural canal for the passage of spinal cord.

These arches may be incomplete, resulting in the condition called spina bifida, where the cord is unprotected by bone.

- Pair of articular processes, on each side, dividing the neural arch into pedicle anteriorly and lamina posteriorly. Mostly these are arranged vertically, except in the cervical region. Hence dislocation can occur without fracture only in the cervical region. Elsewhere, dislocation alone cannot occur.
- Pair of transverse processes, one on each side, attached to neural arch. These are longest in the lumbar region and shortest in the cervical region.
- Spinous process, attached to posterior end of neural arch.
- Ligaments supraspinatous and interspinous ligaments forming posterior ligament complex. If this complex is torn, then the other ligaments offer little resistance, resulting in subluxation or dislocation of spine. Other ligaments and supporting soft tissues are: Intertranseverse, annular, ligamentum flavum, facet joint, and capsule.
- Intervertebral disk, consisting of fibrocartilage, lies between two vertebral bodies, these disks act as buffer zone, absorbing the impact during walking and other movements. These disks share (1/3rd or 1/4th) in the length of vertebral column, and also responsible for the shape of the column. In elderly (post 60 years), these disks start becoming atrophic, resulting in spinal deformities (bowed, or bamboo back).
- Anterior and posterior longitudinal ligaments.
- Movements: Flexion, extension, rotation, and side bending.

## Spinal Injuries

Principles

- Reduction: Perfect anatomical result is indispensable to good function; there is no justification for failure to secure perfect reposition of simple wedge fractures.
- Immobilization: Rigid immobilization is indispensable to perfect union; that till-date inadequate is main cause of nonunion, e.g. immobilization for 4/12 in extreme hyperextension is considered as the proper management for simple wedge fractures—while concession granted to elderly lady patients having fractures thoracic spine with osteoporosis (Watson-Jones). There is no compelling need to strive for anatomical perfection in the thoracolumbar spine.
- Surgical equations: Fracture = Plaster; Deformity = Disability.

Examples:
- All fractures spine to be perfectly reduced and adequately immobilized in a hyperextension plaster.
- All fractures of calcaneum mandatory to have Bohler's angle and other contours perfectly reduced.
- ORIF for fractures spine indicated in case of failure of conservative measures (plaster, splints, jackets, belts, etc.), and for all unstable fractures/fracture dislocations spine.

- Pain: Mandatory to relieve pain (patient's satisfaction) irrespective of restoration of function and to relieve disability (correction of deformity), at the earliest possible.
- Disability and deformity: Causes of residual pain.

Types of injury      A. Stable injuries: Posterior ligament complex and neural arch intact

B. Unstable injuries: Posterior ligament complex torn with/or without fracture of neural arch or facet joints.

MOI      Fall from a height

Diving in shallow water

Fall of heavy weight on the back

RSA

Sports injuries

## Mechanism of injury:

Forces      Flexion, flexion rotation, and extension forces result in sprains, fractures, fracture dislocations, and paraplegia, depending upon the violence

Management      **A. Stable wedge fractures:**

*Conservative treatment:*

Indication:

- Minor disability or derformity
- Fractures of cancellous bone: vertebral bodies

Measures:

- Bedrest
- Analgesics/NSAIDs
- Exercises

**B. Unstable fracture due to flexion/rotation injuries:**

Conservative treatment:

- Apply skull traction, maintaining traction, neck is slowly extended.

After care: Continue with traction.

**Refer:** The patient to the next fracture clinic.

Surgical treatment:

*Surgery:*

- Arthrodesis: If no neurological deficit;

  If paraplegia—then arthrodesis is not required.

  After care: Apply cervical collar after 4/52.

**Sprains of Spine (Whiplash):** These are common injuries of spine.

Described in Chapter of Traumatic affections of Ligaments, tendons, and muscles.

## Fractures of Spine

Types      Complete, incomplete, and compression fractures

## Complete Fractures (Fracture-dislocations) of the Spine

Definition      It is defined as those that interfere with the continuity of the spinal column.

These include:

- Fracture dislocation of the spine.

MOI             Direct trauma: At any level

                Indirect trauma: Flexion and rotation forces: commonly at C5 to C7, and L3 to L5 levels, or at the junction of fixed and mobile portions of the spine.

                Pathogenesis: Separation occurs through an intervertebral disk, that carries with it a portion of the anterosuperior lip of the inferior vertebral body.

Diagnosis       Pain

                Local tenderness

                Crepitus

                Movements: Painful and restricted

                Paraplegia: May be present due to cord involvement.

Investigation   X-ray spine—AP and LAT views.

Management      Conservative treatment:

                Bedrest

                Analgesics/NSAIDs

                SWD/IR

                Epidural block

                Traction: Pelvic

                Surgical treatment:

                Indication:

                Residual pain

                Deformity

                Surgery:

                • ORIF

                • Arthrodesis: If no associated paraplegia.

Prognosis       It is depends upon presence or absence of injury to the spinal cord and nerve root.

## Incomplete Fractures

Definition      It is defined as those that do not interfere with the continuity of the spinal column. These include:
                • Fracture of the spinous and transverse processes
                • Fractures of the laminae
                • Fractures of the vertebral bodies (compression/fissured fractures)

MOI             Direct trauma: Fractures of laminae, and processes
                Indirect trauma: Stress fractures of the spinous processes

Pathogenesis    Fracture of spinous processes of dorsal spine occurs because of relatively long and exposure to trauma; Shoveler's fracture of spinous process occurs in minors due to continuous stress; fracture of the transverse processes of lumbar spine with associated renal injury, occurs because of relatively long and exposure to trauma; fracture of lamina may be associated with bone depression and involvement of the underlying spinal cord.

| | |
|---|---|
| Diagnosis | Pain |
| | Local tenderness |
| | Crepitus |
| | Movements: Painful and restricted |
| Investigation | X-ray spine—AP and LAT views. |
| Management | Conservative treatment: |
| | Bedrest |
| | Analgesics/NSAIDs |
| | SWD/IR |
| | Epidural block |
| | Traction: Pelvic |
| | Closed reduction followed by hyperextensive plaster |

## Compression Fractures of Vertebral Bodies

| | |
|---|---|
| MOI | Direct violence |
| | Fall from a height |
| | RSA |
| | Sports injuries |
| Diagnosis | Pain |
| | Deformity |
| Investigation | X-ray spine—AP and LAT views: wedging of the vertebra; rarefaction |
| Management | Conservative treatment: |
| | Bedrest |
| | Analgesics/NSAIDs |
| | SWD/IR |
| | Traction: Pelvic |
| | Brace |
| | Epidural block |

Surgical treatment:
Indication: Residual pain
Refer the patient to the next orthopedic clinic.
Surgery: Albee's bone grafting
After care: The patient is placed in a hyperextensive plaster bed or on a Stryker frame.

## REGIONAL SPINE INJURIES

## Cervical Spine Injuries

| | |
|---|---|
| Anatomy | Cervical vertebral column formed by seven vertebrae C-1 to C-7); |
| | Cervical joints: |

- Lower five cervical vertebrae unite on the same pattern as the vertebrae in other regions; bodies of the two adjoining vertebrae unite by an intervertebral disk and longitudinal ligaments (anterior and posterior)
- Articular processes unite by capsules
- The laminae unite by a pair of ligamenta flava

- Spines unite by interspinous and supraspinous ligaments
- Transverse processes unite by intertransverse ligaments

Joints of cervical vertebral bodies:
- Median joint: Cartilaginous, between vertebral bodies, connected by disk
- Lateral joints: Synovial, on each side of disk.

Ligaments:
- Anterior longitudinal: Strong, long and wide, on the anterior surfaces of vertebral bodies
- Posterior longitudinal: Long and wide, on the posterior surfaces of vertebral bodies; fixed to the disks and margins of vertebral bodies

Joints of cervical vertebral arches:
- Articular processes: United by fibrous capsule of synovial joints
- Ligamenta flava: Flat bands of yellow elastic tissue, that unite the laminae, widest in the cervical and lumbar regions; too strong to maintain vertebral column.

Ligaments:
- Interspinous: Unite the adjoining spines, very waek in the neck
- Supraspinous: Thick bands, that unite tips of spines; in the neck replaced by ligamentun nuchae
- Intertransverse: Sparsly marked

Joints of atlas, axis, and occipital bone:
- All are synovial joints
- Atlantoaxial joints: Three (pair: between articular processes; dens of axis articulates with back of anterior arch of atlas)
- Atlantooccipital joint: A pair of joints (between occipital condyles and atlas lateral masses.

Ligaments:
- Anterior longitudinal: Unites axis body to the tubercle on the anterior arch of atlas.

**Preface**

Trauma to the cervical spine may result in a variety of lesions (dislocations without fractures or fractures without dislocations); mostly, both fracture and dislocation are sustained; the spinal cord lesion may be present, with negative X-rays, or may be absent, with X-rays showing substantial vertebral displacement; dislocations variable from subluxations to complete dislocation of articular facets; fracture-dislocations variable from small chip fractures of vertebral border to complete separation of the pedicles, fractures of articular processes, or compression fractures of vertebral body.

**Types**

Stable and unstable injuries.
- Stable injuries: Anterior wedge fractures of vertebral bodies, due to flexion injuries
- Unstable injuries: Dislocation and fracture dislocations

## Classification of Cervical Spine Injuries

- Flexion injuries
- Flexion/rotation injuries
- Extension injuries
- Compression injuries.

## Flexion and Flexion/Rotation Injuries

| | |
|---|---|
| MOI | Direct trauma |
| | RSA |
| | Sports injury—rugby football, pole vaulting, and horse riding |
| | Fall from a height |
| | Diving head on into shallow water |
| | Fall of heavy weight on the back of head |
| | Hanging by neck |
| Pathogenesis | Violence force acting on the back of head, resulting in flexion of neck causing stable anterior wedge fracture of vertebral body, while posterior ligament complex and neural arch remain intact. Usually no neurological deficit occurs; in case of flexion/rotation injuries, the rotational force may cause unilateral dislocation of one facet joint-unstable injury |
| Diagnosis | Stable wedge fracture: Pain, stiffness, movements painfull and restricted |
| | Unstable unilateral dislocation: Pain-radiating type, head slightly rotated and tilted away from locked facet |
| Investigation | X-ray cervical spine—AP, LAT, and oblique views |
| | CT scan of cervical spine |
| Management | Stable wedge fractures: |

Conservative treatment: Cervical collar for 6–8/52, followed by physiotherapy.

Unstable unilateral dislocation:

Conservative treatment:

Closed reduction under anesthesia:

Method: Manipulation: Apply traction; maintaining traction, correct the rotation and then flexion, and finally bring the head into midline position followed by cervical collar or by skull traction followed by continuation of traction for 6–8/52.

Surgical treatment:

Indication: Failure of closed reduction and fixation.

Method:

- ORIF (spinal plates and screws)
- Arthrodesis—if no neurological deficit
- Paraplegia: Arthrodesis not required, if paraplegia is present
- Posterior ligament complex rupture: Posterior arthrodesis is the treatment of choice.

Technique of posterior arthrodesis:

- Patient under general anesthesia: Endotracheal intubation

- Patient turned to prone position
- Incision: Midline to expose the cervical spines
- Torn posterior ligament is exposed
- Adjacent spinous processes, laminae, and facet joints rawed
- Spines wired together
- Bone grafts placed on either side of spines.

After care: Continue with skull traction for 6/52, followed by a cervical collar

## Extension Injuries

| | |
|---|---|
| MOI | Direct trauma |
| | RSA: In car accidents, e.g. forehead striking against the front—glass screen, dashboard, etc. |
| | Sports injury: Boxing |
| | Fall downstairs: Forehead striking against ground |
| | Pathogenesis: Hyperextension of neck leads to tearing of the anterior longitudinal ligament, the cord may be stretched or kinked, causing neurological deficit. |
| Diagnosis | History of injury, pain in the neck, weakness |
| Investigation | X-ray cervical spine—AP and LAT views, show wedging of vertebra without narrowing of space |
| Management | Extension injuries are stable. |
| | Conservative treatment: |
| | Heat |
| | Analgesics |
| | Cervical collar. |

## Compression Injuries

| | |
|---|---|
| MOI | Direct violence |
| | Fall from a height (vertex striking ground) |
| | Fall of heavy weights on the head |
| | RSA |
| | Sports injuries (diving into shallow water). |

### Mechanism of neurological involvement:

First of all the motor supply of upper limbs is affected, followed by that of lower limbs, next pain and temperature, and lastly touch sensation.

| | |
|---|---|
| Diagnosis | History of injury |
| | Deformity |
| | Pain in the neck |
| | Local tenderness |
| | Neurological assessment: A complete neurological examination, e.g. |

- Muscle power: Testing of muscle power of upper and lower limbs
- Sensations: Testing of pin prick, touch, and temperature sensations
- Reflexes: Usually return within 4/52.

**Investigation X-ray cervical spine:**

|  |  |
|---|---|
|  | AP and LAT views: Wedging of the vertebra; rarefaction |
| Management | Conservative treatment: Indicated in intact posterior ligament complex: |
|  | Bedrest |
|  | Analgesics/NSAIDs |
|  | SWD/IR |
|  | Traction: Cervical traction for 6–8/52 |
|  | Brace |
|  | Surgical treatment: |
|  | Indications: |

- Impaired posterior ligament complex
- An incomplete cord lesion
- Deteriorating neurological signs
- Myelography: Showing local block

Surgery: Laminectomy: for removal of backward projecting bone fragments compressing cord.

After care: Refer the patient to the orthopedic clinic for follow up.

## Fractures of Atlas (C-1)

|  |  |
|---|---|
| MOI | Direct trauma |
|  | RSA (head striking the roof or dashboard of a car) |
|  | Fall of a weight on the head (mine, construction workers) |
|  | Fall from a height |
|  | Hanging by neck (suicide, or legal punishment/conviction) |
| Pattern | Quadripartite |
| Mechanism of injury | Acute downward forcing of occipital condyles on the atlas |
| Diagnosis | Patient conscious or unconscious |
|  | Supports the head with hands |
|  | Pain: Occipital region |
| Investigation | X-ray cervical spine—AP view through the mouth and LAT view |
|  | CT scanning |
| Management | Conservative treatment: |
|  | Skull traction for 6/52 |
|  | Analgesics/NSAIDs |

**Afer care:**
**Refer:** The patient to the orthopedic clinic.

Surgical treatment:
Indications: Failure of conservative treatment
Surgery: Arthrodesis
After care: Cervical traction for 6/52, followed by collar for 2–3/12.

## Fractures of Axis (C-2)

|  |  |
|---|---|
| MOI | Direct trauma |
|  | RSA |

| | Extension injuries |
|---|---|
| Diagnosis | An elderly patient |
| | Pain in the neck |
| | Local tenderness |
| | Movements: Painful and restricted. |
| Investigation | X-ray cervical spine: AP and LAT views |
| | CT scanning |
| Management | Conservative treatment: |
| | Skull traction for 4–6/52 |
| | Analgesics/NSAIDs |
| | Cervical collar |
| | Minerva plaster jacket |

**Refer:** The patient to the orthopedic clinic for follow up.

Surgical treatment:

Indication: Failure of conservative treatment.

Surgery: Arthrodesis of spine

After care: Refer the patient to the orthopedic clinic for follow up.

## Fractures of Thoracic and Lumbar Spine

| | |
|---|---|
| MOI | Direct trauma |
| | Fall from a height onto the toes |
| | Fall of heavy weight over back of a stooping worker (mines, construction) |
| | Heavy weight lifting |
| | RSA |
| Mechanism of injury | Flexion and rotational forces |
| Diagnosis | History of injury |
| | Backache |
| | Local tenderness |
| | Movements: Painful and restricted |
| Investigation | X-ray—AP and LAT views |
| Management | Conservative treatment: |
| | Bedrest |
| | Analgesics/NSAIDs |
| | Plaster jacket with spine in extension |
| | Physiotherapy |

**Refer:** The patient to the next orthopedic clinic for follow up care.

Surgical treatment:

Indication: Failure of conservative treatment

Surgery:

- ORIF (spinal plates and screws)
- Arthrodesis.

## Neurological Involvement

Preface            Complete neurological examination is conducted to find out any deficit, e.g.
- Muscle power: Testing of muscles below level of injury
- Sensations: Testing of pin prick and touch sensations
- Reflexes.

Lesions
- Neurapraxia (syn. concussion): It is a temporary lesion, fully recoverable
- Axonotmesis: Rupture of axons within an intact sheath
- Neurotmesis: Partial or complete division of nerve
- Cord injury: Recovery possible—if there is any muscle power, and the sensations below level of lesion
- Transaction of cord: Irrecoverable; recovery of reflexes without muscle power, and sensations
- Injury to nerve roots or cauda equina: absence of reflexes.

Prognosis: Potential recovery is there.

## Spinal Cord Injury

Anatomy            Spinal cord ends at the level of lower border of the first lumbar vertebra; fracture-dislocations below this level are associated with injury to the cauda equina. Anatomical factors govern the extent of the cord and nerve lesion at different levels:
- **Cervical spine:** Horizontal articular processes and the large disks, yield high mobility with little resistance to even trivial forces, resulting in the dislocation or fracture-dislocation.
- **Dorsal spine:** Vertical articular processes, yield low mobility with great resistance to major forces resulting in fractures and cord injury as the spinal canal is narrow.
- **Lumbar spine:** Verticular, articular processes with great mobility, causing fracture-dislocations, due to flexion and rotation forces. Nerve lesions are rare, as the spinal canal is spacious.

MOI                Direct trauma
                   RSA
                   Fall from a height

Mechanism          
of injury
- Acute flexion of spine, causing long-axis stretching of cord, resulting in concussion injury of cord
- Nipping of the cord by fractured fragment, resulting in crush injury of cord
- Compression of cord by the protruded disk, due to acute flexion.

Pathogenesis
Lesions
- Partial cord lesions: Show spastic paralysis in extension with exaggerated reflexes and extensor, plantar responses, and return of sensation. Urinary retention may persist for a longer period
- Complete cord lesions: Show spastic paralysis in flexion with flexor spasms, due to absence of inhibition of the spinal flexor reflex arcs. The cord is irreparably damaged in cord transaction.

| | |
|---|---|
| Levels | **Cervical:** |

**Cervical:**
- Above C5 level: Paralysis of respiratory muscles, including diaphragm being supplied by the phrenic nerve ( C4 ); There occurs sudden death
- C5 level: Paralysis of arms, trunk, and legs. Patient breathes only with the aid of diaphragm, arms lie immobile against the trunk
- C6 level: Arms abducted and externally rotated with the forearm flexed and supinated, due to irritation of C5 segment
- C7 level: Arms abducted and internally rotated with the forearm flexed and pronated, due to irritation of C6 segment
- C8 and T1 level: Paralysis of intrinsic muscles of the hand
- Below T1 level: Movements of arm—free down to finger tips.

**Dorsal:**
- D2 level: Contraction of pupils, hyperesthesia along the inner side of arms
- Above D6 level: Paralysis of abdominal muscles.

**Lumbar:**
- Above D12-L1 level: Lumbar enlargement at this level contains center for nervous control of urinary bladder; injury above this level prevents inhibitory impulses from the cortex reaching the center, and there by retention due to spinal shock, reflex micturition starts; injury to this center or to nerves from it supplying the bladder (S2-3) leads to the persistent retention due to paralysis of detrusor muscle.

**Cauda equina:**
- Just below level of cauda equina formation:
  - Paralysis of legs and perineal muscles
  - Anesthesia of perineum (saddle shaped area) and legs
  - Incontinence of urine and feces.

**Diagnosis** **Spinal concussion (spinal shock):**
- Loss of all functions below the level of lesion, e.g.
  - Loss of voluntary movement
  - Loss of muscle tone
  - Loss of pain and temperature sensations
  - Loss of reflexes.

**Spinal contusion:**
- Stage of spinal shock: Complete flaccid paralysis below the level of lesion with urinary retention
- Return of reflex activity.

Stage of septic complications: Urinary infection, bedsores, pneumonia.

**Investigation** **X-ray spine—AP and LAT views show:**
- Wedging of vertebral body
- No narrowing of disk space

MRI/CT scanning

**Management:** First aid treatment:

Position/posture:

- Cervical injuries: Head supported by sand bags
- Dorsal and lumbar injuries: Patient in prone position

Analgesics/NSAIDs

- Inj. Morphine—for relief of pain and anxiety

Prognosis: If no recovery from spinal shock occurs within 48 hours, then the prognosis is grave.

Local treatment:

A. Cervical injuries:
- Reduction: By traction and manipulations, followed by immobilization:
  - Skull traction for 1/52
  - Minerva jacket: apply plaster cast covering head, neck, and upper chest for 4/12.

Surgical treatment:

Surgery: Laminectomy: removal of protruding traumatic disk, pressing upon cord without a fracture

Indication: Relief of pain due to nerve roots compression.

B. Dorsal and lumbar injuries:
- Reduction by hyperextension in prone position.
- Immobilization: Apply plaster from pelvis to axillae for 4–6/12.

Return of reflex activity: The period of spinal shock and flaccid paralysis persists for many days, following which lower motor neuron (LMN) lesion persists, due to injury of anterior horn cells, at level of lesion.

After care:

- Partial or recoverable cord lesion: Adequate immobilization period (2–4/52)
- Complete cord lesion: Removal of plaster cast to avoid formation of bedsores.

**Complications** Death may occur due to following complications:

- Spinal shock
- Respiratory failure: Due to ascending edema
- Hypostatic pneumonia: Due to paralysis of abdominal and intercostals muscles
- Urinary infection: Pyelonephritis
- Bedsores: High protein diet—to combat protein loss from discharging sores

Good nursing care, e.g. regular change of bed sheets, turning to relieve pressure and toilet of skin with spirit and powdering antibiotics

Plenty of fluids

Excision of sloughs, removal of sequestra

- Urinary bladder: Lesions of bladder center cause permanent retention with overflow (incontinence)

Management First aid treatment:

- Patient taught to evacuate the bladder by straining and by pressing the hand above the pelvis (over the bladder)
- Indwelling catheterization: For 3–4/52, followed by automatic evacuation
- Suprapubic cystostomy: Carries the risk of infection and the method is demanding on staff
- Physiotherapy: To commence ASAP:
  - Chest: Deep breathing exercises and postural drainage: To minimize the risks and effects of respiratory distress by infection
  - Joints: Passive exercises with care to avoid risks of myositis ossificance
  - Assistance in sitting, standing, walking, use of wheelchair: To develop unparalysed muscles for support
- Rehabilitation: Helping in return to work at earliest possible:
  - To restore balance for sitting or standing
  - To improve gait in partial lesions with caliper support
  - To overcome dressing problems
  - To permit wheelchair use
  - To restore occupation by business/industrial retraining.

## Bibliography

1. Blount WP. Unequal leg length, American Academy of Orthopedic Surgeons Instructional Course Lectures, vol. XVII, St. Louis, 1960, The C.V. Mosby Co., pp. 218–45.
2. Brooks DM, Seddon HJ. Pectoral transplantation for paralysis of the flexors of the elbow. A new technique, J. Bone and Joint Surg. 41-B:36, 1959.
3. Bunnell S. Tendon transfers in the hand and forearm, American Academy of Orthopedic Surgeons Instructional Course Lectures, vol. VI, Ann Arbor, 1949, J.W. Edwards, p.106.
4. Canale ST, Kay Daugherty K, Jones L. Campbell Operative Orthopaedics 9th Ed. Vol I-IV., Mosby, 1998.
5. Crooks F, Birkett AN. Fractures and Fracture-dislocations of the Cervical Spine. Brit. J. Surg 1944: 31: 252.
6. Kapoor PS. Accident and Emergency: Etiology, Diagnosis and Management. 2nd Ed., CBS, New Delhi, 2016.
7. Love M, Rains AJH, Capper WM. Bailey and Love's Short Practice of Surgery (1965). H.K. Lewis and Co., London.
8. McRae R. Practical Fracture Treatment. 1st Ed. Churchill, Livingstone, 1981.
9. Modern Trends in Orthopedics Fracture Treatment (1962).

# 6

# Delayed Union and Nonunion of Fractures

**Managemernt**
- Preoperative considerations
- Bone graft
  - Autogenous
  - Homogenous
  - Heterogenous
  - Onlay cortical graft
    - Single
    - Dual
  - Inlay
    - Sliding inlay
  - Peg
  - Cancellous
  - Whole bone (transplant)
  - Removal of graft:
    - Tibial
    - Fibular
    - Iliac
    - Phemister

**Regional Nonunions (Specific bones)**
- Femoral neck
- Trochanteric and subtrochanteric
- Femoral shaft
- Patella
- Tibial shaft
- Medial malleolus
- Metatarsals
- Scaphoid
- Clavicle
- Humerus
- Monteggia

| | |
|---|---|
| Preface | The delayed union and nonunion are differentiated mostly of degree. |

## DELAYED UNION

| | |
|---|---|
| Definition | Delayed union is defined as fracture's failure to unite within the expected time (healing fails to advance at the average rate for site and type of a fracture); radiologically may show unexpected bone changes (bone absorption at the fracture site, with gapping bone ends); delayed union implies that spontaneous union, still possible, by continuing the fixation (immobilization). |
| Etiology | Unknown<br>Reduction: Inadequate<br>Immobilization: Inadequate fixation, and for an insufficient time<br>Infective: Compound fractures<br>Overdistraction. |
| Risk factors | Old age; debility; malnutrition; systemic (tuberculosis, syphilis, diabetes). |
| Diagnosis | Pain<br>Swelling<br>Local tenderness<br>Movement: Painful |
| Investigation | X-ray—AP and LAT views shows: unexpected bone changes:<br>Repair: No sign of repair<br>Outline of bone fragments clearly defined<br>Bony absorption at fracture site<br>Gapping: Between bone ends<br>Callus: External bridging callus of poor quality (may be missing) |
| Management | It is difficult as to differentiate between delayed union that may proceed to unite with continued fixation, and delayed union that may lead to nonunion with continued fixation; the only sure arbiter is time factor.<br>Conservative treatment: To be continued for at least 4–10/52.<br>Indication: Spontaneous union<br>Immobilization: Continuing the fixation (proper plaster cast)<br>Exercises of the limb<br>Surgical treatment: A difficult and risky decision:<br><br>Indication:<br>• Failure of conservative treatment as per normal required time for advancing union of fracture<br>• To justify surgery in preference to risk of prolonging convalescence<br><br>Surgery: Phemister graft (onlay bone graft without internal fixation).<br><br>After care: Exercises of the limb. |

## Nonunion

| | |
|---|---|
| Definition | Nonunion is defined as fracturte's failure to unite (permanent end result of the delayed union) spontaneously by the continued fixation; radiologically may show evidence of sclerosis: rounding off of bone |

ends, and closed medullary canal by dense hypertrophic bone (elephant's foot appearance), and clear fracture line.

| | |
|---|---|
| Etiology | Traumatic: Comminuted by major trauma |
| | Reduction: Improper (faulty) |
| | Immobilization: Inadequate fixation, and for an insufficient time |
| | Infective: Compound fractures |
| | Vascular: Impaired blood supply |
| | Overdistraction: By faulty traction, or by internal fixation |
| Interposition | Of soft tissues |
| Pathogenesis | • Traumatic: Comminuted fractures may often lead to nonunion of the fragments (mostly middle or distal ones) |

• Reduction: Improper (faulty) reduction may lead to contact failure of bone fragments (fracture shaft femur/humerus/tibia); interposition of soft tissues between fragments; unnatural mobility; overdistraction.

Repeated manipulations (follow-up) to attain the perfect anatomical reduction may lead to breakage of formed soft callus (cause nonunion).

• Immobilization: Inadequate fixation may lead to continuous unnatural mobility; impaired callus formation foiled by the bony ends becoming insulated from each other by the mature fibrous tissue—resulting in bone ends becoming rounded off and sclerosed (fracture distal third of tibia; fracture shaft femur and humerus).

• Infective: Minor infection may not impair fracture's union; while major infection (osteomyelitis, compound fractures) cause resorption of bone ends (nonunion).

• Vascular: The fracture may cause impaired blood supply to one of the fragments, resulting in nonunion (displaced subcapital fracture of femoral neck; fracture neck of os scaphoid.

• Overdistraction: Excessive skeletal traction may pull apart the bony ends, encouraging the fibrous tissue growth—that insulates the bony ends from each other.

• Interposition of soft tissues may impair callus formation bridging the facture site (fractures of patella, medial malleolus, and olecranon).

| | |
|---|---|
| Diagnosis | Incidence: Variable in long bones: highest to lowest: the tibia, the radius, the femur, the humerus, the ulna, and the clavicle |
| | Unnatural mobility (fracture nonsticky) |
| | Disability: Inability/difficulty in using the limb |
| Investigation | X-ray—AP and LAT views: Hypertrophic and atrophic types: |

• Hypertrophic: Sclerosed bony ends; flated out (elephant's foot) bony ends; clearly visible fracture line; increased bone density (misleading).

• Atrophic: Bony ends narrow, rounded, and osteoporotic.

| | |
|---|---|
| Management | Surgical treatment of choice in established (clinically and radiologically) nonunion |

Hypertrophic nonunion:

Aim: Firm fixation (immobilization)

Surgery:

- ORIF: Plating (compression)

Atrophic nonunion:

Aims and treatment (method):

A. Immobilization: Firm fixation of fractured fragments by:
- ORIF (rigid compression plate)
- Interlocking nailing

B. Interposed soft tissues:
- Open reduction to remove interposed tissue and to oppose widely separated bony fragments
- Bony ends to be freshened by limited excision

C. Decortication of bony ends by:
- Fine interrupted cuts made in the outer surface of bony cortex

D. Bone grafting: To stimulate bony growth (union) by:
- Onlay graft: An autonomous bone graft taken from the normal tibia, thereby screwed across the fracture site; or a sliding graft taken from longer fragment, slide across fracture site, and recessed into the shorter fragment.
- Cancellous iliac bone (of choice because of its greater power of union and its resistance to minor infection) to supplement the cortical graft, is packed circumferentially around the fracture site.

Phemister graft: Indicated in case of little movement in the nonunion.

External fixation: Indicated in infective (compound fractures) nonunion.

### Preoperative considerations:

A. Restoring function of muscles and joints for couple of months, prior to reconstructive surgery:

Method: By fitting a brace that supports the limb as well as allows it to be used, and to allow weight bearing in case of lower limb; improves the patient's health; also indicated extensive physiotherapy for the purpose.
- Evaluation of any nerve injury: Nerve exploration and repair mandatory prior to treating the nonunion. In extreme nerve damage esp. in case of lower limb, amputation to be the treatment of choice.

B. Bony status:
- Osteoporosis of shaft of long bones usually increases chances of union (in old persons, nonunion unites rapidly due to the soft and viable cortex with surplus blood supply).
- Sclerosis: Sclerosed bony ends often associated with formation of poor quality callus, resulting in delayed union post bone grafting; graft may even gets fractured at a later stage. Post cast removal, the limb to be protected with a brace until union confirmed radiologically.

C. Soft tissues status: Correction of complications, e.g. extensive scarring of skin and soft tissues due to infection (compound fractures), sinuses, cavities, foreign bodies, prior to bone grafting for nonunion.

D. Managing cavities, sequestra, sinuses, and skin defects, e.g.

   i. Bone cavities filled with flaps of fat or muscle + coverage with a full thickness skin graft; and then bone grafting post wounds healing.

   ii. Bone defect with wound (compound):

   - Toilet of wound
   - Debridement of wound (saucerization); foreign and infected or devitalized materials removed, under antibiotics coverage
   - Split-thickness skin grafting: Post formation of granulation tissue
   - Full-thickness skin grafting: Post 4–6/52 of wound healing
   - Bone grafting: Deferred until skin graft has fully healed
   - Amputation: Indicated in prolonged/failed treatment.

Shortening and malalignment prevention in compound/infected #s:
- External fixation: Maintains fixation + allows AS dressings of wound.

## Bone grafting
Principles:
- Fixation (cortical graft)
- Osteogenesis (cancellous graft).

Indications:
- To fill up cavities/or defects (due to cysts, tumors, etc.)
- To provide arthrodesis (bridge joints)
- To establish the continuity of a long bone
- To restrict joint movement by providing bone blocks (arthrodesis)
- To establish union in pseudoarthrosis
- To provide fixation; promote union; fill up defects in slow union, delayed union, nonunion, malunion, fresh fractures, and osteotomies.

Structure of grafts expressed in an equation (principles) as:
- Cortical bone to fixation
- Cancellous bone to osteogenesis

Advantages: Bone graft possess both these fundamental principles, however variable with the bone structure: cellular elements in the cortical graft slowly replaced by infiltrating substitution (graft merely acts as a scaffold for new bone formation); while cancellous graft is more osteogenic (unable to provide firm fixation).

Source of grafts:

**Autogenous:** Patient is his/her own bone donor; usually sources are: Tibia: It is a cortical graft, strong, used mainly for bridging a defect in a long bone or for managing pseudarthrosis; subcutaneous anteromedial part of tibia is the usual site; then suturing periosteum over the defect to fill up with callus.

Disadvantages of using tibia as a donor site:
- Normal limb jeopardized
- Prolonged surgical time, being consumed by graft taken
- Prolonged convalescence, and delayed ambulance
- Risk of tibial fracture, at the site, weakened by graft removal.

Fibula: It is a whole bone graft; proximal 2/3rd may be used as a graft, without jeopardizing leg; the proximal rounded end, used as a graft (peg) in fracture neck of femur; as a bony transplant to replace distal 1/3rd of radius or fibula.

Ileum: It is a cancellous bone graft, used mainly for osteogenesis purpose, i.e. to fill up cavities, to promote union of fracture.

**Homogenous**     Donor: The graft is taken from a person other than the patient (a relative; mother/or father preferred for child; other donors including cadavers).

**Heterogenous**     Donor: The graft is taken from another species; often incited an undesirable foreign body reaction.

**Techniques:** Indications for various techniques:

**A. Onlay cortical graft:** Single and dual grafts:
- *Single onlay graft*: It is the simplest and most effective cortical graft used for the management of the ununited shaft fractures; it is usually supplemented by cancellous bone graft for osteogenesis. Indications: New fractures; malunited fractures; and post osteotomies; in bridging joints (arthrodesis).
- *Dual onlay graft*: It is the cortical graft used for the management of the congenital pseudarthrosis, difficult and unusual nonunions (nonunion of shaft near a joint, or of osteoporotic bone in elderly), or for bridging massive shaft defects; two cortical onlay grafts placed opposite each other across nonunion, and are fixed with screws (gripping fragments like a vise); cancellous chips placed around nonunion.

    Advantages:
    - Dual grafts provide more strength and stability
    - Fixation better than by a single onlay bone graft.

    Indications:
    - Congenital pseudarthrosis
    - Difficult and unusual nonunions
    - Nonunion near a joint.

**B. Inlay graft:** The inlay and sliding inlay are cortical grafts used for the management of the shaft nonunions (onlay graft has replaced the inlay graft because of simplicity and efficiency).

*Indications*: Arthrodesis of ankle.

*Inlay graft*: A trough made across the nonunion; a graft of same size removed from the tibia, and placed into the trough made.

*Sliding inlay graft*: Parallel cuts made through the cortex of both the fragments; the shorter graft removed; the longer graft slide across nonunion, into the trough made in the shorter fragment; the shorter graft then deposited in the empty trough of the longer fragment; fix both the grafts with screws.

Disadvantage: Plenty of cortex of both segments removed may hamper union of graft.

C. **Peg graft:** It is a whole bone graft used as an innocuous method of internal fixation, rather than of osteogenesis

Indications: Fractures neck of femur, and nonunion fractures of medial

Malleolus.

Disadvantage: It is a weak graft.

D. **Cancellous graft:** It is a cancellous graft used mainly for osteogenesis purpose

Indications:
   • To fill up cavities or defects (in: cysts, tumors, etc.)
   • To establish bone blocks
   • To promote union in osteotomies.
   • To supplement cortical bone grafting, by promoting healing.

E. **Whole bone graft (transplant):** The fibular graft is commonly used for bridging defects (due to infection or bone tumors) of the shafts of bones of upper limb, except near a joint; also used as a transplant for the distal radius or fibula.

Advantages:
   • Stronger than a full thickness tibial graft
   • Wound over the graft, can be easily closed
   • Disability post removal of graft is less than post removal of a large tibial graft.

**Removal of bone grafts:** To shorten the surgical and tourniquet time; better two teams work simultaneously, i.e. one team manages the nonunion, while the other team removes and prepares the graft; the second team may help the first team in applying and fixing the graft and closing wounds.

Method:
   • Incision: A longitudinal incision over the nonunion, expose it
   • Excise the scar tissue from between the fragments
   • Incise the periosteum of both fragments, for required length of graft to be used
   • Reduction: Appose the fragments in normal alignment
   • Place the graft on the fragments and across the nonunion, hold it with a clamp
   • Drill a hole through the graft and through both cortices of one fragment
   • Insert a screw (allows an impaction of fragments and graft adjustment)
   • Fix the graft by inserting 3–4 screws (engage graft and both cortices) (none should cross junction of fragments); the two central screws to be 2.5 cm from nonunion

- Remove cancellous bone from tibial condyles by a curet, and place it around nonunion.

Postoperative: Apply a cast/or splint for 3/52, followed by:
- In upper limb: A snug cast until complete union
- In lower limb: A walking cast for 2–3/12, then a brace with locked knee joint until firm union.

After care: Exercises.

### Tibial graft:

The tibia may be exposed in its whole length along its subcutaneous anterior border, or its anteromedial surface

Method:

Preoperative: A tourniquet (pneumatic) applied, to avoid blood loss

Procedure:
- Incision: A curved longitudinal over the anteromedial surface of tibia
- Incise the periosteum, and expose the tibia by reflecting periosteum with a periosteal elevator
- Removal of graft through cortex, by an electric saw
- Suturing the periosteum and fascia as a single layer
- Wound closure by interrupted silk stitches.

### Fibular graft:

Method:

Preoperative: A tourniquet (pneumatic) applied, to avoid blood loss

Precautions during surgery:
- To protect the common peroneal nerve (winds round its neck) from operative trauma
- To protect the superficial peroneal nerve (related to upper 2/3rd of the lateral aspect of the shaft, lying between the peronei from operative trauma
- To protect the peroneal muscles from operative trauma
- To preserve the distal 1/4th of the bone to maintain ankle's stability.

Procedure:

Usually the fibular graft made by resecting the middle 1/3rd or middle ½ of the fibula through a Henry approach:
- Incision: From 15 cm proximal to lateral malleolus extend proximally along posterolateral border of the fibula to posterior margin of femoral head, and thence 10 cm proximally along posterior aspect of the biceps tendon divide the fasciae (superficial and deep)
- Isolate the common peroneal nerve along the posteromedial aspect of biceps tendon
- Detach the peroneus longus muscle from the lateral surface of fibular head
- Exposure of fibula by retracting the peronei
- Removal of fibular graft

- Suturing the periosteum and fascia as a single layer
- Wound closure by interrupted silk stitches.

### Iliac graft: Types:

- Multiple sliver or chip grafts: Form and rigidity are non-criteria:
Source: Outer cortex of ilium along with cancellous bone
- Single piece of bone graft: Form and rigidity are criteria:
  *Source*: Posterior or anterior 1/3rd of iliac crest removed
- Wedge grafts: Cuts made at a right angle to the iliac crest
  *Source*: Anterior portion of ilium

Method:

- Incision: Along the subcutaneous border of iliac crest; deepen the incision (subperiosteally) down to the bone.
- Control hemorrhage by packing with gauze.
- Cancellous graft with one cortex: Elevate only the muscles on the outer surface of the ilium (graft peeled up by prying movements with a broad osteotome); for full thickness graft, also elevate the iliacus muscle from the inner surface of the ilium (graft removed by an electric saw); for sliver or chip grafts, remove these by an osteotome parallel to the iliac crest; post removal of iliac crest; sufficient amount of cancellous bone to be taken by a curet inserted into cancellous space between the two intact cortices.
- Appose and suture the periosteum and muscular origins with the interrupted silk sutures.
- To control perfuse hemorrhage: Use Gelfoam and bone wax.
- Wound drainage: By using a rubber drain.

## Phemister Graft

**Definition**

It is an onlay bone graft without internal fixation; the graft is placed subperiosteally across the nonunion, without mobilizing the fragments. Advantages: Simple to perform; hardly disturbs the blood supply of the fragments; does not disturb the impacting forces at the nonunion.

**Source of graft**

- Tibial nonunion: Same bone or ilium (preferred—without impairing opposite leg), or opposite tibia.

Method:

- Incision: A longitudinal incision centered over the nonunion
- Exposure of nonunion, subperiosteally, from one side of the bone
- Prepare flat surface for graft, with a chisel, without disturbing callus and fibrous tissue
- Place a full-thickness onlay graft across the nonunion, and cancellous chips around nonunion
- Suture the periosteum and soft tissues over the grafts, to hold them in position.

Postoperative: Apply a cast/or splint for 2–3/52, followed by a walking cast for 2–3/12, then a brace with locked knee joint until firm union.

After care: Exercises.

## REGIONAL NONUNIONS (SPECIFIC BONES)
### Femoral Neck

Preface        Nonunion occurs often enough inspite of efficient management.

Etiology
- Impaired blood supply: Vascular insufficiency post fracture neck femur is a major factor resulting in nonunion; usually fractures of femoral neck occur through Ward's triangle (weak area bounded by the trabeculae subjected to pressure and tension—in elderly this triangle replaced by fat), damage the retinacula, interrupts main blood supply to femoral head (insufficient blood supply through ligamentum teres—that too impaired in case of fracture dislocation); finally impaired viability of femoral head.
- Imperfect reduction: May lead to impaired callus formation (weak endosteal in place of firm periosteal—because of periosteum absence from femoral neck).
- Inadequate immobilization: Because of improper nailing (continuous mobility at fracture site) nonunion (persisting pain even after 3–4/12) occurs; prematurely nail removal may result in nonunion (that might have united otherwise).
- Inadequate after care: An early weight bearing (prior to new bone consolidation), may lead to impaired union—nonunion.

Pathogenesis: Fracture neck of femur; impaired blood supply to head; nonunion; impaired viability of femoral head; head may atrophy, sequestrated, and its size decreased (by erosion and absorption; secondary osteoarthritic.

Diagnosis      Difficult to predict nonunion post expected/presumed time of union of a particular type of fracture.

Pain: Persisting

Disability: Limp

Lack of endurance

Investigation    X-ray—AP and LAT views shows: Impending nonunion; progressive changes in the femoral head; osteoarthritis of hip joint

Management    Preoperative considerations:
- Crippling: Nonunion usually results in permanent crippling, until and unless managed surgically for relief of pain, stability, and mobility.

  Surgery: Selecting a particular operation is difficult because of factors.
- Age and physical status: Majority of patients are elderly (> 60 years), and debilitated (suffering from disorders of CVS, respiratory, renal, mentally deteriorated, and physical).
- Femoral head status: Femoral head's viability is the most important criteria (usually confirmed radiologically post 2–3 years); other criteria are status of articular cartilage (atrophy), bone density, and mobility of hip joint (head in the acetabulum; and earlier the confirmed diagnosis, easier to select proper operation for nonunion.

- Femoral neck status: Post nonunion, variable degree of neck absorption occurs, resulting in shortening of neck's length, and contracted hip muscles (causing difficulty in regaining limb's length, and reducing the fracture.
- Nonunion duration: Post diagnosis (clinically and radiologically) of the nonunion, best time for any operation is ASAP.

Techniques: Operations for nonunion:

Classification:

A. Viability/nonviability:

Head viable: Treatment of choice is:
- Displacement osteotomy:
- McMurray—no longer in vogue
- Pauwel's valgization osteotomy
- Nailing and bone grafting (Peg graft) in younger patient.

Head nonviable: Either treatment is:
- Prosthesis
- Total Hip Replacement (THR).

B. Anatomical/mechanical:
- Osteosynthesis: To fix a viable head to the neck or trochanter
- Osteotomy: Femur divided close to lesser trochanter, and shifted to provide weight bearing underneath the femoral head
- Arthroplasty: Prosthetic replacement (head or head and neck are substituted by a metallic implant)
- Reconstruction: head removed and remnant of neck or greater trochanter inserted into acetabulum
- Arthrodesis hip fused.

Indications:
- Fractures < 2–3/52: Managed as fresh fractures, e.g. by nailing; while fractures > 3/52 in elderly managed by a prosthetic replacement
- Established nonunions with viable head: Managed by angulation osteotomy
- Established nonunion with absorbed neck, or avascular neck: managed by a prosthetic replacement.
- Crippling disability: Managed by reconstructive or arthrodesis.

Techniques:

Osteosynthesis:

Aims:
- To restore anatomical and physiological status
- To preserve femoral head as an articulating unit
- To induce union between head and the neck or trochanter.

Criteria: Little/or no absorption of neck
- Viable and freely mobile head
- Bone density of both fragments to be normal
- Strong fibrous union with minor proximal displacement of distal fragment.

Disadvantage: Not suitable in case:
- Proximal fragment: Small, atrophic, and nonviable
- Osteoporotic joint bone
- Distal fragment markedly displaced proximally
- Neck absorption significant.

Fixation method: Closed or open.
- Closed osteosynthesis: Bone grafts or metallic implant inserted

Indication: Fibrous nonunion

Method: < 2/52: Nailed as fresh fracture femoral neck; > 2/52 a bone graft + internal fixation.
- Open osteosynthesis: ORIF (open reduction + fixation with bone graft or metal.

Indication: Pseudarthrosis (nonfibrous nonunion); neck markedly absorbed

### Closed osteosynthesis with fibular graft (Henderson):
- Patient placed on a fracture table as per fresh fracture neck
- Incision: Lateral longitudinal centered over base of greater trochanter
- Exposure: Lateral aspect of greater trochanter and proximal shaft
- Insertion of guide wire through center of trochanter, neck and head
- Check position under C-arm scanner
- Tunnel preparation: For the fibular graft by cannulated reamers
- Graft: 10 cm of middle half of fibula
- Threading of graft's medullary canal: Over the guide wire, then graft driven through the tunnel into the head.

### Closed osteosynthesis with metallic implant + grafts:
- Patient placed on a fracture table as per fresh fracture neck
- Incision: Lateral longitudinal centered over base of greater trochanter
- Exposure: Lateral aspect of greater trochanter and proximal shaft
- Insertion of two guide wires through the trochanter, neck and head, parallel with each other and 2 cm apart
- Check position under C-arm scanner
- Threading of SP nail: Over the distal wire, drive in, then remove wire
- Drilling a tunnel over proximal wire: Through the trochanter and neck into the head, remove the wire
- Graft: Taken from middle third of ilium (full thickness graft), or tibia
- Graft insertion: Driven through the tunnel into the head.

After care: Same as for post nailing of fresh fractures of femoral neck; weight bearing allowed after firm union (clinically and radiologically).

Open osteosynthesis:
- Patient placed on a fracture table as per fresh fracture neck
- Incision: Curved lateral longitudinal centered over base of greater trochanter (modified anterior iliofemoral incision)
- Exposure of hip, lateral aspect of greater trochanter and proximal shaft

- Exposure of nonunion; denuding fibrous tissue from fragments ends, that are freshened.
- Fixation of head and neck.

The surgery then completed as per closed osteosynthesis.

After care: Same as for post nailing of fresh fractures of femoral neck; weight bearing allowed after firm union (clinically and radiologically).

Osteotomy:

Preface: Femur divided close to lesser trochanter, and shifted to provide weight bearing underneath the femoral head.

Types: Two types of osteotomy for the nonunion:
- Displacement osteotomy (McMurray): Just proximal to the lesser trochanter
- Angulation osteotomy (Schanz): Just distal to the lesser trochanter

Advantage:
- Greater post angulation osteotomy than post displacement osteotomy
- Line of weight bearing shifted medially
- Shearing strain across nonunion decreased as the fractured surface turns more horizontal.

Disadvantage:
- Mechanical: If femoral head and neck are placed in extreme valgus position (shortened length of lever arm exerts more stress over head)

Pauwels modification: Y osteotomy to maintain length of lever arm.

Indications:
- Viable head with extensive neck absorption

C/I:
- Well preserved head and neck (osteosynthesis + internal fixation + graft/without graft
- Nonviable head (prosthesis preferred because of development of the post arthritic changes)
- Pseudarthrosis.

Displacement osteotomy:

Preface: A displacement or high osteotomy is characterized by the restoration of bony support, either by healing of the nonunion or by changing the line of weight bearing; although nonunion persists, weight borne directly in line underneath femoral head.

**Types:**

McMurray's (modified):
- Bone divided: Just proximal to lesser trochanter; distal fragment displaced directly underneath head
- Neck preserved and fragments reducible: Nonunion fixed with two Knowles pins while osteotomy fixed with Neufeld nail or a reversed Blount

- Neck short: Osteotomy fixed with Neufeld nail or a reversed Blount, while Knowles pins omitted.

Caution: Osteotomy neither to be too oblique, nor to include part of the base of the neck.

Method:
- Patient's fixed on a fracture table, in supine position, with normal limb tied to the foot stirrup
- Check the position of head vs neck by X-ray or C-arm vision
- Incision: 15 cm long along to femoral shaft, from greater trochanter
- Incise vastus lateralis and strip from anterior surface of femur at the site of desirable osteotomy
- Insert guide wire into femur, at surface level with lesser trochanter; advance obliquely—medially and proximally, to emerge medially just proximally to lesser trochanter
- Insert second guide wire proximal to the first one, through greater trochanter, neck, then into the head
- Insert two Knowles pins through greater trochanter, neck, into head
- Divide the femur (by an osteotome or Gigli saw) next to distal guide wire
- Displace medially the distal fragment beneath the femoral head
- Fixation of osteotomy blade plate: Insert the blade through greater trochanter, then fix the osteotomy plate (Neufeld or Blount) to the abducted femoral shaft by 3 screws
- Confirm position by X-ray or C-arm vision.

Postoperative: No immobilization required.
After care: Exercises, and after 8/52 partial weight bearing allowed on crutches, till firm union (appx. 6/12).

Pauwels Y osteotomy:
Indication: Unusual pseudarthrosis of femoral neck (neck absorption + proximal displacement of distal fragment). It is indicated only in case of viable head and in the healthy patient that allows prolonged plaster immobilization to achieve union.

Aims:
- To enlarge femoral neck, so as to increase apposition between neck and the head
- To improve the function of hip abductors, by distal displacement of the greater trochanter.

Method: Pauwels advocates nailing + osteotomy:
- Osteotomy made at the intertrochanteric level
- Lateral wedge—removed
- Fixation of osteotomy—with a plate and screws.

Angulation osteotomy:
Indication: Nonunion with a viable head by shifting line of weight bearing medially, and to change the inclined fracture surfaces to promote union.

Advantage: Over displacement osteotomy: greater trochanter's position more satisfactory; abductor muscles function more effectively; further shortening diminished; improved mobility of the hip; internal fixation maintained more effectively.

Disadvantage: More distal the osteotomy leads to secondary genu valgun.

### Blount's osteotomy:

- Reduction: The fragments reduced by firm, continuous traction, and internal rotation
- Immobilization: Patient's fixed on a fracture table, in supine position, with normal limb tied to the foot stirrup
- Check the position of fragments by X-ray or C-arm vision
- Prepare the skin and drape the patient
- Incision: A curved incision 5 cm centered over greater trochanter; extended distally over lateral surface of thigh parallel with the femur
- Insert guide wire from base of greater trochanter, into femoral neck
- Insert two Knowles pins parallel with guide wire into femoral neck.

Exposure: Circumference of femoral shaft at lesser trochanter

Insert blade of a Blount blade plate (bent to 20 degree neck) into neck and head remove guide wire and cut off ends of Knowles pins insert a screw through most proximal hole in the blade plate to engage the proximal fragment of osteotomy

Osteotomize: Femur at distal angle of the plate

Internally rotate: Distal fragment

Abduct: The shaft until against the plate; attach the plate to shaft with three screws.

After care: Crutch walking may be allowed post 8/52; weight bearing as per progress of union

Osteotomy and osteosynthesis:

Angulation osteotomy + osteosynthesis (Dickson):

- Osteotomy: Changes the weight bearing angle by 45 degree
- Osteosynthesis: Grafts hasten union and prevent fractures impaction.

After care: Same as for angulation osteotomy.

### Prosthesis Replacement (Medullary/Stem) Femoral Endoprosthesis

Principle: For a nonfunctional part, better to substitute another (inert implant).

Indication:

- Age: A frail/elderly patient who is unlikely to have a long/or active life subsequently. The morbidity is appreciable esp. when a posterior approach is used
- Nonunion + absorption of femoral neck
- Avascular necrosis of femoral head (with or without union)
- Secondary osteoarthritis (arthritic degeneration of hip post union).

C/I:
- Avascular necrosis of supporting bone (inevitably loosen)
- Improper size and shape (breakdown, or bone absorption)

Endurance: Depends upon:
- Inertness of substance
- Weight bearing (distribution and pressure)
- Vascular supply (of supporting bone).

Types: Two types:
- Stem prosthesis: Replica of femoral head and a stem to be inserted into the neck and anchored laterally in the femoral shaft's cortex: unsuitable for nonunions of femoral neck.
  Common prosthesis of Judet, Thomson, Rieth.
- Medullary prosthesis: Replica of femoral head (mostly of neck too) and a stem to be anchored in the femoral medullary canal common prosthesis of Thompson and Austin Moore

Method: Excision of the femoral head, and replacement with a:
Thompson or Austin Moore prosthesis:

Specifications:
- Thompson:
  Head dimension: 39; 41; 43; 45; 47; 49; 51; 53 mm
  Stem dimention: 105 mm
- Austin moore:
  Head dimension: 39; 41; 43; 45; 47; 49; 51; 53; 55; 57 mm
  Stem            : 127 ....................; 140 ................; 152 ............ mm

Technique: Preoperative planning:
- Skeletal traction: Any fixed shortening (confirmed by X-ray hip, while traction applied manually to the limb) because of proximal shifting of distal fragment to be corrected prior to surgery.

Procedure:
- Exposure: Lateral, anterolateral, or posterior approach
- Femoral neck resection
- Femoral preparation
- Removal of femoral head
- Measuring of femoral head size
- Acetabular cleaning
- Trial reduction of head into acetabulum
- Femoral cementing
- Stem implantation
- Reduction—by gentle delivery of head into the acetabulum
- Check X-ray
- Closure of wound after putting in a drain.

Post care: Exercises:
- Breathing exercises, starting on the same day of operation
- Quadriceps, toes, ankle exercises—first day onwards

**Refer:** The patient to fracture clinic after 2–3/12. If satisfactory, then next visit post one year and so on for five years, with periodical check X-rays.

## Total Hip Replacement (THR)

Preface: Affords an early immobilization and returning to initial, pre-fracture state is fully justified, provided the patient's condition is satisfactory, for this major surgery.

Technique: Preoperative planning:
- Exposure: Lateral, anterolateral, or posterior approach
- Femoral neck resection
- Femoral preparation
- Acetabular preparation
- Acetabular cementing and pressurization
- Acetabular implantation
- Trial reduction
- Further femoral preparation
- Femoral cementing
- Stem implantation
- Reduction by gentle delivery of head into the acetabulum
- Check X-ray
- Post care: exercises
- Breathing exercises: Starting on the same day of operation
- Quadriceps, toes, ankle exercises: First day onwards.

**Refer:** The patient to fracture clinic after 2–3/12. If satisfactory, then next visit post one year and so on for five years, with periodical check X-rays.

## Reconstructions

Preface: Reconstruction may only provide a bony support by the shortened femoral neck or by the greater trochanter

Indications:
- Reconstruction may be the only possible remedy for removed femoral head or prosthesis postinfection
- Reconstruction may be indicated even in noninfective cases, although results may be comparatively poor.

Disadvantages:
- Displacement of femoral neck or trochanter from the acetabulum
- Weakness of gluteal muscles
- Arthritic changes.

### Method: Whitman reconstruction:

Aims:
- To establish the leverage mandatory for the abductor muscles to balance the pelvis
- To prevent adduction
- To prevent dislocation of proximal femur from acetabulum.

Technique:
- Incision: Curved 2.5 cm from ASI spine, distally and posteriorly to top of greater trochanter.
- Deepen incision between tensor fasciae latae and gluteus medius muscles
- Incise the capsule and remove the femoral head
- Divide obliquely the base of greater trochanter; turn the trochanter and attached muscles posterosuperiorly
- Denude the proximal end of femur of soft tissues; reduce it into acetabulm (in 45 degree of abduction and internal rotation)
- Pull down trochanter and fix it to lateral surface of femur, with a screw, a nail, or wire.

Postoperative: A hip cast applied with affected hip in 45 degree abduction and moderately internally rotated for 4/52; then check up position radiologically; passive exercises of hip and knee; by 8/52, weight bearing with crutches allowed; weight bearing without crutches allowed post 6/12.

## Modified Whitman Reconstruction

Indications
- Necrotic femoral head: Managed by a Whitman reconstruction combined with a mold arthroplasty
- Long femoral neck: May not require transplanting greater trochanter
- Short femoral neck: Managed by transplanting greater trochanter

Distally.

### Albee reconstruction:
Aim:
- To prevent dislocation of hip postreconstruction; managed by establishing a lever to improve action of abductor muscles that hold the proximal femur into the acetabulum.

Technique:
- Incision: An anterior iliofemoral
- Deepen incision and retract muscles from the ilium
- Incise the capsule and remove the femoral head
- Denude trochanter of soft tissues
- Reduce femoral neck into the acetabulum; hold it with sutures through the soft tissues.

Postoperative: A one and a half hip cast applied with affected hip in 30 degree abduction and moderately.

### Colonna reconstruction:
Aims:
- To establish the leverage mandatory for the abductor muscles to balance the pelvis
- To prevent adduction
- To prevent dislocation of proximal femur from acetabulum.

Technique:
- Incision: Curved 2.5 cm from ASI spine, distally and posteriorly for 10–12 cm from the top of greater trochanter.
- Deepen incision between tensor fasciae latae and gluteus medius muscles
- Denude the trochanter of soft tissues and divide attached muscles
- Incise the capsule
- Adduct and externally rotate the limb
- Remove the femoral head
- Pull down the femur and adduct it; transplant trochanter into the acetabulum
- Fix abductor muscles into a trough made into femoral shaft with sutures through the holes.

Postoperative: A one and a half hip cast applied with affected hip in 30 degree abduction and moderately.

## Modified Colonna Reconstruction

Indications
- Nonunion femoral neck (with nonviable femoral head and absorbed neck): Managed by transplanting distally greater trochanter and its attached muscles
- To prevent subluxation of proximal of femur from acetabulum while abducting the limb
- To prevent impinging of acetabulum on anterior lip of cotyloid notch: managed by deepening the acetabulum.

Arthrodesis:
Indications: Rarely indicated, because of difficulty in achieving fusion; to be used in combination with the muscle pedicle bone grafts
Aims in managing nonunion of femoral neck:
- To relieve from pain
- To provide stability in weight bearing
- To be an effective salvage operation for infected trochanteric mold arthroplasty
- To be indicated for failed prosthetic replacement.

## Trochanteric and Subtrochanteric

Preface
Mostly delayed union proceed eventually to union, but in the meantime the risk of late mechanical complication has increased, while in some cases nonunion results (1–2%); the problem of nonunion of trochanteric and subtrochanteric region is never an easy one. esp. post conservative treatment, and sometimes even post ORIF; cortical bone grafts fail to prevent fragments angulation; fragments to be fixed in valgus with a nail/nail-plate besides cancellous grafting across the nonunion.

Management:
Surgical treatment:

Preoperatively: Skeletal traction to restore length and alignment, for severe angulation

Surgery: ORIF + bone grafting

Technique:
- Position: Supine on the fracture table
- Reduction: Under C-arm
- Incision: Lateral approach
- Exposure: Lateral and anterior aspects of greater trochanter and the proximal third of femoral shaft
- Denude and freshen: Fragments ends made to be in contact in a valgus position
- Bend: A nail as per position of the aligned fragments in valgus position
- Fixation: Insert nail and fix plate part of nail to the femoral shaft with screws
- Grafting: Place iliac grafts across nonunion
- Suturing: Vastus lateralis.

Postoperatively: Immobilization by a balanced splint in abduction for 2/52.

After care: Exercises

## Femur Shaft

Preface

Mostly delayed union proceed eventually to union, but in the meantime the risk of late mechanical complication has increased, while in some cases nonunion results; the problem of nonunion of femoral shaft is never an easy one esp postconservative treatment, and sometimes even post ORIF; nonunion occurs more often at the junction of middle and distal thirds of femoral shaft, thereby medullary nailing is unsatisfactory here, and plating, or interlocking nailing preferred; compound fractures with nonunion may be managed with external fixator.

### Management:

Conservative treatment:

Indication: Uncomplicated closed fracture femoral shaft

Method: Traction in a Thomas splint for 4/12.

After care: Check up radiological for firm union.

Surgical treatment:
- Most nonunions of middle third and distal part of proximal third of femoral shaft may be treated with bone grafting and a medullary nail; while nonunions at junction of middle and distal thirds may better be treated with interlocking nailing with cancellous grafts.

Technique:

Bone grafting + medullary nailing:
- The technique of inserting a medullary nail is similar to the one for fresh fractures

- The type of graft indicated based on the type of nonunion and quality of fixation of fragments with the nail:

A. Fracture < 12/52 old, and the fragments unopposed and vascular: managed by medullary nailing + cancellous grafts around nonunion

B. Complicated nonunion (sclerosed fragment ends): Managed by medullary nailing + Phemister graft

C. Inadequate fixation with medullary nailing: Managed by onlay grafts with nailing

D. Sclerosed fragments; a defect to be bridged; failed previous grafting: managed with onlay grafts.

Method: Post nail insertion, a cortical graft fixed with four or more screws to the bone across nonunion (only through lateral cortex) + cancellous bone chips around nonunion.

After care:
- Uncomplicated nonunion: Same as for fresh fracture
- Complicated nonunion: A long leg cast for few weeks.

Plate and grafting:

Indications: Nonunion too distal to permit medullary nailing

Technique: Managed by a compression plate applied on lateral surface + iliac onlay grafts applied on medial surface.

After care: A spica cast applied from the nipple line to the toes on affected side, with knee and hip flexed to 30 degree, and up to knee on the opposite side, for 10/52; followed by removal of cast; exercises; weight bearing on crutches till firm union.

## Patella
Preface

Mostly delayed union proceed eventually to union, but in the meantime the risk of late mechanical complication has increased, while in some cases nonunion results; the problem of nonunion of patellar fracture is never an easy one esp. postconservative treatment, and sometimes even post ORIF; nonunion occurs more often when the fragments are separated; severity of late arthritic changes proportional to irregular articular surfaces of patella; fibrous union may be compatible with good function.

Management:

Conservative treatment:

Indication: Uncomplicated closed fracture patella

Method: Cylindrical POP cast for 4/12.

After care: Check up radiological for firm union.

Surgical treatment:

Surgery: Patellectomy (partial or complete)

Indication: Separated fragments

Surgery: Reconstruction

Indication: To re-establish quadriceps mechanism tension periosteum from the bony fragments must be marginal (if mandatory for procedure); bone grafting alone or in combination with internal fixation is treatment of choice for **tibial shaft's** nonunion

Management: Bone grafting alone or in combination with internal fixation is treatment of choice for **tibial shaft's** nonunion.

Indications and methods:

- Delayed or nonunion (fragments in position with slight mobility of fracture site): Phemister grafting
- Uncomplicated nonunion of middle third: Nailing or compression plate
- Failure of two consecutive treatments: Bone grafting (sliding onlay or iliac onlay)
- Nonunion with bone loss: Sliding bone graft + cancellous bone grafts
- Unstability: Osteotomy or resection of a fibular segment
- Compound fractures with delayed/nonunion: External fixator (ilizarov).

After care:

- Phemister grafting: A long leg cast applied from toes to the groin for 2–3/52; followed by weight bearing (walks) with aid of walking casts until firm union
- Bone grafting (sliding onlay or iliac onlay): A long leg cast applied from toes to the groin for 8/52; followed by weight bearing (walks) with aid of walking casts and crutches until firm union
- Bone grafting + fixation (nailing or plating) of unstable fractures: same treatment as per fresh fractures.

## Medial Malleolus

Preface    Nonunion is a common feature postconservative treatment (closed reduction) of fracture medial malleolus.

Management: Nonunion may be treated by one of the following methods:

- Minor fracture in a sedentary patient: Managed by conservative treatment (arch support; heel wedging; ankle corset/support)
- Sclerosed adjacent bone with large proximal malleolus: managed by resecting the distal fragment
- Failure of two consecutive conservative measures: Managed by bone grafting.

### Technique:

Resecting distal fragment:

- Incision: 5 cm curved incision centered over medial malleolus
- Divide periosteum and deltoid ligament
- Removal of distal fragment subperiosteally
- Wound closure by interrupted silk stitches.

After care: Weight bearing in an ankle corset for 3/52.

Sliding bone grafting:

- Incision: 10 cm curved incision centered over medial malleolus

- Subperiosteally remove the fibrous tissue from nonunion; freshen fragments ends
- Removal of graft (3–4 cm long) from proximal fragment; displace the graft distally across nonunion into distal fragment; transfix both fragments and graft with a screw
- Place cancellous bone chips around the graft
- Wound closure by interrupted silk sutures.

Postoperative: Apply a cast from toes to below knee for 4/52; followed by partial weight bearing for 2–3/52; and then full weight bearing; cast usually removed post 8–10/52 ( radiologically nonunion healed).

Bone grafting:

- Incision: 10 cm curved incision centered over medial malleolus
- Subperiosteally remove the fibrous tissue from nonunion; freshen fragments ends
- Reduce fragments; fix with a 4 cm long screw
- Removal of graft (3–4 cm long) from proximal fragment
- Place cancellous bone chips at the nonunion
- Replace cortex
- Wound closure by interrupted silk sutures.

Postoperative: Apply a cast from toes to below knee for 4/52; followed by partial weight bearing for 2–3/52; and then full weight bearing; cast usually removed post 8–10/52 ( radiologically nonunion healed).

## Metatarsals

Preface

Nonunions of metatarsals are rare; usually caused by either inadequate apposition of the fragments or sepsis; usually occur in the distal third of the bone.

Management: Conservative treatment:
Measures:

- Support: Minor fracture in a sedentary patient: managed by arch support; heel wedging; ankle corset/support; POP walking cast
- Heat therapy: SWD/IR
- Analgesics and NSAIDs.

### Surgical treatment
Surgery:

Indication: Failure of conservative measures
Technique:

- Incision: Dorsal longitudinal incision centered over metatarsal
- Exposure: Fragments, denude and freshen ends
- Reaming: Medullary canal/s
- Reduction: And alignment of fragments
- Fixation: Fragments with a medullary bone peg graft or a Kirschner wire
- Grafting: Cancellous bone chips across nonunion
- Suturing of wound.

Postoperative: Apply a cast from toes to below knee for 4/52; followed by partial weight bearing for 2–3/52; and then full weight bearing; cast usually removed post 8–10/52 ( radiologically nonunion healed).

After care: Exercise.

## Scaphoid

**Preface**

Delayed union and nonunion of fractured scaphoid are common; when treated inadequately for an erroneous diagnosis of a sprained wrist, a fracture through the waist of the bone may pass inevitably into nonunion, resulting in permanent weakness of the wrist and subsequent osteoarthritis; this is a preventable tragedy (medical negligence) esp. in a working man/woman.

Management: Conservative treatment (ASAP):

Immobilization: The hand to be fixed in a 'Cock up' POP cast that should include thumb (metacarpal) and embrace sides of wrist and forearm (to prevent lateral slide); cast for 8/52

After care:
- Support (cock up splint for 3–6/12 for delayed union)
- Heat therapy: SWD/IR
- Analgesics and NSAIDs

Surgical treatment:

Indication: Failure of conservative measures

Surgery: Excision of short fragment

Indication: Nonunion within 5 cm of either end

Surgery: Bone grafting

Indication: Nonunion

Surgery: Excision of fragments

Postoperative:
- Immobilization: The hand to be fixed in a 'Cock up' POP cast that should include thumb (metacarpal) and embrace sides of wrist and forearm (to prevent lateral slide); cast for 8/52.

After care:
- Support (cock up splint for 3–6/12 for delayed union)
- Heat therapy: SWD/IR
- Analgesics and NSAIDs.

## Clavicle

**Preface**

Nonunion of fractured clavicle is rare; usually symptomless and thereby needs no specific treatment; except those resulting in disability require treatment.

Indication:
- Inadequate apposition of the fragments or sepsis
- Disability

Management: Conservative treatment:

Measures:
- Support: Minor fracture in a sedentary patient: managed by arm support; clavicle brace
- Heat therapy: SWD/IR
- Analgesics and NSAIDs.

Surgical treatment:
Indication: Failure of conservative measures
Surgery: Excision of short fragment
Indication: Nonunion within 5 cm of either end
Surgery: Bone grafting
Indication: Nonunion of middle 3/4th of clavicle
Surgery: Onlay graft + cancellous bone graft
Indication: Apposing fragments ends

Technique:
- Incision: 15 cm long, parallel and just distal to the clavicle
- Incise: Periosteum and strip it from anterior half of the bone
- Exposure: Fragments, denude and freshen ends
- Reduction: And alignment of fragments
- Fixation: Fragments with an onlay graft across the nonunion, fix it with screws
- Grafting: Cancellous bone chips across nonunion
- Suturing of wound.

Postoperative: Apply a cast from toes to below knee for 4/52; followed by partial weight bearing for 2–3/52; and then full weight bearing; cast usually removed post 8–10/52 ( radiologically nonunion healed).
After care: Exercises.

## Humerus Proximal Third

Preface

Nonunions of fractures of proximal third of the humerus are rare; usually caused by either inadequate apposition of the fragments or sepsis; usually occur just distal to the surgical neck of the humerus.
Management: Conservative treatment:
Measures:
- Support: Minor fracture in a sedentary patient: managed by arm support, brace, or POP U-slab
- Heat therapy: SWD/IR
- Analgesics and NSAIDs

Surgical treatment:
Surgery: Bone grafting (onlay + intraosseous graft).
Indication: Failure of conservative measures

Technique:
- Incision: Anterior approach
- Exposure: Fragments, denude and freshen ends
- Reduction: Appose the fragments of the nonunion

- Fixation: Fragments with a medullary bone peg graft
- Grafting: Cancellous bone chips across nonunion
- Suturing of wound.

Postoperative: Apply a cast from toes to below knee for 4/52; followed by partial weight bearing for 2–3/52; and then full weight bearing; cast usually removed post 8–10/52 (radiologically nonunion healed).

After care: Exercises

## Shaft

Preface

Nonunions of humeral shaft are common; usually caused by either inadequate apposition of the fragments or sepsis; usually occur in the middle third of the bone.

Management: Conservative treatment:

Measures:
- Support: Minor fracture in a sedentary patient: managed by the arm support, brace; POP splint
- Heat therapy: SWD/IR
- Analgesics and NSAIDs.

Surgical treatment:

Surgery: ORIF (medullary nail or plate) + bone grafting

Indication: Failure of conservative measures

Technique:
- Incision: Henry approach
- Exposure: Fragments, denude and freshen ends
- Reaming: Medullary canal/s
- Reduction: And alignment of fragments
- Fixation: Fragments with a medullary nail or plating with screws
- Grafting: Iliac bone grafts + cancellous bone chips across nonunion
- Suturing of wound.

Postoperative: Apply a cast from toes to below knee for 4/52; followed by partial weight bearing for 2–3/52; and then full weight bearing; cast usually removed post 8–10/52 ( radiologically nonunion healed).

After care: Exercises.

## Condyles of Humerus

Preface

Nonunion of the medial humeral epicondyle may occur post inadequate management of an acute fracture. A fibrous union occurs between the small fragment and the medial condyle, although the fragments are widely separated and the function is usually normal. For associated ulnar neuritis, an attempt is made to achieve bony union between the epicondyle and the condyle; enough to free the ulnar nerve and transfer it anteriorly, and to excise the bony fragment from the common origin of the flexor group of muscles; these myscles are freed and attached to the medial condyle with nonabsorable silk sutures.

| Management | In children: Nonunion of humeral condyles causes disability (cubitus valgus deformity and instability of the elbow). |
|---|---|

In children: Nonunion of humeral condyles causes disability (cubitus valgus deformity and instability of the elbow).

Surgery for established nonunion is contraindicated, as the symptoms are minimal, and the results of surgery are poor.

In adults: Surgery is not indicated for asymptomatic elbow other than anterior transfering of ulnar nerve for relief of ulnar neuritis. Surgery is indicated for painful and unstable elbow.

Technique:
- Incision: Lateral incision over distal third of humerus and extend it 10 cm distally to the radial head
- Exposure: Subperiosteally the anterior and posterior aspects of the nonunion
- Denude and freshen the surfaces
- Remodel: The large condylar fragment
- Freshen and appose the fractured surfaces
- Fixation: Fragments with two screws
- Grafting: Cancellous bone chips across nonunion
- Transfer: Ulnar nerve to the anteromedial aspect of the forearm for persistent ulnar neuritis.
- Postoperative: Apply a cast from knuckles to above elbow for 2/25; followed by support by an arm pouch or brace.

After care: Exercises.

## Monteggia

**Preface**

Postmonteggia fractures, delayed and nonunion of the ulna either with or without persistent dislocation of the radial head is common; usually caused by either inadequate apposition of the fragments or sepsis.

**Management**

Surgical treatment of chjoice.
Surgery: ORIF + Bone graft (cancellous bone strips)
Indication: Delayed union (small or no sclerosis at fracture site)
Surgery: Excision of sclerosed bone + reduction + bone graft
Indication: Nonunion (sclerosed bone ends)

Technique:
- Incision: Posterior longitudinal incision centered over posterior aspect of elbow
- Exposure: Fragments, denude and freshen ends
- Exposure radial head by incising capsule; resect radial head
- Denude and freshen: Coronoid process and ulnar shaft
- Engage: Coronoid process and olecranon against trochlea
- Fixation: Ulnar fragments with dual onlay grafts
- Grafting: Cancellous bone chips across nonunion.
- Suturing of wound.

Postoperative: Apply a cast from palm to axilla with elbow at 90 degree and forearm in midpronation for 8/52
After care: Exercises.

## Bibliography

1. Abbott LC. The use of iliac bone in the treatment of ununited fractures, American Academy of Orthopaerdic Surgeons Instructional Course Lectures, vol. Ii, Ann Arbor, J.W. Edwards, p. 13, 1944.
2. Albee FH. Principles of the treatment of nonunion of fracture, Surg., Gynec. and Obst. 51:289, 1930.
3. Armstrong JR. Bone grafting in ther treatment of fractures, Williams and Wilkins Co., Baltimore, 1945.
4. Banks SW. The treatment of nonunion of fractures of the medial malleolus, J. Bone and Joint Surg. 31-A:658, 1949.
5. Blount WP. Proximal osteotomies of the femur, American Academy of Orthopaedic Surgeons Instructional Course Lectures, vol. IX, Ann Arbor, J.W. Edwards, p.1, 1952.
6. Boyd HB, Lipinski SW. Nonunion of trochanteric and subtrochanteric fractures, Surg., Gynec. and Obst. 104:463, 1957.
7. Campbell WC, Boyd HB. Fixation of onlay bone grafts by means of Vitallium screws in the treatment of ununited fractures, Am. J. Surg. 51:748, 1941.
8. Canale ST, et al. Campbell's Operative Orthopaedics 9th Ed. Vol I-IV, C.V. Mosby Co., Saint Louis, 1998.
9. Clark JMP. Modern Trends in Orthopedics Fracture Treatment, Butterworths, London, 1962.
10. Colonna PC. The trochanteric reconstruction operation for ununited fractures of the upper end of the femur, J. Bone and Joint Surg. 42-B:5, 1960.
11. Gibson A, Loadman B. The bridging of bone defects, J. Bone and Joint Surg. 30-A:381, 1948.
12. Gill AB. Arthrodesis of the hip for ununited fractures J. Bone and Joint Surg. 29:305, 1947.
13. Henderson MS. Treatment of ununited fractures of the hip, S. Clin. North America 24:751, 1944.
14. Hermann OJ. The McMurray osteotomy for nonunited hip fractures, New England J. Med. 2342:186, 1945.
15. Kapoor PS. Fractures treatment. Kapoor's Accident and Emergency, 2nd Ed. CBS, New Delhi.
16. Krida A. The Whitman reconstruction operation for complications of fracture of the neck of the femur, J. Bone and Joint Surg. 29:310, 1947.
17. Love M, Rains AJH, Capper WM. Bailey & Love's Short Practice of Surgery, 1965.
18. McMurray TP. Fracture of the neck of the femur treated by oblique osteotomy Brit. M. J. 1:330, 1938.
19. McRae R. Practical Fracture Treatment, 1st Ed., Mc Rae R, Churchill Livingstone, 1981.
20. Murray CR. Delayed and nonunion in fractures in the adult, Ann. Surg. 93:961, 1931.
21. Phemister DB. Treatment of ununited fractures by onlay bone grafts without screw or tie fixation and without breaking down of the fibrous union, J. Bone and Joint Surg. 29:946, 1947.

# 7

# Malunited Fractures

**Malunions of lower limb**
- Pelvis
- Trochanteric fractures of femur
- Femoral shaft
- Proximal shaft
- Patella
- Tibial condyles
- Shafts of tibia and fibula
- Ankle
- Calcaneus
- Talus
- Metatarsals
- Spine

**Malunions of upper limb**
- Clavicle
- Humerus
- Neck
- Proximal third
- Middle third
- Distal third
- Supracondyler
- Condylar fractures
- Olecranon
- Monteggia fracture dislocation
- Shafts of radius and ulna
- Colles' fracture
- Smith's fracture
- Hand

Preface — Majority of malunited fractures can be prevented by perfect treatment of fresh frctures/fracture dislocations; in certain instances, however, malunion occurs inspite of best treatment provided.

Definition — It is defined as a fracture that has united in an abnormal position; the deformity (fracture united in a position of persistent angulation or rotation) is often displeasing; may impair function in one or many ways; movement of the adjoining joint may be impaired; may cause traumatic arthritis; may disturb balance/gait; may result in shortening.

| | |
|---|---|
| Etiology | Imperfect reduction of fracture/fracture dislocation |
| | Inadequate immobilization |
| Pathogenesis | Deformity: Angulation results in incorrect transmission of force (weight—in lower limb) through joints above and below the fracture; shortening results in impaired gait (limp); secondary osteoarthritis. |
| Diagnosis | Deformity: |

Diagnosis  Deformity:
- Angulation
- Shortening

Gait: Limp

| | |
|---|---|
| Investigation | X-ray—AP and LAT views |
| Management | Aim of treatment: To correct deformity: |

Conservative treatment:

Shortening:
- Gross shortening can be corrected by raised shoe
- 2.5 cm shortening by raising shoe heel by 1.25 cm.

  > 2.5 cm shortening to be corrected surgically.

Angulation:
- Cannot be corrected by conservative measures; to be corrected surgically

Surgical treatment:

Indication:
- Failed conservative measures
- Deformity:
  - Shortening: > 2.5 cm
  - Angulation

Surgery: Osteotomy.

Regional malunited fractures/fracture dislocations:

## LOWER LIMB

## Malunited Fractures/fracture Dislocation of Pelvis

| | |
|---|---|
| Preface | Majority of malunited fractures/fracture dislocations of pelvis involving the acetabulum are to be corrected surgically; however the surgery (correction) may not be required in certain exceptional cases. |
| Definition | It is defined as (a fracture/fracture dislocation of pelvis that has united in an abnormal position; fracture of acetabulum with central dislocation; fracture acetabular's superior rim with posterior dislocation; acetabular comminuted fracture) that may impair function in one or many ways; movement may be impaired; may cause traumatic arthritis; may disturb balance/gait; may result in shortening. |
| Etiology | • Imperfect reduction of fracture/fracture dislocation |
| | • Inadequate immobilization |
| Pathogenesis | Deformity: Malunited acetabular fracture with central dislocation; traumatic arthritis (secondary osteoarthritis); shortening results in impaired gait (limp). |

| | |
|---|---|
| Diagnosis | Deformity:<br>• Contracted pelvis<br>• Shortening<br>• Gait: limp |
| Investigation | X-ray pelvis—AP and LAT views |
| Management | Aims of treatment:<br>• To correct deformity<br>• To relieve pain |

Conservative treatment:

Shortening:
• Gross shortening can be corrected by raised shoe
• 2.5 cm shortening by raising shoe heel by 1.25 cm.
> 2.5 cm shortening to be corrected surgically.

Angulation:
• Cannot be corrected by conservative measures to be corrected surgically

Surgical treatment:

Indication:
• Failed conservative measures
• Deformity:
  – Malunited fracture dislocation (central)
  – Comminuted acetabulum with traumatic arthritis
  – Fracture acetabular superior rim with posterior dislocation
  – Shortening: > 2.5 cm.

Surgery:
• Arthrodesis:
Indication: Hip movements painful and restricted
• Arthroplasty (mold)
Indication: Sedentary life
• Prosthesis:
Indication: Elderly persons

## Malunion of Trochanteric Fractures of Femur

| | |
|---|---|
| Preface | Malunited fractures of the trochanteric region may include:<br>• Rotated malunited fractures (internally or externally)<br>• Coxa vera<br>• Shortening > 5 cm.<br><br>Fresh fractures in certain instances, however, malunion occurs inspite of best treatment provided. |
| Definition | It is defined as a fracture that has united in an abnormal position; the deformity (fracture united in a position of rotation (internally or externally) is often displeasing; may impair function in one or many ways; movement of the hip joint may be impaired; may cause traumatic arthritis; may disturb balance/gait; may result in shortening. |

| | |
|---|---|
| Etiology | • Imperfect reduction of fracture<br>• Inadequate immobilization |
| Pathogenesis | Deformity: Malunited fracture (internally/or externally) results in impaired weight bearing; traumatic shortening results in impaired gait (limp); secondary osteoarthritis of hip and knee joints. |
| Diagnosis | Deformity:<br>• Internally or externally rotated<br>• Coxa vara<br>• Shortening<br>• Gait: Limp |
| Investigation | X-ray hip—AP and LAT views |
| Management | Aim of treatment: To correct deformity:<br>A. Shortening:<br>  Conservative treatment:<br>  • Gross shortening can be corrected by raised shoe<br>  • 2.5 cm shortening by raising shoe heel by 1.25 cm<br>    > 2.5 cm shortening to be corrected surgically: |

Surgical treatment:
Surgery: Angulating the bone at the osteotomy.

B. Rotation and coxa vara:
• Cannot be corrected by conservative measures; to be corrected surgically

Surgical treatment:
Indication:
• Failed conservative measures
• Deformity:
  – Shortening: > 2.5 cm
  – Rotation and coxa vara
Surgery: Osteotomy (subtrochanteric).

## Malunion of Femoral Shaft Fractures

| | |
|---|---|
| Preface | Malunion of femoral shaft fractures are common; majority of malunited fractures can be prevented by perfect treatment of fresh fractures; incertain instances, however, malunion occurs inspite of best treatment provided. |
| Definition | It is defined as a fracture that has united in an abnormal position; the deformity (fracture united in a position of persistent angulation or rotation) is often displeasing; may impair function in one or many ways; movement of the adjoining joints may be impaired; may cause traumatic arthritis; may disturb balance/gait; may result in shortening. |
| Etiology | • Imperfect reduction of fracture/fracture dislocation<br>• Inadequate immobilization. |
| Pathogenesis | Deformity: Angulation results in incorrect transmission of force (weight – in lower limb) through joints above and below the fracture; shortening results in impaired gait (limp); secondary osteoarthritis. |

Diagnosis        Deformity:
                 • Angulation
                 • Shortening (overlapping)
                 • Rotation
                 Gait: Limp
Investigation    X-ray femur—AP and LAT views
Management       Aim of treatment: To correct deformity:
                 A. Shortening:
                    Conservative treatment:
                    • Gross shortening can be corrected by raised shoe
                    • 2.5 cm shortening by raising shoe heel by 1.25 cm
                      > 2.5 cm shortening to be corrected surgically.
                 B. Angulation and overlapping:
                    Closed reduction: Malunion of short duration may be broken up
                    manually; angulation and overlapping corrected by skeletal traction
                    • Malunion of long duration cannot be corrected by manipulation;
                      to be corrected surgically.
                 Surgical treatment:
                 Indication:
                 • Failed conservative measures
                 • Deformity:
                   − Shortening: > 2.5 cm
                   − Angulation
                   − Rotation
                 Surgery: ORIF + iliac bone grafts.
                 • Malunion of proximal third of femoral shaft:
                   ORIF (medullary nailing; interlocking nailing; plating).

                 Specific indications:
                 i. Malunion with angulation and rotation:
                    Etiology: Early weight bearing

                    Treatment:
                    • Malunion of short duration: Closed reduction with skeletal
                      traction
                    • Malunion of long duration: ORIF ASAP; osteotomy for solid
                      malunion in bad position.
                 ii. Malunion with massive overlapping:
                     Etiology: Early weight bearing
                     Treatment:
                     • Young children (shortening < 4 cm): Wait and watch for recovery
                       (may be compensated by overgrowth); > 4 cm may require
                       correction.
                     • Young adults (shortening > 4 cm): Surgery indicated, but with
                       caution of impaired functioning of knee joint
                     • Elderly: Surgery unjustified because of danger of nonunion or
                       shock.

  iii. Malunion with massive overlapping, angulation, or rotation:

   Etiology: Early weight bearing

   Treatment:

    • Young adults (shortening > 4 cm and marked angulation): surgery.

    (shortening < 4 cm): Closed reduction with skeletal traction

    Nonunion: Bone grafting.

  iv. Severe deformity of long duration:

   Treatment:

    • Osteotomy; then skeletal traction (to restore length); reduction; fixation with a medullary nail; external fixator; or a plate; and bone grafting.

## Proximal Shaft Fractures of Femur

| | |
|---|---|
| Preface | Majority of malunited fractures can be prevented by perfect treatment of fresh frctures/fracture dislocations; in certain instances, however, malunion occurs inspite of best treatment provided. |
| Definition | It is defined as a fracture that has united in an abnormal position; the deformity (fracture united in a position of persistent angulation or rotation) is often displeasing; may impair function in one or many ways; movement of the adjoining joint may be impaired; may cause traumatic arthritis; may disturb balance/gait; may result in shortening. |
| Etiology | Imperfect reduction of fracture/fracture dislocation |
| | Inadequate immobilization |
| Pathogenesis | Deformity: Angulation results in incorrect transmission of force (weight—in lower limb) through joints above and below the fracture; shortening results in impaired gait (limp); secondary osteoarthritis. |
| Diagnosis | Deformity: |
| | • Angulation |
| | • Shortening |
| | Gait: Limp |
| Investigation | X-ray—AP and LAT views |
| Management | Aim of treatment: To correct deformity: |
| | Conservative treatment: |
| | Shortening: |
| | • Gross shortening can be corrected by raised shoe |
| | • 2.5 cm shortening by raising shoe heel by 1.25 cm |
| | > 2.5 cm shortening to be corrected surgically. |
| | Angulation: |
| | • Cannot be corrected by conservative measures to be corrected surgically |
| | Surgical treatment: |
| | Indication: |
| | • Failed conservative measures |

- Deformity:
  - Shortening: > 2.5 cm.
  - Angulation

Surgery: Osteotomy.

## Malunion of Patellar Fractures/Fracture Dislocations

| | |
|---|---|
| Preface | Majority of malunited patellar fractures undergo degenerative changes; can be prevented by perfect treatment of fresh frctures/fracture dislocations; in certain instances, however, malunion and degenerative changes occur inspite of best treatment provided. |
| Definition | It is defined as a fracture that has united in an abnormal position; the deformity (fracture united in a position of persistent angulation or rotation) is often displeasing; may impair function in one or many ways; movement of the adjoining joint may be impaired; may cause traumatic arthritis; may disturb balance/gait; may result in shortening. |
| Etiology | Imperfect reduction of fracture/fracture dislocation |
| | Inadequate immobilization |
| Pathogenesis | Irregular articular surface of the patella; roughened contiguous surface of the femur; traumatic arthritis. |
| Diagnosis | Pain: Subpatellar |
| | Swelling |
| | Disability: Proportionate to irregular articular surface |
| | Crepitus |
| | Movements of knee painful |
| | Gait: Limp |
| Investigation | X-ray knee—AP and LAT views |
| Complication | Chondromalacia of patella |
| Management | Aim of treatment: To relieve pain and disability: |
| | Conservative treatment: |
| | Rest |
| | Analgesics |
| | Surgical treatment: |
| | Indication: |

- Failed conservative measures
- Disability

Surgery: Patellectomy: treatment of choice.

## Malunion of Tibial Condyles Fractures

| | |
|---|---|
| Preface | Malunited fractures of tibial condyles heal with moderate/or severe displacement; changed weight bearing position; increased joint space; relaxed knee ligaments; valgus or varus weight bearing alignment; rotational deformity; and disability from traumatic arthritis; can be prevented by perfect treatment of fresh fractures/fracture dislocations; in certain instances, however, malunion occurs inspite of the best treatment provided. |

| Definition | It is defined as a fracture that has united in an abnormal position; the deformity (fracture united in a position of persistent rotation) is often displeasing; may impair function in one or many ways; movement of the knee joint may be impaired; may cause traumatic arthritis; may disturb balance/gait. |
|---|---|
| Etiology | Imperfect reduction of fracture/fracture dislocation<br>Inadequate immobilization |
| Pathogenesis | Deformity: Fracture united in a position of persistent rotation) is often displeasing; may impair function in one or many ways; movement of the knee joint impaired; traumatic arthritis. |
| Diagnosis | Deformity:<br>• Displacement<br>Disability: Axial malalignment post depressed condyle<br>Gait: Limp<br>Movements: Painful and restricted |
| Investigation | X-ray—AP and LAT views |
| Management | Aim of treatment to correct deformity:<br>Conservative treatment:<br>Displacement: |

• Cannot be corrected by conservative measures; to be corrected surgically

Surgical treatment:
Indication:
• Failed conservative measures
• Disability by axial malalignment postcondylar depression
Surgery:
• Osteotomy (transverse subcondylar) + wedge grafting

Malunited lateral condyle fracture:
Technique:
• Incision: 10 cm longitudinal over anterolateral aspect of knee and an inverted across lateral condyle, down the tibial crest
• Detach: Subperiosteally origin of extensors from bone
• Osteotomy: Transversally just distal to tibial tuberosity
• Tilting of upper fragment of bone proximally, and angulate distal tibial shaft medially (to restore normal transverse plane of condyles)
• Filling of wedge shaped osteotomy space with bone graft (taken from same tibial shaft).

Malunited medial condyle fracture:
Technique: Similar procedure as for lateral codyle.

## Malunion of Shafts of Both Bones (Tibia and Fibula) of Leg

| Preface | Majority of malunited fractures can be prevented by perfect treatment of fresh fractures/fracture dislocations; in certain instances, however, malunion occurs inspite of best treatment provided. |
|---|---|

| | |
|---|---|
| Definition | It is defined as a fracture that has united in an abnormal position; the deformity (fracture united in a position of persistent angulation or rotation) is often displeasing; may impair function in one or many ways; movement of the adjoining joint may be impaired; may cause traumatic arthritis; may disturb balance/gait; may result in shortening. |
| Etiology | Imperfect reduction of fracture/fracture dislocation |
| | Inadequate immobilization |
| Pathogenesis | Deformity: Angulation results in incorrect transmission of force (weight– in lower limb) through joints above and below the fracture; shortening results in impaired gait (limp); secondary osteoarthritis. |
| Diagnosis | Deformity: |

Diagnosis — Deformity:
- Rotational
- Angulation: lateral and posterior
- Shortening

Gait: Limp

Investigation — X-ray leg—AP and LAT views

Management — Aim of treatment to correct deformity:

Conservative treatment:

Shortening:
- Gross shortening can be corrected by raised shoe
- 2.5 cm shortening by raising shoe heel by 1.25 cm
  > 2.5 cm shortening to be corrected surgically.

Angulation:
- Cannot be corrected by conservative measures; to be corrected surgically

Surgical treatment:

Indication:
- Failed conservative measures
- Deformity:
  - Shortening: > 2.5 cm
  - Angulation

Surgery: Osteotomy + internal fixation (plating) + bone grafting.

Technique:
- Incision: 2.5 cm long longitudinal centered over apex of angulation on the anteromedial aspect of the tibia; divide periosteum
- Osteotomy of tibia
- Fracturing of fibula
- Apposition of fragments into proper position
- Fixation: Internal fixation
- Grafting: Strips of cancellous bone graft across osteotomy site
- Wound closure.

Postoperative: Similar to that post open reduction of a fresh fracture.

## Malunion of Ankle

| | |
|---|---|
| Preface | Majority of malunited fractures can be prevented by perfect treatment of fresh fractures/fracture dislocations; in certain instances, however, malunion occurs inspite of best treatment provided; disability post malunited ankle fracture is mostly so much that only surgery may provide relief; a minor valgus or varus deformity of the ankle joint may impair weight bearing alignment, that the knee joint being a hinge type, fails to compensate for; damaged articular surface; prognosis for the malunion of ankle is poor. |
| Definition | It is defined as a fracture that has united in an abnormal position post reduction of the ankle fractures (Pott's or bimalleolar fracture; fibular fracture plus ruptured deltoid ligament; reversed Pott's fracture; tibia-fibular diastasis from ruptured interosseous ligament; explosion fracture; and Cotton's or the trimalleolar fracture, i.e. fractured medial and lateral malleoli and the fractured posterior part of tibial articular surface); deformity is often displeasing; may impair function in one or many ways; may cause traumatic arthritis; may disturb balance/gait. |
| Etiology | Imperfect reduction of fracture/fracture dislocation |
| | Inadequate immobilization |
| Pathogenesis | Pathological changes in the articular cartilage; deformity results in incorrect transmission of force (weight—in lower limb) through knee joint; shortening results in impaired gait (limp); secondary osteoarthritis. |
| Diagnosis | Disability |
| | Swelling |
| | Gait: Limp |
| Investigation | X-ray ankle—AP and LAT views |
| Management | Aim of treatment to correct deformity: |

**Conservative treatment:**

Indication:
- Deformity of short duration:
  Procedure: Closed reduction (manipulation)
- Duration of long duration: Cannot be corrected by conservative measures; to be corrected surgically

**Surgical treatment:**

Indication:
- Failed conservative measures
- Deformity: Impaired weight bearing alignment
- Diastasis of tibia and fibula
- Equinus deformity
- Advanced traumatic arthritis

Surgery:
- Osteotomy: Restoration of weight bearing alignment
- Arthrodesis: Advanced traumatic arthritis

### Osteotomy for malunited Pott's fracture:

Indication:
- Faulty weight bearing alignment
- Minimal traumatic arthritis

Technique:
- Incision: 5 cm long longitudinal, centered over old fibular fracture
- Refracture fibula by oblique osteotomy; freshen and engage fragments
- Incision: 5 cm long longitudinal, centered over old tibial fracture
- Refracture tibia by oblique osteotomy; freshen and engage fragments
- Fixation of medial malleolus with a screw
- Bimalleolar osteotomy + TA lengthening for equinus deformity (via a third incision posteriorly).

Postoperative: A long cast applied from the groin to the toes, with knee flexed to 20 degree and the foot at right angle or in little equinus
Check X-ray/or reduction under C-arm to confirm reduction
Removal of cast post 6/52; then walking cast for 4/52; then by an ankle brace with arch support for 3–6/12.

### Arthrodesis (compression) for malunited ankle's fracture

Indication:
- Malunited bimalleolar fractures with marked deformity and advanced traumatic arthritis
- Malunited trimalleolar fractures of long duration with talus dislocation
- Deformity: Equinus, medial and lateral angulations
- Malunited fractures: Failed conservative measures.

Technique (Charley):
- Incision: 5 cm longitudinal incision centered over anterior aspect of ankle joint
- Exposure of extensor tendons
- Divide: Between sutures the tendons of tibialis anterior, extensor hallucis longus, extensor digitorum communis, peroneus tertius
- Divide and ligate: Anterior tibial vessels and nerve
- Incise: Capsule transversely
- Exposure: Subperiostealy the distal tibia and posterior surfaces of the malleoli
- Divide: Tibial and fibular collateral ligaments; plantarflex the foot
- Osteotomy of distal ends of tibia and fibula horizontally
- Pass a Steinmann pin: Transversally through talus anterior to body axis, and transversally through the tibial shaft
- Apply: Compression clamps to the pins
- Tie: The tendon sutures and close the wound.

Postoperative: Apply a below knee cast to the toes for 4–6/52.

After care: Post 4–6/52, removal of cast, pins, clamp, and sutures; then a walking boot cast for 4/52 followed.

## Malunion of Calcaneus

| | |
|---|---|
| Preface | Majority of malunited fractures can be prevented by perfect treatment of fresh fractures, in certain instances, however, malunion occurs inspite of best treatment provided (pain and disability persist post fractures of the calcaneus); esp. amongst walking over rough ground. |
| Definition | It is defined as a fracture that has united in an abnormal position; the deformity (fracture united in a position of persistent angulation or rotation) is often displeasing; may impair function in one or many ways; movement of the adjoining tarsal joints may be impaired; may cause traumatic arthritis; may disturb balance/gait. |
| Etiology | Imperfect reduction of fracture |
| | Inadequate immobilization |
| Pathogenesis | Deformity: Angulation results in incorrect transmission of force (weight—in lower limb) through joints above and below the fracture; shortening results in impaired gait (limp); traumatic arthritis. |
| Diagnosis | Pain |
| | Disability |
| | Gait: Limp |
| Investigation | X-ray—AP and LAT views |
| Management | Aim of treatment to correct deformity: |

Conservative treatment:

Analgesics, NSAIDs

Weight bearing with arch supports

Deformity:
• Cannot be corrected by conservative measures; to be corrected surgically

Surgical treatment:
Indication:
• Failed conservative measures
• Severe crushed fracture

Surgery:
• Triple arthrodesis
• Subtalar arthrodesis (to be limited to subtalar arthrodesis; midtarsal joints to be preserved as the mobility increases with activity).

Tripple arthrodesis:
Indication: Malunion of midtarsal joints (talonavicular and the calcaneocuboid)

Subtalar arthrodesis:
Indication: Malunion of subtalar joint

Technique:
• Incision: Kocher U, from proximal and posterior to lateral malleolus, over to anterolateral surface of foot, distally to the malleolus

- Displace and retract: peroneal tendons from posterior to lateral malleolus
- Resect: Surfaces of subtalar joint (to correct eversion of the calcaneus)
- Restore: Peroneal tendons in original position
- Suture: The tendon sheaths.

Postoperative: Same as for triple arthrodesis.

## Malunion of Fracture of Talus

| | |
|---|---|
| Preface | Malunion of fracture of talus results in marked disability; malunion may involve both the neck or body or both together; may result in irregular surfaces of ankle joint, subtalar, and talonavicular joints; malunited fractures of the talar neck may be analogous to intracapsular fractures of femoral neck in that they impair vascular supply, thereby causing degeneration/or sequestration of talar head or body, and irregularity of articular surfaces; may cause valgus or varus deformity due to rotation or deviation (medial or lateral). |
| Definition | It is defined as a fracture that has united in an abnormal position; the deformity (fracture united in a position of persistent angulation or rotation) is often displeasing; may impair function in one or many ways; movement of the adjoining joint may be impaired; may cause traumatic arthritis; may disturb balance/gait; may result in shortening. |
| Etiology | Imperfect reduction of fracture/fracture dislocation<br>Inadequate immobilization |
| Pathogenesis | Deformity: Valgus or varus (distal fragment united in rotation or deviated medially or laterally); the deviation results in incorrect transmission of force (weight—in lower limb) through joints above and below the fracture; impaired gait (limp); secondary osteoarthritis. |
| Diagnosis | Pain<br>Deformity:<br>• Angulation<br>• Blockaged ankle joint<br>Disability<br>Gait: Limp |
| Investigation | X-ray foot including Ankle joint—AP and LAT views |
| Management | Aim of treatment to correct deformity:<br>Conservative treatment:<br>Analgesics, NSAIDs<br>Braces, anklet, shoe with arch support<br>Deformity:<br>• Cannot be corrected by conservative measures; to be corrected surgically<br><br>Surgical treatment:<br>Indication:<br>• Failed conservative measures<br>• Deformity |

Surgery:
- Excision of protruding bone

Indication: Displaced distal fragment
- Arthrodesis or

Indication: Malunited subtalar or ankle joint or both; traumatic arthritis
- Posterior arthrodesis of ankle: Arthritis of superior and inferior surfaces of talus; arthritic subtalar joint
- Calcaneotibial arthrodesis: Nonviable talar body

Pantalar arthrodesis: Malunited comminuted fracture of body or neck

Ankle arthrodesis: Traumatic arthritis of ankle joint

Subtalar arthrodesis: Traumatic arthritis of subtalar joint
- Tripple arthrodesis: To correct heel inversion and forefoot varus
- Talectomy: Infective (compound fracture)

Talectomy:
Technique: Similar to that described for tuberculosis of talus, in chapter of inflammatory affections of bones and joints.

## Malunion of Fractures of Metatarsals

| | |
|---|---|
| Preface | Majority of malunited fractures can be prevented by perfect treatment of fresh fractures/fracture dislocations; in certain instances, however, malunion occurs inspite of best treatment provided. |
| Definition | It is defined as a fracture that has united in an abnormal position; the deformity (fracture united in a position of persistent angulation plantarwards; producing a bony mass on the sole; mass may simulate a tumor; may impair function in one or many ways; movement may be impaired; may cause traumatic arthritis. |
| Etiology | Imperfect reduction of fracture/fracture dislocation |
| | Inadequate immobilization |
| Pathogenesis | Deformity: Angulation plantarwards results in formation of a bony mass on the sole—that may simulate a tumor. |
| Diagnosis | Deformity: |

Deformity:
- Angulation

Swelling: Bony mass on the sole

Gait: Limp

| | |
|---|---|
| Investigation | X-ray foot—AP and LAT views |
| Management | Aim of treatment: To correct deformity: |

Conservative treatment:
Analgesics, NSAIDs

Physiotherapy: IR, SWD

Angulation:
- Malunion of short duration: Closed reduction post breaking of malunion
- Malunion of long duration: Cannot be corrected by conservative measures to be corrected surgically

Surgical treatment:

Indication:
* Failed conservative measures
* Deformity:
  - Angulation

Surgery: ORIF + bone grafting

Technique:
* Incision: Over dorsum of forefoot, parallel with the shaft of affected bone/s
* Exposure of old fractures
* Osteotomy: Divide malunited fractures with an osteotome
* Reduction: By manipulation (elevating fragments)
* Fixation of fragments with medullary Kirschner wires/pins.

Postoperative:
* A cast applied from tibial tubercle to the toes for 3/52
* Cast and the pin/s removed after 3/52
* A walking boot cast applied for 6/52
* Walking in a sturdy shoe fitted with an arch support and metatarsal bar.

After care: Physiotherapy: wax bath therapy.

## Malunion of Spinal Fractures

| | |
|---|---|
| Preface | Compression fractures of the vertebral bodies often overlooked and consequently result in malunion; majority of malunited fractures can be prevented by perfect treatment of fresh fractures/fracture dislocations; in certain instances, however, malunion occurs inspite of the best treatment provided (at times, some compression of the vertebral body may persist inspite of good reduction and cast immobilization); any prolonged disability post compression fractures of the spine occurs due to inadequate rehabilitation rather than to residual deformity of the vertebral bodies. |
| Definition | It is defined as a fracture that has united in an abnormal position; the deformity (fracture united in a position of persistent compression is often displeasing; may impair function in one or many ways; that may disturb balance/gait; may result in shortening. |
| Etiology | Imperfect reduction of fracture/fracture dislocation |
| | Inadequate immobilization |
| Pathogenesis | Deformity: Compression results in incorrect transmission of force through joints above and below the fracture; shortening; secondary osteoarthritis. |
| Diagnosis | Malunion of short duration: |

Malunion of short duration:
* Pain: Persisting
* Swelling
* Local tenderness
* Movements: Painful and restricted

Malunion of long duration:
- Pain: Persisting
- Deformity: Angulation
- Shortening
- Gait: Limp

Investigation    X-ray spine—AP and LAT views

Management    Aim of treatment: To correct deformity:

Conservative treatment:

Rest

Analgesics, NSAIDs

Shortening:
- Gross shortening can be corrected by raised shoe
- 2.5 cm shortening by raising shoe heel by 1.25 cm
  > 2.5 cm shortening to be corrected surgically.

Angulation:
- Cannot be corrected by conservative measures; to be corrected surgically

Surgical treatment:

Indication:
- Failed conservative measures
- Deformity:
  – Shortening: > 2.5 cm
  – Angulation

Surgery:
- Arthrodesis of affected vertebrae

Indication: Persisting pain post 10/52 of rehabilitation

Arthrodesis spine + posterior nerve root resection

Indication: Nerve root pain restricted to distribution of 1–2 segments (post fractures of spine involving pedicles or articular facets).

## MALUNION OF UPPER LIMB FRACTURES

### Malunion of Clavicle Fractures

Preface    Majority of malunited fractures can be prevented by perfect treatment of fresh fractures/fracture dislocations; in certain instances, however, malunion occurs inspite of best treatment provided; malunions of the clavicle usually require no treatment unless massive overlapping of the fragments either causes shortening of the shoulder girdle, or nerve (brachial plexus) compression; disabling malunions are of medial or lateral thirds of clavicle

Definition    It is defined as a fracture that has united in an abnormal position; the deformity (fracture united in a position of persistent angulation or overlapping) is often displeasing; may impair function in one or many ways; movement of the adjoining joints may be impaired; may result in shortening of the shoulder girdle.

| | |
|---|---|
| Etiology | Imperfect reduction of fracture<br>Inadequate immobilization |
| Pathogenesis | Deformity: Angulation results in incorrect transmission of force through adjoining; shortening results in disability. |
| Diagnosis | Deformity:<br>• Angulation<br>• Shortening<br>Disability: Cosmetic<br>Movements of shoulder painful and restricted. |
| Investigation | X-ray clavicle—AP view<br>Management:<br>Aim of treatment: To correct deformity:<br>Conservative treatment:<br>Shortening:<br>• Cannot be corrected by conservative measures; to be corrected surgically |

Surgical treatment:

Indication:
• Failed conservative measures
• Deformity:
  – Shortening: > 2.5 cm
  – Angulation

Surgery:
• Excision: Excessive bone from posterior and inferior surfaces of clavicle
  Indication: Massive overlapping of fragments causing shortening
• Open reduction:
  Indication: Rarely indicated for cosmetic reasons
• Osteotomy:
  Indication: To lengthen the shortened clavicle due to overlapping of the fragments

Technique:
• Clavicle divided through the plane of the malunion/or an oblique osteotomy

ORIF:
• Reduction: Open reduction of fragments by manipulation followed by
• Fixation with a plate or a heavy threaded pin
• Bone grafting: Cancellous bone strips placed across osteotomy.

After care: Exercises.

## MALUNION OF HUMERUS FRACTURES

### Malunion of Humerus Neck (Anatomical and Surgical)

| | |
|---|---|
| Preface | Majority of malunited fractures can be prevented by perfect treatment of fresh fractures/fracture dislocations; in certain instances, however, |

malunion occurs inspite of best treatment provided; major fractures of the shoulder often result in restricted mobility, esp. in elderly persons; malunion of the anatomical neck of the humerus with painful traumatic arthritis may require shoulder athrodesis, or acromioplasty; major deformity of the surgical neck may be compatible with reasonable function, while major disability due to the anteriorly displaced distal fragment, may require surgical management.

| | |
|---|---|
| Definition | It is defined as a fracture that has united in an abnormal position; the deformity (fracture united in a position of persistent angulation or rotation) is often displeasing; may impair function in one or many ways; movement of the adjoining joint may be impaired; may cause traumatic arthritis. |
| Etiology | Imperfect reduction of fracture/fracture dislocation |
| | Inadequate immobilization |
| Pathogenesis | Deformity: Angulation results in incorrect transmission of force through joints above and below the fracture; shortening; traumatic arthritis. |
| Diagnosis | Deformity: |

Deformity:

- Angulation
- Shortening
- Movements: Painful and restricted.

| | |
|---|---|
| Investigation | X-ray humerus—AP and LAT views |
| Management | Aim of treatment: To correct deformity: |

Conservative treatment:

A. Malunion of short duration:

Analgesics, NSAIDs

Closed reduction: By manipulation

Immobilization: By splint, arm pouch

B. Malunion of log duration:

- Deformity: Shortening and angulation cannot be corrected by the conservative measures; to be corrected surgically

Surgical treatment:

Indication:

- Failed conservative measures
- Deformity:
  - Shortening
  - Angulation
  - Traumatic arthritis

Surgery:

- Osteotomy
- ORIF
- Bone grafting

Osteotomy + ORIF + Bone grafting:

Technique:

- Incision: Over the anterolateral aspect of the shoulder; from lateral third of the clavicle, then distally 10 cm along the anterior border of the deltoid

- Deepen incision and separate deltoid and pectoralis major muscles
- Exposure and divide the malunited bone
- Reduction of the fragments in position
- Fixation: Internal fixation with:
  - Two long screws in younger persons
  - A blade plate in older persons: Plate fixed to distal fragment, while blade (angled 30–40 degree) driven into the humeral head

Postoperative:
- An abduction splint applied with traction to immobilize the limb for 4/52
- Physiotherapy: Exercises; heat therapy: IR or SWD for 2/52.

## Malunion of Proximal third of Humeral Shaft

Preface — Majority of the malunited fractures of the proximal third of the humeral shaft, angulated medially and anteriorly/or posteriorly; while the medial angulation restricts the elbow to touch the chest, the shoulder mobility restricted in abduction and external rotation.

Management — Surgical treatment:
Surgery: Osteotomy + ORIF (compression plate) + bone grafting

Technique:
- Incision: 8 cm long anterolateral, centered over the apex of angulation
- Exposure of the malunited bone by incising the eriosteun
- Osteotomy: Divide the malunited bone, through apex of angulation
- Reduction of the fragments in position
- Fixation: Internal fixation with:
  - A compression plate
  - Bone grafting: With cancellous bone chips placed

Postoperative:
- An abduction splint applied with traction to immobilize the limb for 4/52
- Physiotherapy: Exercises; heat therapy: IR or SWD for 2/52.

## Malunion of Middle Third of Humerus

Preface — Majority of malunited fractures can be prevented by perfect treatment of fresh fractures/fracture dislocations; in certain instances, however, malunion occurs inspite of best treatment provided; rarely requires correction as the deformity (angulation, rotation, and shortening) of this bone impair function less than when the femur and the tibia are similarly affected.

Definition — It is defined as a fracture that has united in an abnormal position; the deformity (fracture united in a position of persistent angulation or rotation) is often displeasing; may impair function in one or many ways; movement of the adjoining joint may be impaired; may cause traumatic arthritis; may result in shortening.

Etiology — Imperfect reduction of fracture/fracture dislocation
Inadequate immobilization

| | |
|---|---|
| Pathogenesis | Deformity: Angulation results in incorrect transmission of force through joints above and below the fracture; shortening results in disability: traumatic arthritis. |
| Diagnosis | Deformity: |

Deformity:
* Angulation
* Rotation
* Shortening

Disability

| | |
|---|---|
| Investigation | X-ray humerus/arm—AP and LAT views |
| Management | Aim of treatment: To correct deformity: |

Conservative treatment:
* Malunion of short duration:
  Closed reduction: By manipulation followed by immobilization.
* Malunion of long duration:

Deformity: Angulation, rotation, shortening: cannot be corrected by conservative measures; to be corrected surgically

Surgical treatment:

Indication:
* Failed conservative measures
* Deformity:
  - Shortening
  - Angulation
  - Rotation

Surgery: Osteotomy + ORIF (compression plate) + bone grafting

Technique:
* Incision: 8 cm long anterolateral, centered over the apex of angulation
* Exposure of the malunited bone by incising the eriosteun
* Osteotomy: Divide the malunited bone, through apex of angulation
* Reduction of the fragments in position
* Fixation: Internal fixation with:
  - A compression plate
  - bone grafting: With cancellous bone chips placed

Postoperative:
* An abduction splint applied with traction to immobilize the limb for 4/52
* Physiotherapy: Exercises; heat therapy: IR or SWD for 2/52.

## Malunion of Distal Humerus

| | |
|---|---|
| Preface | Any surgical correction for malunion of distal humerus may increase the disability (massive scarring of the elbow joint, or exuberant callus; advisable to avoid extensive excision of soft tissues to correct malunion, unless the deformity and the disability are remarkable. Elbow trauma demand respect; they generate a vast variety of malunited fractures, |

and are often associated with the neurovascular injury as compared to any other region of the body.

Types            Malunions of the distal humerus are classified as:
- Supracondylar fracture
- Condylar fractures
- Olecranon fractures
- Epicondylar fractures

## Malunion of Supracondylar Fractures

Preface          Majority of malunited fractures can be prevented by perfect treatment of fresh fractures/fracture dislocations; in certain instances, however, malunion occurs inspite of best treatment provided.

Definition       It is defined as a fracture that has united in an abnormal position; the deformity (fracture united in a position of persistent angulation or rotation) is often displeasing; may impair function in one or many ways; movement of the elbow joint may be impaired; may cause traumatic arthritis of elbow.

Types            
- Malunion with posterior displacement
- Malunion with anterior displacement
- Malunion with medial or lateral angulation of the bone with or without rotation

Etiology         Imperfect reduction of fracture
                 Inadequate immobilization

Pathogenesis     Deformity: Angulation results in incorrect transmission of force through adjoining joints of the fracture; traumatic arthritis.

Diagnosis        Deformity:
- Angulation: Medial or lateral
- Rotation
- Displacement: Anterior or posterior

                 Disability

Investigation    X-ray arm including elbow—AP and LAT views

Management       Aim of treatment to correct deformity:
                 Mamagement of malunion of the supracondylar fractures based upon the grade of displacement including rotation of the fragments, restricted range of elbow mobility, and the age of the patient.

                 ### Malunion with posterior displacement:
                 Surgery:
                 Indication in children, malunited supracondylar fractures with major deformity (angulation and posterior displacement of distal fragment) to be treated surgically (osteotomy + ORIF).

                 Technique:
- Incision: Posterolateral incision centered over the malunion
- Exposure of triceps aponeurosis, incise a tongue shaped flap of triceps tendon, reflected distally
- Osteotomy: Divide the bone

- Excision of callus from fragments ends
- Reduction of fragments in position
- Fixation: With Kirschner wire drilled through lateral condyle, directed proximally and medially; then drill a similar wire through medial condyle, directed proximally and laterally
- Confirm the reduction radiologically or conducted under C-arm
- Wound closure.

Postoperative:
- Immobilize: The arm in a posterior right angle splint or arm sling
- Exercises: Post 3/52.

Malunion with anterior displacement:
Surgery:
Indication in children, malunited supracondylar fractures with major deformity (angulation and anterior displacement of distal fragment) is relatively infrequent; usually mobility in extension restricted; to be treated surgically (osteotomy + ORIF).

Technique:
- Incision: Posterolateral incision centered over the malunion
- Exposure of triceps aponeurosis, incise a tongue shaped flap of triceps tendon, reflected distally
- Osteotomy: Divide the bone
- Excision of callus from fragments ends
- Reduction of fragments in position
- Fixation: With Kirschner wire drilled through lateral condyle, directed proximally and medially; then drill a similar wire through medial condyle, directed proximally and laterally
- Confirm the reduction radiologically or conducted under C-arm
- Wound closure

Postoperative:
- Immobilize: The arm in a posterior right angle splint or arm sling for 3/52
- Physiotherapy: Active and passive exercises.

## Malunion of Condylar Fractures

Preface        Majority of malunited fractures can be prevented by perfect treatment of fresh fractures/fracture dislocations; in certain instances, however, malunion occurs inspite of best treatment provided; in children, the severity of the deformity, may increase with growth; malunion of lateral humeral condyle is more disabling than that of medial condyle; surgery is based upon the age of the patient and duration of the malunion.

Definition     It is defined as a fracture that has united in an abnormal position; the deformity (fracture united in a position of persistent angulation or rotation) is often displeasing; may impair function in one or many ways; movement of the adjoining joint may be impaired; may cause traumatic arthritis.

| Etiology | Imperfect reduction of fracture/fracture dislocation |
| --- | --- |
| | Inadequate immobilization |
| Pathogenesis | Deformity: Angulation results in incorrect transmission of force through joints above and below the fracture; traumatic arthritis. |
| Diagnosis | Deformity: |

- Angulation
- Rotation

Disability

| Investigation | X-ray elbow—AP and LAT views |
| --- | --- |
| Management | Aim of treatment: To correct deformity: |

Malunited medial condyle:

Surgical treatment:

Indication:

- Failed conservative measures
- Deformity:
  – Angulation
  – Rotation

Surgery:

- Osteotomy + ORIF
- Arthroplasty

Malunited lateral condyle:

Surgical treatment:

Indication:

- Failed conservative measures
- Deformity:
  – Valgus
  – Rotation

Surgery:

Malunion of short duration:

Technique: ORIF

Malunion of long duration:

Technique: Excision and remodeling of lateral condyle.

## Malunion of Olecranon

| Preface | Majority of malunited fractures can be prevented by perfect treatment of fresh fractures/fracture dislocations; in certain instances, however, malunion occurs inspite of best treatment provided. |
| --- | --- |
| Definition | It is defined as a fracture that has united in an abnormal position; the deformity (fracture united in a position of persistent angulation or displacement) is often displeasing; may impair function in one or many ways; movement of the elbow joint may be impaired; may cause traumatic arthritis. |
| Etiology | Imperfect reduction of fracture |
| | Inadequate immobilization |
| Pathogenesis | Deformity: Angulation; impaired elbow mobility; traumatic arthritis |

| | |
|---|---|
| Diagnosis | Deformity: Angulation |
| | Movements of elbow painful and restricted. |
| | Loss of power of extension |
| Investigation | X-ray elbow—AP and LAT views |
| Management | Aim of treatment: To correct deformity: |

Conservative treatment:

Malunion of short duration:

• Closed reduction and immobilization in a cast

Malunion of long duration:

• Cannot be corrected by conservative measures; to be corrected surgically

Surgical treatment:

Angulation:

• Cannot be corrected by conservative measures; to be corrected surgically

Surgical treatment:

Indication:

• Failed conservative measures

• Deformity: Angulation

Surgery: Osteotomy + ORIF + Bone grafting.

## MALUNION OF FOREARM BONES (RADIUS AND ULNA)

## Malunion of Monteggia Fracture Dislocation

| | |
|---|---|
| Preface | Majority of malunited fractures can be prevented by perfect treatment of fresh fractures/fracture dislocations; in certain instances, however, malunion occurs inspite of best treatment provided; malunion of Monteggia fracture dislocation may often result in deformity that is often so disabling that requires a reconstruction surgery. |
| Definition | It is defined as a fracture that has united in an abnormal position; the deformity (fracture united in a position of persistent anterior or posterior angulation) is often displeasing; may impair function in one or many ways; movements (flexion of elbow and supination and ponation) of the adjoining joints may be impaired; may cause traumatic arthritis. |
| Etiology | Imperfect reduction of fracture dislocation |
| | Inadequate immobilization |
| Pathogenesis | Deformity: Angulation of ulnar shaft; dislocation of radial head; callus formed about radial head; ankylosed radioulnar and elbow joints; traumatic arthritis. |
| Diagnosis | Deformity: |

• Angulation: Posterior: angulation of ulna with head dislocated posteriorly, anterior: angulation of ulna with head dislocated anteriorly

• Shortening of forearm

Movements: Painful and restricted (radioulnar and elbow)

| Investigation | X-ray forearm including elbow and wrist—AP and LAT views |
| Management | Aim of treatment: To correct deformity: |

Conservative treatment:

Malunion of short duration:

Closed reduction and immobilization in a cast

Malunion of long duration:

- Cannot be corrected by conservative measures; to be corrected surgically

Surgical treatment:

Indication:

- Failed conservative measures
- Deformity:
  - Angulation
  - Ankylosed joints

Surgery: Osteotomy + ORIF + Bone grafting.

Technique:

- Incision from 2.5 cm proximal to elbow and lateral to triceps tendon; distally over to lateral side of olecranon tip; then along ulnar border; ending at junction of proximal and middle thirds of ulna.
- Deepen the interval between ulna and anconeus and extensor carpi ulnaris
- Exposure of radial head by stripping and reflecting the anconeus
- Divide: The radial neck just proximal to bicipital tuberosity
- Exposure of ulnar malunion by stripping and reflecting the supinator
- Osteotomy: Divide the malunited ulna
- Reduction of ulnar fragments in position
- Fixation of ulnar fragments by passing an intramedullary nail
- Bone grafting: Place cancellous bone strips about the osteotomy

Postoperative:

- Immobilization: Apply an above elbow cast, with elbow at right angle, and the forearm in neutral position, for 12/52

After care: Physiotherapy: active exercises.

## Malunion of Shafts of Radius and Ulna

| Preface | Majority of malunited fractures can be prevented by perfect treatment of fresh fractures; in certain instances, however, malunion occurs inspite of best treatment provided; disability in children from malunited shafts of radius and ulna, often corrects itself with growth; overlapping in children rarely requires correction; angular deformity usually requires correction; malunion of both bones of the forearm in adults usually not to be treated surgically unless deformity (angulation and overlapping) and disability are markedly severe. |
| Definition | It is defined as a fracture that has united in an abnormal position; the deformity (fracture united in a position of persistent angulation or |

rotation) is often displeasing; may impair function in one or many ways; movement of the adjoining joint may be impaired; may cause traumatic arthritis; may result in shortening.

| | |
|---|---|
| Etiology | Imperfect reduction of fracture |
| | Inadequate immobilization |
| Pathogenesis | Deformity: Angulation results in incorrect transmission of force through joints above and below the fracture; shortening; traumatic arthritis. |
| Diagnosis | Deformity: |

- Angulation
- Shortening

Disability

| | |
|---|---|
| Investigation | X-ray forearm including elbow and wrist—AP and LAT views |
| Management | Aim of treatment: To correct deformity: |

Conservative treatment:

Shortening:

- 2.5 cm shortening: Rarely requires correction
- > 2.5 cm shortening: To be corrected surgically.

Angulation:

- Cannot be corrected by conservative measures; to be corrected surgically

Surgical treatment:

Indication:

- Failed conservative measures
- Deformity:
  - Shortening: > 2.5 cm
  - Angulation

Surgery:

- Children: Osteotomy + ORIF
- Adults: Osteotomy + ORIF + Bone grafting

Technique (in adults):

- Incision: Two longitudinal incisions (medial and lateral) each centered over malunion
- Exposure of malunited radial and ulnar shafts
- Osteotomy: Divide radius and ulna, through malunion plane
- Reduction of fragments in position
- Fixation of radius with compression plate and screws; of ulna with intramedullary nailing (ulnar nailing first)
- Bone grafting: Place cancellous bone strips about osteotomies
- Wounds closure.

Postoperative: An above elbow cast applied with elbow at right angle and forearm in neutral position for 2/52; reduction checked radiologically; a snug cast applied for 12/52.

After care: Physiotherapy: exercises.

## Malunited Colles' Fracture

**Preface**      Majority of malunited fractures can be prevented by perfect treatment of fresh fractures; in certain instances, however, malunion occurs inspite of best treatment provided; malunion occurs more often post Colles' fracture than any other, and may result in considerable disability; until signs and symptoms are relatively static or an apparent improvement, surgery delayed may be beneficial.

**Definition**      It is defined as a fracture that has united in an abnormal position; the deformity (fracture united in a position of persistent angulation or rotation) is often displeasing (esp. in ladies); may impair function in one or many ways; movement of the adjoining joint may be impaired; may cause traumatic arthritis.

**Etiology**      Imperfect reduction of fracture

Inadequate immobilization

Comminuted fracture

**Pathogenesis**      Deformity: Dinner fork: angulation (backwards and radially) and rotated; radial and ulnar styloid processes at same level; traumatic arthritis; Sudeck's atrophy.

**Diagnosis**      Deformity:
- Angulation
- Rotation

Disability

**Investigation**      X-ray forearm including hand—AP and LAT views: malunited fracture; osteoporotic bones

**Management**      Aim of treatment: To correct deformity:

Conservative treatment:

Physiotherapy: Active exercises

Angulation:
- Cannot be corrected by conservative measures; to be corrected surgically

Surgical treatment:

Indication:
- Failed conservative measures
- Deformity:
  - Angulation
  - Rotation

Surgery:
- Osteotomy of radius + reconstructions + bone grafting
- Resection of distal ulna + division of deep transverse carpal ligament
- Arthrodesis of the wrist
- Resection of distal ulna + arthrodesis

**Resection of distal ulna + division of deep transverse carpal ligament:**
Indication:
- More often than other surgical procedures, because bony union post surgery not required nonunion and recurrent malunion are

insignificant; radial deformity (angulation up to 30 degree and shortening) may be acceptable by resecting distal ulna

- To improve functioning of wrist and hand: by decompressing the carpal tunnel.

Technique:

- Incision: A medial longitudinal incision
- Exposure of distal ulna subperiosteally
- Osteotomy: Divide ulna about 2.5 cm proximal to distal end
- Divide: Capsule and styloid process at its base; spare it attached to the ulnar collateral ligament
- Reef and plicate: Periosteum and ligament

Postopertive: No immobilization required.

After care: Active exercises.

### Osteotomy of radius + reconstructions + bone grafting

Indication: Rarely indicated for malunited Colles' fracture, esp. past age of fifty years; an attempt to restore radial length is impractical

- To restore position of distal articular surface of radius

Technique:

- Incision: A dorsal curvilinear, beginning at Lister's tubercle; extending proximally 5–7 cm
- Deepen: The incision between extensor carpi radialis longus and brevis laterally and extensor pollicis longus and extensor digitorum communis medially
- Exposure of bone subperiosteally
- Osteotomy Divide the bone at the level of malunion
- Reduction of distal fragment by manipulation to restore its articular surface
- Fixation of distal fragment with a Kirschner wire, drilled through radial styloid, across the osteotomy, through the proximal fragment; cut off the wire underneath the skin
- Bone grafting: About the osteotomy with cancellous bone strips
- Resect: Distal ulna if required
- Wound closure.

Postoperative: An above elbow splint applied, with forearm in neutral and wrist in little flexion; discard the splint post 6/52.

After care: Active exercises.

### Malunited Smith's Fracture

Preface        Majority of malunited fractures can be prevented by perfect treatment of fresh fractures/fracture dislocations; in certain instances, however, malunion occurs inspite of the best treatment provided; extreme of angulation requires surgery.

Definition     It is defined as a fracture that has united in an abnormal position; the deformity (fracture united in a position of persistent flexion of the distal radial fragment) is often displeasing; may impair function in one or many ways; movement of the adjoining joint may be impaired; may cause traumatic arthritis.

| | |
|---|---|
| Etiology | Imperfect reduction of fracture |
| | Inadequate immobilization |
| Pathogenesis | Deformity (distal end of radius displaced anteriorly): traumatic arthritis. |
| Diagnosis | Deformity: |

- Angulation

Disability.

| | |
|---|---|
| Investigation | X-ray forearm including wrist—AP and LAT views |
| Management | Aim of treatment: |

- To restore radial length
- To shorten the ulna
- To resect the distal ulna

Conservative treatment:

Malunion of short duration:

Closed reduction and immobilization

Angulation:

- Cannot be corrected by conservative measures; to be corrected surgically

Surgical treatment:

Indication:

- Failed conservative measures
- Deformity: angulation
- Shortening
- Traumatic arthritis

Surgery:

Resection of ulna

Technique:

- Incision: Medial incision 8 cm long

Exposure of distal ulna

Osteotomy: Resect a segment of bone, to correct discrepancy

Reduction of fragments in position

Fixation of fragments with a screw/or wire loop

Postoperative: A long arm cast applied for 6/52

After care: Active exercises.

## Malunion of Hand

| | |
|---|---|
| Preface | Majority of malunited fractures can be prevented by perfect treatment of fresh fractures/fracture dislocations; in certain instances, however, malunion occurs inspite of best treatment provided; malunited fractures of hand result in weakened grasp and pinch, esp. in case of metacarpals and proximal phalanges being involved; functioning of fingers and hand are the determining factors for requirement of necessary treatment or not; majority of malunited fractures of metacarpal neck (esp. of 5th) |

not to be treated as the carpometacarpal joint permits displacement of the distal end of the bone (exception is that of 2nd and 3rd metacarpals).

**Definition**          It is defined as a fracture that has united in an abnormal position; the deformity (fracture united in a position of persistent angulation or rotation) is often displeasing (deviation of digits); may impair function in one or many ways; movement of the adjoining joint may be impaired; may cause traumatic athritis.

**Etiology**          Imperfect reduction of fracture/fracture dislocation
Inadequate immobilization

**Pathogenesis**          Deformity: Angulation; traumatic arthritis.

**Diagnosis**          Deformity:
- Angulation

**Investigation**          X-ray hand—AP and LAT views

**Management**          Malunion of metacarpal neck:
Aim of treatment: To correct deformity:

Conservative treatment:
- Mostly malunited fractures of the metacarpal neck not to be treated, esp. those of neck of 5th metacarpal, as the carpometacarpal joint usually permits dorsal displacement of the distal end of the bone; exception: of 2nd and 3rd metacarpals—as the carpometacarpal joints lack mobility and require surgery (osteotomy).
- Angulation: Cannot be corrected by conservative measures; to be corrected surgically.

Surgical treatment:
Indication:
- Failed conservative measures
- Deformity: Angulation

Surgery: Osteotomy.
Technique:
- Incision: A dorsal longitudinal, proximal and lateral to metacarpal head
- Exposure of extensor hood and retract it laterally
- Dissect: Free neck of muscles
- Osteotomy of bone at level of malunion
- Bone grafting: A peg bone graft (ulnar or tibial), fitted int ends of proximal and distal fragments; pack cancellous bone chips about the osteotomy
- Capsulotomy: For contracted collateral ligaments
- Sururing of lateral expansion of extensor hood in position
- Wound closure.

Postoperative: Apply a volar splint with flexed joints of the finger
Malunion of metacarpal shaft or a phalanx:

Surgery: A medullary cortical bone peg or Kirschner wire + bone graft

## Bibliography

1. Armstrong JR. Bone grafting in ther treatment of fractures, Williams and Wilkins Co., Baltimore, 1945.
2. Blount WP. Proximal osteotomies of the femur, American Academy of Orthopedic Surgeons Instructional Course Lectures, Vol. IX, Ann Arbor, J.W. Edwards, p.1, 1952.
3. Boyd HB. The treatment of malunited fractures of the ankle, American Academy of Orthopedic Surgeons Instructional Course Lectures, vol. II, Ann Arbor, 1944, J.W. Edwards, p. 60.
4. Campbell WC. Malunited colles' fractures, J.A.M.A. 109:1105, 1937.
5. Campbell WC. Malunited fractures and unreduced dislocations about the elbow, J.A.M.A. 92:122, 1929.
6. Campbell WC. Malunited fractures, Surg., Gynec. and Obst. 66:466, 1938.
7. Campbell's Operative Orthopaedics (1998) 9th Ed. Vol I-IV. Canale S. Terry, Daugherty K, and Jones Linda. Mosby.
8. Charnley J. Malunion: Bailey and Love's Short Practice of Surgery, ed. 13th, H.K. Lewis and Co., London, 1965.
9. Clark JMP. Modern Trends in Orthopedics Fracture Treatment, Butterworths, London, 1962.
10. Darrach W. Colles' fracture, New England J. Med. 226:594, 1942.
11. Dingman PVC. Resection of the distal end of the ulna (Darrach operation), Bone and Joint Surg. 34-A:893, 1952.
12. French PR. Vasrus deformity of the elbow following supracondylar fractures of the humerus in children, Lancet 1:439, 1959.
13. Hallock H. Arthrodesis of the ankle joint for old painful fractures, J. Bone and Joint Surg. 27:49, 1945.
14. Kapoor PS. Malunion: Kapoor's Accident and Emergency, 2nd Ed., CBS, New Delhi, 2016.
15. McRae R. Malunion: Practical Fracture Treatment, ed. 1st, Churchill Livingstone, 1981.
16. Mukopadhaya B. Treatment of malunited Colles' fracture, (A new method with a report on 40 cases), Indian J. Surg. 20:95, 1958.
17. Practical Fracture Treatment 1st Ed., Mc Rae R, Churchill Livingstone, 1981.
18. Smith H. Malunited fractures: Campbell's Operative Orthopaedics, ed. 9th, vol. I, C.V. Mosby Co., Saint Louis, 1998.
19. Speed JS, Knight RA. The treatment of malunited Colles' fractures, J. Bone and Joint Surg. 27:361, 1945.

# 8

# Traumatic Affections of Joints

**Acute traumatic synovitis of knee**
Internal derangements of joints
- Of knee joints
- Of ankle joints
- Of talofibular joints
- Of radioulnar joints
- Of temporomandibular joints

Old ruptures of ligaments
- Of knee

Osteochondritis dissecans
- Of hip
- Of knee
- Of patella
- Perthes' disease
- Osgood Schlatter's disease
- Sever's disease
- Kohler's disease
- Freiberg's disease
- Scheuermann's disease
- Calve's disease
- Kienböck's disease

Chondromalacia of patella
Coccygodynia
Baseball Pitcher's shoulder
Baseball Pitcher's elbow

| Preface | Trauma is the main cause of majority of joint affections (traumatic arthritis, synovitis; arthropathies; rheumatoid arthritis (atrophic); gout; syphilis; low backache; epiphysitis; osteoarthritis (hypertrophic; tuberculosis; metabolic, and may be the chief cause of many other disorders. |

## ACUTE TRAUMATIC SYNOVITIS OF KNEE

| Definition | It is defined as the synovium (synovial membrane) response to the trauma |
| Etiology | Traumatic |

| | |
|---|---|
| Pathogenesis | Pathological changes that occur in the knee immediately post injury depend upon the nature, site, and severity of the injury; hypersecretion of synovial fluid; synovial effusion; distended knee; may be hemarthrosis (injured bone, cruciate ligaments, menisci, or synovium and capsule; blood clots (I/A fractures); synovial fluid becomes acidic (pH decreased); fibrosed; adhesions formed; chronic synovitis with hypertrophy and proliferation of synovial folds. |
| Diagnosis | Pain |
| | Swelling |
| | Local tenderness |
| | Movements: Painful and restricted |
| | Fever: May or may not be present |
| | Weakness, lethargy, anorexia |
| D/d | Acute suppurative arthritis |
| | Hemophilic joints |
| | Internal derangement of knee (IDK) |
| Investigation | CBC, ESR |
| | Synovial fluid analysis: Culture and serological tests |
| | X-ray knee: AP and LAT views |
| | MRI |
| | CT scan |
| Management | As per precise diagnosis based on detailed history, adequate physical examination and investigations including X-rays. |
| | Conservative treatment: |
| | Rest |
| | Cold therapy: Ice packs |
| | Traction: Buck's |
| | Analgesics/NSAIDs |
| | Surgical treatment: |
| | Surgery: Aspiration of knee. |

Aims:
- To relieve pain
- To prevent stretching of (synovium, capsule, and ligaments)
- To analyze synovial fluid.

After care:
- Apply an elastic crepe bandage
- Rept. aspiration every 3rd or 4th day
- Exercises.

## INTERNAL DERANGEMENTS OF JOINTS

| | |
|---|---|
| Definition | Internal derangement of joints is mainly applied to various affections (intra-articular or extra-articular or both, mostly caused by trauma, that interferes with the joint's functioning; internal derangements of knee are much more common than those of other joints. |
| Pathogenesis | Disturbed joint mechanics |

## Internal Derangements of Knee (IDK)

| | |
|---|---|
| Preface | Internal derangements of knee are common and mostly disabling until and unless diagnosed promptly and managed perfectly. |
| Anatomy | Knee joint is formed by the distal end of femur, the patella, and the proximal end of tibia; is the largest and most complicated body's joint; in all positions: the patella remains in contact with the femur, and the femur with the tibia; the bones do not interlock with one another; dislocation of the knee is rare because of large articular surfaces, strong ligaments and adjoining muscles; femoral condyles partly separated from tibial condyles by the two menisci / semilunar cartilages; two strong bands (cruciate ligaments) cross each other like letter X, ascend from upper surface of tibia to femoral condyles, and the fibrous capsule that envelops the joint incompletely. |

Mobility of knee joint:

- Rotary locking: With knee fully extended; the menisci compressed between articular surfaces; tight ligaments: restrict mobility (rotation, forward and backward gliding, medial and lateral side movements of tibia on the femur.
- Rotary motion of femur on tibia: In walking
- Hyperextension: Prevented by the collateral ligaments, cruciate ligaments, oblique popliteal ligament, posterior portion of capsule, the anterior portions of menisci, contour of the femoral condyles, and the muscles controlling the knee joint.
- Hyperflexion: Prevented by cruciate ligaments, posterior portions of menisci, posterior capsule attachment to femur, contour of the femoral condyles, and the muscles controlling the knee joint.

Stability of knee joint: By the following structures:

- Muscles and tendons
- Ligaments
- Capsule
- Menisci
- Contours of bones

| | |
|---|---|
| Frequency | Internal derangements of the knee joint are much more common than those of other joints. |
| Movements | Flexion and exension |
| Classification | IDK includes following: |

- Injury to collateral ligaments—commonly medial
- Injury to meniscus or cartilage—commonly medial
- Cysts of lateral meniscus
- Injury to cruciate ligaments
- Injury to infrapatellar pad of fat
- Fracture of tibial spine
- Loose bodies

## Injury to Collateral Ligaments

| | |
|---|---|
| Preface | Ligaments and capsule of knee are significant passive stabilizers of joint; aid in preventing hyperextension and hyperflexion of knee; commonly the medial collateral ligament is injured; aid in preventing. |

## Injury to Medial (Tibial) Collateral Ligament

| | |
|---|---|
| Anatomy | Long, flat band (wider in the middle); originates from medial epicondyle of femur just below adductor tubercle of femur, descends, attached to margin of medial tibial condyle and to upper tibial shaft; fused with the fibrous capsule opposite femoral-tibial space; related to tendons of semitendinosus, sartorius, gracilis, semimembranosus; and oblique popliteal ligament. |
| MOI | Forcible abduction strain, on the extended leg, due to: |
| | RSA |
| | Sports injury |
| | Fall downstairs |
| | Direct violence |
| Types of injury | Tear of anterior portion of deep layer; and avulsion/or rupture. |
| Pathogenesis | Usually associated with injury to the medial meniscus, due to attachment of its deeper fibers to the meniscus. By further continued strain, the cruciate ligament esp. the anterior one may rupture. |
| Diagnosis | Pain on the medial side of knee |
| | Local tenderness |
| | Movements of knee: Painful and restricted, esp. abduction |
| Investigation | X-ray knee—AP and LAT views, to rule out any bony lesion |
| Management | Conservative treatment: |
| | Analgesics |
| | Elastic crepe bandage or knee cap |
| | SWD/IRD |
| | Local massage |
| | Rest |
| | Surgical treatment: |

Surgery:
- Repair of collateral ligament
- Meniscectomy
- Repair of anterior cruciate ligament (ACL)

Technique: Repair of medial (tibial) collateral ligament:
- Incision: A longitudinal incision centered over medial aspect of knee
- Exposure of entire ligament: focus on the injured part (hematoma)
- Inspection of any associated meniscus tear, or cruciate ligament tear
- Separate superficial layer from deeper layer at site of injury
- Repair deeper layer first with nonabsorbable interrupted sutures, then repair of superficial layer

- Reattach (if detached from bone) with bone through drilled holes in the bony cortex
- Wound closure with interrupted silk sutures.

Postoperative: A long leg cast applied with knee flexed to 10–15 degree; active exercises (quadriceps and hamstrings); cast and stitches removed after 2/52; a walking cylindrical cast applied from groin to above ankle; walking with aid of crutches; post 6/52 walking cast removed, followed by active exercises.

Technique: Repair of medial collateral ligament, anterior cruciate ligament, and medial meniscus (triad of O'Donoghue):

- Incision: A long curved incision from medial epicondyle of femur, descends, crossing anteromedial aspect of knee joint, to 7 cm distal from knee joint over to anteromedial aspect of leg
- Exposure of entire ligament: Focus on the injured part (hematoma)
- Inspection of any associated meniscus tear, or cruciate ligament tear
- Separate superficial layer from deeper layer at site of injury
- Exposure of joint through incision in the capsule
- Excision of medial meniscus (torn body)
- Repair of medial meniscus (torn peripheral attachment)
- Inspection of any associated cruciate rupture (mostly ACL):
- Repair of ACL
- Repair deeper layer first with nonabsorbable interrupted sutues, then repair of superficial layer
- Reattach (if detached from bone) with bone through drilled holes in the bony cortex
- Wound closure with interrupted silk sutures.

Postoperative: A long leg cast applied with knee flexed to 10–15 degree; active exercises (quadriceps and hamstrings); cast and stitches removed after 2/52; a walking cylindrical cast applied from groin to above ankle; walking with aid of crutches; post 6/52 walking cast removed, followed by active exercises.

### Injury to Medial Meniscus

| | |
|---|---|
| Preface | Commonest cause of internal derangement of knee joint is traumatic injury to one of the menisci (tear, rupture/or vertical splitting of medial meniscus); often occur in partly flexed knee due to sudden, forcible lateral rotation or abduction of the tibia (sports injury, e.g. football playing); torn displaced. |
| MOI | RSA |
| | Sports injury—esp. common in footballers |
| Mechanism of injury | The flexed knee is subjected to rotational and abduction strains. The knee momentarily opens upon the medial side, the meniscus is sucked inside and gets nipped between the condyles of femur and tibia, resulting in a tear. Repeated strains lead to a 'Bucket handle' tear. |
| Diagnosis | Usuall a footballer |

|                | History of locking of knee, followed by sudden unlocking and effusion |
|----------------|-----------------------------------------------------------|
|                | Local tenderness |
|                | McMurray's test—positive |
| Investigation  | X-ray knee—AP and LAT views, to rule out any bony lesion |
| Management     | Conservative treatment: |
|                | Rest |
|                | Analgesics, elastic crepe bandage or knee cap |
|                | SWD/IRD |
|                | Local massage. |
|                | Surgical treatment: Refer the patient to the orthopedic team for surgery. |
| Surgery        | Meniscectomy. |

## Injury to Lateral Meniscus

|            | It is a rare injury. |
|------------|----------------------|
| MOI        | Sports injury |
| Management | Conservative treatment: |
|            | Analgesics |
|            | SWD/or IRD |
|            | Knee cap. |

## Cysts of Lateral Meniscus

| Diagnosis  | Pain on the lateral side of knee |
|------------|----------------------------------|
|            | Swelling: A round hard swelling over lateral side of knee. |
| Management | Surgical treatment of choice. |
|            | Surgery: Excision of cyst. |

**Refer:** The patient to the orthopedic team for surgery

## INJURY TO CRUCIATE LIGAMENTS

### Anterior Cruciate Ligament (ACL) Injury

| MOI | Direct violence |
|-----|-----------------|
| Pathogenesis | Isolated tears are uncommon, and usually associated with tears of medial collateral ligament and/or medial meniscus |
| Diagnosis | Abnormal forward movement of tibia over femur |
|  | Knee can be hyperextended |
| Investigation | X-ray knee—AP and LAT views, for any bony lesion |
| Management |  |
| Conservative treatment | Plaster cylinder for 6 weeks—If anterior tibial spine is intact |
| After care | Physiotherapy |
| Surgical treatment | Refer the patient to the orthopedic team for surgery |
| Surgery | ORIF (screw fixation)—if anterior tibial spine is fractured |
|  | Reattach/or ACL replacement (tendon of semitendinosus) is the treatment of choice—if ACL is avulsed |

Repair of associated tears of medial collateral ligament and medial meniscus.

## Posterior Cruciate Ligament (PCL) Injury

| | |
|---|---|
| MOI | Direct violence |
| Pathogenesis | Tibia is forced backwards |
| Diagnosis | Abnormal backward movement of tibia over femur |
| Investigation | X-ray knee—AP and LAT views, for any bony lesion |
| Management | Same as for ACL injury |

## Injury to Infrapatellar Pad of Fat

| | |
|---|---|
| MOI | When hypertrophied, may be nipped in between the femur and tibia during extension of the knee |
| Diagnosis | History of pain and locking of knee without being followed by sudden unlocking (cf. medial meniscus injury) |
| | Local tenderness over sides of ligamentum patellae |
| Investigation | X-ray knee—AP and LAT views, for any bony lesion |
| Management | Refer the patient to the orthopedic team for surgery |
| Surgery | Excision of hypertrophied fat |

## FRACTURE OF TIBIAL SPINE

### It is a Rare Injury, Common in Children

| | |
|---|---|
| MOI | Fall on the bent knee with a violent twist of tibia over the femur |
| Diagnosis | Local tenderness underneath ligament patellae |
| | Extension knee—painful and restricted |
| Investigation | X-ray knee—AP and LAT views |
| Management | |

## Conservative Treatment

| | |
|---|---|
| Indication | Undisplaced fracture |
| Treatment | Aspiration of knee and plaster cylinder |
| Surgical treatment | Refer the patient to the orthopedic team for surgery |
| Indication | Displaced fracture |
| Surgery | ORIF of fragment with a screw, or |
| | Excision of fragment |

## Loose Bodies

| | |
|---|---|
| MOI | Direct violence |
| Diagnosis | History of locking at different angles each time |
| Investigation | X-ray knee—AP and LAT views |
| Management | Refer the patient to the orthopedic team for surgery |
| Surgery | Sugical removal |

## Internal Derangement of Ankle Joints (Chronic Sprain of Ankle)

| | |
|---|---|
| Preface | Internal derangements of the ankle joint is common and mostly disabling until and unless diagnosed promptly and managed perfectly. |
| Anatomy | Ankle joint is a synovial joint of the hinge type; formed by talus and distal ends of tibia and fibula; joint of great strength; its stability is provided by its strong ligaments and tendons around it, and by the closed interlocking of the articular surfaces; talus articulates with bones of leg (tibia and fibula forming a socket-mortice). |
| | Ligaments: Medial (deltoid), lateral, anterior and posterior. |
| MOI | Direct trauma: violence |
| | RSA |
| | Sports injury |
| | Fall downstairs |
| Predisposing factors | Traumatic: |
| | • Injured deltoid ligament |
| | • Ruptured lateral ligament |
| | • Dislocation/or subluxation |
| | Deformed: |
| | • Angulated tibia or fibula. |
| Pathogenesis | Torn capsule/synovia; ruptured deltoid and lateral ligaments |
| Diagnosis | Pain |
| | Local tenderness |
| | Clicking joint: On moving of ankle |
| | Weakness |
| | Movements: Painful and restricted. |
| Investigation | X-ray ankle—AP and LAT views, to rule out any bony lesion |
| | MRI of ankle |
| Management | Surgical treatment: |
| | Indications: |
| | Ruptured ligaments: |
| | Management: Repair |
| | Dislocation/subluxation: |
| | Management: Reduction (closed or open) |
| | Angulated tibia or fibula |
| | Management: Osteotomy |

## Internal Derangement of Talofibular Joint

| | |
|---|---|
| Preface | Internal derangements of the talofibular joints is common and mostly disabling until and unless diagnosed promptly and managed perfectly. |
| Anatomy | The fibula articulates with the tibia by both of its ends; proximal tibio-fibular joint is a synovial joint, while the distal joint is a syndesmosis, i.e. bones held together by ligaments, that do not enclose a cavity. |
| | Movements: Only possible are those permitted by slight stretching and twisting of the ligaments; interosseus membrane common—to both |

joints; ligaments are: interosseus ligament, anterior and posterior inferior tibiofibular ligaments, transverse tibiofibular ligament.

| | |
|---|---|
| MOI | Direct trauma: Violence |
| | RSA |
| | Sports injury |
| | Fall downstairs |
| Predisposing factors | Traumatic: |

- Injured interosseus ligament
- Ruptured tibiofibular ligaments
- Dislocation/or subluxation

Deformed:

- Angulated tibia or fibula.

| | |
|---|---|
| Pathogenesis | Torn ulnar interosseus ligament; ruptured tibiofibular ligaments |
| Diagnosis | Pain |
| | Local tenderness |
| | Weakness. |
| | Movements: Painful and restricted. |
| Investigation | X-ray ankle – AP and LAT views, to rule out any bony lesion |
| | MRI of ankle |
| Management Indications: | Surgical treatment: |
| | Ruptured ligaments: |
| | Management: Repair |
| | Dislocation/subluxation: |
| | Management: Reduction (closed or open) |
| | Angulated tibia or fibula: |
| | Management: Osteotomy |

## Internal Derangement of Radioulnar Joints

| | |
|---|---|
| Preface | Internal derangements of the radioulnar joints is common and mostly disabling until and unless diagnosed promptly and managed perfectly. |
| Anatomy | Radioulnar joints are two: proximal radioulnar joint: formed by the medial part of radial head and the radial notch of the ulna-articular disk; its ligaments: annular and quadrate |

- Distal radioulnar joint: Formed by the ulnar head and the ulnar notch of the radius; united by fibrous capsule and the articular disk (real bond of union)

| | |
|---|---|
| MOI | Direct trauma: Violence |
| | RSA |
| | Sports injury |
| | Fall downstairs |
| Predisposing factors | Traumatic: |

- Injured articular disk
- Injured ulnar collateral ligament
- Ruptured distal radioulnar ligaments
- Dislocation/or subluxation

Deformed:
- Angulated radius or ulna
- Enlarged ulnar head

| | |
|---|---|
| Pathogenesis | Torn articular disk; torn ulnar collateral ligament; ruptured distal radioulnar ligaments |
| Diagnosis | Pain |
| | Local tenderness |
| | Clicking joint: On rotation of forearm |
| | Ulnar head: Prominent |
| | Weakness of grip and of wrist |
| Investigation | X-ray wrist—AP and LAT views, to rule out any bony lesion |
| | MRI of wrist |
| Management | Surgical treatment: |

Indications:
- Torn articular disk:

Management: Excision of disk

Ruptured ligaments:
Management: Repair

Dislocation/subluxation:
Management: reduction (closed or open)

Angulated radius or ulna:
Management: osteotomy

## Internal Derangement of Temporomandibular Joint

| | |
|---|---|
| Preface | Internal derangements of the temporomandibular joint is rare, but disabling until and unless diagnosed promptly and managed perfectly. |
| Anatomy | Temporomandibular joint is the articulation of mandibular head with the articular fossa and articular tubercle of the temporal bone; is a synovial joint; its cavity is separated into an upper and a lower part by an articular disk; fibrous capsule attached superiorly to the temporal bone around margins of articular fossa and tubercle, and inferiorly to the mandibular neck; its lateral part  thickened to form the triangular temporomandibular/or lateral ligament—attached by its base to the zygoma and tubercle of the zygoma's root, and by its apex to the lateral side of the mandibular neck; muscles of mastication mainly keep the mandible in its place. |
| | Movements are depression, elevation, protraction, retraction, and side to side or chewing. |
| MOI | Direct trauma: Violence |
| | RSA |
| | Sports injury |
| | Fall downstairs |
| | Degeneration of disk or degenerative arthritis. |
| Pathogenesis | Degenerated articular disk—torn or wrinkled; degenerative arthritic changes |

| Diagnosis | Pain |
|---|---|
| | Local tenderness |
| | Snapping or popping of joint |
| | Movements: Painful and restricted |
| Investigation | X-rays of TM joint—AP and LAT views, to rule out any bony lesion |
| | MRI of TM joint |
| Management | Conservative treatment: |
| | Rest |
| | Analgesics/NSAIDs |
| | Warm fomentation |
| | Immobilization: Mandibular splint |
| | Surgical treatment: Usually contraindicated, unless pian severe—not relieved by conservative measures |

Indications:
- Torn articular disk:

Management: Excision of disk

Ruptured ligaments:

Management: Repair

Dislocation/subluxation:

Management: Reduction (closed or open)

Degenerative arthritis or recurrent subluxation:

Management: Resection of mandibular condyle.

## OLD RUPTURES OF LIGAMENTS

### Old Ruptures of Ligaments of Knee

| Definition | Old ruptures of the collateral and cruciate ligaments are diagnosed with the help of same tests meant for acute ruptures, while the tests are easier to perform and diagnosis more precise as per reactions to acute trauma are absent |
|---|---|
| Etiology | Traumatic |
| Pathogenesis | Damaged articular surfaces; torn ligaments; torn menisci; arthritic changes; degenerative joint |
| Diagnosis | Pain: May or may not be present |
| | Swelling+– |
| | Local tenderness |
| | Muscle: Weakness |
| | Movements: Painless but restricted |
| Investigation | X-rays knee—AP and LAT views |
| Management | Surgical treatment: |
| | Surgery: Reconstruction |
| | Preoperative: Criteria to be considered: |

- Age and general health of the patient: Elderly patients too much debilitated to achieve much strength in the stabilizing muscles, may better be managed in a brace/or with a cane or crutches.

- Condition of the articular surfaces of the joint; with the damaged articular surfaces, reconstruction of the ligaments is of little practical value.
- Strength of muscles controlling the joint: Quadriceps, hamstring, and gastrosoleus groups—to be strong enough, otherwise joint will be unstable/flail.
- Particular ligaments ruptured: Collateral ligament with an old rupture causing valgus or varus instability and recurrent episodes of IDK, are to be reconstructed; cruciate ligament with an old rupture causing anterior or posterior instability—unjustify reconstruction; for persisting instability, ACL may be reconstructed.
- Limitations of reconstruction procedures: Surgery cannot restore fully the structure and function of the original ligaments; the reconstructions of collateral ligaments are more satisfactory than those of the cruciates.

### Reconstruction of old ruptured tibial collateral ligament:

Many procedures been advocated from extensive excision of supporting tissues, i.e. tendons/or fascia, to form an inadequate replica of original ligament:

Technique:

A. Transferring (Mauck): Distal attachment of the ligament to a further distal point on the tibia (to restore its tension)
   Indication: Only for tibial collateral ligament.
B. Transferring (Lange, et al.): Proximal attachment of the ligament to a further proximal point on the femur (to restore its tension)
   Indication: For tibial collateral ligament
C. Transferring (Edwards—modified): Attachment of flaps from fascia lata and biceps tendon.

### Reconstruction of old ruptured anterior cruciate and tibial collateral ligaments (Hey Groves—modified):

Technique:

- Incision: Anteromedial incision to expose the knee joint; a second longitudinal incision over lateral aspect of thigh ending distal to fibular head, to expose fascia lata
- Explore: Flex the knee and explore the knee joint
- Strip: Through 2nd incision, free a strip of fascia lata (20 × 8 cm), and reflect it distal ward, leaving it anchored to fibular head
- Drill: An olique hole through the lateral femoral condyle, opening posteriorly into intercondylar notch; drill a 2nd oblique hole through tibia (from anteromedial prominent part of medial tibial condyle, opening just anterior to the tibial spine
- Passage of fascia strip through the holes in the tibia and femur; with knee flexed to right angle, pull the fascial strip taut; fix its proximal end to the medial femoral condyle with silk sutures/or steel staples.

After care: Apply a long leg cast with the knee flexed to 15 degree; begin exercises from 1/52; removal of cast post 4/52; then walking in a brace for 3/12.

### Reconstruction of old ruptured fibular collateral ligament (Edwards—modified):

Technique:
* Incision: Longitudinal over lateral aspect of distal thigh and proximal leg, centered over fibular head
* Exposure of fascia lata, biceps femoris tendon, lateral femoral condyle, and the fibular head
* Isolate and protect: The peroneal nerve
* Flap: Raise a facial flap of ligament girth; then raise a similar flap from the tibial tendon
* Grooves: Make grooves in the lateral femoral condyle and fibular head
* Fixation of biceps tendon flap into the femoral groove, and fascia lata flap into the fibular groove

Modification: For avulsed biceps tendon from the fibula:
* Drill: An anteroposterior hole through fibular head
* Flap: Raise a rectangular flap of fascia lata; pass it through fibular hole; then suture it to the biceps tendon under tension.

After care:
* Apply a long leg cast with knee slightly flexed for 3/52
* Active exercises (quadriceps and hamstring)
* Weight bearing allowed post 4/52.

## OSTEOCHONDRITIS DISSECANS

| | |
|---|---|
| Definition | It is defined as an area of subchondral bone that undergoes avascular necrosis, and degenerative changes that occur usually in the overlying cartilage, until and unless interrupted by surgical or conservative measures, the necrotic bone and the overlying cartilage separate gradually from adjacent bone and cartilage, thereby forming a loose body. |
| Types | Synovial chondromatosis |
| | Traumatic loose bodies: By fracture |
| | Detached osteophytes: Due to degenerative changes |
| Etiology | Traumatic: Intra-articular fracture |
| | Degenerative: Osteoarthritis |
| Pathogenesis | Avascular necrosis of subchondral bone, overlying cartilage degenerated, loose body formation. |
| Diagnosis | Joints: Knee, elbow, shoulder, ankle, hip |
| | Swelling |
| | Local tenderness |
| | Movements: Painful and restricted |
| | Disability: Difficulty in walking |

| Investigation | X-ray of affected joint: Loose body(s) seen |
| Management | Conservative treatment: |

Conservative treatment:
- Weight bearing to be restricted: May help in the revascularization of the avascular bone and preservation of the overlying cartilage
- Immobilization of knee in 30 degree flexion by plaster cast
- Walking with crutches, without weight bearing on the affected leg

Surgical treatment:
Indications: Detached osteochondritic area.

Surgery:
- Excision of osteochondric lesion
- Removal of loose bodies:
Postoperative: Immobilization for 2–3/52.
After care:
Physiotherapy:
Exercises

## Osteochondritis Dissecans of Hip

Definition    It is defined as an osteochondritis characterized by the lesion that is the same as that of the knee except that the cartilage overlying the avascular fragment of bone usually remains intact, and ultimately a loose body is not formed; weight bearing area of the head usually affected; without treatment the area collapses, and osteoarthritis develops.

Etiology    Traumatic: Intra-articular fracture
Degenerative: Osteoarthritis

Pathogenesis    Avascular necrosis of subchondral bone, overlying cartilage degenerated, loose body formation.

Diagnosis    Pain
Local tenderness
Movements: Painful and restristed
Disability: Difficulty in walking.

Investigation    X-ray pelvis—AP view: Loose body(s) seen

Management    Conservative treatment:
- Weight bearing to be restricted: May help in the revascularization of the avascular bone and preservation of the overlying cartilage
- Immobilization: By traction
- Walking with crutches, without weight bearing on the affected leg.

Surgical treatment:
Indication: Small osteochondritic lesion
Surgery: Drilling to restore revascularization of area
Indication: Large lesion
Surgery: Drilling + packing with cancellous bone to maintain contour of the articular surface
Indications: Detached osteochondritic area.
Surgery:
- Excision of osteochondric lesion

- Removal of loose bodies:
    Postoperative: Immobilization for 2–3/52.
After care:
Physiotherapy:
Exercises

## Osteochondritis Dissecans of Knee

Definition | It is defined as an osteochondritis characterized by the lesion that is usually found on the medial femoral condyle near the attachment of the posterior cruciate ligament, but may occur anywhere on the articular surface of medial condyle, and sometimes on that of the lateral femoral condyle or the inferomedial surface of the patella.

Etiology | Traumatic: Intra-articular fracture
Degenerative: Osteoarthritis

Pathogenesis | Avascular necrosis of subchondral bone, overlying cartilage degenerated, loose body formation.

Diagnois | Joints: Knee
Swelling
Local tenderness
Movements: Painful and restricted
Disability: Difficulty in walking

Investigation | X-ray of knee joint: Loose body(s) seen

Management | Conservative treatment:
- Weight bearing to be restricted: May help in the revascularization of the avascular bone and preservation of the overlying cartilage
- Immobilization of knee in 30 degree flexion by plaster cast
- Walking with crutches, without weight bearing on the affected leg

Surgical treatment:
Indications: Detached osteochondritic area.
Surgery:
- Excision of osteochondric lesion
- Removal of loose bodies:
    Postoperative: Immobilization for 2–3/52.
After care:
Physiotherapy:
Exercises

## Osteochondritis of Patella

Definition | It is defined as an osteochondritis characterized by the lesion that is usually found anywhere on the patella esp. on its femoral surface.

Etiology | Traumatic: Fracture; fracture-dislocation
Degenerative: Osteoarthritis

Pathogenesis | Avascular necrosis of bone; degenerated, loose body formation.

Diagnois | Joints: Knee
Swelling

Local tenderness
Movements: Painful and restricted
Disability: Difficulty in walking

**Investigation** X-ray of knee joint: Loose body(s) seen

**Management** Conservative treatment:
- Weight bearing to be restricted: May help in the revascularization of the avascular bone and preservation of the overlying cartilage
- Immobilization of knee in 30 degree flexion by plaster cast
- Walking with crutches, without weight bearing on the affected leg.

Surgical treatment:
Indications: Detached osteochondritic area.

Surgery:
- Excision of osteochondric lesion
- Removal of loose bodies:
  Postoperative: Immobilization for 2–3/52.
After care:
Physiotherapy:
Exercises

## Perthes' Disease (Syn. Coxa Plana, Pseudocoxalgia)

**Definition** It is defined as a disability characterized by limping, muscular wasting, restricted movements of hip joint, present mostly in boys between the age of 5–15 years.

**Etiology** Unknown
Genetic
Traumatic

**Pathogenesis** Femur head flattened, fragmented, and condensed

**Diagnosis** Sex: Commoner in boys than girls
Age: 5–15 years.
Pain and limp: Early symptoms
Deformity: Limb adducted and externally rotated
Muscular westing
Movements: Abduction and internal rotation restricted, while flexion and extension are free and painless

**Investigation** X-ray pelvis: AP view: shows marked incongruity, flattening of femoral head, femur displaced upwards, confirmed by Shenton's line.

**Management** Conservative treatment:
Bedrest
Traction
Diathermy: SWD, Infrared
Analgesics, NSAIDs
Surgical treatment:
Indications: Failure of conservative measures.
Surgery:
Drilling of proximal femoral epiphysis

Correction of disturbed soft tissues

Osteotomy: Trochanteric

Arthrodesis: Hip fixed in flexion and adduction.

## Osgood-Schlatter's Disease (Syn. Epiphysitis of Tibial Tuberosity)

| | |
|---|---|
| Definition | It is defined as a disability characterized by pain, limping, undualy prominent tibial tubercle, restricted sports activities, mostly in boys between the ages of 10–15 years. |
| Etiology | Unknown |
| | Genetic |
| | Traumatic: Sports trauma |
| | Infective |
| Pathogenesis | Tibial epiphyseal separated (partial) |
| Diagnosis | Sex: Commoner in boys than girls |
| | Age: 10–15 years. |
| | Pain |
| | Deformity: Prominent tibial tubercle |
| | Local tenderness |
| | Walking/running: Painful |
| Investigation | X-ray: Shows partial separation of the tongue shaped portion of the epiphysis from the shaft |
| Management | Conservative treatment: |
| | Bedrest |
| | Avoid strenuous exercises |
| | Diathermy: SWD, Infrared |
| | Strapping |
| | Analgesics, NSAIDs, Antibiotics |
| | Cylinder walking cast for 8–10 weeks |
| | Surgical treatment: Rarely indicated. |
| | Indications: Failure of conservative measures. |
| | Surgery: |
| | Excision of bony prominence (Thomson) |
| | Insertion of bone pegs (Bosworth) |
| | Postoperative: Cylinder walking cast (groin to toes) × 2/52. |
| | After care: |
| | Physiotherapy: |
| | Exercises |
| | SWD/IR therapy. |

## Sever's Disease (Syn. Apophysitis of os Calcis)

| | |
|---|---|
| Definition | It is defined as a disability characterized by pain, limping, undualy prominent heel, restricted sports activities, mostly in boys between the ages of 10–15 years. |
| Etiology | Unknown |
| | Genetic |

|  | Traumatic: Sports trauma |
|---|---|
|  | Infective |
|  | Endocrinal |
| Pathogenesis | Fragmented, irregular epiphysis |
| Diagnosis | Sex: Commoner in boys than girls |
|  | Age: 10–15 years. |
|  | Pain |
|  | Deformity: Prominent heel |
|  | Local tenderness |
|  | Walking/running: Painful |
| Investigation | X-ray: Shows fragmentation and irregularity of epiphysis |
| Management | Conservative treatment: |
|  | Bedrest |
|  | Avoid strenuous exercises |
|  | Diathermy: SWD, Infrared, wax bath |
|  | Analgesics, NSAIDs |
|  | Shoe: Cut away at the back to relieve pressure, and raised heel to relax the calf muscles. |
|  | Surgical treatment: Rarely indicated. |
|  | Indications: Failure of conservative measures. |
|  | Surgery: Excision |

## Kohler's Disease (Syn. Osteochondritis of os Scaphoid Tarsal)

| Definition | It is defined as a disability characterized by pain, disability, restricted sports activities, mostly in boys between the ages of 5–10 years, due to osteochondritis of navicular epiphysis. |
|---|---|
| Etiology | Unknown |
|  | Genetic |
|  | Traumatic: Sports trauma |
| Pathogenesis | Fragmented, irregular navicular epiphysis, flattened head of the talus |
| Diagnosis | Sex: Commoner in boys than girls |
|  | Age: 5–10 years. |
|  | Pain |
|  | Deformity: Prominent foot (dorsum near ankle) |
|  | Local tenderness |
|  | Walking/running: Painful |
| Investigation | X-ray: Shows fragmentation and irregularity of epiphysis, disk like scaphoid |
| Management | Conservative treatment: |
|  | Bedrest |
|  | Avoid strenuous exercises |
|  | Diathermy: SWD, Infrared, wax bath |
|  | Analgesics, NSAIDs |
|  | Strapping support |

Shoe: Cut away at the back to relieve pressure, and raised heel to relax the calf muscles.

Surgical treatment: Rarely indicated.

Indications: Failure of conservative measures.

Surgery: Arthrodesis of midtarsal joints (talonavicular and calcaneocuboid).

## Freiberg's Didease

| | |
|---|---|
| Definition | It is defined as a disability characterized by pain, disability, restricted sports activities, mostly in young adults, due to osteochondritis of head of second or third metatarsal. |
| Etiology | Unknown |
| | Genetic |
| | Traumatic: Sports trauma |
| Pathogenesis | Flattened articular surface and irregular sclerosed head of the metatarsal. |
| Diagnosis | Sex: Commoner in boys than girls |
| | Age: 10–15 years. |
| | Pain |
| | Deformity: Prominent foot (dorsum near metatarsal head) |
| | Local tenderness |
| | Walking/running: Painful |
| Investigation | X-ray: Shows flattened articular surface and irregular sclerosed head of the metatarsal |
| Management | Conservative treatment: |
| | Bedrest |
| | Avoid strenuous exercises |
| | Diathermy: SWD, Infrared, wax bath |
| | Analgesics, NSAIDs |
| | Shoe: Provision of metatarsal bar |
| | Surgical treatment: Rarely indicated. |
| | Indications: Failure of conservative measures. |
| | Surgery: Excision of the metatarsal head. |

## Scheuermann's Disease

| | |
|---|---|
| Definition | It is defined as epiphysitis, affecting the epiphysis, usually of one single or multiple vertebrae in the thoracic region, mostly in adolescents, characterized by deformity, pain, and disability. |
| Etiology | Unknown |
| | Genetic |
| | Traumatic: Sports trauma |
| Pathogenesis | Flattened articular surface and irregular sclerosed head of the metatarsal. |
| Diagnosis | Sex: Commoner in boys than girls |
| | Age: 10–15 years. |
| | Pain |

Deformity: Kyphosis (round) of thoracic spine, compensated by lordosis of the lumbar spine below it, round shoulders

Local tenderness

Walking/running: Painful

| | |
|---|---|
| Investigation | X-ray: Shows irregular anterosuperior and anteroinferior angles of the vertebral bodies at the site of normal epiphysis |
| Management | Conservative treatment: |

Bedrest

Analgesics, NSAIDs

Diathermy: SWD, Infrared, wax bath

Brace

Active exercise

Surgical treatment: Rarely indicated.

Indications: Failure of conservative measures.

Arthrodesis of spine

## Calve's Disease

| | |
|---|---|
| Definition | It is defined as epiphysitis, affecting the epiphysis, usually of one single vertebra, mostly in infants or very small children, characterized by deformity, pain, and disability. |
| Etiology | Unknown |
| | Genetic |
| | Traumatic: Birth trauma |
| Pathogenesis | Flattened and irregular sclerosed articular surface of vertebra. |
| Diagnosis | Sex: Commoner in boys than girls |
| | Age: Infants and very young children |
| | Pain |
| | Deformity: Prominent spine |
| | Local tenderness |
| | Walking/running: Painful |
| Investigation | X-ray: Shows flattened and irregular sclerosed articular surface |
| D/d | Tuberculosis. |
| Management | Conservative treatment: |

Bedrest

Diathermy: SWD, Infrared

Analgesics

Strapping: Adhesive plaster

Surgical treatment: Rarely indicated, as hardly any deformity or disability occurs in later life.

After care:

Physiotherapy

Exercises

SWD/IR.

## Kienböck's Disease

| | |
|---|---|
| Definition | It is defined as epiphysitis, affecting the epiphysis, usually of one single vertebra, mostly in infants or very small children, characterized by deformity, pain, and disability. Disability characterized by pain, disability, restricted sports activities, mostly in young adults, due to osteochondritis of head of second or third metatarsal. |
| Etiology | Unknown |
| | Genetic |
| | Traumatic: Sports trauma |
| Pathogenesis | Flattened articular surface and irregular sclerosed head of the metatarsal. |
| Diagnosis | Sex: Commoner in boys than girls |
| | Age: 10–15 years. |
| | Pain |
| | Deformity: Prominent foot (dorsum near metatarsal head) |
| | Local tenderness |
| | Walking/running: Painful |
| Investigation | X-ray: Shows flattened articular surface and irregular sclerosed head of the metatarsal |
| Management | Conservative treatment: |
| | Bedrest |
| | Avoid strenuous exercises |
| | Diathermy: SWD, Infrared, wax bath |
| | Analgesics, NSAIDs |
| | Shoe: Provision of metatarsal bar |
| | Surgical treatment: Rarely indicated |
| | Indications: Failure of conservative measures |
| | Surgery: Excision of the metatarsal head. |

## CHONDROMALACIA OF PATELLA

| | |
|---|---|
| Definition | Chondromalacia of patella is defined as degeneration of its articular cartilage; usually frequent and results in osteoarthritis of the knee joint; the patellofemoral joint is usually the first body joint to undergo degenerative changes |
| Etiology | Direct trauma: Violence, recurrent subluxation or dislocation of patella, fractured patella, IDK |
| Predisposing | Obesity, disturbed quadriceps mechanism (knee lockings) factors |
| Pathogenesis | Degenerative changes; arthritic; ankylosed |
| Diagnosis | Pain: Deep seated subpatellar |
| | Swelling |
| | Local tenderness |
| | Crepitus |
| | Locking: Knee |
| | Movements of knee and patella painful and restricted |

| | |
|---|---|
| Investigation | X-rays knee—AP and LAT views: May show fracture, dislocation, degenerative changes |
| Management | Symptomatic: |

Conservative treatment:

- Analgesics/NSAIDs
- Closed reduction of fracture, fracture dislocation

Surgical treatment:

Indication: IDK, arthritic lesions

Surgery:
- Exploration of knee joint

Shaving of involved cartilage

Arthroplasty

Patellectomy or patellaplasty

Technique of patellaplasty:

- Incision: Medial parapatellar incision to expose the knee joint
- Explore: The knee thoroughly; meniscectomy—if required
- Excision: Turnover patella with its articular surface facing anteriorly, separate patella from the attached synovial membrane, quadriceps expansion and patellar tendon, from its edges; with an electric saw cut one-fourth of the patella in a frontal plane
- Flap: Prepare a flap from infrapatellar pad of fat; turn the flap proximally to cover the raw surface of the patella
- Suture: Its flap's edges to the adjoining synovium and tendinous cuff; return the thinned patella to its original position
- Wound closure: In layers.

After care: Elastic crepe bandage for 1/52.
- Exercises: Quadriceps and hamstrings
- Weight bearing with crutches ASAP.

Technique of patellectomy:

- Incision: Transverse incision at level of lower third of patella; incise the quadriceps expansion in line with incision
- Excision of patella by sharp dissection
- Overlap: Edges of quadriceps mechanism (to restore tension)
- Wound closure: In layers.

After care: Quadriceps exercises ASAP.

## COCCYGODYNIA (COCCYDYNIA)

| | |
|---|---|
| Definition | Coccygodynia is defined as painful coccyx; may be of functional origin, or may be organic and results either from rigidity of the sacrococcygeal joint or from traumatic arthritis of this joint without rigidity. |
| Etiology | Traumatic: Violence |
| | Fall from a height |
| | Sports injury |
| | Functional |

|  | Organic |
|  | Spasmodic |
| Pathogenesis | Arthritic changes |
| Investigation | X-rays pelvis—AP view |
| Management | Conservative treatment: |
|  | Rest |
|  | Warm fomentation; SWD; IR |
|  | Analgesics/NSAIDs |

Local infiltration: Inj. Lignocaine 1% (1–5 ml) plain mixed with 1 ml of triamcinolone, hydrocortisone acetate, or methylprednisolone

Surgical treatment:
Indication:
- Organic coccygodynea: Rarely indicated for rigid sacrococcygeal joint and painful sitting due to pressure on the bone
- Traumatic arthritis: Developed in a movable sacrococcygeal joint

Contraindication:
- Functional coccygodynea: Highly nervous persons often the pain decreases without treatment or increased by any treatment
- Traumatic arthritis: With low backache
- Acute injuries of sacrococcygeal joint

Surgery: Coccygectomy
Preoperatively: Local infiltration with lignocaine + steroid (relieve pain)

Technique:
- Incision: Longitudinal centered over sacrococcygeal joint
- Excision of coccyx, by separating the sacrococcygeal joint
- Suturing of wound.

After care: Toilet of the wound with full care to prevent infection.

## BASEBALL PITCHER'S SHOULDER

| Definition | Baseball pitcher's shoulders are often occupational and are caused by repeated severe strains of the joint. |
| Etiology | Occupational: Repeated strains |
|  | Sports injury |
| Pathogenesis | Injured single structure or multiple structures; degenerated arthritic changes; irritated capsule and synovium cause irritation of radial nerve; exostosis formed on the glenoid; frayed or degenerated rotator cuff tendons caused by repeated snubbing of the cuff over the humeral head and greater tuberosity. |
| Diagnosis | Pain: Referred to deltoid region |
|  | Local tenderness |
|  | Movements of shoulder painful and restricted. |
| Investigation | CBC, ESR |
|  | X-ray shoulder—AP and LAT views |

| | |
|---|---|
| Management | Conservative treatment: |
| | Warm fomentation |
| | Analgesics/NSAIDs |
| | Local infiltration: Inj. Lignocaine 1% 2 ml with hydrocortisone |
| | Surgical treatment: |
| | Surgery: Exploration |

## BASEBALL PITCHER'S ELBOW

| | |
|---|---|
| Definition | Baseball Pitcher's shoulders are often occupational and are caused by repeated severe strains of the joint. |
| Etiology | Occupational: Repeated strains |
| | Sports injury |
| Pathogenesis | Traumatic arthritis; thickened synovial membrane; fibrillated cartilage; spurred junction of bone and cartilage; loose bodies in the joint. |
| Diagnosis | Pain: Over front of medial humeral condyle |
| | Swelling |
| | Local tenderness |
| | Movements of elbow painful and restricted |
| Investigation | CBC, ESR |
| | X-ray elbow—AP and LAT views |
| Management | Conservative treatment: |
| | Warm fomentation |
| | Analgesics/NSAIDs |
| | Local infiltration: Inj. Lignocaine 1% 2 ml with hydrocortisone |
| | Surgical treatment: |
| | Surgery: |
| | • Excision of osteophytes from origin of the common flexor group of muscles, olecranon, and olecranon fossa. |
| | Dividing the deep fascia covering the pronator teres. |

## Bibliography

1. Advanced Paediastric Life Support: Advanced Life Support Group, the practical approach, 3rd Ed., BMJ Books, London, 2001.
2. Aritomi H, Yamamoto M. A method of Arthroscopic Surgery. Clinical evaluation of Synovectomy with the Electric Resectoscope and Removal of Loose bodies in the Knee Joint, Orthopedic Clinics of North America 10: 565–84, 1979.
3. Chatterjee CC. Human Physiology, 5th Ed., Books and Allied Pvt. Ltd., Calcutta, 1963.
4. Clark JMP. Modern Trends in Orthopaedics: Fracture Treatment, 3, Butterworths, London, 1962.
5. Cunningham's Manual Of Practical Anatomy, vol. I-III, 12th Ed., Oxford University Press, London, 1961.
6. Das K. Clinical Methods In Surgery, 6th Ed., Lakshman Chandra Sil, Calcutta, 1962.
7. Gilltes H, Seligson D. Arthrograpgy and Arthroscopy: Precision in the Diagnosis of Meniscal Lesions: A Comparison of Clinical Evaluation, J. Bone and Joint Surg. 61-A: 343–6, 1979.
8. Hargreaves DJ, Seedhom BB. On the 'bucket-handle' tear: Partial or total meniscectomy? A quantitative study. J Bone and Joint Surg. 61-B: 381, 1979.
9. Huckstep RL. A Simple Guide to Trauma, 5th Ed., Churchill Livingstone, Edinburgh, 1995.
10. McGinty JB, Matza RA. Arthroscopy of the Knee: Evaluation of an out-Patient Procedure under Local Anesthesia, J Bone and Joint Surg. 60-A: 787–9, 1978.

11. Jenkins JL, Braen R, Richard G. Manual of Emergency Medicine, 4th Ed., Lippincott Williams and Wilkins, Philadelphia, 1999.

12. Johnstone RW. A Text Book of Midwifery, 20th Ed., Adam and Charles Black, London, 1965.

13. Kapoor PS. Accident and Emergency: Etiology, Diagnosis, and Management, 2nd Ed., CBS, New Delhi, 2016.

14. Keele CA, Neil E. Samson Wright's Applied Physiology, 10th Ed., Oxford University Press, London, 1963.

15. Krupp MA, Chatton MJ. Current Medical Diagnosis and Treatmernt, Maruzen Asian Edition, Bombay, 1975.

16. Mattox KL. Complications of Trauma, Churchill Livingstone, Edinburgh, 1994

17. McGREGOR AL. A Synopsis of Surgical Anatomy, 9th Ed., John Wright and Sons Ltd., Bristol, 1963.

18. McRae R. Practical Fracture Treatment, 3rd Ed., Churchill Livingstone, Edinburgh, 1994.

19. Mirvis SE, Young JWR. Imaging in Trauma and Critical Care, Williams and Wilkins, Baltimore, 1992.

20. Operative Principles of Ilizarov: Fracture Treatment—Nonunion, Osteomyelitis—Lengthening, Deformity correction, A.S.A.M.I. Group, Williams and Wilkins, Milan, Italy, 1991.

21. Raby N, Berman L, de Lacy G. Accident and Emergency Radiology, W.B. Saunders Co., Philadelphia, 1997.

22. Shaw's Textbook of Gynaecology, 8th Ed., Howkins J., J. and A. Churchill Ltd., London, 1962.

23. Trunkey DD, Lewis FR. Current Therapy of Trauma, 4th Ed., Mosby Year Book, St Louis, 1998.

24. Watanabe M, Takeda S, Ikeuchi H. Atlas of Arthroscopy, 2nd Ed., Igaku Shoin Ltd., Tokyo, 1969.

# 9

# Amputations

**Types**
- Closed amputation
- Open amputation

Regional amputations
- Upper limb
  - Fingertip amputation
  - Wrist amputation
  - Wrist disarticulation
  - Forearm
  - Elbow disarticulation
  - Upper arm amputation
    ◊ Above elbow
    ◊ Mid-shaft
  - Shoulder amputations
    ◊ Surgical neck
    ◊ Shoulder disarticulation
    ◊ Forequarter amputation
- Lower limb
  - Toes
  - Forefoot
  - Midfoot
  - Ankle
  - Syme
  - Boyd
  - Leg
  - Knee disarticulation
  - Thigh
  - Epicondylar tendoplastic
  - Supracondylar tendoplastic
  - Hip disarticulation
  - Hindquarter amputation
  - PVD amputations

**Definition**      It is defined as the removal of a limb through the continuity of the bone, while disarticulation is the resection through a joint.

**Principles**      Anatomical factors governing selection of site for amputation:
- Extent and nature of trauma or disease
- Certain anatomical principles

- Nature of stump (length and shape): In the leg a long stump is inferior to 15 cm one, whereas a short stump may be difficult/impossible to fit in a prosthesis, so that, it is better in certain cases to loose a joint above rather than to be handicapped by a very short stump.
- An arthritic (knee) joint above the projected stump: Advisable to do above knee rather than below knee amputation.

Weight bearing: May be:

- End bearing: Skin at the end of stump unable to bear pressure of the body weight, without developing trophic ulcers and pressure sores
- Lateral bearing (tibial, ischial): Weight bearing at the accessible bony points of the joint above the amputation.

Exception: Syme amputation.

- Diffuse bearing: Due to friction between skin and prosthesis, only a part of the weight taken in this way, otherwise a tendency exist for the skin to be pulled upwards. A well fitted prosthesis for the lower limb bears weight all round that part of the limb above the amputation site that is embraced by the bucket.

Stump: A good healthy stump requires to be:

- Covered by healthy skin that is nonadherent to the stump
- Skin flaps to be free of muscles or tendons
- Tissues covering bone end, must not be bulky ones
- Scar to be painless, nonadherent, and free from pressure in the prosthesis.

**Types**

- Closed amputation
- Open amputation

**Closed amputation**

It is a final amputation performed for the aim of producing a stump that may be used effectively with a prosthesis.

**Principles**

- Tourniquet: To be avoided, because its use may impair circulation by initiating vascular spasm and thrombosis formation.
- Skin and deeper tissues to bleed freely at the site of amputation
- Skin flaps to be highly vascular, so as to avoid atrophic damage
- To avoid excessive muscle damage, and to be trimmed off in such a fashion as to give a cone-shaped appearance to the stump, distally severed about 1 cm below the bone end, not to be sutured over the end of the stump.
- Periosteum to be incised at the amputation level, and to be stripped distally
- Bone to be divided through intact periosteum and smoothed
- Nerve not to be pulled while sectioned
- Blood vessels to be doubly ligated before dividing.

**Emergency (temporarily) closed amputation:** It is not a final amputation for the purpose of using in an artificial limb, but rather is a method for providing loose skin closure, and adequate drainage for the traumatized tissues and can be easily convertible into an open amputation, in case of developing infection. It is indicated in acute injuries, wherein debridement would permit closure of the wound, if no amputation were present, provided: reasonable tissue viability, infection not imminent, eliminated dead space.

Procedure: Closing of the flaps of a circular open amputation, by interrupted sutures to ensure skin viability and obliteration of dead space, or debridement of all soft tissues of doubtful viability, obliteration of dead space, bone resection at the site whereby the bone is ensheathed with muscle, and easy closure of available flaps.

**Surgical amputation:** To save the life or to preserve the health of patient, by severing from the body a harmful limb, to improve function, by resecting wholly or partially, a deformed or useless limb, and thereby substituting for it an artificial prosthesis from the functional point of view, and to remove an unsightly part for cosmetic reasons. In case of impaired blood supply of the limb, amputation is mandatory, to safeguard the life from release of toxins from destroyed tissues.

Specific indications for removal:
- Uncontrolled infection
- Malignant tumor (necrosed, infected, fungating mass)
- Deformity: Congenital, awkward, deformed, useless limb.

Drawbacks

Mental hazard: Some patients unable to surmount psychologically for amputation, as readjustment post surgery is more difficult as compared to any other available orthopedic procedure.

Principles of final amputation technique:
- Mandatory clean operative field: Skin free of foreign matter, crusts, and blemishes. In case of closing an open wound, effort to be made to prevent tissue contamination and destruction. Old open wounds must be clean, firm, red granulating surface, that are usually prepared by debridement, eliminating deep infections.
- Mandatory provision of a good skin coverage over the end of the stump, the skin must have normal sensation and free mobility and an adequate subcutaneous fat. The healed surgical scar to be flat, thin, and nonadherent, and to be placed over the site least subjected to any undue pressure or tension.
- Skin flaps consist of skin and fascia only; to be sutured under normal tension, as tight flaps tend to breakdown due to tension and avascularity, while loose skin folds fit poorly in a prosthesis.

## Rules for Length of Flap

Upper limb
- Above the level of wrist: Anterior and posterior flaps of equal length, so as to ignore pressure from the prosthesis on the sides of the stump.
- Distal to wrist: A long anterior and short posterior flap, so as to provide thick, tough palmar skin for stump coverage.

Lower limb:
- Hip: Through racquet incisions, the scar on the anterior or lateral aspects of the stump, to keep scar away from weight bearing ischial tuberosity.

- Thigh: An anterior flap 2.5 cm longer than the posterior one, so that the scar to be 2.5 cm above the bone end.
- End bearing amutations of lower end of femur: A long anterior and a short posterior flap, so that suture line lie posteriorly and above the weight bearing end of the stump.
- Below knee: An anterior flap 1.0 cm longer than the posterior one, so that the scar lies 1.0 cm above the bone end.
- Syme amputation: A long posterior heel anterior used, so that the scar lies anteriorly above the weight bearing area.

**Open amputation** Skin is not sutured over the end of the wound. It is a temporary procedure, must always be followed by a secondary amputation, as final repair of the stump.

Aim: To control and eliminate infection, so that the final amputation performed without any risk of wound's breakdown.

Indications:
- Presence of a traumatic wound with extensive tissue damage
- Infection made probable by unavoidable delay
- Controlled or uncontrolled sepsis present.

Principles of open amputation:
- To be carried out at the lowest possible level consistent with control of infection, so that maximum tissue available for the final repair.

Types:
- Circular open amputation
- Open amputation with skin flaps.

Circular open amputation: It is method of choice, meets all the requirements—affords generous open drainage, eliminates dead space, eliminates necrotic tissue, precludes osteomyelitis and soft tissue infection, preserves bone length, and the procedure can be performed rapidly and easily, by using a tourniquet, and the bone to be divided at the most distal site so as to eliminate the risk of actuator potential sepsis.

Postoperative: Skin traction to be applied (stockinet), and continued until the granulating area is fixed by cicatrix or healed by scar.

Open amputation with skin flaps: Skin is cut like formal flap, secondary closure carried out early to avoid an open granulating wound with minimal subsequent dressings, often sacrifices valuable skin that may be required in future repair.

Open disarticulation: Simple, rapid, and easy procedure, the tissues proximal to the joint undisturbed, to be used inlater on in the final revision. The skin flaps to be cut longer due to great elasticity and contractibility of the skin around joints.

Indication: Joint level most distal, where sepsis can be controlled

Procedure: Knee and hip joints.

## Regional Amputations

Upper limb  Aim: To maintain or to substitute for the functional elements of the part. In case of fingers and metacarpals, amputations aimed to preserve the function of left over parts, and to retain the essential elements, i.e. grasp, pinch, and hook; and at proximal levels, aimed to create a stump that is capable of supporting and activating a prosthesis—substitute effectively for the amputated hand.

Preoperative factors to be evaluated:
- Function/s that injured digits fulfill
- Extent to which loss of each amputated segment affects the hand
- Relative importance of each basic hand function to an individual, i.e. appearance, occupation, and use of the hand.
- Number of digits and metacarpals: Their length, power, sensation, mobility.

Importance of hand:
- Thumb: Most essential digit of the hand.
  Function: Grasp and pinch, due to its length and mobility, its wide range movement of circumduction depends upon balanced motor elements, integrated first metacarpal hinge, and free movement allowed by the skin and the muscles in the web space between thumb and the index finger.
- Index: 2nd most important digit next to thumb.
  Function: Forms the lateral pole of finger elements in grasp and pinch. Its metacarpal loss including loss of transverse metacarpal ligament results in loss of grasp and stability.
- Middle finger: Fills the span in grasp and prevents objects from falling through the fingers of the clentched hand.
  Function: In conjunction with index finger, provides strength and stability to grasp and pinch. Its metacarpal's loss results in impaired strength and mobility.
- Ring finger: Fills the span in grasp, and prevents objects from falling through the fingers of the clentched hand.
  Function: In conjunction with little finger provides the palmar arch with mobility. Its metacarpal's loss results in rotator deviation of adjacent fingers.
- Little finger: Mainly important because of its ulnar position.
Function: Provides breadth and stability to grasp, and provides palmar arch with mobile dexterity. Its metacarpal provides stability by sharing breadth of the palm in grasp.

## Fingertip Amputation

| | |
|---|---|
| MOI | Crushing, avulsing, or slicing injuries. |
| Pathogenesis | Involve skin alone, skin and bone, or skin, bone, and fingernail. |
| Diagnosis | Wound: Tender, painful |
| | Scar: Tender, breakdown with mild trauma |
| | Length: Loss |
| Management | Surgical repair (graft) or reamputation at higher level. |
| | Aim: To provide skin coverage to maintain length to achieve good function to provide skin with sensation |

Procedures:
- Split thickness skin graft: Maintains maximum possible length, and excellent coverage, esp. for injued finger (dorsal aspect)
- Full-thickness skin graft: Maintains maximum possible length, and provide more durable skin than split thickness graft
- Skin flap: Provides an excellent coverage of skin and subcutaneous tissue; indicated for denuded bone or for extensive subcutaneous tissue loss.

Drawback: Prolonged disability because of two stage procedure
- Cross finger graft: Valuable in covering the defect of an adjacent finger. A split thickness skin graft used to cover the base of the skin flap and the raw surface left over by its elevation.

Recepient: Injured thumb

Donor: Middle, ring, or little finger
- Regional flaps: Obtained from the thenar eminence and base of the palm. Defect covered with a split thickness skin graft.
  Drawback: Scarring in the palm
- Sliding-flap graft: Provides sensation by swinging a skin flap over the denuded area, thereby indicated in transverse fingertip amputations, wherein area of sensitive skin lost. Donor area covered with a split thickness skin graft.
- Plastic closure: Indicated in transverse fingertip amputations

Procedure of making two V-shaped incisions through the skin and subcutaneous tissue, one on each side of the finger with the apex of the V pointing proximally, the two triangular skin flaps created are shifted distally to cover the end of the stump, and are sutured in the midline.

## Amputations Through Fingers and Metacarpals

Aims:
- To maintain, restore, or re-establish function
- To achieve best cosmetic results.

Principles:
- Up to PIP joint, loss of function is in direct contrast to loss of length
- No shortening of bone
- Coverage of terminal wound with a skin graft, the skin over the bone and denuded areas to be well circulated and sensory, and well padded to bear the trauma of use.
- Mobility of hand to be maintained by avoiding development of soft tissue contracture.
- To prevent injury to the intrinsic muscles, so as to safeguard medial and lateral movements of the adjacent fingers and extension of their IP joints.
- Amputation through proximal phalanx forms a useless stump, may be helpful in grasping by index and little fingers.
- Metacarpal amputation forms a useless stump, that may contribute to breadth of the hand.

Surgery: Long palmar and short dorsal skin flaps made in the ratio of 2:1

Free skin grafts: Split thickness or full thickness, provide excellent coverage for the dorsal, terminal, and lateral wounds in the freshly amputated finger, an early graft to avoid inevitable infection.

## Amputations and Disarticulations of Wrist

Advantages: Have advantages over forearm amputation:
- No elbow joint in the prosthesis, and no cuff above elbow to restrict flexion or to cause discomfort in the cubital fossa arm retains supination and pronation

Criteria: Stump to be covered with palmar skin, and without any protruding bony prominences, and intact radioulnar joint, and unimpaired vascularity and sensation of the stump.

## Amputation of Wrist

Criteria: A long palmar and a short dorsal flap in the ratio of 2:1 mandatory.

Procedure:
- Flaps dissected proximally to expose the soft tissues to the bone level
- Flexors and extensors of fingers pulled down and sectioned, so as to retract into forearm, whereas flexors and extensors of the wrist reflected above bone level, and later on reattached to bone end, to preserve wrist movements
- Nerves (ulnar, median and radial, drawn downward and sectioned to retract above the wrist joint
- Bone divided with an electric saw and smoothened
- Skin flaps under normal tension, approximated over bone end by interrupted sutures.

## Disarticulation of Wrist

Criteria: A long palmar and a short dorsal flap in the ratio of 2:1 mandatory.

Procedure
Skin incision: 1 cm distal to styloid processes, extended downwards into palm and dorsum of hand, to form a long palmar and a short dorsal flap:
- Expose radiocarpal joint
- Radial and ulnar arteries divided and doubly ligated
- Nerves (ulnar, median and radial, drawn downward and sectioned to retract above the wrist joint
- Carpus and hand freed
- Skin flaps under normal tension, approximated over bone end by interrupted sutures.

## Amputation Through Forearm

Criteria:
- Site of amputation: Junction of middle and distal thirds, length of stump is adequate for powerful activation of the artificial limb, as short forearm stumps are less effective in activating prosthesis and are difficult to fit
- End of the stump is smoothened with terminal scar
- Pronation and supination preseved

## Disarticulation of Elbow

Criteria:
- Preferred in children, as the distal humeral epiphysis is preserved

Upper arm amputation:
Above elbow (supracondylar) amputation

Criteria:
- Fitted best with standard prosthesis, as the length of stump is well sufficient
- Prosthesis consists of an upper arm piece and forearm piece with an elbow joint, that may be fixed in many positions, socket of its upper arm piece is a firm triangular cylinder, extending to axilla on inside and higher laterally over deltoid region, and being powered by a single control cable.

Procedure:
- Flaps (anterior and posterior or medial and lateral) of equal length employed, at supracondylar level
- Flexor muscles of the arm sectioned 1 cm distal to saw line to retract
- Triceps tendon divided from its insertion into olecranon
- Bone divided transversely
- Brachial artery isolated and doubly ligated
- Nerves (ulnar, median and radial, drawn downward and sectioned to retract above
- Triceps tendon brought forwards to cover the end of the bone, and sutured to the brachialis and biceps
- Skin flaps approximated with interrupted sutures.

## Mid-shaft Arm Amputation

Criteria:
- Flaps (anterior and posterior or medial and lateral) of equal length employed
- Flexor muscles of the arm sectioned 1 cm distal to saw line to retract
- Triceps tendon divided 3 cm below
- Bone divided transversely
- Brachial artery isolated and doubly ligated
- Nerves (ulnar, median and radial, drawn downward and sectioned to retract above
- Triceps tendon brought forwards to cover the end of the bone, and sutured to the brachialis and biceps
- Skin flaps approximated with interrupted sutures.

## SHOULDER AMPUTATIONS

## Amputation Through Surgical Neck of Humerus

Criteria:
- Stump is of little functional value, with or without a prosthesis
- Cosmetically, this amputation is superior than disarticulation of shoulder, as the head of humerus fills up the glenoid cavity, thereby provides shoulder a rounded form, exception: Malignant growth of middle and upper thirds of humerus, necessitating shoulder disarticulation.

Drawback:

Tends to produce deformity of spine due to:
- Weight loss of the limb
- Functional loss due to muscles atrophy
- Gait disturbance

Procedure:
- Skin incision from level of coracoids process, along anterior border of deltoid to its insertion, then along the posterior border of the deltoid to axillary fold, then connecting two ends of incision by an incision through axilla
- Pectoralis major muscle sectioned at its insertion
- Exposure of neurovascular bundle between pectoralis minor and coracobrachialis
- Axillary artery and vein divided below pectoralis minor muscle
- Nerves (ulnar, median, radial, and musculocutaneous) drawn downward and sectioned to retract above
- Deltoid muscle divided at its insertion
- Teres major and latissimus dorsi divided near their insertions
- Biceps tendon, triceps and coracobrachial divided
- Bone sectioned at level of humeral neck
- Muscles sutured over bone end
- Skin flaps approximated with interrupted sutures.

## Disarticulation of Shoulder

Criteria:
- Indicated in case of malignant tumor of middle and upper thirds of humerus.

Procedure:
- Skin incision: From level of coracoids process, along anterior border of deltoid to its insertion, then along the posterior border of the deltoid to axillary fold, then connecting two ends of incision by an incision through axilla
- Pectoralis major muscle sectioned at its insertion
- Exposure of neurovascular bundle between coracobrachialis and short head of biceps
- Axillary artery and vein divided below pectoralis minor muscle
- Nerves (ulnar, median, radial, and musculocutaneous) drawn downward and sectioned to retract above
- Deltoid muscle divided at its insertion
- Teres major and latissimus dorsi divided near their insertions
- Biceps tendon, triceps and coracobrachial divided
- Capsule divided to complete severance of the limb
- Muscles reflected into glenoid cavity and sutured
- Skin flaps approximated with interrupted sutures.

## Forequarter Amputation

Criteria:
- It is a mutilating procedure, performed for the removal of malignant tumors extending into shoulder joint or infiltrating muscles (deltoid, pectoralis or subscapular
- Combined with excision of regional lymph nodes

- Atypical skin flaps formed
- Prosthesis not advisible/possible at this level.

Procedure:

- Skin incision from lateral border of sternocleidomastoid muscle, to anterior aspect of clavicle, to the acromioclavicular joint, to the top of shoulder, to the spine of scapula, then along its vertebral border to its angle. Lower limb of incision extends from middle third of clavicle, downwards in the deltopectoral groove, cross the axilla, joins upper incision at the angle of scapula. Clavicle limb of incision deepened to bone
- Clavicular part of pectoralis muscle resected
- External jugular vein retracted/or sectioned
- Clavicle divided and removed by division of acromioclavicular joint
- Pectoralis major and minor divided to expose neurovascular bundle
- Subclavian vessels isolated and doubly ligated
- Brachial plexus sectioned
- Latissimus dorsi divided to free limb from chest wall, scapular muscles divided to remove the limb, remaining muscle mass sutured over lateral chest wall
- Flaps approximated with skin sutures.

Postoperative: A drainage tube inserted into the wound, for 2–3/7.

## Amputations of Lower Limb

Functions of stump and prosthesis: Walking and static weight bearing

Criteria:

- Skin coverage, able to withstand weight bearing pressure
- Scar pacement
- Bony base of weight bearing surface: To be broad and smooth.

Tissues subjected to pressure:

- Cancellous bone enveloped by thin cortex and covered by hyaline cartilage or periosteum
- Tendinous origins and insertions of muscles
- Joints and bursae
- Scar: To be away from pressure area.

Limitations: Abovesaid criteria limit use of end bearing stump to:

- Distal end of femur, tibia, and calcaneus
- Certain prosthetic objections.

## Amputation Through Toes

Criteria:

- A long plantar and a short dorsal skin flap formed.

Procedure:

- Skin incision: From intended bone level, on the midpoint, over medial side of toe, curved over dorsal aspect, ending at similar point on lateral aspect.
- Skin flaps dissected upward to saw line
- Flexor and extensor tendons sectioned to retract just above bony end
- Digital nerves isolated and sectioned

- Digital vessels sectioned and ligated with catgut
- Bone divided and toe removed
- Skin flaps approximated with interrupted sutures.
Transmetatarsal amputation.

Criteria:
- A long plantar and a short dorsal skin flap formed.

Procedure:
- Skin incision: Dorsal incision from level of saw line, on the anteromedial aspect, curved below to midpoint of lateral aspect of foot. Plantar incision from a similar point, curved downward below the metatarsal heads
- Skin flaps dissected upward to saw line
- Tendons sectioned to retract
- Nerves isolated and sectioned
- Vessels sectioned and ligated with catgut
- Metatarsals sectioned transversely
- Skin flaps approximated with interrupted sutures.

Postoperative: Posterior plaster slab to prevent foot drop.

## Amputations of Forefoot

Criteria:
Length conservation: Possibly to bases of metatarsals
- Greater toe amputation: Does not affect standing or walking (normal pace), but limps while brisk walking or running—due to loss of take-off from greater toe.
- 2nd toe amputation: Results in hallux valgus due to tendency of this toe to drift toward 3rd toe, so as to fill the gap left by amputation.
- 5th toe amputation: Removed because of overriding upon 4th toe, as being simple and final procedure.

  Relief: Using a stuffed shoe
- All toes amputation: Slightly disturbed slow walking, while being manifest on brisk walk, usually no prosthesis required, with just padding of shoes in the front region meant for toes.

Levels:
- Through metatarsals: Disabling vide height of the amputation, limping due to loss of positive fulcrum in the ball of foot

  Relief: Using a stuffed shoe
- At tarsometatarsal joints (Lisfranc's): Highest, that allows all functions of the foot, although disturbed walking due to loss of support.

  Relief: Using a stuffed shoe
- Midtarsal joint (Chopart's): Amputations through tarsus remain unsatisfactory due to development of equinovalgus deformity that is uncomfortable while walking and standing

  Exception: Amputation combined with arthrodesis of calcaneus to the tibia.

## Amputations Through Middle of Foot

Surgery: Include:
- Tarsometatarsal disarticulation: Discarded because of development of equines deformity
- Chopart's amputation: Discarded because of development of equino-valgus deformity
- Pirogoff's amputation: Calcaneus rotated forward to fuse to the tibia
- Burgess's amputation: Tendocalcaneus sectioned to salvage midtarsal and tarsometatarsal amputations, whereby equines deformity developed.

Relief: More proximal amputation or reconstruction operation.

Criteria:
- A long plantar and a short dorsal skin flap formed.

Procedure:
- Tendocalcaneus sectioned subcutaneously above its insertion
- Ankle and hind foot stretched into dorsiflexion
- Stump immobilized in a cast B/K for 2/56
- Weight bearing allowed on the plantar heel skin.

## Ankle Amputations

Criteria:
- To provide an end bearing stump
- To leave adequate space between end of the stump and ground, for production of ankle joint of prosthetic foot.

Procedures:
- Syme amputation
- Boyd amputation
- A long plantar and a short dorsal skin flap formed.

## Syme Amputation

Criteria: It is the classical example of an end-bearing stump, enjoyed great popularity, but from permanent efficiency point of view, is not a good amputation. Skin forms a firm non-mobile pad, scar is anterior, life span of 5–10 years, thereafter reamputation with a 15 cm tibial stump mandatory. Can be performed, in case of sound tissues round the heel. End of stump formed by the skin of the heel, used to weight bearing.

Indication: Fulfills all criteria, bone level: Sistal end of tibia, 0.5 cm above ankle joint

Procedure:
- Skin flaps: A single, long, posterior heel flap utilized.
- Skin incision: Incision from tip of lateral malleolus, across front of ankle joint, to one finger below tip of medial malleolus, down to the bottom of foot, across sole to lateral aspect, ending at lateral malleolus (starting point).
- All structures divided to the bone
- Tarsus excised
- Foot planterflexed
- Anterior capsule of ankle divided
- Ligaments (deltoid) on medial side and (calcaneofibular) on lateral side of ankle divided
- Posterior capsule of ankle divided

- Tendocalcaneus divided at its insertion
- Entire foot except heel flap removed
- Periosteum incised circumferentially 0.5 cm above joint line, bone divided at this level, and smoothened
- All tendons pulled down and sectioned, to retract above bone level
- Plantar nerves (medial and lateral) isolated and sectioned
- Vessels (posterior and anterior tibial) sectioned and ligated with catgut
- Metatarsals sectioned transversely
- Skin flaps approximated with interrupted sutures
- Drain tube placed in the wound for 2/7.

Postoperative:
- Sutures removed after 2/56
- Walking cast applied till shrinkage is complete.
- Using an 'elephant boot'.

## Boyd Amputation

Criteria: It is the method of choice, in case a prosthesis not used. It is performed on the principle of talectomy, i.e. shifting of calcaneus forward and arthrodesis of calcaneotibial arthrodesis, and can afford more length vs Syme's amputation, and a wider weight bearing surface, utilizing a bulky prosthesis rather than an 'elephant boot'.

Procedure:
- Skin flaps: A long plantar and a short dorsal flap utilized
- Skin incision: Incision from tip of lateral malleolus, across dorsum of foot at level of talonavicular joint, to one finger below tip of medial malleolus, down to the bottom of foot, across sole to lateral aspect, ending at lateral malleolus (starting point)
- All structures divided to the bone
- Talus excised
  Front part of calcaneus, distal to peroneal tubercle divided
- Ligaments (deltoid) on medial side) and calcaneofibular on lateral side of ankle divided
- Calcaneus shifted anteriorly vs ankle joint
- Calcaneotibial arthrodesis performed
- All tendons pulled down and sectioned, to retract above bone level
- Plantar nerves (medial and lateral) isolated and sectioned
- Vessels (posterior and anterior tibial) sectioned and ligated with catgut
- Skin flaps approximated with interrupted sutures
- Drain tube inserted in the wound for 2/7.

Postoperative:
- Sutures removed after 2/56
- Internal fixator removed after 4/56
- Weight bearing upon stump allowed after 8/56
- Walking cast applied till arthrodesis is complete.

## Amputation Through Leg

Criteria: Ideal amputation below knee is at level of 15 cm below medial tibial condyle, length of bone varies between 12–18 cm, based upon height of the individual, stump affords an excellent leverage, healthy skin, and adequate circulation, and fits well in a prosthesis, while longer stumps are poorly adapted to a prosthesis, mostly breakdown due to poor circulation, and weight may be transferred to ischial tuberosity by the extended thigh corset. A short below knee stump cannot be fitted comfortably and becomes inefficient, and may equire excision of fibula and additional muscle bulk.

Procedure:
- Skin flaps: A long anterior and a short posterior flap utilized.
- Skin incision: Incision from intended level of bone section, downward to a similar point on the opposite side of leg, posterior skin flap incision downward to estimated point, then upward to level of bone division
- All structures divided to the bone
- Periosteum incised at this level
  Front part of calcaneus, distal to peroneal tubercle divided
- Ligaments (deltoid on medial side) and calcaneofibular on lateral side of ankle divided
- Calcaneus shifted anteriorly vs ankle joint
- Calcaneotibial arthrodesis performed
- All tendons pulled down and sectioned, to retract above bone level
- Superficial peroneal nerve isolated and sectioned
- Muscles of anterior compartment divided just distal to saw line
- Anterior tibial vessels sectioned and ligated with catgut
- Bones (tibia and fibula) divided by transverse section, smoothened
- Gastrocnemius divided
- Posterior tibial vessels and nerves isolated and sectioned
- Skin flaps approximated with interrupted sutures
- Drain tube inserted in the wound for 2/7.

Postoperative:
- Sutures removed after 2/56
- Internal fixator removed after 4/56
- Weight bearing upon stump allowed after 8/56
- Walking cast applied.

## Disarticulation of Knee

Criteria:
- Preservation of intact femoral condyles
- Reattachment of thigh muscles to stump's end
- Coverage of weight bearing end of stump by a wider full thickness anterior skin flap, that may bear weight during kneeling
- Anterior flap to be wider than posterior skin flap, so as to cover the condyles, and extend by 2.5 cm below level of tibial tuberosity, thus rendering suture line posterior to weight bearing zone.
- Posterior flap to extend to level of 2.5 cm below the popliteal flexor crease.

Procedure:
- A tourniquet to be applied.
- Skin flap: A long, wider anterior and a short posterior flap utilized.

- Skin incision: Anterior skin incision deepened to the bone, dissected from tibia and patellar tendon capsule of knee joint dissected from anterior and lateral margins of tibia, exposing knee joint cruciate ligaments divided posterior capsule of knee joint dissected from tibia popliteal nerve isolated and divided, to retract politeal vessels isolated, clamped, divided, and doubly ligated biceps tendon separated from fibula amputation completed through posterior skin flap leg removed synovium resected (except in case of gangrene) tourniquet released, and bleeders ligated/cauterized patellar tendon sutured to the cruciate ligaments.
- Skin flaps approximated with interrupted sutures.
- A drain inserted in the wound for 2–3/7.

Postoperative:
- Sutures removed after 2/56.
- Prosthesis fitted after 6/56.

## Amputation Through Thigh

Criteria: End bearing amputation at level of distal end of femur is ideal, provided stump's end covered by suitable weight bearing, that provides a long leverage and a direct end bearing surface, eliminates pressure from prosthesis on perineum, thus preferred over the amputation at higher level.

Drawback: Bulky knee, and prosthesis's hinges fails to control rapid swing of shin during gait, due to friction.

Types:
- Tendoplastic: Weight transmitted to distal end of femur via a layer of tendinous tissue (supracondylar amputation): osteotomy site is 3 cm above articular surface of femur
- Osteoplastic: Weight transmitted through a bone (patella) that is arthrodesed to the distal end of femur.

Site: Ideal site is upper margin of rounded edges of bone at the epicondylar level, wherein weight bearing surface is the transcondylar region.

Advantages of length, better weight bearing surface, good muscular control, minimal thigh atrophy, and abundant circulation, and method of choice in children, by preserving the distal femoral epiphysis.
- Above knee, ischial bearing amputation, is to be 10–12 cm above the joint line of knee, affords minimum of clearance required in fitting of artificial joint, providing a leverage of 30 cm below tip of greater trochanter, based upon height of individual, thus control of stump in all directions.
- In shorter stumps, muscle balance lost, and stump's control less efficient.

## Procedure

### Epicondylar tendoplastic amputation:
- Skin flap: A long anterior and a short posterior flap utilized.
- Skin incision: Anterior skin incision from adductor tubercle of medial epicondyle, downward, crossing front of knee at level of patellar insertion, then upwards to along lateral border of knee, ending at lateral epicondyle of femur, posterior incision forms an arc between ends of anterior incision and anterior incision deepened
- Soft tissues reflected, synovium resected
- Periosteum incised

- Bone divided and smoothed
- Vessels isolated and doubly ligated with catgut
- Sciatic nerve and other nerves isolated and divided, allowed to retract
- Skin flaps approximated with interrupted sutures
- A drain inserted in the wound for 2–3/7
- Sutures removed after 2/56.

## Supracondylar tendoplastic amputation:

- Osteotomy site is 3 cm above articular surface of femur
- Skin flap: A long anterior and a short posterior flap utilized
- Skin incision: From midportion of medial aspect of thigh, downward below upper margin of patella, then upwards to midlateral aspect of thigh, anterior incision deepened to bone
- Quadriceps tendon severed at its patellar insertion
- Soft tissues reflected, synovium resected
- Posterior fascia and soft tissues sectioned to bone
- Periosteum incised
- Bone divided
- Vessels isolated and doubly ligated with catgut
- Sciatic nerve and other nerves isolated and divided, allowed to retract
- Skin flaps approximated with interrupted sutures
- A drain inserted in the wound for 2–3/7
- Sutures removed after 2/56.

## Hip and pelvis amputations

Indications:
- Malignant tumors of middle and upper thigh, that cannot be removed by wide excision
- Malignant tumors of middle and upper femur, that cannot be cured by high thigh amputation
- Malignant melanoma of skin of lower limb
- Chronic osteomyelitis with discharging sinuses
- Diabetes mellitus.

## Disarticulation of Hip

Criteria:
- Amputations above level of lesser trochanter
- Length of bone to be conserved as much as possible
- Socket of the artificial limb to be fitted with the stump fixed to a right angle, weight is thereby on the ischial tuberosity.

Indications:
- Removal of a malignant tumor or disorder

Procedure:
- Skin flap: A long anterior and a short posterior flap utilized.
- Skin incision: An anterior racquet skin incision from anterosuperior iliac spine, curved downward and medially parallel with inguinal ligament to inner aspect of thigh, 5 cm below origin of adductor muscles, then curved around posterior aspect of thigh, distal

to ischial tuberosity, along lateral aspect of thigh distal to greater trochanter, then curved upwards, to original incision (ASIS).

- Femoral vessels isolated and ligated
- Femoral nerve isolated and divided
- Sartorius muscle detached from ASIS
- Rectus femoris detached from AIIS
- Pectinus divided from pubis
- Thigh rotated externally to expose lesser trochanter and iliopsoas tendon – divide
- Adductor and gracilis detached from pubis and ischium
- Obturator vessels isolated and ligated
- Obturator externus detached from femur
- Thigh rotated internally, glutei muscles detached from greater trochanter
- Fascia lata divided below insertion of tensor fasciae latae
- Sciatic nerve isolated and divided
- Short rotators of hip (piriformis, gemelli, obturators, quadrates femoris) divided from femur
- Hamstrings detached from ischial tuberosity
- Capsule of hip joint incised from acetabulum, along with division of
- Ligamentum teres, limb separated
- Glutei muscles distal parts sutured with origin of pectineus and adductors
- Skin flaps approximated with interrupted sutures
- A drain inserted into the wound for 2/7
- Sutures removed after 2/56.

## Hindquarter Amputation

Synonyms:
- Interinnominoabdominal amputation
- Interilioabdominal amputation
- Ilioabdominal amputation
- Interpelviabdominal amputation
- Transiliac amputation
- Transpelvic amputation.

Preoperative care:
- Medically fit to withstand major procedure
- Bowel enema/purgative: Previous night
- Bladder empty: Indwelling catheter
- Skin prepared: From costal margins to both knees
- Antibiotic coverage
- IV fluids
- Blood arranged for transfusion.

Procedure:
- Skin flap: A long anterior and a short posterior flap utilized.
- Skin incision: Anterior skin incision from pubic tubercle, upward, along inguinal ligament to ASIS, posteriorly along iliac crest.

- Abdominal muscles and inguinal ligament detached from liac crest
- Iliac fossa opened between iliacus and peritoneum
- Rectus abdominis tendon and inguinal ligament excised from pubis
- Cord retracted medially
- Bladder retracted into pelvis
- External iliac vessels isolated and ligated
- Femoral nerve isolated and divided
- Perineal incision: Carried down and outward from pubic tubercle, along pubic and ischial rami to ischial tuberosity
- Symphysis pubis divided
- Posterior incision from iliac crest to PSIS, then outward to greater trochanter, then posteriorly into perineum, to join perineal incision
- Gluteus medius and rotators of hip excised
- Sciatic nerve exposed and divided
- Obturator vessels and nerve ligated and divided
- Psoas muscle divided
- Levator ani divided from pubis
- Skin flaps approximated with interrupted sutures
- A drain inserted in the wound for 2–3/7
- Sutures removed after 2/56.

### Amputations in Peripheral Vascular Disease (PVD)

Preface: Failure of medial and surgical procedures to furnish adequate nutrition to the limb, irreparable tissue damage occurs; salvage amputation to save the life of the person and to preserve the remaining functional limb, ignoring the etiologiocal factors like arteriosclerosis, diabetes, thromboangitis oblitrans.

Indications for amputation:
- Pain: Ischemic, unrelieved by rest, position, sedation
- Infection
- Gangrene.

Technique:
- Skin flap: A long anterior and a short posterior flap utilized.
- Skin incision: Anterior skin incision from adductor tubercle of medial epicondyle, downward, crossing front of knee at level of patellar insertion, then upwards to along lateral border of knee, ending at lateral epicondyle of femur, posterior incision forms an arc between ends of anterior incision and anterior incision deepened
- Soft tissues reflected, synovium resected
- Periosteum incised
- Bone divided and smoothed
- Vessels isolated and doubly ligated with catgut
- Sciatic nerve and other nerves isolated and divided, allowed to retract
- Skin flaps approximated with interrupted sutures
- A drain inserted in the wound for 2–3/7
- Sutures removed after 2/56.

## Bibliography

1. Advisory Committee on Artificial Limbs, National Research Council: Biceps cineplasty and prosthesis for below elbow amputations, 1950.
2. Aitken GT. Amputation as a treatment for certainlower-extremity congenital abnormalities. J. Bone and Joint Surg. 41-A:1267, 1959.
3. Alldredge RH, Thompson TC. The technique of Syme amputation, J. Bone and Joint Surg. 28:415, 1946.
4. Batch JW, et al. Advantages of the knee disarticulation over amputations through the thigh, J. Bone and Joint Surg. 36-A:921, 1954.
5. Bennett RJ. Major amputations of extremities due to trauma, Am. J. Surg. 78:597, 1949.
6. Brittain HA. Hindquarter amputations, J. Bone and Joint Surg. 31-B:404, 1949.
7. Campbell's Operative Orthopaedics, ed. 9th, Vol I-IV., Slocum DB, CV Mosby Co., Saint Louis, 1998.
8. Canale ST, et al. Campbell's Operative Orthopaedics, ed. 9th, Vol I-IV. C.V. Mosby Co., Saint Louis, 1998.
9. Chatterjee CC. Human Physiology, 5th Ed., Books and Allied Pvt. Ltd., Calcutta, 1963.
10. Clark JMP. Modern Trends in Orthopaedics: Fracture Treatment, 3, Butterworths, London, 1962.
11. Cunningham's Manual of Practical Anatomy, vol. I-III, 12th Ed., Oxford University Press, London, 1961.
12. Das K. Clinical Methods In Surgery, 6th Ed., Lakshman Chandra Sil, Calcutta, 1962.
13. Gordon T, Gordon, Monro RS. Technique and management of hindquarter amputation, Brit. J. Surg. 39:536, 1952.
14. Grimes OF, Bell HG. Shoulder girdle amputation, Surg. Gynec. and Obst. 91:202, 1950.
15. Holden WD. Technique of low thigh amputation, Surg. Gynec. and Obst. 87:739, 1948.
16. Huckstep RL. A Simple Guide to Trauma, 5th Ed., Churchill Livingstone, Edinburgh, 1995.
17. Jenkins JL, Braen R, Richard G. Manual of Emergency Medicine, 4th Ed., Lippincott Williams and Wilkins, Philadelphia, 1999.
18. Kapoor PS. Amputations: Kapoor's Accident and Emergency: Etiology, Diagnosis, and Management, 2nd Ed., CBS, New Delhi, 2016.
19. Keele CA, Neil E. Samson Wright's Applied Physiology, 10th Ed., Oxford University Press, London, 1963.
20. Krupp MA, Chatton MJ. Current Medical Diagnosis and Treatmernt, Maruzen Asian Edition, Bombay, 1975.
21. Kutler W. New method for finger tip amputation, J.A.M.A. 133:29, 1947.
22. Love M, et al. Bailey and Love's Short Practice of Surgery, ed. 13th, H.K. Lewis and Co., London, 1965.
23. Mattox KL. Complications of Trauma, Churchill Livingstone, Edinburgh, 1994.
24. McGREGOR AL. The Anatomy Governing Amputations: A Synopsis of Surgical Anatomy, 9th Ed., John Wright and Sons Ltd., Bristol, 1963.
25. McKeever FM. Upper extremity amputations and prostheses, J. Bone and Joint Surg. 26:660, 1944.
26. McLatchie GR. Essentials of Sports Medicine, 2nd Ed., Churchill Livingstone, Edinburgh, 1993.
27. McRae R. Practical Fracture Treatment, 3rd Ed., Churchill Livingstone, Edinburgh, 1994.
28. Mirvis SE, Young JWR. Imaging in Trauma and Critical Care, Williams and Wilkins, Baltimore, 1992.
29. Pack GT, Ehrlich HE, Gentil F. Radical amputation of extremities in treatment of cancer, Surg., Gynec. and Obst. 84:1105, 1947.
30. Perkins G. Amputations, Brit. J. Surg. 31:377, 1944.
31. Raby N, Berman L, de Lacy G. Accident and Emergency Radiology, W.B. Saunders Co., Philadelphia, 1997.
32. Robertson C, Redmond AD. Management of Major Trauma, 2nd Ed., Oxford University Press, Oxford, 1996.
33. Shumacker HB, Jr, Moore TC. Leg and thigh amputations in obliterative arterial disease, A.M.A. Arch. Surg. 63:458, 1951.
34. Silbert S. Mid-leg amputations for gangrene in the diabetic, Ann. Surg. 127:503, 1948.
35. Slocum DB. Major amputations, GP 3:55, 1951
36. Trunkey DD, Lewis FR. Current Therapy of Trauma, 4th Ed., Mosby Year Book, St Louis, 1998.

# 10

# Peripheral Nerve Trauma

Peripheral nerve injuries
- Neurapraxia
- Axonotmesis
- Neurotmesis

Cervical rib

Scalene syndrome

Brachial plexus injuries:
- Complete
- Incomplete
- Upper arm lesion (Erb-Duchen)
- Lower arm lesion (Klumpke)
- Axillary (circumflex) nerve injury
- Nerve of Bell injury
- Ulnar nerve injury
- Tardy ulnar nerve injury
- Median nerve injury
- Radial nerve injury
- Sciatic nerve injury
- Lateral popliteal nerve injury
- Medial politeal nerve injury

Bibliography

## PERIPHERAL NERVE INJURIES

Preface
: The degree of peripheral nerve injury may be variable from mild contusion (incomplete ischemia) to complete severance of the nerve, with loss of substance; for evaluating peripheral nerve lesions, a precise anatomical knowledge of the pathway of the nerve, level at which these motor branches originate, muscles supplied by its branches, and various dermatomes of sensation; motor loss evaluation very important.

MOI
: Direct violence (stretch injuries): Trauma: fractures, dislocations, wounds
RSA
Sports injuries
Malignant growth: Involving nerve

| | |
|---|---|
| Diagnosis | Loss of motor and sensory functions (temporary): |

Sensory:

- Mixed peripheral nerve injury: Paresthesia, sensory loss (small area)
- Sensory nerve: Paresthesia, sensory loss (large area).

Motor: Loss of all motor functions (tone, power) distal to injury level:

- Concussion: Weakness of muscle groups (lasting for days)
- Compression or severance: Distal to injury level: muscles paralyzed, atrophy, fibrosed, die.

Reflex: Mostly normal in concussion injuries, while in complete severance or compression, all reflex activity abolished.

Autonomic: Interrupted sweating:

- Loss of sweating (autonomus zone)
- Reduced sweating (intermediate zone)
- Skin: Shining in concussion, while in compression or severance skin: pale, cyanotic, or mottled; thin, shining, disuse atrophy, ulcerated.
- Nails: Distorted, may fall out
- Bones: Osteoporotic
- Joints: Ankylosed.

Pathogenesis   Variable from mild contusion, incomplete ischemia to complete severance of nerve with substance loss

Types: Three types of injuries: as per extent of damage to the nerve fibers and sheath:

- Neurapraxia (concussion): There is a momentary loss of conduction, without any organic damage. The nerve fibers and nerve sheath remain intact; incomplete paralysis, sensory loss, and autonomic functional loss; and the recovery is almost complete.
- Axonotmesis: Axons injured, Wallerian degeneration occurs, Schwann tubules preserved
- Neurotmesis: Nerve partially or completely severed, neuroma and glioma formed.

Managememt   Aim: Early diagnosis and management of nerve injuries:

Preoperative:

Continuous immobilization: Alone contraindicated.

Indication: Associated fracture, and then should not including joints

Surgery:

Primary suture:

Indication: Sharply incised wounds

Contraindication: Gunshot wounds, fracture, or severe trauma

Débridement and closure of wound:

Indication: Severed ends of nerve visible in the wound, that can be easily approximated without further dissection, so that neurorrhaphy may be carried out easily later on.

Neurapraxia   It is defined as a concussion injury.

MOI   Direct violence (stretch injuries): Trauma: fractures, dislocations, wounds
Fall from height

| | |
|---|---|
| | RSA |
| | Sports injuries |
| | Malignant growth: Involving nerve. |
| Pathogenesis | There is a momentary loss of conduction, without any organic damage. The nerve fibers and nerve sheath remain intact; incomplete paralysis, sensory loss, and autonomic functional loss; and the recovery is almost complete. |
| Diagnosis | Loss of motor and sensory functions (temporary): |
| | Sensory: Paresthesia, sensory loss (lasting for days) |
| | Motor: Weakness of muscle groups (lasting for days) |
| | Reflex: Mostly normal |

Autonomic:
* Loss of sweating (autonomus zone) reduced sweating (intermediate zone)
* Skin: Shining
* Nails: Brittle, shining

| | |
|---|---|
| Investigation | Blood sugar—for diabetes mellitus |
| | Electrical reactions: No reaction of degeneration (RD). |
| Management | Conservative treatment: |

* Immobilizing the limb in the position of relaxation of the affected muscle, by the use of splints, braces, etc.
* Analgesics and NSAIDs.

After care:
* Physiotherapy: Active and passive exercises
* Muscle stimulators.

| | |
|---|---|
| **Axonotmesis** | It is defined as rupture of axons within an intact nerve sheath. |
| MOI | Direct violence (stretch injuries): Trauma: fractures, dislocations, wounds |
| | Fall from height |
| | RSA |
| | Sports injuries |
| | Malignant growth: Involving nerve |
| Pathogenesis | Rupture of axons occurs within an intact neural sheath; degeneration of ruptured axons occurs in distal segments, leading further to intraneural fibrosis, thereby affecting the conduction functions, followed by incomplete recovery. |
| Diagnosis | Loss of motor and sensory functions, e.g. |
| | Sensory: Paresthesia, sensory loss (incomplete recovery) |
| | Motor: Weakness of muscle groups (incomplete recovery) |
| | Reflex: Abolished activity |
| | Autonomic: Abolished sweating (autonomus zone) reduced sweating (intermediate zone) |
| | Skin: Thin, shining, atrophic, ulcerated |
| | Nails: Brittle, shining |
| | Bones: Osteoporotic |
| | Joints: Ankylosed |

| | |
|---|---|
| Investigation | Blood and urine: To rule out diabetes. |
| | Electrical reactions: Reaction of degeneration (RD) appears in the denervated muscles in 4–5 days and fully established within 3/56. The muscle fibers no longer respond to rapid make-and-break of faradic stimulation (F = 0), and weak galvanic response with reversal of polar formula, i.e. ACC becomes stronger than KCC (normally KCC stronger than ACC). |
| Management | Conservative treatment: |
| | Splints support to the paralyzed muscles of the affected limb |
| | Passive exercises—to built up tone and muscle power |
| | Massage |
| | Analgesics and NSAIDs. |
| | Surgical treatment: |
| | Indications: Failure to recover, or regression post initial recovery. |
| | Surgery: |
| | Local exploration of traumatized site; to remove a scar or an intraneural fibroma. |
| | Results: Based on rates of nerve regeneration (1–2 mm/day) calculated by: |
| | • Tinel's sign: Nerve's course percussed with a percussing hammer from below upwards, a tingling sensation felt on reaching the level of the regeneration. |
| | • Rate of return of pain and touch sensation |
| | • Rate of return of muscle's function. |
| **Neurotmesis** | It is defined as partial or complete division of the neural sheath and fibers. |
| MOI | Direct violence: Trauma, e.g. fractures, dislocations, gunshot wounds, cut wounds; stab wounds, pressure (tight plaster/splint), and traction. |
| | RSA |
| | Fall from a height. |
| | Sports injuries |
| | Malignant growth: Involving nerve |
| Pathogenesis | In partial division, a lateral neuroma is formed at the site of injury, whereas in complete division a terminal neuroma is formed at the proximal segments end. |
| Diagnosis | Loss of motor and sensory functions: |
| | Sensory: Paresthesia, sensory loss (deceptive recovery) |
| | Motor: Weakness of muscle groups (deceptive recovery) |
| | Reflex: Abolished activity |
| | Autonomic: Abolished sweating (autonomus zone) reduced sweating (intermediate zone) |
| | Skin: Thin, shining, atrophic, ulcerated |
| | Nails: Brittle, shining |
| | Bones: Osteoporotic |
| | Joints: Ankylosed |

| Investigation | Electrical reactions: Reaction of degeneration (RD) appears in the denervated muscles in 4–5 days and fully established within 3/56. The muscle fibers no longer respond to rapid make-and-break of faradic stimulation (F = 0), and weak galvanic response with reversal of polar formula, i.e. ACC becomes stronger than KCC (normally KCC stronger than ACC). |
|---|---|
| Management | Conservative treatment:<br>Use of splints<br>Analgesics<br>Antibiotics. |

Surgical treatment:
* Exploration of injured nerve:
  Indication: Complete physiological lesion
* Primary suturing:
  Indication: Sharply incised wounds
* Débridement and closure if possible:
  Indication: Open wounds
* Neurorrhaphy
  Indication: Severed nerve: repair of injured nerve: nerve suturing.

Technique:
* Incision: A long incision to expose the injured nerve, without too much interfering with adjoining anatomical structures, obscured by scar tissue later on.
* Free: The two ends of nerve freed and freshened by a sharp BP knife
* Mobilization: By dissecting from adjoining structures
* Posture: Limb held in a suitable position
* Transposition: Ulnar nerve in front of medial condyle; while radial nerve in front of humerus
* Nerve anchoring: The two ends approximated as closely as possible by the tension stitches
* Nerve sheath: Post approximation of nerve ends, suturing through nerve sheath with silk or tantalum wire.
* Fracture: Nonunion: ORIF + grafting

Postoperative: Immobilize the limb by a plaster cast for 8/56.
After care: Physiotherapy.

## Complications of Nerve Suture

| Preoperative: | * Nerve injured: Disappointing results in suturing of ulnar nerve for palmar muscles<br>* Infection: Delayed recovery, neuritis<br>* Time factor: Early secondary suture yields better results, while further delay yields poor results<br>* Muscle tone: Recovery chances diminished, if tone not maintained. |
|---|---|

Operative:
* Poor hemostasis, failure to prevent torsion and tension, use of irritating suture material

Postoperative:
- Infection
- Non cooperating patient
- Vicarious movements: Adjoining muscles fail to share functions of the paralysed.

## CERVICAL RIB

| | |
|---|---|
| MOI | Direct trauma: Stretching or pressing injury |
| Pathogenesis | Trauma: The lower trunk (C-8, D-1) formed at the anterior border of the scalenus medius muscle, immediate above the 1st rib, stretches or pressed upon, at this point, by an elevated cervical rib pushing it between the nerve and the 1st rib. |
| Diagnosis | Incidence: Rare (1%)<br>Unilateral (more frequent on right side)<br>Gender: Female > male<br>Age: Youner (puberty) and older (disease or weakness)<br>Symptomless, or<br>Swelling: Lump (bony hard) in the lower part of neck<br>Sensory: Tingling, numbness, pain along medial side of forearm and hand<br>Motor: Wasting of thenar or hypothenar eminence, powerless<br>Vasomotor: Sweating of hand, gangrene |
| Investigation | X-ray neck: AP and Lateral views: mostly rib nonvisible<br>CT Scan |
| Management | Conservative treatment:<br>Posture: Relief from elevation of arm by use of an arm support<br>SWD or Infrared therapy<br>Analgesics, NSAIDs<br>Surgical treatment:<br>Surgery: Timely extraperiosteal excision of cervical rib and its periosteum. |

## SCALENE SYNDROME

| | |
|---|---|
| Definition | It is defined as a syndrome characterized by the clinical picture of the cervical rib, while there is no cervical rib. |
| MOI | Trauma: Stretching injury. |
| Pathogenesis | Pulled scalenus anticus muscle stretching lower trunk or subclavian artery against the 1st rib. |
| Diagnosis | Age: Usually after 40 years<br>Pain: Supraclavicular region; radiating inner aspect of forearm, hand and fingers (little and ring)<br>Swelling in lower neck<br>Local tenderness<br>Sensory: Tingling, numbness, pain along inner aspect of forearm and hand<br>Motor: Wasting of thenar or hypothenar eminence, powerless<br>Vasomotor: Sweating of hand, gangrene. |

| Investigation | X-ray neck: AP and Lateral views: mostly rib nonvisible |
| --- | --- |
| | CT Scan |
| | Arteriography: May show subclavian artery compression |
| Management | Conservative treatment: |
| | Posture: Relief from elevation of arm by use of an arm support |
| | SWD or Infrared therapy |
| | Analgesics and NSAIDs |
| | Surgical treatment: |
| | Surgery: Excision: timely division of the muscle. |

## BRACHIAL PLEXUS INJURIES

| Anatomy | The brachial plexus is a plexus of cords, formed by the union of the anterior rami of C-5, C-6, C-7, C-8, and D-1; C-5 usually receives some fibres from C-4 (prefixed) and D-1 from D-2 (postfixed). It consists of roots, trunks, divisions, cords, and branches. The roots and trunks lie in the neck, the divisions behind the clavicle, and the cords and branches in the axilla. Thus, the subclavian artery related to roots and trunks, while axillary to cords and branches. Cords end by giving off terminal branches, at the lower border of pectoralis minor; the 1st and 2nd parts of axillary artery related tocords, and 3rd part to branches; terminal branches of the cords, long nerves to arm and forearm begin at the lower border of pectoralis minor. |
| --- | --- |

Plan of plexus:
C-5 and C-6 roots unite to form upper trunk
C-7 forms the middle trunk
C-8 and D-1 unite to form lower trunk
Each trunk divides into an anterior and a posterior division
All posterior divisions unite to form posterior cord
Upper two anterior divisions unite to form lateral (outer) cord
Lowest anterior division forms medial (inner) cord

Branches:
From roots:

| | |
| --- | --- |
| Long thoracic (Bell) nerve | C-5, C-6, C-7 |
| Dorsalis scapulae nerve | C-5 |

Muscular branches to three scaleni and longus colli

From trunks: From upper trunk only:

| | |
| --- | --- |
| Suprascapular nerve | C-5, C-6 |
| Subclavius nerve | C-5, C-6 |

From cords:
Medial cord:

| | |
| --- | --- |
| Ulnar nerve | C-8, D-1 |
| Medial head of median nerve | C-8, D-1 |
| Medial anterior thoracic (medial pectoris) | C-8, D-1 |

| | |
|---|---|
| Medial cutaneous of forearm | C-8, D-1 |
| Medial cutaneous of arm | D-1 |
| Lateral cord: | |
| Lateral head of median nerve | C-5, C-6, C-7 |
| Musculocutaneous nerve | C-5, C-6, C-7 |
| Lateral anterior thoracic (lateral pectoris) | C-5, C-6, C-7 |
| Posterior cord: | |
| Radial nerve | C-5, C-6, C-7, C-8, D-1 |
| Circumflex (Axillary) nerve | C-5, C-6 |
| Subscapular nerve | C-5, C-6 |
| Thoracodorsal | C-6, C-7, C-8 |

Erb's point: It is the point meeting of six nerves:
5th and 6th cervical roots unite to form the upper trunk, very short, that supplies the suprascapular nerve and nerve to subclavius muscle, then divides into an anterior and a posterior divisions

Trauma: The upper trunk usually stretches or tears, at this point, as in upper arm (Erb's) lesion of obstetric birth injury.

Types — Complete and incomplete Brachil plexus injuries:

## Complete Brachial Plexus Injury

It is a rare injury, as a major trauma required to damage all the roots of the plexus, may inflict fatal injuries on adjoining vital structures.

| | |
|---|---|
| MOI | Direct violence. |
| Pathogenesis | Tearing of all the nerve roots, associated with fatal injuries of the adjoining vital structures. |
| Diagnosis | Complete paralysis of upper limb (arm and scapular muscles) with wasting and degeneration of muscles |
| | Complete anesthesia of hand, forearm, and distal part of arm. |
| Investigation | X-ray—to rule out any fracture-dislocation. |
| Management | Conservative treatment: |
| | • Use of splints and physiotherapy. |

## Incomplete Bracheal Plexus Injury

| | |
|---|---|
| MOI | Direct violence: Cuts, stabs, gunshots, and by blows with sticks, etc. |
| | Fall from a height |
| | Fall of heavy weight over shoulder |
| | Obstructed labor—traction injury. |
| Pathogenesis | Usually the injury leads to traction or pressure lesions of the upper or lower parts of the plexus, i.e. |
| | • Upper lesion (Erb Duchen) |
| | • Lower lesion (Klumpke). |

**Segmental innervations of arm muscles:** (Table 10.1) summarizes a distribution of segmental innervation of arm muscles.

**Table 10.1:** Segmental innervations of arm muscles

| Nerve root | Muscles | Movements impaired |
|---|---|---|
| C. 5 | Deltoid, spinati, rhomboids, teres minor, Biceps, brachialis, brachioradialis, supinator | Abduction at shoulder |
| C. 6, 7 | Pectoralis major (clavicular head) and minor, subscapularis, coracobrachialis, teres minor, serratus anterior, latissimus dorsi, triceps, pronator teres and quadrates, extensors of fingers, extensor carpi ulnaris, pectoralis major (sternal head) | Adduction at shoulder Extension at wrist and fingers |
| C. 5, 6 | Deltoid, spinati, biceps, brachioradialis, brachialis, supinator brevis | Abduction at shoulder Lateral rotation shoulder Flexion at elbow Supination elbow |
| C. 7, 8 | Extensors of fingers, extensor carpi ulnaris, pectoralis major (sterna head), triceps, anconeus, extensor carpi radialis longus and brevis | Extension at elbow wrist and fingers |
| C. 8, T. 1 | Intrinsic muscles of hand, flexors of fingers, flexor carpi ulnaris | Flexion at wrist and fingers |

## Upper arm lesion (Erb–Duchen)

| | |
|---|---|
| Definition | It is defined as the upper lesion of brachial plexus, due to involvement of C5 and C6 nerve roots. |
| MOI | Trauma: |

- Obstructed labor: Traction force—during forced delivery of fetus
- RSA
- Fall of a heavy weight on the shoulder
- Direct violence: hit by a stick, gunshot injury

Pathogenesis    Traction or pressure trauma, resulting in injury, i.e. increased angle between the neck and shoulder, as may occur during forced delivery of fetus, in obstructed labor, and also by fall of a heavy weight over the shoulder. The 5th and sometimes 6th cervical roots involved. Muscles affected: deltoid, spinati, biceps, brachioradialis, supinator brevis.

Diagnosis    Deformity:
- Arm hanging by the side of body, adducted  and internally rotated
- Elbow fully extended
- Forearm fully pronated
- Wrist and fingers flexed

Muscular wasting: Thin, soft, and flabby—in lesions of long duration
Muscle power and tone: Loss
Sensations and reflexes: Loss
Skin: Cold, glazed, and smooth (paralysis), excessive sweating in case of incomplete lesion; vasomotor changes: pallor, cyanosis, redness, shiny, and scaly skin, brittle nails in case of irritating lesion.

| Management | Conservative treatment: As soon as possible: |
|---|---|

Management — Conservative treatment: As soon as possible:
Immobilization of arm in relaxation position (right angled, by use of splints to relax deltoid and spinati), (forearm flexed and supinated to relax biceps, brachialis, and supinator).
Physiotherapy
Surgical treatment:
Indication: Neurotmesis lesions.

Surgery:
- Exploration of brachial plexus: Little recovery due to difficulty in the approximation (retraction) of torn nerve ends
- Suturing: Difficult procedure, thus better to suture two nerve roots to one trunk.

## Lower Arm lesion (Klumpke)

Definition — It is the lower lesion of brachial plexus due to involvement of C8 and T1 nerve roots.

MOI — Trauma:
- Fracture-dislocation of cervical spine, sholder joint
- RSA
- Fall from height
- Direct violence: Hit by a stick, gunshot injury
- Operative trauma: Rarely damaged while operating excising elbow.

Pathogenesis — Avulsion or stretching trauma exerted on 8th cervical and 1st dorsal nerve roots and sometimes also the 7th cervical. resulting in injury, i.e. due to forced hyperabduction of the arm, when a falling person tries to hold an object, e.g. failing to obtain a foothold on a moving train or bus, thus avulsing the nerve roots from the spinal cord. Usually the 1st dorsal root involved, resulting in paralysis of intrinsic muscles of hand, anesthesia of inner three and half fingers in front, and inner one and half behind, and oculopupillary fibers passing along 1st dorsal nerve root impaired.

Diagnosis — Deformity:
- Clawhand: Extended first phalanx with flexed 2nd and 3rd phalanges, with
Forearm flexed at the elbow
Muscular wastings (late cases) of hand muscles (hypothenar)
Muscle power and tone: Loss
Sensations and reflexes: Loss of sensations and reflexes (anesthesia along inner side of forearm, hand, and little finger
Muscular wasting: Thin, soft, and flabby—in lesions of long duration
Skin: Cold, glazed, and smooth (paralysis), excessive sweating in case of incomplete lesion; vasomotor changes: pallor, cyanosis, redness, shiny, and scaly skin, brittle nails in case of irritating lesion.
Horner's syndrome: Due to paralyzed cervical sympathetic:
- Partial tosis of upper eyelid (paralyzed levator palpebrae superioris)
- Enophthalmos (paralyzed Müllers muscle)

- Myosis (unopposed action of oculomotor nerve)
- Anhydrosis (loss of sweating on the affected side of face).

Management  Conservative treatment:

Immobilization of arm in relaxation position (right angled, by use of splints to relax deltoid and spinati), (forearm flexed and supinated to relax biceps, brachialis, and supinator).

Physiotherapy

Surgical treatment:

Indication: Neurotmesis lesions.

Surgery:
- Exploration of brachial plexus: Little recovery due to difficulty in the approximation (retraction) of torn nerve ends
- Suturing: Difficult procedure, thus better to suture two nerve roots to one trunk.

## Axillary (Circumflex) Nerve Injury

Anatomy  Composed of nerve fibers from C-5 and C-6, is a branch of posterior cord of the brachial plexus, passes through the quadrilateral space, then winds around the neck of the humerus, about finger's breadth below center of deltoid muscle, supply the deltoids and teres minor muscles, may got injured by fractures or dislocations of shoulder, or by penetrating wounds.

MOI  Direct trauma: Blow, gunshot injury, penetrating stab wounds

Fall from height

RSA

Fracture-dislocation of humerus

Pathogenesis  Deltoid muscle paralysed and wasted; paralysed teres minor

Diagnosis  Deformity: Arm hanging by side of chest

Muscular wasting: Deltoid thin, soft, flabby (old lesion)

Power: Deltoid paralysed: unable to raise flexed elbow

Sensations and reflexes: Loss of sensations and reflexes (anesthesia along outer side of arm

Skin: Cold, glazed, and smooth (paralysis)

Investigation  Testing deltoid: Asking patient to raise the flexed elbow from the side, while resistance to arm offered

Test: Electrical stimulation of nerve *in situ*, by inserting needles along the posterior border of the deltoid.

X-ray shoulder

Management  Conservative treatment:

Immobilization of arm in relaxation position (right angled—by use of splints to relax deltoid and spinati), (forearm flexed and supinated to relax biceps, brachialis, and supinator).

Physiotherapy

Surgical treatment:

Indication: Compression factor: Fracture dislocation

Surgery:
- Exploration of nerve: Best exposed through the same incision as for distal parts of brachial plexus, or to expose nerve in the axilla
- Suturing: As in case of brachial plexus, sutures to be inserted in the nerve ends, and the wound/s closed as much as possible prior to completion of neurorrhaphy.

Results of suturing: Usually unsatisfactory.

Postoperative: Immobilization with POP cast for 6–8/56.

Stitches removed after 2/7, through window in the plaster cast

Physiotherapy: Exercises in abduction brace.

Occupational therapy.

## Nerve of Bell (Syn. External Respiratory Nerve, Long Thoracic Nerve) Injury

| | |
|---|---|
| Anatomy | Composed of nerve fibers from C-5, C-6, and C-7, sometimes from C-8 also, runs downward behind the cervical part of the brachial plexus, then runs on the outer surface of serratus anterior muscle, giving off twigs to each of its digitations |
| MOI | Direct trauma: Blow, gunshot injury, penetrating stab wounds |
| | Carrying a heavy weight on the shoulder |
| | RSA |
| | Operative complications: Procedures on the breast or chest wall. |
| Pathogenesis | Serratus anterior muscle paralysed and wasted by the stretching of long thoracic nerve or of severing of this nerve during operation. |
| Diagnosis | Deformity: 'Winging' of scapula, i.e. vertebral border and inferior angle unduly prominent |
| | Muscular wasting: Serratus anterior thin, soft, flabby (old lesion) |
| | Power: Serratus paralysed: unable to raise arm above shoulder |
| | Sensations and reflexes: Loss of sensations and reflexes (anesthesia along outer side of arm |
| | Skin: Cold, glazed, and smooth (paralysis). |
| Investigation | Testing serratus: Asking patient to raise the arm, scapula wings and the vertebral body and inferior angle become unduly prominent. |
| | • Also unable to exert forward pushing forward |
| | Electrical stimulation of nerve *in situ*, by inserting two needles through the skin, one on each side of nerve, and connecting these needles to a stimulator—motor response (distal nerve) to the stimulation at level of lesion (intact nerve). |
| | X-ray chest |
| Management | Conservative treatment: |
| | Immobilization of arm in relaxation position (right angled—by use of splints to relax deltoid and spinati), (forearm flexed and supinated to relax biceps, brachialis, and supinator). |
| | Physiotherapy |
| | Surgical treatment: |
| | Indication: Compression factor: fracture dislocation |

Surgery:
- Exploration of nerve: Best exposed through the same incision as for distal parts of brachial plexus, or to expose nerve in the axilla
- Suturing: As in case of brachial plexus, sutures to be inserted in the nerve ends, and the wound/s closed as much as possible prior to completion of neurorrhaphy.
  Results of suturing: Usually unsatisfactory.
- Scapula fixing: Steadied by a slip of pectoralis major muscle, that is detached from the humerus and fixed to the inferior angle of the scapula.

Postoperative: Immobilization with POP cast for 6–8/56.

Stitches removed after 2/7, through window in the plaster cast

Physiotherapy: Exercises in abduction brace.

Occupational therapy.

## Ulnar Nerve Injury

| | |
|---|---|
| Anatomy | Composed of nerve fibers from C-8 and D-1, from the medial cord of the brachial plexus. After supplying one and half muscles in the forearm flexor carpi ulnaris and medial half of flexor digitorum profundus, it gives branches to short muscles of the hand (Palmaris brevis, abductor digiti inimi, opponens, flexor digiti minimi, 3rd and 4th lumbricals, palmar and dorsal interossei, and two parts of the adductor pollicis). |
| MOI | Trauma at the elbow: |
| | Supracondylar fractures of humerus in children |
| | Fractures of medial epicondyle of humerus |
| | Dislocations of elbow |
| | Monteggia fracture dislocation |
| | Direct trauma: Blow, gunshot injury, penetrating stab wounds |
| | RSA |
| | Operative complications: Excision of the elbow joint |
| | Deformity of elbow: Cubitus valgus—nerve stretched (tardy palsy) |
| | Trauma at the wrist: |
| | Cuts: Stab, blow, gunshot injury |
| | Fractures of lower end of radius: Colles fracture |
| Pathogenesis | Flexor carpi ulnaris and flexor digitorum profundus, and short muscles of hand paralysed and wasted by the stretching of ulnar nerve or of severing of this nerve during operation. |
| Diagnosis | Deformity: 'Claw hand' (clawing of little and ring fingers) |

Motor:
- Muscular wasting: Hypothenar eminence and intermetacarpal spaces
- Power: Flexor carpi ulnaris and medial half of flexor digitorum profundus, and short muscles of the hand paralysed.

Sensory:
- Deep:
- Loss of muscle pain: In all above said muscles

- Loss of joint sense: All joints of little finger and IP joints of ring finger
- Loss of pressure sense: On ulnar border of hand and whole little finger
- Cutaneous: Loss of light touch, pin prick, temperature (little finger)

Skin: Cold, glazed, and smooth (paralysis)

**Investigation**

Testing muscles:

Interossei: Dorsal and palmar are abductors and adductors of fingers, and are extensors of middle and terminal phalanges, fail in following:

Test:
- Ask patient to spread out (abduct) and close (adduct) fingers.
- Ask patient to straighten 2nd and 3rd phalanges of fingers, while 1st phalanges are steadied by the physician.
- Ask patient to grip (adduction) a card (card test).

Adductor pollicis and 1st palmar interosseus:
- Ask patient to grasp a book between thumbs and fingers of both hands: Terminal phalanx of thumb flexed immediately (ulnar palsy)
- Ask patient to grip a card between thumb and palm (unable to grip in ulnar palsy).

Electrical stimulation of nerve *in situ*, by inserting two needles through the skin, one on each side of nerve, and connecting these needles to a stimulator—motor response (distal nerve) to the stimulation at level of lesion (intact nerve).

Tinel's sign: To determine about regeneration that occurred or not in the nerve (injured or sutured); to be elicited after about a couple of months, by tapping over the course of the nerve, from below upwards, until a sensation of tingling or of pins and needles felt in the area supplied by the nerve: that is level of regeneration which shifts distally as regeneration progresses

X-ray forearm includes Elbow and wrist

X-ray hand

**Management**

Conservative treatment:

Immobilization of arm: Universal arm pouch

Analgesics, NSAIDs

Physiotherapy: Exercises

Surgical treatment:

Indication: Compression factor: fracture dislocation, wounds

Surgery:
- Exploration of nerve: To expose nerve in the line of incision, to isolate ends of divided nerve.
- Suturing: Sutures to be inserted in the nerve ends, and the wound/s closed as much as possible prior to completion of neurorrhaphy.

Results of suturing: Usually unsatisfactory.

Postoperative: Immobilization with POP cast for 4–6/56.

Stitches removed after 2/7, through window in the plaster cast

Physiotherapy: Exercises

Occupational therapy.

## Tardy (Syn. Delayed) Ulnar Nerve Palsy

| | |
|---|---|
| MOI | Malunited fractures of lateral condyle of humerus in children |
| | Fracture of medial epicondyle of humerus |
| | Fracture head of radius |
| | Dislocation of elbow joint |
| Pathogenesis | Increased carrying angle (cubitus valgus), ulnar nerve stretched in its groove, behind the medial epicondyle of humerus, resulting in an irritable syndrome or incomplete nerve paralysis. |
| Diagnosis | Deformity: Cubitus valgus |

Motor:

- Muscular wasting: Hypothenar eminence and intermetacarpal spaces
- Power: Flexor carpi ulnaris and medial half of flexor digitorum profundus, and short muscles of the hand paralyzed.

Sensory:

- Deep:
- Loss of muscle pain: In all above said muscles
- Loss of joint sense: All joints of little finger and IP joints of ring finger
- Loss of pressure sense: On ulnar border of hand and whole little finger
- Cutaneous: Loss of light touch, pin prick, temperature (little finger)

Skin: Cold, glazed, and smooth (paralysis)

| | |
|---|---|
| Investigation | X-ray elbow |
| Management | Surgical treatment |

- Transposition (anterior) of ulnar nerve:
  Indication: Tardy ulnar nerve palsy.

Procedure:

- Skin incision: Curved incision with concavity forwards
- Muscle: Humeral head of flexor carpi ulnaris divided/excised
- Medial intermuscular septum divided, to expose the nerve
- Nerve transferred anteriorly in front of medial epicondyle
- A bed prepared amongst flexor group of muscles, to burry the nerve therin.

Postoperative: Immobilization with POP cast for 4–6/56.

Stitches removed after 2/7, through window in the plaster cast

Physiotherapy: Exercises

Occupational therapy.

## Median Nerve Injury

| | |
|---|---|
| Anatomy | Composed of nerve fibers from C-6, C-7, C-8 and D-1, from the medial and lateral cords of the brachial plexus in the axilla. After supplying muscles in forearm (pronator teres, flexor carpi radialis, palmaris longus, flexor digitorum sublimis, flexor pollicis longus, lateral half of flexor digitorum profundus, and pronator quadratus) it gives branches |

|  | in the hand to (abductor pollicis brevis, flexor pollicis brevis, opponens pollicis, and 1st and 2nd lumbricals) |
| MOI | Trauma at the elbow: |
|  | Supracondylar fractures of humerus in children |
|  | Dislocations of elbow joint |
|  | Direct trauma: Blow, gunshot injury, penetrating stab wounds |
|  | RSA |
|  | Operative complications: excision of the elbow joint |
|  | Trauma at the wrist: |
|  | Cuts: Stab, blow, gunshot injury |
|  | Fractures of lower end of radius: Colles fracture |
|  | Dislocation of semilunar bone |
|  | Carpal tunnel syndrome |
| Pathogenesis | Pronator teres, flaxor carpi radialis, palmaris longus, flexor digitorum sublimis, flexor pollicis longus, lateral half of flexor digitorum profundus, and pronator quadratus, it gives branches in the hand to (abductor pollicis brevis, flexor pollicis brevis, opponens pollicis, and 1st and 2nd lumbricals), paralyzed by the stretching of median nerve or of severing of this nerve during operation. |
| Diagnosis | Deformity: 'Ape thumb' (thumb being in line with other metacarpals) |

Motor:

- Muscular wasting: thenar eminence
- Power:
  - Flexor carpi radialis paralyzed: hand deviates to ulnar side when being flexed against resistance
  - Flexor longus pollicis paralyzed: unable to flex terminal phalanx of the thumb

Sensory:

- Deep:
- Loss of muscle pain: In all above said muscles
- Loss of joint sense: All joints of little finger and IP joints of ring finger
- Loss of pressure sense: On ulnar border of hand and whole little finger
- Cutaneous: Loss of light touch, pin prick, temperature (ends of the thumb, index, middle fingers).

Skin: Cold, glazed, and smooth (paralysis), trophic changes in the terminal phalanx of index finger).

|  | |
| Investigation | Testing muscles: |

Interossei: Dorsal and palmar are abductors and adductors of fingers, and are extensors of middle and terminal phalanges, fail in following:

Test:

- Ask patient to spread out (abduct) and close (adduct) fingers
- Ask patient to straighten 2nd and 3rd phalanges of fingers, while 1st phalanges are steadied by the physician.
- Ask patient to grip (adduction) a card (card test).

Abductor pollicis brevis:

- Ask patient to lay his/her hand flat upon the table with the palm facing upwards and touch with his/her thumb a pen held in front of it (pen test): unable to touch.

Opponens pollicis:

- Ask patient to touch ends of the fingers with the tip of the thumb (unable to touch in median palsy).

Flexor pollicis longus:

- Ask patient to bend the terminal phalanx of the thumb, while proximal phalanx being held firmly by the physician to eliminate action of short flexors (unable to touch in median palsy).

Electrical stimulation of nerve *in situ*, by inserting two needles through the skin, one on each side of nerve, and connecting these needles to a stimulator—motor response (distal nerve) to the stimulation at level of lesion (intact nerve).

Tinel's sign: To determine about regeneration that occurred or not in the nerve (injured or sutured); to be elicited after about a couple of months, by tapping over the course of the nerve, from below upwards, until a sensation of tingling or of pins and needles felt in the area supplied by the nerve: that is level of regeneration which shifts distally as regeneration progresses

X-ray forearm including Elbow and wrist

X-ray hand.

**Management**

Conservative treatment:

Immobilization of arm: universal arm pouch

Analgesics, NSAIDs

Physiotherapy: Exercises

Surgical treatment:

Indication: Compression factor: fracture dislocation, wounds

Surgery:

- Exploration of nerve: To expose nerve in the line of incision, to isolate ends of divided nerve.
- Suturing: Sutures to be inserted in the nerve ends, and the wound/s closed as much as possible prior to completion of neurorrhaphy.
  Results of suturing: Usually unsatisfactory.
- Carpal tunnel decompression:
  Indication: Unrelieved symptoms of carpal tunnel syndrome
- Excision lunate, with/without prosthetic replacement:

Indication: Avascular necrosis, with median nerve compression

Postoperative: Immobilization with POP cast for 4–6/56.

Stitches removed after 2/7, through window in the plaster cast

Physiotherapy: Exercises

Occupational therapy.

## Radial (Syn. Musculospiral) Nerve Injury

| | |
|---|---|
| Anatomy | Composed of nerve fibers from C-6, C-8 and D-1, from the posterior cord of the brachial plexus. It is primarily a motor nerve and supplies muscles in the arm (triceps, anconeus, brachioradialis, lateral fourth of brachialis anticus, extensor carpi radialis longus and brevis), and in the forearm (supinators of forearm, and extensors of the wrist, fingers, and thumb). |
| MOI | Trauma:<br>Fractures of the middle of shaft of humerus<br>Fractures and dislocations of the upper end of humerus<br>Supracondylar fracture of humerus<br>Fracture dislocations of lower end of humerus<br>Direct trauma: Blow, gunshot injury, penetrating stab wounds<br>RSA<br>Operative complications: Excision of malignant tumors of humerus, prolonged application of tourniquet |
| Pathogenesis | Triceps, supinators, and extensors of the wrist, fingers, and thumb paralyzed and wasted by the stretching of radial nerve or of severing of this nerve during operation. |
| Diagnosis | Deformity: 'Wrist drop' |

Motor:
- Muscular wasting
- Power: Triceps, and extensors of wrist and fingers paralyzed

Sensory:
- Deep:
- Loss of muscle pain: in all above said muscles
- Loss of joint sense: usually unaffected
- Loss of pressure sense: on ulnar border of hand and whole little finger
- Cutaneous: Loss of light touch, pin prick, temperature (dorsum of forearm, back of hand (2nd and 3rd metacarpals and proximal phalages).

Skin: Cold, glazed, and smooth (paralysis), trophic changes usually trivial.

| | |
|---|---|
| Investigation | Testing muscles:<br>Triceps:<br>Test: |

- Ask patient to place forearm mid prone position, and then to flex it against resistance (unable to extend wrist, thumb and MP joints of the fingers.
- Ask patient to place forearm mid prone position, and then to flex it against resistance, muscle seen and felt as it stands out (unable to flex it against resistance)

Electrical stimulation of nerve *in situ*, by inserting two needles through the skin, one on each side of nerve, and connecting these needles to a stimulator—motor response (distal nerve) to the stimulation at level of lesion (intact nerve).

Tinel's sign: To determine about regeneration that occurred or not in the nerve (injured or sutured); to be elicited after about a couple of months, by tapping over the course of the nerve, from below upwards, until a sensation of tingling or of pins and needles felt in the area supplied by the nerve: that is level of regeneration which shifts distally as regeneration progresses

X-ray arm including Shoulder and elbow

X-ray hand including wrist

| Management | Conservative treatment: |
|---|---|

Immobilization of arm: Universal arm pouch

Physiotherapy: Exercises

Surgical treatment:

Indication: Compression factor: fracture dislocation, wounds

Surgery:
- Exploration of nerve: To expose nerve in the line of incision, to isolate ends of divided nerve.
- Suturing: Sutures to be inserted in the nerve ends, and the wound/s closed as much as possible prior to completion of neurorrhaphy.

Results of suturing: Usually unsatisfactory.

Postoperative: Immobilization with POP cast for 4–6/56.

Stitches removed after 2/7, through window in the plaster cast

Physiotherapy: Exercises

Occupational therapy.

## Sciatic Nerve Injury

| Anatomy | Composed of nerve fibers from L-4, L-5, S-1, S-2, and S-3, from the sacral plexus. It is the thickest nerve in the body, initially in form of a flattened band, then sooner becomes oval or round one, traverses the gluteal region between greater trochanter of femur and ischial tuberosity, ends half-way down back of thigh by dividing into lateral and medial popliteal (in popliteal fossa) nerves, and also as common peroneal nerves (in leg and their relation to its bones), primarily a motor nerve and supplies muscles (all hamstrings, i.e. all flexors of knee, except sartorius, all leg, and all foot). |
|---|---|
| MOI | Trauma: |

Fractures of the pelvis and upper end of femur

Dislocations of hip

Direct trauma: Blow, gunshot injury, penetrating stab wounds

RSA

Operative complications: Excision of malignant tumors of femur, hindquarter amputations

| Pathogenesis | Flexors of knee paralyzed, complete paralysis below knee, by the truma of stretching, or severance of this nerve during operation. |
|---|---|

| | |
|---|---|
| Diagnosis | Deformity: 'Foot drop' |
| | Motor: |

- Muscular wasting
- Power: All hamstrings (all flexors of knee) paralyzed

Sensory:
- Deep:
- Loss of muscle pain: In all paralyzed (above said) muscles
- Loss of joint sense: Ankle, foot, and toe joints
- Loss of pressure sense: Beyond metatarsal heads
- Cutaneous: Loss of light touch, pin prick, temperature, below knee

Skin: Cold, glazed, and smooth (paralysis), trophic changes usually trivial.

| | |
|---|---|
| Investigation | Testing muscles: |

Doriflexion of ankle:

Test:
- To be tested: With the foot on its lateral border; with the leg hanging down from end of bed; and against resistance (unable to dorsiflex foot).

Electrical stimulation of nerve *in situ* is difficult as—is deeply placed, electromyography is helpful in evaluating this nerve—by inserting two needles through the skin, one on each side of nerve, and connecting these needles to a stimulator—motor response (distal nerve) to the stimulation at level of lesion (intact nerve).

Skin resistance test: Confirmatory

Tinel's sign: To determine about regeneration that occurred or not in the nerve (injured or sutured); to be elicited after about a couple of months, by tapping over the course of the nerve, from below upwards, until a sensation of tingling or of pins and needles felt in the area supplied by the nerve: that is level of regeneration which shifts distally as regeneration progresses.

X-ray pelvis, knee, and ankle.

| | |
|---|---|
| Management | Conservative treatment: |

Immobilization of leg
Physiotherapy: Exercises

Surgical treatment:
Indication: Compression factor: fracture dislocation, wounds

Surgery:
- Exploration of nerve: Exposed from its emergence from the sciatic notch to the point of its division into tibial and peroneal nerves
- Suturing: Sutures to be inserted in the nerve ends, and the wound/s closed as much as possible prior to completion of neurorrhaphy.

Results of suturing: Usually satisfactory, when tibial nerve is affected than when peroneal is the nerve involved.

Postoperative: Immobilization with splints for 4–6/56.

Stitches removed after 2/7, through window in the plaster cast

Physiotherapy: Exercises

Occupational therapy.

## Lateral Popliteal (Common Peroneal) Nerve Injury

Anatomy  Composed of nerve fibers from L-4, L-5 and S-1, S-2, is the smaller of the two terminal divisions of the sciatic nerve, arises from middle of the thigh, and terminates at the lateral side of fibular neck, under cover of peroneus longus muscle, dividing into superficial peroneal (musculo-cutaneous) nerve, and deep peroneal (anterior tibial) nerve, supplies two cuteneous and three articular branches, no muscular branch, except occasionally 1st branch to peroneus longus.

MOI  Trauma:

Fracture or excision of upper end of fibula

Fracture dislocations of knee

Lateral collateral ligament injury

Direct trauma: Blow, gunshot injury, penetrating stab wounds

RSA

Operative complications: Multiple ligation of varicose veins

Subcutaneous tenotomy of biceps tendon

Pressure from tight plasters/or splints.

Pathogenesis  Complete paralysis of extensor and peroneal groups of muscles, resulting talipes equinovarus, by the stretching of nerve or of severing of this nerve during operation.

Diagnosis  Deformity: 'foot drop', i.e. ankle fully plantar flexed and cannot be dorsiflexed, foot adducted and inverted, 2nd and 3rd phalanges can be extended by interossei, being supplied by tibial nerve.

Motor:
- Muscular wasting
- Power: Paralyzed extensor and peroneal groups of muscles.

Sensory:
- Deep:
  - Loss of muscle pain: In all above said muscles
  - Loss of joint sense: Usually unaffected
  - Loss of pressure sense: On ulnar border of hand and whole little finger
  - Cutaneous: loss of light touch, pin prick, temperature (dorsum of foot and outer surface of leg)

Skin: Cold, glazed, and smooth (paralysis), trophic changes usually trivial.

Investigation  Testing muscles:

Doriflexion of ankle:

Test:
- To be tested: With the foot on its lateral border; with the leg hanging down from end of bed; and against resistance (unable to dorsiflex ankle).

Electrical stimulation of nerve *in situ*, by inserting two needles through the skin, one on each side of nerve, and connecting these needles to a stimulator—motor response (distal nerve) to the stimulation at level of lesion (intact nerve).

Tinel's sign: To determine about regeneration that occurred or not in the nerve (injured or sutured); to be elicited after about a couple of months, by tapping over the course of the nerve, from below upwards, until a sensation of tingling or of pins and needles felt in the area supplied by the nerve: that is level of regeneration which shifts distally as regeneration progresses.

X-ray knee and ankle

Management                  Conservative treatment:

Immobilization: For fracture dislocation

Physiotherapy: Exercises

Surgical treatment:

Indication: Compression factor: fracture dislocation, wounds

Surgery:
- Exploration of nerve: To expose nerve in the line of incision, to isolate ends of divided nerve.
- Suturing: Sutures to be inserted in the nerve ends, and the wound/s closed as much as possible prior to completion of neurorrhaphy.

Results of suturing: Usually unsatisfactory.
- Fracture dislocation: Closed or open reduction
- Ligament repair:

Indication: Tear lateral collateral ligament with injury nerve

Postoperative: Immobilization in a double spica cast from nipple line to the toes on affected side, and to above knee on the normal side, for 6/56.

Stitches removed after 2/7, through window in the plaster cast

Physiotherapy: Exercises

Occupational therapy.

## Medial Popliteal Nerve Injury

Anatomy                     Composed of nerve fibers from L-4, L-5, S-1, S-2, and S-3, is the larger of the two terminal branches of the sciatic nerve, begins a little above the popliteal fossa about middle of back of thigh, enters fossa at its upper angle, emerging from under cover of biceps femoris, bisects fossa and continuous below at its distal angle as the posterior tibial nerve. It is primarily a motor nerve and supplies muscles in the lower part of fossa (gastrocnemius, plantaris, soleus, and popliteus), three articular branches, and cutaneous (sural nerve) branch.

MOI                         Trauma:

Fracture dislocations of knee

Direct trauma: Blow, gunshot injury, penetrating stab wounds

RSA

|  |  |
|---|---|
|  | Operative complications: Excision of malignant tumors<br>Subcutaneous tenotomy of biceps tendon<br>Pressure from tight plasters/or splints. |
| Pathogenesis | Paralysis of calf muscles and muscles of the sole, resulting in talipes calcaneovalgus, by the stretching of nerve or of severing of this nerve during operation. |
| Diagnosis | Deformity: 'Talipes calcaneovalgus', foot held dorsiflexed at ankle and everted<br>Motor: |

Diagnosis

Deformity: 'Talipes calcaneovalgus', foot held dorsiflexed at ankle and everted

Motor:
- Muscular wasting
- Power: Popliteus, soleus, gastrocnemius, tibialis posterior, flexor longus digitorum, flexor longus hallucis, all muscles of foot except extensor brevis digitorum paralyzed, sole paralyzed.

**Sensory:**
- Deep:
- Loss of muscle pain: In all above said muscles
- Loss of joint sense
- Loss of pressure sense: On sole
- Cutaneous: Loss of light touch, pin prick, temperature (plantar surface of toes and on dorsal aspect of last phalanges.

Skin: Cold, glazed, and smooth (paralysis), trophic changes usually trivial.

Investigation

Testing muscles:

Muscles of foot:

Test:
- Ask patient to flex the foot or toes, or to stand on tiptoe (unable to flex the foot or toes, or to stand on tiptoe).

Electrical stimulation of nerve *in situ*, by inserting two needles through the skin, one on each side of nerve, and connecting these needles to a stimulator—motor response (distal nerve) to the stimulation at level of lesion (intact nerve).

Tinel's sign: To determine about regeneration that occurred or not in the nerve (injured or sutured); to be elicited after about a couple of months, by tapping over the course of the nerve, from below upwards, until a sensation of tingling or of pins and needles felt in the area supplied by the nerve: that is level of regeneration which shifts distally as regeneration progresses

X-ray knee and arm including shoulder and elbow

X-ray hand including wrist

Management

Conservative treatment:

Immobilization

Physiotherapy: Exercises

Surgical treatment:

Indication: Compression factor: fracture dislocation, wounds

Surgery:

- Exploration of nerve: To expose nerve in the line of incision, to isolate ends of divided nerve.
- Suturing: Sutures to be inserted in the nerve ends, and the wound/s closed as much as possible prior to completion of neurorrhaphy.

Results of suturing: Usually unsatisfactory.

Postoperative: Immobilization in a double spica cast from nipple line to the toes on affected side, and to above knee on the normal side, for 6/56.

Stitches removed after 2/7, through window in the plaster cast

Physiotherapy: Exercises

Occupational therapy.

## Bibliography

1. Abbott LC. Injuries of the median nerve in fractures of the lowewr end of the radius, surg., Gynec. and Obst. 57:507, 1933.
2. Adson AW. The surgical treatment of progressive ulnar paralysis, Med. 1:455, Minnesota, 1918.
3. Allbritten FF, Jr. Method for repair of posterior tibial nerve, Am. J. Surg. 73:588, 1947.
4. Calandruccio A. Orthopaedic reconstruction for paralysis due to injury of brachial plexus, Campbell's Operative Orthopaedics, ed. 9th, Vol I-IV. C.V. Mosby Co., Saint Louis, 1998.
5. Canale ST, et al. Campbell's Operative Orthopaedics, ed. 9th, Vol I-IV. C.V. Mosby Co., Saint Louis, 1998.
6. Cannon B, Love JG. Tardy median palsy, median neuritis, median thenar neuritis amenable to surgery, Surgery 20:210, 1946.
7. Davidsopn AJ, Horwitz MT. Late or tardy ulnar-nerve paralysis, J. Bone and Joint Surg. 17:844, 1935.
8. Davis L, Martin J, Perret G. The treatment of injuriesw of the brachial plexus, Ann. Surg. 125:647, 1947.
9. Haymaker W, Woodhall B. Peripheral nerve injuries. Principles of diagnosis, ed. 2, W.B. Saunders Co., Philadelphia, 1953.
10. Kapoor PS. Peripheral nerve injuries. Accident and Emergency, ed. 2nd, Part I, CBS, New Delhi, 2016.
11. Kirklin JW, et al. Suture of peripheral nerves, Surg., Gynec. and Obst. 88:719, 1949.
12. Love M, et al. Bailey and Love's Short Practice of Surgery, ed. 13th, H.K. Lewis and Co., London, 1965.
13. Lyons WR, Woodhall B. Atlas of peripheral nerve injuries, W.B. Saunders Co., Phildelphia, 1949.
14. Mayfield FH, Devine JW. Causalgia, Surg., Gynec. and Obst. 80:631, 1945 Pollard C. Jr., and Grantham E.G.: Peripheral nerve surgery: incisions for exposures of peripheral nerves, Am. J. Surg. 86:61, 1953.
15. Murphy F. Peripheral nerve injuries, Campbell's Operative Orthopaedics, ed. 9th, Vol I-IV. C.V. Mosby Co., Saint Louis, 1998.
16. Pollock LJ, Davis L. Peripheral nerve injuries, Paul B. Hoeber, Inc., New York, 1933.
17. Scarff JE. Peripheral nerve injuries: principles of treatment, M. Clin. North America 42:611, 1958.
18. Seletz E. Surgery of peripheral nerves, Charles C Thomas , Publisher, Springfield, III, 1951.
19. Woodhall B. The surgical repair of acute peripheral nerve injury, S. Clin. North America 31:1369, 1951.

# 11

# Peripheral Vascular Trauma

Affections of arteries:
- Traumatic:
  – Acute arterial injury
  – Volkmann's ischemic contracture (VIC)
  – Acute arterial arrest
  – Aneurysm
- Infective:
  – Gangrene
  – Infective gangrene
  – Diabetic gangrene
- Arterial occlusive diseases:
  – Arteriosclerotic occlusive disease
  – Arterial embolism
  – Fat embolism
  – Arterial thrombosis
- Vasospastic disorders:
  – Raynaud's disease
  – Thromboangitis oblitrans (Buerger's disease)
- Vasomotor disorders:
  – Cervical rib (Scalenus anticus syndrome)
  – Causalgia
  – Sudeck's atrophy

Affections of veins:
- Venous occlusive dieases:
  – Superficial vein thrombosis (Thrombophlebitis)
  – Deep vein thrombosis (DVT) (Phlebothrombosis)
  – Varicose veins
  – Venous insufficiency.

## Acute Arterial Injury

Definition     It is defined as an injury to the artery in form of contusion, laceration, or division, resulting in arterial hemorrhage, hematoma, ischemia of the muscles and nerves, paresthesiae, paralysis, gangrene of the part; the contusion and simple laceration are most common arterial injuries encountered in the management of trauma involving the limbs.

MOI     Direct trauma: Violence
Fractures/fracture dislocations

Infective: Compound fractures, wounds

Suicidal trauma

Endocrinal: Diabetes mellitus

Metabolic: Growths esp. malignant one penetrating artery.

**Pathogenesis**  Arterial contusion; arterial laceration; arterial division; hemorrhage; hematoma; muscle/nerve ischemia; paresthesia; paralysis

**Diagnosis**  Pain

Swelling: May pulsate (pulsating hematoma)

Local tenderness

Paresthesia

**Complications**
- Anterior compartment of leg syndrome
- Aneurysm (penetration/or rupture)
- Arteriovenous fistula
- VIC
- Gangrene

**Investigation**  X-ray for fracture/fracture dislocation—pressing/perforating artery
- Color doppler

**Management**  Aim: To arrest hemorrhage, and reconstruction of damaged artery.

Conservative treatment:
- Analgesics, NSAIDs
- Vasodilators: Methods:
  - Buerger's position: HOB raised (cause hydrostatic congestion that may result in vasodilatation)
  - Buerger's exercises: Elevating and lowering leg, each for two mts.; repeat for half an hour b.i.d. or t.i.d.
- Vasodilator drugs: Role controversial:
  - Alcohol (whisky, brandy, sherry)
  - Barbiturate: To induce vasodilation and sleep
  - Paravertebral block: For lower limb: 20 mL of 1% lignocaine injected beside bodies of 2nd, 3rd, and 4th lumbar vertebrae.
- Anticoagulants:
  - Heparin 5 KA units IV four hourly, or by continuous infusion of 3 KA units in 1.5 KL of normal saline in 24 hours
  - Phenindione (Dindevan) 200 mg, and Dicoumarol (Warfarin) 30 mg: lower blood level of prothrombin.

Surgical treatment:

*Surgery*:
- Exploration of the affected blood vessel; further treatment depends upon the type of injury
- Contusion (arterial spasm): Massage; irrigation with Papaverine
- Lacerated (intimal damage): Resection of the affected segment and grafting
- Divided: Direct (an end to end) anastomosis
- Gaped: Graft or prosthesis to bridge the gap.

Management of complications:
- Traumatic anterior compartment leg syndrome: Splitting of the roof ASAP, to drian the hematoma.

## Volkmann's Ischemic Contracture (VIC)

| | |
|---|---|
| Preface | It is a progressive degeneration of muscle tissue resulting from an interrupting vascular supply to a limb or part of a limb, resulting in ischemic necrosis of muscles and nerves; fibrosis; ischemic contractures |
| Definition | It is defined as a progressive degeneration of muscle tissue resulting from an interruption of arterial blood supply distal to the obstruction, usually caused by trauma (fracture/fracture dislocation); resulting in ischemia of muscles and nerves, paresthesia, and finally muscle replaced by fibrous tissue causing ischemic contractures and/or paralysis; the roughened bony edge may cause arterial laceration, resulting in the formation of a hematoma; fracture/fracture dislocation may also cause severe arterial spasm, aneurysm, or intimal damage. |
| Etiology | Direct trauma: Violence, fractures, fracture dislocations |
| | Upper limb: Usually post supracondylar fractures of the humerus; post fractures of radius and ulna |
| | Lower limb: Post tibial fractures |
| | RSA |
| | Fall from a height |
| | Sports injuries |
| | Exposure: To cold or heat |
| | CVS: Arteriosclerosis, embolism, thrombosis |
| Precipitating factors | Smoking, exposure to extreme of cold (frost bite) or heat. |
| Pathogenesis | Impaired blood supply distal to a fracture, by displaced fracture/or dislocation; hematoma; arterial spasm; muscle ischemia; nerve ischemia; degenerated and necrosed muscle tissue replaced by fibrous tissue causing Volkmann's contracture. |
| Diagnosis | Pain: Severe persisting post reduction of fracture |
| | Pulse: Loss of distal pulses (radial, popliteal, and dorsalis pedis) |
| | Skin: White or dusky |
| | Sensation: Anesthesia |
| | Deformity: Fingers held in flexion (claw hand); surgeon unable to straighten the patient's fingers, and to extend the wrist (+ve sign) |
| | Muscle: Paralytic |
| Investigation | CBC, ESR, blood sugar, cholesterol |
| | WR for syphilis |
| | Color doppler: Arteriography |
| | X-ray—plain: May show arterial calcification |
| D/d | • Arteriosclerosis in elderly persons |
| | • Cervical rib in middle and elderly persons |
| | • Raynaud's disease: Commonly the upper limbs esp. finger tips |
| | • Buerger's disease: Commonly the lower limbs |

- Senile gangrene: Commonly the lower limbs
- Superficial gangrene of fingers/toes (cervical rib; Morvan's disease).

**Management**    Aim: An early diagnosis and management may relieve the agony.

Preventive treatment:
- To protect ischemic parts: Peripheral vascular disorders require cautious chiropody
- To avoid: Heating or freezing an ischemic part.

Specific treatment:
- Analgesics, NSAIDs
- Vasodilator drugs: Role controversial:
- Alcohol (whisky, brandy, sherry)
- Barbiturate: To induce vasodilation and sleep
- Paravertebral block for lower limb: 20 mL of 1% lignocaine injected beside bodies of 2nd, 3rd, and 4th lumbar vertebrae
- Anticoagulants:
- Heparin 5 KA units IV four hourly, or by continuous infusion of 3 KA units in 1.5 KL of normal saline in 24 hours
- Phenindione (Dindevan) 200 mg, and dicoumarol (Warfarin) 30 mg: lower blood level of prothrombin.

Surgical treatment:
Surgery: Procedures indicated in:
Impending VIC: Fasciotomy and arteriectomy.

Established VIC:
- Lengthening of tendons: Preferable over other procedures
- Transferring distally of muscles origins
- Shortening bones of forearm
- Carpectomy.

## Fasciotomy and arteriectomy
Technique:
- Anesthesia: General
- Incision: An anterior curvilinear incision centered over the elbow, medial to biceps tyendon
- Incise: Deep fascia, lacertus fibrosus, drain any hematoma present; mostly that is sufficient to relieve the impaired vascularity
- Exposure of brachial artery; ligate if lacerated; incise arterial wall if spasmodic and remove if any thrombus present, repair the arterial wall incision
- Arteriectomy: To relieve reflex spasm of collateral vessels
- Exposure of flexor muscle bellies (ischemic, grey): Incise deep fascia; divide intermuscular septa
- Suturing of damaged median nerve for repair later on
- Suturing: Skin with loose sutures

Postoperative: Immobilization of arm.
After care: Exercises.

## Acute Arterial Arrest

| | |
|---|---|
| Preface | Trauma plays an important role in interrupting vascular supply to any part of the body, resulting in necrosis or gangrene, unless there is an alternative pathway to by-pass the obstruction (collateral circulation); end artery obstruction due to trauma may cause necrosis (no collateral circulation); factors that help in establishing an adequate collateral circulation including normal cardiac output, no atherosclerosis, tissues with abundant vascular network; adverse factors including CHF, atherosclerosis, embolism/thrombosis, and joints without muscle coverage, e.g. knee joint; time factor is vital for opening up of collateral circulation. |
| Definition | It is defined as an interruption of arterial blood supply distal to the obstruction, usually caused by trauma (fracture/fracture dislocation); resulting in ischemia of muscles and nerves, paresthesia, and finally muscle paralysis; roughened bony edge may cause arterial laceration, resulting in formation of a hematoma; fracture/fracture dislocation may also cause severe arterial spasm, aneurysm, or intimal damage. |
| Etiology | Direct trauma: Violence<br>RSA<br>Fall from a height<br>Sports injuries<br>Exposure: To cold or heat<br>CVS: Arteriosclerosis, embolism, thrombosis |
| Precipitating factors | Smoking, exposure to extreme of cold (frost bite) or heat. |
| Pathogenesis | Blood supply distal to a fracture, interrupted by displaced kinking of artery by displaced fracture/or dislocation; hematoma; arterial spasm; muscle ischemia; nerve ischemia. |
| Diagnosis | History: (Interrogation and clinical examination): |

Age:
- Raynaud's disease: Common in young women
- Buerger's disease: In men of 30–40 years
- Diabetes and Syphilis in middle age
- Arteriosclerosis: In elderly persons
- Cervical rib: In middle and elderly persons.

Limbs:
- Raynaud's disease: Commonly the upper limbs esp. finger tips
- Buerger's disease: Commonly the lower limbs
- Senile gangrene: Commonly the lower limbs
- Superficial gangrene of fingers/toes (cervical rib; Morvan's disease).

MOI:
- Traumatic: Fractures, dislocations
- Infective: Compound fractures
- CVS: Embolism, thrombosis
- Endocrinal: Diabetic
- Metabolic: Growths.

Unilateral/bilateral:

- Unilateral: Senile gangrene
- Bilateral: Raynaud's disease, Buerger's disease (frequently)
- Both: Senile gangrene

Pain: Types:

- Exercise-pain (intermittent claudication): Cramplike pain that may occur in the calf muscles on exertion; localization of pain depends upon the level of obstruction.
- Rest-pain: Due to nerve ischemia (cry of dying nerve); mostly occurring at night, aggravated by elevating limb and relieved by lowering the leg.

Pulse: Loss of distal pulses

Skin: Pale, cold

Sensation: Paresthesiae

Muscle: Paralytic, green or black (gangrene), characteristic odor.

| | |
|---|---|
| **Investigation** | CBC, ESR, blood sugar, cholesterol<br>WR for syphilis<br>Color doppler: Arteriography<br>X-ray—plain: May show arterial calcification |
| **Management** | Conservative treatment: |

Preventive treatment:

- To avoid smoking: Esp. in case of patients with intermittent claudication (atherosclerosis; Buerger's disease; senile gangrene)
- To protect ischemic parts: Peripheral vascular disorders require cautious chiropody
- To avoid: Heating or freezing an ischemic part
- To reduce muscular activity: Walking within patient's claudication distance.

Specific treatment:

- Analgesics, NSAIDs
- Vasodilators: Methods:
- Buerger's position: HOB raised (cause hydrostatic congestion that may result in vasodilatation)
- Buerger's exercises: Elevating and lowering leg, each for two mts.; repeat for half an hour b.i.d. or t.i.d.
- Vasodilator drugs: Role controversial
- Alcohol (whisky, brandy, sherry)
- Barbiturate: To induce vasodilation and sleep
- Paravertebral block: For lower limb: 20 mL of 1% lignocaine injected beside bodies of 2nd, 3rd, and 4th lumbar vertebrae
- Anticoagulants:
- Heparin 5 KA units IV four hourly, or by continuous infusion of 3KA units in 1.5 KL of normal saline in 24 hours
- Phenindione (Dindevan) 200 mg, and Dicoumarol (Warfarin) 30 mg: Lower blood level of prothrombin

Surgical treatment

Surgery:

* Embolectomy and thrombectomy:

Technique:

* Anesthesia: Local or general
* Incision: Centered over the artery bulging with clot
* Exposure of artery bulging with clot, and its branches, exposed and isolated
* Divide: A longitudinal incision over the obstructed artery
* Removal of clot along with thrombus/embolus; extension-thrombus extracted by milking artery, or by a catheter
* Toilet of the wound with heparin saline solution, to wash out clots
* Perfusion of artery with papaverine sulphate 1% solution, to lessen spasm
* Perfusion of artery with fibrinolysins to control extension-thrombus.

## Aneurysm

**Definition**  It is defined as a sac (filled with blood) that is in direct communication with the interior of an artery; may be true (fusiform, saccular, dissecting) and false or arteriovenous fistula (congenital and acquired).

**Types**  True (fusiform, saccular, dissecting): due to dilatation of an artery:

* Fusiform: Commonest type; lumen more or less equally expanded; usually the artery weakened by hypertension and atheroma

Example:

* Mycotic aneurysm: Arterial wall weakened by bacterial and not fungal infection
* Syphilitic aneurysm: Aortic arch weakened by end arteritis of the vasa vasorum
* Saccular: Due to stretching of arterial wall because of trauma
* Dissecting: Occurs in aorta and its large branches due to separation of an atheromatous plaque, that permits blood insinuation between inner and outer layers of the media; rupture/or obstruction of arterial lumen may occur; mimics an embolus or thrombosis.

False: Due to trauma; extravasated blood enclosed in a condensed sac of cellular tissue

Arteriovenous fistula: Communication between an artery and a vein may be congenital or acquired by trauma sharp blow or a penetrating wound.

* Congenital: Structural effect of arterial blood shunting into veins, resulting in veins becoming dilated, tortuous, and thick walled (arterialized).
* Acquired: Physiological effect of arterial blood shunting into veins, resulting in high pulse pressure, left ventricular enlargement, and cardiac failure.

**Etiology**  Traumatic

Inflammatory

Infective: Bacterial, syphilitic

| | |
|---|---|
| Pathogenesis | Weakened arterial wall; dilatation; rupture; hemorrhage; inflammation; infective; thrombosis; embolism; termination: Consolidation (spontaneous cure), rupture, infection. |
| Diagnosis | Intrinsic: |

Intrinsic:
- Swelling: Pulsatile in the course of an artery; reducible
- Thrill: Palpable
- Bruit: Auscultated

Extrinsic:
- Pressure effects: Adjoining or distal structures affected, e.g. edema or altered sensation due to pressure on veins or nerves; bones, joints, or trachea, and esophagus, may be affected
- Backache

| | |
|---|---|
| D/d | Cervical rib |
| | Pancreatic cyst |
| | Abscess |
| | Tumor: Pulsating, e.g. osteosarcoma, osteoclastoma, meta |
| Investigation | CBC: Anemia |
| | ESR: Inceased, blood sugar |
| | Color doppler |
| | Arteriography (confirmatory) |
| Management | Surgical treatment of choice |
| | Indication: As per arteriography findings. |
| | Surgery: Various techniques: |

- Ligation and excision
- Exclusive + grafting
- Excision + grafting
- Reconstructive aneurysmorrhaphy

Ligation and excision:

Indication: Aneurysms of secondary arteries: Ligation of proximal and distal vessels; excision may be obligatory

Example: Hunterian ligation: Indicated in limb aneurysms esp. the popliteal aneurysm: Ligature to be placed above the main collateral nearest the aneurysm (above descending geniculate artery)

Exclusive + grafting: Excision undesirable (to safeguard adjoining vital structures; excluded aneurysm thromboses, shrinks into fibrous mass

Example: Abdominal vena cava aneurysm

Excision + grafting:

Indication: Excision desirable + grafting (end to end or end to side)

Reconstructive aneurysmorrhaphy: Excision of the sac + arterial reconstruction

Indication: Femoral or popliteal aneurysms.

## Infective Gangrene

| | |
|---|---|
| Definition | It is defined as death with putrefaction of macroscopic portions of tissue; usually affects the distal part of a limb, the appendix, small intestine, gallbladder, pancreas, or testis |
| Etiology | Traumatic: Direct trauma: crush injuries, pressure sores |
| | Infective: Boils, carbuncles, gas gangrene, scrotal gangrene |
| | Physical agents: Burns, scalds, frostbite, trench feet, acids, alkalies, electricity, and X-rays radiations |
| | Secondary: Classical mnemonic RESTED (Raynaud, ergot, senile, thrombosis, embolism, diabetes |
| Pathogenesis | Arterial obstruction; ischemic necrosis; death of tissue; slough; sequestrum formation; line of demarcation (between viable and dead tissue) appears quickly in dry gangrene compared to that in moist gangrene (due to infection); in atherosclerosis and embolism, line of demarcation is very slow; gangrene spreads by local extension; infection; and skipping. |
| Diagnosis | Clinical types: Dry and moist: |

- Dry gangrene: Part becomes dry, wrinkled, discolored, greasy; manifested in traumatic gangrene and frostbite; line of demarcation appears between
  Skin: Color changes (Table 11.1): Due to hemoglobin breakage and formation of iron sulphide.
- Moist gangrene: Part becomes swollen, discolored, and the epidermis raised in blebs; crepitus on palpation (gas formed); manifested in acute appendicitis, strangulated intestine and hernia.

Pain: Rest pain or intermittent claudication: senile gangrene
Swelling: Gas gangrene
Fever: Infective gangrene
Muscles: Brick red, green, or black

| | |
|---|---|
| Investigation | CBC, ESR |
| | WR (for syphilis) |
| | Urine: For diabetes |
| | Color Doppler |
| | X-ray neck |
| Management | As per type of gangrene, site, the organ affected, and the vascularity of the adjoining tissues. |
| | Preventive treatment: |

- Refrain from smoking, alcohol consumption, and cold exposure
- To protect pressure areas

**Table 11.1:** Color changes in gangrene

Purple → Mottled → Pale → Dusky grey
↓
Black ← Dark brown ← Black ← Greenish black

Conservative treatment

General measures:

- Analgesics, NSAIDs
- Vasodilators: Papaverine, methyldopa, reserpine

Local measures:

- Care of the affected part: To keep part dry with spirit, well aerated
- Toilet of the gangrenous part, by lifting of a crust, or removal of the dessicated skin.

Surgical treatment

Surgery:

- Amputation

Indication: As a life-saving measure

### Regional amputations

Amputations of leg:

Types: Conservative, semiconservative, and radical (definitive).

- Conservative amputation:

Aim: No urgency to remove a dry, painless, gangrenous toe, with adequate final line of demarcation

Indication: Diabetic or frostbitten gangrenous part be left to separate

Technique:

- Incision: Through line of demarcation
- Excision of bone and tendons at higher level, through cuff of skin and soft tissue
- Wounds: Left open to heal by granulation excision
- Semiconservative (compromise) amputation:

Aim: To compromise, when conservative amputation of the foot of no avail (failed), and there is an adequate blood supply

Indication: Below knee, through knee, or supracondylar

- Radical (definitive) amputation:

Aim: To overcome an impossible conservative amputation; to amputate high enough to ensure sound wound healing

Indication: Mid-thigh amputation, when there is failure of demarcation, spread of gangrene, failure of direct arterial salvage surgery or sympathectomy.

Technique:

- Incision: Above line of demarcation
- Excision of muscles at bone level (quadriceps divided with the knee flexed, and hamstrings with the knee extended)
- Femoral vessels isolated and ligated in the Hunter's canal
- Sciatic nerve: Isolated and divided sharply
- Dvide: Bone with bony stump of 15–20 cm below greater trochanter
- Skin flaps: Equal anterior and posterior flaps of skin, subcutaneous tissue and deep fascia; flaps sutured
- Drainage of the wound.

Postoperative: Immobilization of stump for 2/7

After care: Exercises

## Diabetic Gangrene

| | |
|---|---|
| Definition | It is defined as death with putrefaction of macroscopic portions of tissue; usually affects the distal part of a limb, the appendix, small intestine, gallbladder, pancreas, or testis. |
| Etiology | Due to three factors: |
| | Peripheral neuritis: Resulting in trophic changes |
| | Atheroma of arteries: Resulting in ischemia |
| | Hyperglycemia: Resulting in lowering of tissues resistance to infection |
| Pathogenesis | Arterial obstruction; ischemic necrosis; death of tissue; slough; sequestrum formation; line of demarcation (between viable and dead tissue) appears quickly in dry gangrene compared to that in moist gangrene (due to infection); in atherosclerosis and embolism, line of demarcation is very slow; gangrene spreads by local extension; infection; and skipping. |
| Diagnosis | Clinical types: dry and moist: |

- Dry gangrene: Part becomes dry, wrinkled, discolored, greasy; manifested in traumatic gangrene and frostbite; line of demarcation appears between
- Moist gangrene: Part becomes swollen, discolored, and the epidermis raised in blebs; crepitus on palpation (gas formed); manifested in acute appendicitis, strangulated intestine and hernia.

Pain: Diffuse

Sensation: Impaired, followed by vasomotor disturbances

Reaction of hyperemia: Absent

Muscles: Brick red, green, or black

Reflexes: Loss

Deformities: Claw toes with callosities

| | |
|---|---|
| Investigation | CBC, ESR |
| | Blood sugar |
| | Urine sugar |
| | Color Doppler |
| | X-ray: For any osteomyelitis |
| Management | As per type of gangrene, site, the organ affected, and the vascularity of the adjoining tissues. |

Preventive treatment:

- Refrain from smoking, alcohol consumption, and cold exposure
- To protect pressure areas

Conservative treatment

General measures:

- Control of diabetes by diet, exercise, and insulin or antidiabetic drugs
- Analgesics, NSAIDs
- Vasodilators: Papaverine, methyldopa, reserpine

Local measures:
* Care of the affected part: To keep part dry with spirit, well aerated
* Toilet of the gangrenous part, by lifting of a crust, or removal of the dessicated skin.

Surgical treatment
Surgery:
* Amputation

Indication         As a life-saving measure
### Regional amputations

Amputations of leg:
Types: Conservative, semiconservative, and radical (definitive).
* Conservative amputation:
Aim: No urgency to remove a dry, painless, gangrenous toe, with adequate final line of demarcation
Indication: Diabetic or frostbitten gangrenous part be left to separate

Technique:
* Incision: Through line of demarcation
* Excision of bone and tendons at higher level, through cuff of skin and soft tissue
* Wounds: Left open to heal by granulation excision
* Semiconservative (compromise) amputation:

Aim: To compromise, when conservative amputation of the foot of no avail (failed), and there is an adequate blood supply

Indication: Below knee, through knee, or supracondylar
* Radical (definitive) amputation:
Aim: To overcome an impossible conservative amputation; to amputate high enough to ensure sound wound healing
Indication: Mid-thigh amputation, when there is failure of demarcation, spread of gangrene, failure of direct arterial salvage surgery or sympathectomy

Technique:
* Incision: Above line of demarcation
* Excision of muscles at bone level (quadriceps divided with the knee flexed, and hamstrings with the knee extended)
* Femoral vessels isolated and ligated in the Hunter's canal
* Sciatic nerve: Isolated and divided sharply
* Divide: Bone with bony stump of 15–20 cm below greater trochanter
* Skin flaps: Equal anterior and posterior flaps of skin, subcutaneous tissue and deep fascia; flaps sutured
* Drainage of the wound.

Postoperative: Immobilization of stump for 2/7
After care: Exercises

## Arteriosclerotic Occlusive Disease

| | |
|---|---|
| Definition | It is defined as a spasmodic condition usually occurs in women, that affects the upper limb more than the lower; the digital arteries respond excessively to the vasospastic stimuli |
| Etiology | Unknown |
| | Direct trauma: Exposure to extreme cold |
| | Emotional distress |
| | Sympathetic nervous system: Abnormal |
| Pathogenesis | Exposure to cold; spasmodic arterioles; part blanched; accumulated metabolites in the capillaries; dilated capillaries; part swollen; recovery: relaxed arterioles, capillaries filled with oxygenated blood, part reddish and warm. |
| Diagnosis | Family history of a vasospastic phenomenon |
| | Sex: Women usually affected |
| | Age: 15 to 40 years |
| | Pain: Precipitated by cold; relieved by warmth |
| | Raynaud's phenomenon: Intermittent attacks of pallor or cyanosis in the fingers (rarely in toes), precipitated by cold or by emotional stress;  fingers usually involved; thumbs rarely affect; recovery usually takes place near base of fingers (red return of color to cyanotic or pale digit) |
| | Skin: Cold, pale, numbness of fingers, trophic changes (ulceration) |
| | Muscle: Wasting |
| D/d | Buerger's disease (thromboangitis obliterance) |
| | Arteriosclerosis |
| | Thoracic outlet syndrome |
| Investigation | CBC, ESR |
| | WR (for syphilis) |
| | Urine: For diabetes |
| | Color doppler |
| | X-ray neck |
| Management | Conservative treatment: |
| | Preventive: Refrain from exposure to cold |
| | Warmth: Body to be kept warm |
| | Analgesics, NSAIDs |
| | Vasodilators: Papaverine, methyldopa, reserpine |
| | Surgical treatment: |
| | Surgery: |
| | • Sympathectomy |
| Indication | Frequent severe attacks |

## Arterial Embolism

| | |
|---|---|
| Definition | An embolism is defined as a foreign body that circulates in the bloodstream, and may become lodged in the vessel, thereby cause an obstruction |

| | |
|---|---|
| Etiology | Atheromatous plaque |
| | Blood clots: From thrombosed veins or auricular appendage (MS or AF), mural thrombosis (MI) |
| | Vegetations from cardiac valves |
| Pathogenesis | An embolus blocking vessel; ischemic part; necrotic tissue; gangrene |
| Diagnosis | Pain: Sudden or gradual onset |
| | Coldness |
| | Numbness |
| | Pulsations: Absent in arteries distal to block |
| | Skin: Coldness, pallor, mottling, anesthesia/or hyperesthesia, blebs, necrosis, gangrene |
| | Muscles: Weakness, or paralyzed |
| | Superficial veins: Collapsed |
| | Regional effects: |
| | Brain: Hemiplegia (temporary or permanent), due to blockage of middle cerebral artery |
| | Eyes: Flash of light followed by blindness (total and permanent) due to the blockage of central artery supplying retina |
| | Lungs: Pulmonary embolism due to phlebothrombosis |
| | Mesentery: Engorgement and gangrene of the intestinal loop |
| | Kidneys: Pain in the loin and hematuria due to blockage of renal artery |
| | Spleen: Pain and splenomegaly due to blockage of splenic artery |
| | Limbs: Pain, pallor, loss of pulses, anesthesia, paresis, congestion and gangrene (legs: due to blockage of femoral artery, popliteal artery, or common iliac artery; arm: due to blockage at bifurcation of brachial artery). |
| Investigation | CBC, ESR, blood sugar |
| | Color doppler: Arterial |
| | Arteriography |
| Management | Conservative treatment: |
| | Rest: Reducing muscular activity |
| | Buerger's position |
| | Buerger's exercises |
| | Smoking: Abstinence |
| | Reflex heating |
| | Drugs: |
| | • Vasodilators: Papaverine 60 mg IV every 2–3 hours |
| | • Heparin: 5 KA units IV |
| | Paravertebral sympathetic block |
| | Protection of ischemic parts: By chiropody |
| | Exposure of ischemic parts: To well aerated, ambient temperature |
| | Analgesics, NSAIDs |
| | Surgical treatment: |
| | Surgery: Embolectomy |

## Fat Embolism

| | |
|---|---|
| Definition | Fat embolism is defined as a clinical entity, that occur following severe polytrauma (multiple fractures); characterized by signs and symptoms of involvement of multiple systems; is due to appearance of fat droplets (act as emboli) in the circulation, that may become lodged in the vessel, thereby cause an obstruction. |
| Etiology | Traumatic: Injury to bone marrow or adipose tissue; fractures of the osteoporotic bone |
| | Atheromatous plaque |
| | Blood clots: From thrombosed veins or auricular appendage (MS or AF), mural thrombosis (MI) |
| | Vegetations: From cardiac valves |
| Pathogenesis | Emboli blocking vessels of any part of the body (brain, heart, lungs); ischemic part; necrotic tissue |
| Diagnosis | Types: Cerebral and pulmonary: |

Cerebral:
- Drowziness, restlessness, delirium tremens
- Pupils: Narrow
- Fever
- Comatosed

Pulmonary:
- Dyspnea
- Cyanosis
- Chest pain: Sudden or gradual onset
- Retina: Striate hemorrhages
- Petechial hemorrhages: Anterior chest, conjunctival sac, hard palate
- Mouth: Frothy

Numbness

Pulse: Rising

Respiration: Rising

Skin: Coldness, pallor, mottling, anesthesia/or hyperesthesia, blebs, necrosis, gangrene

Muscles: Weakness, or paralyzed

Superficial veins: Collapsed

Regional effects:

Brain: Hemiplegia (temporary or permanent), due to blockage of middle cerebral artery

Eyes: Flash of light followed by blindness (total and permanent) due to the blockage of central artery supplying retina

Lungs: Pulmonary embolism due to phlebothrombosis

Mesentery: Engorgement and gangrene of the intestinal loop

Kidneys: Pain in the loin and hematuria due to blockage of renal artery

Spleen: Pain and splenomegaly due to blockage of splenic artery

Limbs: Pain, pallor, loss of pulses, anesthesia, paresis, congestion and gangrene (legs: due to blockage of femoral artery, popliteal artery, or

| | |
|---|---|
| | common iliac artery; arm: due to blockage at bifurcation of brachial artery). |
| Investigation | CBC, ESR, blood sugar |
| | Sputum: For fat droplets |
| | Urine: For fat droplets |
| | Color Doppler: Arterial |
| | Arteriography |
| Management | Emergency measures: |
| | Admit the patient in A&E unit |
| | Maintenance of imput/output charts |
| | IV fluids: 5% dextrose sol. |

Drugs:

- Vasodilators: papaverine 60 mg IV every 2–3 hours
- Heparin: 5 KA units IV
- Antibiotics IV
- Analgesics, NSAIDs

Surgical treatment:
Surgery: Closed reduction or ORIF of fractures.
Aim: To attain the best fixation of fractures with least manipulation and surgery.

## Acute Arterial Thrombosis

| | |
|---|---|
| Definition | An arterial thrombosis is defined as a foreign body that circulates in the bloodstream, and may become lodged in the vessel, thereby cause an obstruction |
| Etiology | Atheromatous plaque |
| | Blood clots: From thrombosed veins or auricular appendage (MS or AF), mural thrombosis (MI) |
| | Vegetations: From cardiac valves |
| Pathogenesis | An inflammatory vessel wall; atherosclerotic lumen; trauma; the thrombosed vessel; ischemic part; necrotic tissue; gangrene |
| Diagnosis | Pain: Sudden or gradual onset |
| | Coldness |
| | Numbness |
| | Pulsations: Absent in arteries distal to block |
| | Skin: Coldness, pallor, mottling, anesthesia/or hyperesthesia, blebs, necrosis, gangrene |
| | Muscles: Weakness, or paralyzed |
| | Superficial veins: Collapsed |

Regional effects:
Brain: Hemiplegia (temporary or permanent), due to blockage of middle cerebral artery
Eyes: Flash of light followed by blindness (total and permanent) due to the blockage of central artery supplying retina
Lungs: Pulmonary embolism due to phlebothrombosis

Mesentery: Engorgement and gangrene of the intestinal loop

Kidneys: Pain in the loin and hematuria due to blockage of renal artery

Spleen: Pain and splenomegaly due to blockage of splenic artery

Limbs: Pain, pallor, loss of pulses, anesthesia, paresis, congestion and gangrene (legs: due to blockage of femoral artery, popliteal artery, or common iliac artery; arm: due to blockage at bifurcation of brachial artery).

Investigation    CBC, ESR, blood sugar

Color Doppler: Arterial

Arteriography

Management    Conservative treatment:

Rest: Reducing muscular activity

Buerger's position

Buerger's exercises

Smoking: Abstinence

Reflex heating

Drugs:
- Vasodilators: Papaverine 60 mg IV every 2–3 hours
- Heparin: 5 KA units IV

Paravertebral sympathetic block

Protection of ischemic parts: By chiropody

Exposure of ischemic parts: To well aerated, ambient temperature

Analgesics, NSAIDs

Surgical treatment:

Surgery: Thrombectomy

## Raynaud's Disease

Definition    It is defined as a spasmodic condition usually occurs in women, that affects the upper limb more than the lower; the digital arteries respond excessively to the vasospastic stimuli

Etiology    Unknown

Direct trauma: Exposure to extreme cold

Emotional distress

Sympathetic nervous system: Abnormal

Pathogenesis    Exposure to cold; spasmodic arterioles; part blanched; accumulated metabolites in the capillaries; dilated capillaries; part swollen; recovery: relaxed arterioles, capillaries filled with oxygenated blood, part reddish and warm.

Diagnosis    Family history of a vasospastic phenomenon

Sex: Women usually affected

Age: 15 to 40 years

Pain: Precipitated by cold; relieved by warmth

Raynaud's phenomenon: Intermittent attacks of pallor or cyanosis in the fingers (rarely in toes), precipitated by cold or by emotional stress; fingers usually involved; thumbs rarely affected; recovery usually takes place near base of fingers (red return of color to cyanotic or pale digit)

Skin: Cold, pale, numbness of fingers, trophic changes (ulceration)

Muscle: Wasting

| | |
|---|---|
| D/d | Buerger's disease (thromboangiitis obliterance) |
| | Arteriosclerosis |
| | Thoracic outlet syndrome |
| Investigation | CBC, ESR |
| | WR (for syphilis) |
| | Urine: For diabetes |
| | Color Doppler |
| | X-ray neck |
| Management | Conservative treatment: |
| | Preventive: Refrain from exposure to cold |
| | Warmth: Body to be kept warm |
| | Analgesics, NSAIDs |
| | Vasodilators: Papaverine, methyldopa, reserpine |
| | Surgical treatment: |
| | Surgery: |
| | • Sympathectomy |
| Indication | Frequent severe attacks. |

## Buerger's Disease (Thromboangiitis Obliterans)

| | |
|---|---|
| Definition | It is defined as an episodic and segmental inflammatory and thrombotic disorder of the arteries and veins, mostly in the limbs esp. the lower; usually terminates in gangrene. |
| Etiology | Unknown |
| | Collagen disorder |
| | Smoking: Tobacoo/cigarette |
| | Sympathetic nervous system: Abnormal |
| Pathogenesis | Inflammatory occlusion of distal arteries; vascular insufficiency of toes or fingers; thrombotic superficial veins. |
| Diagnosis | Signs and symptoms: Mainly those of arterial insufficiency. |
| | Family history of a vasospastic phenomenon |
| | Sex: Men usually affected |
| | Age: 20 to 40 years |
| | Limbs: Mostly legs |
| | Pain: |
| | • Rest pain: Persisting, aching or gnawing |
| | • Intermittent claudication |
| | Skin: Cold, pale, numbness of fingers, trophic changes (ulceration) |
| | Muscle: Wasting |
| | Sensations: Diminished, numbness |
| | Pulses: Absent or impaired |
| D/d | • Arteriosclerosis obliterance: Occurs in comparatively older age; with associated hyperlipidemia; blood vessel calcification; no phlebitis |

- Scleroderma: Skin involvement prior to vascular changes
- Raynaud's disease: Symmetrical, bilateral color changes; mostly in the young women; arterial pulsations not affected
- Frostbite: History of cold exposure; may cause superficial gangrene; arterial pulsations proximal to gangrene not affected.

| | |
|---|---|
| Investigation | CBC, ESR |
| | WR (for syphilis) |
| | Urine: For diabetes |
| | Color doppler |
| | X-ray leg |
| Management | Conservative treatment: |
| | Preventive: Refrain from smoking (can have cigarettes or legs) |
| | Avoid trauma to the feet |
| | Warm stockings |
| | Analgesics, NSAIDs |
| | Vasodilators: Papaverine, methyldopa, reserpine |
| | Exercises |

Surgical treatment:

Surgery:

- Sympathectomy

Indication: Frequent severe attacks

Aim
- To eliminate the vasospasm
- To aid in establishing collateral circulation
- To relieve rest pain and intermittent claudication
- To precede amputation (may aid in wound healing).
- Amputation

Indication: Gangrene.

## Cervical Rib (Scalenus Anticus Syndrome)

Preface
The brachial plexus and the subclavian artery may be compressed in the neck by a rudimentary cervical rib, 1st thoracic rib, fibrous band, or tight scalene muscle, resulting in sensory, motor, or vascular symptoms in one or both upper limbs.

Anatomy
A cervical rib arises from the 7th cervical in about 0.5% of persons; mostly unilateral; more frequent on the right side; mostly symptomless; troublesome when pressing upon structures (subclavian artery and brachial plexus), passing through a triangle in the neck.

Types: Four main types:
- Complete rib: Articulates with the manubrium sterni
- Rib with expanded free end
- Rib with tapering end, connected by a fibrous band to the scalene tubercle of the first rib
- Rib (fibrous band), incorporated in the scalenus medius; not infrequent.

| | |
|---|---|
| Etiology | Congenital |
| | Traumatic: Weight lifting or straining |
| | Muscle tone: Loss of muscle tone of shoulder girdle muscles. |
| Pathogenesis | Interposition of cervical rib into base of triangle; lowest trunk of the brachial plexus (carrying sympathetic fibers and subclavian artery, compressed or angulated, while passing over cervical rib, instead of 1st thoracic rib; arterial angulation cause constriction, thrombus formation; that leads to embolism; 1st dorsal nerve angulates, and then fibrosed. |
| Diagnosis | Mostly asymptomatic |
| | Sex: Women usually affected |
| | Age: Young age group |
| | Pain: On exertion (ischemic), relieved by rest |
| | Skin: Cold, pale, numbness of fingers, trophic changes (ulceration) |
| | Swelling: Prominence in the lower part of neck |
| | Local tenderness |
| | Pulsation: Decreased |
| | Muscle: Wasting |
| | Horner's syndrome: Damaged cervical sympathetic |
| | Adson's test: +ve |
| Investigation | CBC, ESR |
| | WR (for syphilis) |
| | Urine: For diabetes |
| | Color doppler |
| | X-ray neck |
| Management | Clinical course variable; remissions or slow progression occur frequently |
| | Conservative treatment: |
| | Rest in bed |
| | Arm support/sling |
| | Cervical traction |
| | Diathermy: IR or SWD |
| | Analgesics, NSAIDs |
| | Physiotherapy: Exercises |
| | Surgical treatment: |
| | Surgery: |
| | • Excision (extraperiosteal) of the cervical rib |
| | • Sympathetic denervation of the upper limb. |

## Causalgia (Post-traumatic Sympathetic Dystrophy)

| | |
|---|---|
| Definition | It is defined as a burning or aching pain in an injured limb; characterized by the disparity between severity of the injury and the degree of pain. |
| Etiology | Traumatic: Direct violence, crush injuries |
| | RSA |
| | Fall from a height |

|  |  |
|---|---|
|  | Sports injuries |
|  | Burns |
|  | Operations: Elective |
| Pathogenesis | Lacerated; destroyed soft tissues |
| Diagnosis | Pain: Mild/moderate/severe; diffuse; worst at night |
|  | Swelling |
|  | Local tenderness |
|  | Skin: Warm, dry, red/or cyanotic |
|  | Nails: Ridged |
|  | Sensation: Hyperesthesia |
|  | Muscles: Holding limb in a splinted position |
| Investigation | CBC, ESR, blood sugar, lipid profile, TFT |
|  | X-ray of the part of the limb |
| Management | Aim: To diagnose and manage the condition at the earliest possible, in order to avoid development of secondary changes. |

Conservative treatment:

Mild, early cases:
- To protect the limb from irritating stimuli
- Physiotherapy: Active and passive exercises
- Drugs: Analgesics/NSAIDs and sedatives (diazepam).

Surgical treatment:
Indications: Failure of conservative treatment

Surgery:
- Sympathetic blocks (stellate or lumbar) + physiotherapy
- Sympathectomy.

## Sudeck's Atrophy

|  |  |
|---|---|
| Definition | It is defined as an acute atrophy of the bones of a limb, that frequently occurs post trauma, esp. of wrist (Colles fractures) or ankle (Pott's fractures); may be due to vasomotor hyperactivity (sympathetic). |
| Etiology | Unknown |
|  | May be sympathetic response to trauma |
| Pathogenesis | Diffuse osteoporotic mottling of the carpus/or tarsus |
| Diagnosis | S/S of vasomotor hyperactivity: |
|  | Pain: Burning; mobility worsens pain |
|  | Swelling |
|  | Skin: Shining, brittle, warm |
|  | Local tenderness |
|  | Limb: Later on become cold, cyanotic |
|  | Pulses: Diminished |
|  | Muscles: Wasted |
|  | Movements: Painful and restricted |
| Investigation | X-ray—shows: United fracture, osteoporosis, mottled carpus/tarsus. |
| Management | Preventive: Adequate early treatment of sprains, etc. |

Conservative treatment:
Analgesics/NSAIDs
Physiotherapy: Heat therapy (IR, SWD, Wax bath); massage; exercises.

Surgical treatment:
Indication: Failure of conservative treatment
Surgery: Sympathectomy.

## AFFECTIONS OF VEINS

### Vein Thrombosis

| | |
|---|---|
| Types | Superficial and deep vein thrombosis: |

### Superficial Vein Thrombosis (Syn. Thrombophlebitis)

| | |
|---|---|
| Definition | It is defined as an inflammatory condition resulting in formation of a hard thrombus firmly adherent to the venous wall; usually the varicose veins and a vein being cannulated for IV transfusion are affected; mostly idiopathic. |
| Etiology | Idiopathic: Mostly spontaneous occurring:<br>• Pre/or postpartum<br>• Varicose veins<br>Direct trauma: Local trauma of any kind; violence<br>Inflammatory: Damaged endothelium with vessel wall changes<br>Sedentary: Immobility<br>PUO: Debilitating illness: typhoid fever; myocardial degeneration<br>Surgery: Prolonged immobilization postoperatively. |
| Predisposing factors | • Increased blood coagulability: Postinfection or hemorrhage<br>• Decreased blood flow: During and postoperatively or typhoid fever |
| Pathogenesis | Clot organized into fibrous tissue; calcification; phlebolith formed; suppuration that forms an abscess/or pyemia:<br>• Distally: Edema may occur; venous collateral circulation established evinced by varicosed superficial veins<br>• Proximally: Thrombosis may extend upwards into larger veins; parts of clot liable to be detached (emboli); resultant emboli may cause pulmonary infarcts; infected clot may cause pylephlebitis. |
| Diagnosis | Pain: Dull ache<br>Vein: Indurated, red, tender, hard cord like; long saphenous vein usually involved<br>Skin: Dusky, inflamed<br>Constitutional reaction: Absent. |
| Investigation | CBC, ESR, blood sugar<br>Color doppler: Venous |
| D/d | Erythema induratum<br>Erythema nodosum<br>Lymhangitis |
| Management | Conservative treatment:<br>Symptomatic measures: |

Rest
Position: Leg elevated
Analgesics/NSAIDs
Elastic crepe bandage
Antibiotics
Anticoagulants: Usually not indicated

Surgical treatment:
Indication: Thrombus that gets detached (rare)—resultant emboli.
Surgery:
- Ligation of the vein.
- Ligation and division of vein.

## Deep Vein Thrombosis (DVT) (Syn. Phlebothrombosis)

| | |
|---|---|
| Preface | Deep vein thrombosis is characterized by minimal inflammatory element; is much more serious as the thrombus is soft and loose; thus there is more chance of breaking off and causing pulmonary embolism; there may be partial or complete occlusion of a vein by a thrombus with a secondary inflammatory reaction in the venous wall; usually the deep veins of legs (calf) and pelvis are affected; mostly idiopathic. |
| Etiology | Traumatic: Local trauma of any kind |
| | Surgical: Postoperative immobility |
| | Sedentary: Physical inactivity |
| | Delivery: Childbirth |
| | Debilitating: Typhoid fever |
| | CVS: Hypertension, MI, CHF |
| | CVA: Stroke |
| | Metabolic |
| Predisposing factors | Age |
| | Infection |
| | Obesity |
| | Prolonged immobilization |
| | Anemia |
| | Dehydration |
| | Shock |
| | IV drug usage |
| | Metabolic |
| Pathogenesis | Virchow's triad: Vessel wall trauma; venous stasis, and hyper-coagulation; thrombus originates in a venous tributary of a main vein (eddying currents around a valve); extends into main deep vein; portion of the thrombus breaks (by faster current); form emboli (pulmonary embolus); occluded deeper veins; pelvic, femoral, and calf veins usually affected. |
| Diagnosis | Symptomless: Early stages |
| | Pain: Dull ache/tight feeling/or frank pain; increased on exertion |
| | Edema: Swollen calf |

|                | Distended: Peripheral veins |
|----------------|------------------------------|

Distended: Peripheral veins
Local tenderness
Fever
Pulse rate: Rise
Homans sign: +ve
Vein: Tender, hard cord like
Skin: Pale or cyanotic, cool (reflex arterial spasm)

**Investigation**
CBC, ESR, blood sugar
Ultrasound
Color doppler: Venous
CXR
MRI.

**Complications**
Pulmonary embolism: Obstructing pulmonary circulation; lung infarction
Chronic venous insufficiency

**Management**
Preventive:
- During surgery: Legs, well padded/stockings, and elevated by 20 Degrees
- Postoperative: Massage the legs, exercises of legs

Medical:
- Adequate hydration
- Analgesics/NSAIDs
- Anticoagulants to be continued for 10/7
- Oral (PO): Aspirin

   Warfarin:    Day 1 : 30–50 mg o.d.
                Day 2 : 10–20 mg o.d.
                Day 3 : 5–15 mg o.d.

- Parentral:
- Unfractionated heparin (UFH) 7.5–10 K IU as initial bolus dose IV, followed by 1 K IU/hour as continuous infusion.
- Low molecular weight heparin (LMWH) comparatively safe as less incidence of thrombocytopenia s.c.; agents:
- Enoxaparin 1.5 mg/kg o.d. or 1 mg/kg b.i.d. s.c., Alt:
- Delteparin 200 IU/kg b.i.d. s.c.
- Thrombolytics: Urokinase or streptokinase I/A, through a catheter until a clot dissolved:

Dose: Urokinase 50 K IU in 5% dextrose/saline
Streptokinase 0.75–1.5 million IU, IV in 1 hour.
- Elastic crepe bandage
- Antibiotics

Surgical treatment:
Indication: Thrombus that gets detached (rare)—resultant emboli.

Surgery: Procedures:
- Ligation of the femoral vein:

Indication: Anticoagulants C/I

Thrombectomy and embolectomy:

Indication: Failure of conservative measures

## Varicose Veins

| | |
|---|---|
| Definition | Defined as a disorder of veins, whereby the vein is dilated, lengthened, and tortuous; usually occurs in connection with the veins of the leg; also the spermatic, esophageal, and hemorrhoidal veins are affected frequently. |
| Etiology | Congenital: Arteriovenous fistula |
| | Traumatic |
| | Inflammatory |
| | Postural: Erect (animals spared) |
| | Pregnancy: Venous obstruction |
| | Metabolic: Venous obstruction |
| Pathogenesis | Impaired venous pump (congenital paucity of non-return valves esp. saphenofemoral valve at junction of internal saphenous and common femoral veins and sapheno-popliteal valve; muscle weakness/ wasting; stretched deep fascia); resulting in dilated external saphenous system; may occur at the site of any incompetent communicating vein; under high pressure leakage of blood into superficial system. |
| Diagnosis | Symptoms: Occur only in case of retrograde flow, and depend on extent of back pressure: |

- Discomfort: Aching or burning
- Fatigue/or pain: In legs on prolonged standing, cramps
- Itching
- Eczematoid dermatitis.

Signs:

- Bilateral: Usually
- Veins: Dilated, tortuous, elongated, visible underneath skin of thigh and leg
- Skin: Pigmented, thinned
- Swelling: Postphlebitic.

Trendelenberg's test: Aims:

- To determine the competency of valves in the superficial and the communicating systems (valves at the proximal end of the long saphenous vein adjoining the saphenofemoral junction; in the long saphenous vein in the thigh and leg, and in the communicating veins between the superficial and deep vessels).

Test:

- Position: Patient supine, elevate the leg to empty veins:
  Result: Varicosities empty in case of no organic venous obstruction

- Place a rubberband around the upper thigh, or compress the proximal end of long saphenous vein with thumb and ask the patient to stand:

Result:

A. Pressure released: Varices fill up rapidly by a column of blood from above: Shows incompetency of superficial system (+ve test)

B. Pressure not released but maintained for 1–2 mts.
   Result: Gradual filling of veins: shows incompetency of communicating veins—blood flowing from deep to superficial veins (+ve test)

Perthes' test: Aim:

- To determine the competency of deep veins.

Test:

- Tie firmly a tourniquet around upper thigh, to prevent any reflux down the vein; ask patient to have a brisk walk for a while with the tourniquet in place:

Result: Varices become more distended due to obstruction (+ve test)

| | |
|---|---|
| D/d | Chronic venous insufficiency of deep venous system |
| | Arteriovenous fistula |
| Investigation | CBC, ESR, blood sugar |
| | Color doppler: Venous |
| | Ultrasound |
| | MRI |
| Complications | • Ulceration from direct trauma |
| | • Hemorrhage from ulcerating varix |
| | • Thrombophlebitis of superficial veins |
| | • Eczema |
| Management | Conservative treatment: |

- Elastic stockings
- Exercises: Elevation of legs
- Injection therapy:

Indication: Cosmetic reasons; failure of stripping technique

Action: Sclerosing solutions (Sodium tetradecyl) damage the intima of the vein, so as to form the thrombosis of venous segment.

Technique:

- Position: Patient lie supine
- Sterile: Site with spirit
- Insert: Needle into the vein, withdraw blood in syringe containing the sclerosant; then injection is made
- Rpeat: At weekly intervals.

Surgical treatment:

Principle: Ligation and division of those veins into which occurred high pressure leak from deep venous system (ligation of internal saphenous vein at its entry into femoral vein—saphenofemoral flush ligation); flush ligation proximal to any tributaries mandatory, to avoid recurrence; incompetent superficial saphenous vein requires exposure and ligation in the popliteal fossa.

Indication: Failure of conservative measures

Surgery: High ligation of long saphenous vein at the saphenofemoral junction + removal (stripping) of the saphenous vein + ligations of secondary veins + ligation of short saphenous vein at sapheno-popliteal junction.

## Chronic Venous Insufficiency

| | |
|---|---|
| Definition | Chronic venous insufficiency is characterized by progressive edema of the leg (esp. lower leg), and secondary changes in the skin and the subcutaneous tissues; usually occurs from changes secondary to deep thrombophlebitis; may also occur from neoplastic obstruction of the pelvic veins. |
| Etiology | Congenital<br>Traumatic<br>Inflammatory: Thrombophlebitis<br>Endocrinal: Diabetic |
| Pathogenesis | Damaged valves of deep venous channels by thrombotic process; progressive edema of legs; secondary changes in the skin and the subcutaneous tissues (fibrosed). |
| Diagnosis | Pain: Dull ache, made worse by prolonged standing<br>Itching<br>Skin: Thin, shiny, atrophic, pigmented, cyanotic, and eczematous<br>Subcutaneous tissues: Thick and fibrosed<br>Ulcerations of leg<br>Varicosities: Often present (incompetent perforating veins) |
| Investigation | CBC, ESR, blood sugar |
| D/d | • CHF and renal failure: Bilateral edema of lower limbs; sacral edema<br>• Lymphedema: Brawny, thickened subcutaneous tissue; varicosities absent; H/o cellulitis<br>• Arterial insufficiency<br>Erythema induratum: Bilateral<br>Fungal infections: No varices, no swelling, specific cultures. |
| Management | Conservative treatment:<br>Bedrest: With raised legs (to control edema)<br>Avoid prolonged standing or sitting<br>Braces/leg supports<br>Dermatitis: Wet compresses; hydrocortisone cream, zinc oxide oint.<br>Ulceration: Toilet with isotonic saline sol.<br>Secondary varicosities: Excision of varices<br><br>Surgical treatment<br>Surgery: Excision of ulcer with skin graft of the defect + ligation of veins<br>Indication: Large, chronic ulcer<br><br>Secondary varicosities:<br>Conservative: Elastic stockings, antibiotics, analgesics/NSAIDs.<br>Surgery: Excision of varices + ligation of incompetent perforations |

## Bibliography

1. Brown H, et al. Thromboangitis oblitrans. Brit J Surg 56:59, (1969).
2. Canale ST, et al. Campbell's Operative Orthopaedics, ed. 9th, Vol I-IV. C.V. Mosby Co., Saint Louis, 1998.
3. Cranley JJ, et al. Chronic venous insufficiency of the lower extremity. Surgery 49:48, (1961).
4. Darling RC, et al. Arterial embolism. Surg Gynec Obst 124:106, (1967).
5. Deterling RA Jr. Acute arterial occlusion. S Clin North America 46:587, (1966).
6. Erskine JM. Blood vessels and Lymphatics, Current Medical Diagnosis and Treatment. Maruzen (1975).
7. Freeark RJ, et al. Posttraumatic venous thrombosis. Arch Surg 95:567, (1967).
8. Gifford RW jr. The cical significance of Raynaud's phenomenon and Raynaud's disease. M Clin North America 42:963, (1958).
9. Gray FD Jr. Pulmonary embolism. Lea and Febiger, (1966).
10. Home M, et al. Venous thrombosis and pulmonary embolism. Harvard Univ Press, (1970)
11. Kapoor PS. Deep vein thrombus: Accident and Emergency, ed. 2nd, CBS, New Delhi, 2016.
12. Kapoor PS. Peripheral vascular disease: Accident and Emergency, ed. 2nd, CBS, New Delhi, 2016.
13. Kleinert HE, et al. Post-traumatic sympathetic dystrophy. Orthop Clin North America 4:917, (973).
14. Lofgren K.A, et al. Extensive ulcerations in the postphlebitic leg. S Clin North America 44:1383, (1964).
15. Love M, et al. Bailey and Love's Short Practice of Surgery, ed. 13th, H.K. Lewis and Co., London, 1965.
16. Sherman RS. Varicose veins. S Clin North America 44: 1369, (1964).
17. Smith H. Management of Arterial Injuries: Campbell's Operative Orthopaedics, 9th Ed., Vol I., C.V. Mosby Co., Saint Louis, 1998.
18. Wheat MW Jr, Palmar RF. Dissecting aneurysms of aorta. Curr Probl Surg, (July 1971).

# 12

# Orthopedic Practical Procedures

Reduction, fixation, and rehabilitation
- Reduction: Closed and open
- Fixation (immobilization): External and internal
- Rehabilitation

Punctures
- Joint puncture
- Lumbar puncture
- Cisternal puncture
- Sacral puncture

Joint and soft tissue injection

Aspiration and drainage

Surgical approaches to joints and long bones

Arthroplasty
- Evolution of prosthesis design
- Total hip replacement

Arthrodesis

Osteotomy

Synovectomy

Arthroscopy (endoscopy) and arthroscopic surgery

Amputations

## REDUCTION, FIXATION, AND REHABILITATION

### Reduction

- Fractures
- Dislocations

### Reduction of Fracture

Aims: To reduce a displaced fracture, so as to unite in good functional position, and the reduction is usually easier if performed without unnecessary delay, prior to surrounding soft tissues becoming swollen and turgid. Often unreduced fractures unite rapidly, but may yield to malunion. Repeated manipulations to achieve perfect radiological reduction may lead to hazards (malunion/nonunion). Slight/little displacement esp. in children and old, weak patient may often be accepted (to outweigh undesirable risks).

Indication: Correction of deformities: displacement, angulation, and rotation (cosmetic and functional issues).

**Anesthesia:** General, regional, or local:
- General: Provides muscle relaxation, duration, and versatility.
- Regional: Safer for minor procedures
- Local: Safer for minor procedures.

**Types of reduction:** Closed or open.
**Closed reduction:** Majority of fractures are reduced by this method.

Advantages:
- Relatively safe method—chances of infection are less.
- Relatively much cheaper.

Disadvantages:
- Failure of reduction sometimes—due to interposition of soft tissues between fragments.
- Failure to maintain reduction.
- Prolonged immobilization.

Technique:
- Most of fractures reduced manually by using longitudinal traction, angulation, or hingeing. Ideally postreduction, the limb should look similar to its fellow in length and appearance. Frequently X-ray picture may be deceptive, thereby alarming inexperienced surgeon to resort to repeated manipulations or unnecessary open reduction, that may lead to undesirable results, as loss of alignment is of more serious consequences than lacking end to end apposition, esp. in weight bearing bones.
- By continuous traction (fractures of femur and dislocation of cervical spine). In fractures of femur shaft, overlapping does not prevent union, although some shortening may occur.

Types: Skin and skeletal tractions:

- _ Skin traction (by using an adhesive strapping): Mostly indicated in children and young adults for fractures femur and fractures of lower end of humerus.

Method:
- _ Toilet of skin with spirit/alcohol/betadine scrub, post skin-shaving
- _ Apply adhesive tape (of traction kit) on both sides of leg, extending beyond foot for spreader bar
- _ Place foam/cotton over malleoli (protection)
- _ To secure adhesive tapes throughout with encircling elastic crepebandage:
  - ▪ Apply desired weights to the cord.

Skeletal traction (by using a Steinmann pin through tibial tuberosity): Indicated in an older patient, that require a heavy traction, but often complications like pin track infection do occur.

**Open reduction:** Should always be undertaken by a surgeon highly skilled in fracture management. Better to be avoided in children.

Indications:
- Failure of closed reduction (fractures of medial malleolus)
- Particular fractures in need of perfect reduction and fixation, e.g. fracture neck of femur.
- To reduce mortality and morbidity (internal fixation of trochanteric fractures)
- To achieve acceptable reduction—not possible by closed methods (depressed comminuted fractures of tibial condyle)
- To prevent occurrence of displacement, angulation, or deformity, common after closed reduction (Monteggia fracture dislocation, fracture patella, olecranon fracture)
- Compound fractures, complicated fractures
- Early mobilization required esp. in elderly patients.

Disadvantages:
- Relatively unsafe method, as chances of infection are more. Sometimes disastrous one: resulting in gangrene, requiring amputation, or even death may occur.
- To impair vascularity by stripping of soft tissues for exposure of fragments, and insert implants (risk of nonunion), being absent in closed methods
- To produce scar that may impair muscle function (fractures of femur)
- To produce foreign body reaction (metallic implants)
- Relatively much costlier method.

**Fixation (immobilization) of fracture** (external and internal fixation): Attention must be given not only to the broken bone, but also to the soft parts, while considering the correct method of fixation of each type of fracture.

## External Fixation

A. **Plaster fixation:** It is the most widely used form of fixation, and has superseded all other forms external fixation, e.g. splints (wooden, metallic), braces for treatment of majority of fractures.

Aims:
- To retain the limb/part in the desired comfortable position, by its adaptation, and not by traction or pressure.
- To be light in weight, but strong enough to be effective in use, and to be easily removable.
  Method: Plaster slabs: available in readymake packs, or may be prepared from desired size plaster bandages, by dry method (prepared beforehand); wet method (prepared from wet bandage); pattern method (shapes prepared from wide bandages).
- Dry method: Water to be tepid (neither cold or hot), slab gripped by hands and emersed in water till no air bubbles, then held slab vertically and slightly squeezed to drain out surplus water, then placed over a flat surface and smoothed out with the palm, then apply over the desired fractured part.
- Wet method: Commonest, unroll bandage a little, immerse in water till no bubbles, squeezed, then prepare the desired sized slab, and finally apply over the desired fractured part.
- Pattern method: Unroll plaster bandage to desired size and make 4–6 layered slab, then hold the slab, immerse in water, squeeze, and apply over the desired fractured part, often to the proximal parts first, so that moulding be carried out more profitably

against a set or nearly set cuff of plaster on the calf or forearm (B/K plaster at tibial tubercle, and forearm plaster at the elbow).

- Ridging plaster slabs: To reinforce a plaster, for providing resistance to strain and stress, by ridging (central part of wet slab raised along its length, and applied to the cast, while in girdering, an additional slab, shorter than first slab is ridged and superimposed.
- Cast-bracing: Sometimes indicated in the failed initial conservative treatment of a fracture (delayed union):

  Example: Fractures of femur ant tibia in same limb: separate support for each, linked together by hinges at the side of the knee, allowing early ambulation.

  Post care: Should be taken of swelling, change in the skin color, numbness, etc. following application of plaster—if present, then: Immediately loosen the plaster by splitting, or removing/changing the plaster.
- Elevation: To wear an arm sling in case of upper limb, while in case of lower limb, elevate the leg on pillows or RBE
- Active exercises.

**B. Traction:** Fixed traction in a thomas splint or by continuous traction for couple of weeks, holding a reduced fracture. It is often used for treating fracture femoral shaft (skin traction by adhesive strapping, or skeletal traction by using a Steinmann pin).

C. Braces, splints, jackets, collars, belts, knee caps, anklets

D. Elastic crepe bandaging, adhesive strapping

E. External fixator and ring fixator: Bone fragments held in alignment by skeletal pins (Ilizarov method):

## *Operative Principles of Ilizarov*

Indications          Congenital deformity:
- Upper limb
- Lower limb
- Congenital pseudoarthrosis of tibia

Traumatic            • Fractures
- Nonunion

Lengthening          • Bone lengthening
- Limbs lengthening

Arthrodesis: local

Operative Principles of Ilizarov

Principles

Indication:

Congenital deformities: Correction:
- Upper limb
- Lower limb
- Pseudarthosis of tibia

Traumatic:
- Fractures (transosseous osteosynthesis):
  - Upper limb

– Lower limb
– Nonunion

Infective:
- Compoud fractures: Wherein condition of skin and other soft tissues, disapprove use of internal fixation devices
- Pin track (skeletal traction) infections.

Lengthening: Bone lengthening:
- Upper limb
- Lower limb.

Achondroplastic dwarfism: Limb lengthening
- Compound fractures, wherein condition of skin and other soft tissues, disapprove use of internal fixation devices
- Pin track (skeletal traction) infections.

Specific:
- Angular deformities: Correction
- Contractures Joints
- Arthrodesis: Local
- Widening and recontouring of leg.

Method: (Ilizarov): It is mostly a nonsurgical procedure, except for the insertion of wires/pins, performedin an operation theater.

Insertion of wires/pins:
- Wires/pins (bayonet type for hard cortical bone, while trocar type for metaphyseal cancellous bone), 1.5 to 1.8 mm in diameter for insertion: central part of each pin in the bone, with the ends protruding from the skin
- Drilling through both cortices, then hammer wires/pins
- Set of wires/pins (1–3) inserted in each bone fragment, with care to protect neurovascular structures (precise anatomical insertion of wires/pins.

Reduction of fracture: Fracture reduced with the aid of pins *in situ* (by an open reduction or by using an image intensifier).

Fixation of wires/pims to rings: Pins held in position by a firm external support rings (made of two half rings), as per maximal diameter of the limb (space to be kept between inner part of the ring and the limb all around).

Ring assembly: To place limb centrally in the ring, so as to avoid the postoperative edema, pain, and pressure ulcers. The wires on the rings to be tensioned by a pair of dynamometers or by turning wire fixation bolt, as any movement between the wires and soft tissues may cause continuous irritation and infection. Ring attachments (cannulated bolt for a wire passing centrally through ring hole; slotted bolt used for a wire passing eccentrically to ring hole; and washers used for a wire passing above or below the ring surface.)

Rods assembly to connect rings: Rods (threaded or telescopic) placed  parallel to one another and to bone axis, and the rods (3–4) to be  placed at equidistance from each other on the ring's circumference.

## Postoperative care

| | |
|---|---|
| Early | • Bedrest |
| | • Elevate the limb |
| | • ASD |
| | • Physiotherapy: Exercises |
| Late | • Wires checking: To remain tight |

## Internal Fixation

Principles of internal fixation of fractures: Anatomical and physiological factors involved in the healing of a fracture are essential to perfect management, esp. in the case of treatment by open methods, using implants like plates and screws, screws, intramedullary nailing and interlocking nailing, tension wires, percutaneous wires, etc.

Aims:
- Clinical: To achieve proper union (primary object): as function of the adjoining soft tissues and joints depends upon it
- Anatomical: To restore normal anatomical position of the bones after healing: as function of the adjoining soft tissues and joints depends upon it
- Physiological: To restore normal function of the limb, relative to early mobilization of soft tissues and adjoining joints.

Circulation: To maintain/re-establish the local circulation
Example: Fracture femoral neck, or fracture scaphoid.

## Principles

- Freedom from foreign body reaction: Implant should be biological inert, free from toxic reactions, inflammatory response, fibrous and giant cell reactions. These usually cause pain, swelling, and loss of function
- Freedom from rust: Implant should be made of high quality stainless steel, etc. to avoid rusting of implant esp. in compound fractures.
- Reedom from mechanical failure: Implant should be lighter in weight, of great strength and of suitable design to match the shape and size of donor bone.

### Materials commonly used are:
- Stainless steel
- Vitallium—alloys of chromium, cobalt, and molybdenum
- Titanium.

### Advantages of internal fixation:
- Firm fixation
- Early weight bearing
- Early return to work.

### Disadvantages of internal fixation:
- Infection
- Failure: Due to faulty technique or faulty (wrong) selection of implant.
- Failure: Due to faulty selection of treatment (closed or internal fixation) for needs of each and every particular case.

**Implants:**
- Screws: Cortical and cancellous screws, available in large range of lengths but restricted in range of diameters.

Types of screws:
- Self tapping screws: The screw cuts its own thread in the bone.

Example: Sherman and Lanes screws.

The screw has an OD (outside diameter) and a slot single, cruciate, or combination.

Insertion: A hole is drilled through the bone, followed by driving in the screw, cutting its hread into the bone by its flutted end.

Screws which require bone to be tapped prior to insertion:
- AO series screws: AO cortical screw has: an OD; a hexagonal socket; a buttress thread with pitch

  Insertion: A hole is drilled through the bone, followed by tapping with a corresponding tap and finally the screw is driven through.

  Screws which does not require bone tapping prior insertion.
- Single cortical screw is a week internal support and requires external support, e.g. plaster of paris or splint.
- Cancellous screws: Indicated in cancellous bone.
- Locking screws: Cannulated, self-drilling, self-tapping screws.
- Dynamic hip screw (DHS).

Plates and Screws:
- Sherman plate is a light weight, comparatively of weaker strength plate, and requires external support.
- Eggar plate is slotted, so that the screws are not fully tightened, allowing the bone ends to remain in contact. Requires external support.
- Dynamic compression plate (DCP) is slotted and tightening of plate is achieved by pinching of plate by the heads of screws.
- Nail/blade plate is being used in a fracture closer to a long bone's end.

  Insertion: Nail or blade part is driven through the cancellous part, while the plate part is fixed with the cortical screws, to the shaft of the long bone.
- Buttress plates, Y plates, fracture plates, LC plates, cervical spine locking plates
- Intramedullary nailing: For fractures of shafts of long bones, e.g.
  Kuntscher nail for fracture shaft femur.
- Interlocking Nails:
  - Antegrade Femoral Nail (AFN)
  - Proximal Femoral Nail (PFN)
  - Distal Femoral Nail (DFN)
  - Universal Femoral Nail (UFN)—Titanium solid nail
  - Cannulated Femoral Nail (CFN)
- Rush pins (nails) for fracture humerus, ulna, etc.
- Spine system (Schanz screws)—for cervical spine surgery
- Pedicle screw system—for low back surgery.

## Rehabilitation

Principle and aim:
- To return the trauma (injured) person to work ASAP with the minimal residual disability
- To relieve pain as well as to prevent muscle wasting
- To discard fixed splints in favor of unpadded POP of minimal weight, and that exercises, not only of the injured limb but also of the whole body, should take place; exercises to be designed to imitate normal natural movements, i.e. walking; these exercises to be based on the postural reflexes, thus ensuring maintenance of maximum tone.
- Instructions towards patient's behavior: Exercises, occupational therapy
- Preventive and corrective methods: To avoid teethering of muscles, while passion wires through
- Rehabilitation methods and physiotherapy: Based upon a strategy to overcome resistance of powerful muscles that create deformities due to joint contractures.

## PUNCTURES

- Joint puncture
- Lumbar puncture
- Cisternal puncture
- Sacral puncture

Anatomy
It is a routine medical procedure to withdraw fluid from a joint or a body cavity, for purpose of examination, diagnosis, or therapeutic. For that purpose, a sterile needle puncture is made. The anatomy of the part administers the site of insertion of the needle. It is usually presumed that the joint or cavity being to be puncured is distended with fluid/blood/or pus.

## Joint Puncture

Indications
Diagnostic:
- Aspiration of joint and physical, microscopical and bacteriological examination of the aspirated fluid

Therapeutic:
- To administer intra-articular drugs
- To relieve tension by withdrawing:
  - Fluid: Synovitis
  - Blood: Hemophilia trauma
  - Pus: Septic

Joints
Shoulder joint:
- Enter the needle just lateral to the tip of the coracoid process and push in a direction backwards, upwards, and outwards
- Enter the needle just lateral to the angle formed by the junction of the acromion with the spine of the scapula, and push it upward and inward.

Elbow joint
- Flex the elbow joint to a right angle, with the forearm semi-pronated
- Enter the needle just proximal to the radial head, and push it, in a direction directly forwards (anteriorly). An elbow joint distended

with pus, that bulges the capsule on either side of triceps tendon, can be easily and efficiently drained.

| | |
|---|---|
| Wrist joint | • Enter the needle just below the ulnar (usually) or radial styloid process (risk: radial artery passes just distal to radial styloid) and push in at right angle to the process. |
| Hip joint | • Enter the needle at a point 5 cm below the anterior inferior iliac spine and push in upwards, backwards, and medially |
| | • Enter the needle from the side just above the upper border of the greater trochanter and push in direction of inwards and upwards in a line parallel with femoral neck. |
| Knee joint | • Enter the needle into the suprapatellar bursa through the vastus lateralis, and push in direction of inward and backward |
| | • Enter the needle on either side of the ligamentum patellae below the patella, and push in directly backwards and upward direction. |
| Ankle joint | • Enter the needle just below the tip of medial or lateral malleolus and push in an upward direction, so as to enter the joint between the malleolus and articular surface of the talus. |

## Lumbar Puncture

| | |
|---|---|
| Anatomy | It is the procedure whereby spinal subarachnoid space is punctured below the level of the spinal cord, to spare cord from injury (cord ends at L-2 vertebra, while subarachnoid space ends at of S-2 vertebra). |
| Site | L-3 and L-4 intervertebral space (at level of highest point of iliac crest) is usually 5–7 cm from the surface |
| Indication | Diagnostic (manometric readings mandatory to assess IDP): |

• Traumatic: Intradural hemorrhage: Raised pressure, crystal clear fluid
• Inflammatory: Acute infective meningitis, syphilis (Wassermann reaction, gold test), intracerebral abscess (reduced number of cells, increased protein content)
• Neoplastic: Raised CSF pressure, increased protein content.

Therapeutic:
• To relieve pain: Intrathecal injection of bupivacaine HCl
• To introduce drugs: Penicillin for acute meningitis.

Anesthetic:
• To induce anesthesia: Caudal, epidural, lumbar: lignocaine HCl 5%, sensorcaine heavy 0.5%.

| | |
|---|---|
| C/I | • Raised pressure |
| | • Papilledema—may cause herniation of medullary cone (fatal) |
| | • Lumbar spine disorders |
| | • Skin infections |
| Method | • Hold the patient in sitting/or lateral recumbent position, with neck flexed to the chest and knees flexed to abdomen (to separate spinous processes and vertebral arches) |
| | • Sterile the area (3rd–4th intervertebral space) |
| | • Local anesthesia (1% Xylocain) given |

- Introduce a lumbar puncture needle with stillet in position, through skin, between spines, through lig. flavum
- Withdraw the stillet
- Collect the CSF
- Replace the stylet and then withdraw the needle
- Seal the puncture site with Tinc. Benzoin co.

## Cisternal Puncture

| | |
|---|---|
| Anatomy | It is the procedure performed, whereby spinal subarachnoid space is punctured in the midline, above the level of the 1st palpable cervical spinous process (axis or 2nd vertebra). |
| Site | Above the level of the 1st palpable cervical spinous process (axis or 2nd vertebra). |
| Indication | Diagnostic (manometric readings mandatory to assess IDP): |

- Traumatic: Intradural hemorrhage: raised pressure, crystal clear fluid
- Inflammatory: Acute infective meningitis, syphilis (Wassermann reaction, gold test), intracerebral abscess (reduced number of cells, increased protein content)
- Neoplastic: Raised CSF pressure, increased protein content.

Therapeutic purposes:
- To relieve pain: Intrathecal injection of bupivacaine HCl
- To introduce drugs: Penicillin for acute meningitis.

| | |
|---|---|
| C/I | |

- Raised pressure
- Papilledema—may cause herniation of medullary cone (fatal)
- Cervical spine disorders
- Skin infections

| | |
|---|---|
| Method | |

- Hold the patient in sitting /or lateral recumbent position, with neck flexed to the chest (to separate spinous processes and vertebral arches)
- Sterile the area (1st–3rd) intervertebral space)
- Local anesthesia (1% Xylocain) given
- Introduce a lumbar puncture needle with skillet in position, through skin, just above 2nd cervical spinous process, directed forwards and upwards, advanced to a depth of 5 cm, at level to an imaginary line joining the external auditory meatus with the nasion, to the occipito-atlantoid ligament, pierces the ligament to enter the cistern, with the caution that medulla is 2.5 cm from this ligament.
- Withdraw the stillet
- Collect the CSF
- Replace the stylet and then withdraw the needle
- Seal the puncture site with Tinc. Benzoin co.

## Sacral Puncture

| | |
|---|---|
| Anatomy | It is the procedure performed, whereby spinal subarachnoid space is punctured through the large triangular opening on the dorsum of the sacral bone. |

| | |
|---|---|
| Site | Large triangular opening on the dorsum of the sacral bone. |
| Indication | Diagnostic (manometric readings mandatory to assess IDP): |

- Traumatic: Intradural hemorrhage: raised pressure, crystal clear fluid
- Inflammatory: Acute infective meningitis, syphilis (Wassermann reaction, gold test), intracerebral abscess (reduced number of cells, increased protein content)
- Neoplastic: Raised CSF pressure, increased protein content.

Therapeutic purposes:
- Obstetric: To relieve pain of child birth, without affecting the infant
- Surgical: Operations on the lower gut and anal margin, performed painlessly

| | |
|---|---|
| C/I | |

- Raised pressure
- Papilledema—may cause herniation of medullary cone (fatal)
- Lumbosacral spine disorders
- Skin infections.

| | |
|---|---|
| Method | |

- Hold the patient in prone/or lateral recumbent position (with neck flexed to the chest)
- Sterile the area
- Local anesthesia (1% Xylocain) given
- Palpate the median crest of sacrum, to trace the depression caused by sacral opening
- Introduce a lumbar puncture needle with skillet in position, through skin, through the large triangular opening on the dorsum of sacral bone just above 2nd cervical spinous process, directed forwards till ligaments covering opening being pierced, then change the direction of the needle, i.e. pass vertically upwards within the sacral canal, within the epidural space
- Withdraw the stillet
- Collect the CSF
- Replace the stylet and then withdraw the needle
- Seal the puncture site with Tinc. Benzoin co.

## JOINT AND SOFT TISSUE INJECTION

| | |
|---|---|
| Preface | The current era of corticosteroids has resulted in the useful and effective treatment for the panful, inflammed musculoskeletal lesions that commonly involve soft tissues and joints. Corticosteroid are extensively used for their anti-inflammatory (glucocorticoid) and anti-allergic actions, although anti-inflammatory activity is not of much advantage until and unless it happens with low mineralocorticoid activity, i.e. the effect on water and electrolytes not increased, resulting in fluid retention, hypertension and potassium loss. Corticosteroids should not be used unless the benefits justify clearly the hazards, in any case the lowest dose that produce the desired response, to be utilized. |
| Anatomy | Mandatory knowledge of the clinical (functional) anatomy, along with comprehensive knowledge and an illustrative way of skills, to impart |

an RMP the ability to inject a corticosteroid with confidence. An accurate anatomical diagnosis, justifies a strong indication for management by corticosteroid injection, thereby assuring the patient prompt relief.

**Precautions**   General principles (prior to giving injection of steroids):
- Clinical diagnosis: Precise history and detailed examination mandatory, e.g. patient with tendoachillis (hereditary)—unethical to inject steroid into tendon, because of danger of tendon rupture later on
- Mandatory knowledge of the anatomy of joint, capsule, ligaments, muscles, etc. to achieve good response
- Mandatory aseptic technique to be used for giving an injection, as steroids in presence of infection, may result in disaster.
- Toilet (sterilize) of the site with methyl alcohol (surgical spirit)
- Sterile syringe (gamma-irradiated) to be used
- Inject carefully and slowly.

**Indication**   Traumatic: Rotator cuff lesions, traumatic effusion (RSA, sports injuries, fall from height

Inflammatory: Rheumatoid arthritis, gouty arthritis, CTS, bursitis, tendinitis, plantar facitis, polyarteritis nodosa

Chronic arthritis: Chronic serous synovitis, tuberculosis, syphilis, gonorrhea

Infective: Acute Suppurative arthritis

Degenerative: Osteoarthritis, frozen shoulder

Hemophilic joints.

**C/I**
- Skin Infection: Boils, cellulitis, abscess
- Herpes: Ocular
- Acute psychosis
- Diabetes
- Hypertension
- Hyperthyroidism
- Osteoporosis
- Prosthetic joint
- Hypersensitivity: To steroid/local (ingredients of injection)
- Pregnancy (1st trimester)
- Tendon: Substance

**Steroid**   Intra-articular steroids: Insoluble, non-systemic, longer lasting: glucocorticoids

Hydrocortisone acetate 25 mg/ml

Triamcinolone acetonide 40 mg/ml

Methylprednisolone acetate (Depo-Medrol) 20–40 mg/ml

Sodium hyaluronate I/A once a week for 3–5 week

**Anesthetic**   Local anesthetic mixed with the steroid:
- Lignocaine (xylocaine) plain 1%, rapid onset, lasts for 2–4 hours
- Bupivacaine plain 0.25% or 0.5% (Marcain plain), longer lasting

Procedure

Regional:

Shoulder:

Clinical anatomy: It is a synovial joint of the ball and socket variety, i.e. socket is the glenoid cavity of the scapula, whereas the ball is the head of the humerus, topping all other joints of the body, in free and varied range of movements, due to large size of the head of humerus, compared to small, shallow glenoid cavity, and greater laxity of the joint's capsule, while its strength lies in the powerful surrounding muscles (supraspinatus, infraspinatous, teres minor, subscapularis); the overhanging coracoacromial arch; and gravitational pressure, that keeps opposing surfaces in contact with each other. Below, the capsule is unsupported by muscles (weakest spot—prone to the dislocation of head of humerus downwards into axilla, may injure circumflex (axillary) nerve and vessels.

Technique:

Anterior approach:
- Position: Patient to sit with the arm held by the side and externally rotated
- Toilet (sterilize) of the site with methyl alcohol (surgical spirit)
- Syringe: 2 ml with a 2.5 cm needle
- Ingredient: 1 ml steroid sol. mixed with 1 ml of 1% lignocaine plain
- Direction: Insert the needle slowly, then advance horizontally and little laterally under the acromion process, to the tip of coracoids process and medial to humeral head (easily palpable), enters the capsule, inject into the steroid into the capsule and not into the narrow joint.

Posterior approach:
- Position: Patient to sit with the arm held by the side and externally rotated
- Toilet (sterilize) of the site with methyl alcohol (surgical spirit)
- Syringe: 2 ml with a 2.5 cm needle
- Ingredient: 1 ml steroid sol. mixed with 1 ml of 1% lignocaine plain
- Direction: Insert the needle 2.5 cm below the tip of acromion slowly, then advance horizontally and medial to humeral head, enters the capsule, inject into the steroid into the capsule and not into the narrow joint.

### Acromioclavicular Joint

Technique

Anterior approach:
- Position: Patient to sit with the arm held by the side
- Toilet (sterilize) of the site with methyl alcohol (surgical spirit)
- Syringe: 2 ml with a 2.5 cm needle
- Ingredient: 1 ml steroid sol. mixed with 1 ml of 1% lignocaine plain
- Direction: Palpate the joint and insert the needle slowly, then advance horizontally, anteriorly, and little medially, enters the joint/capsule, inject into the steroid into the joint or capsule.

### Bicipital tendinitis

Technique:

- Position: Patient to sit with the arm held by the side and externally rotated
- Toilet (sterilize) of the site with methyl alcohol (surgical spirit)
- Syringe: 2 ml with a 2.5 cm needle
- Ingredient: 1 ml steroid sol. mixed with 1 ml of 1% lignocaine plain
- Direction: Insert the needle slowly, then advance upwards into the bicipital groove (palpable), enters the substance of tendon, inject steroid into the synovial sheath and not into the substance of the tendon.

### Elbow

Clinical anatomy: It is a synovial joint of the hinge variety, formed by the distal end of humerus with the radius and the ulna, the trochlea of the humerus articulates with trochlear notch of the ulna, while capitulum of the humerus articulates with the upper surface of the radial head.

Ligaments: Fibrous capsule envelops the joint and is thickened at sides to form collateral ligaments (strong radial and radiating ulnar); strong, thin membranous, anterior ligament, that is attached to the humeral epicondyles and ulnar's coronoid process and to annular ligament of radius; weak posterior ligament, attached to humeral epicondyles to the olecranon.

Synovial membrane: Lines the deeper surface of fibrous capsule.

Movements:

Flexion: Muscles: biceps, brachialis, brachioradialis, and pronator teres, aided by muscles attached to the medial epicondyle.

Extension: Muscles: triceps and anconeus, aided by muscles attached to the lateral epicondyle.

### Tennis elbow (syn. lateral epicondylitis)

Technique:

- Position: Patient to sit with the arm held by the side and elbow flexed at right angle, and mid prone
- Toilet (sterilize) of the site with methyl alcohol (surgical spirit)
- Syringe: 2 ml with a 2.5 cm needle
- Ingredient: 1 ml steroid sol. mixed with 1 ml of 1% lignocaine plain
- Direction: Insert the needle slowly into the point of maximum tenderness over the lateral epicondyle, then infiltrate the tender points, with the steroid sol.

### Golfer's elbow (syn. medial epicondylitis)

Technique:

- Position: Patient to sit with the arm held by the side and elbow flexed at right angle, and mid prone
- Toilet (sterilize) of the site with methyl alcohol (surgical spirit)
- Syringe: 2 ml with a 2.5 cm needle

- Ingredient: 1 ml steroid sol. mixed with 1 ml of 1% lignocaine plain
- Direction: Insert the needle slowly into the point of maximum tendernes, then infiltrate the tender points, with the steroid sol.

### Olecranon bursitis

Technique:
- Position: Patient to sit with the arm held by the side and elbow flexed at right, and mid prone
- Toilet (sterilize) of the site with methyl alcohol (surgical spirit)
- Syringe: 2 ml with a 2.5 cm needle
- Ingredient: 1 ml steroid sol. mixed with 1 ml of 1% lignocaine plain
- Direction: Insert the needle slowly into the distended bursa, aspirate the fluid using a 10 ml syringe, then inject the steroid sol. slowly.

### Wrist (radiocarpal)

Clinical anatomy: It is a synovial joint of condyloid variety, formed by the lower articular surface of the radius and the articular disk (proximal face); and by the scaphoid, lunate and triquetral bones (distal face), with interosseus ligaments.

Ligaments: Fibrous capsule retains in apposition the opposing surfaces of the joint, by its attachment to radius, articular dik, and proximal row of carpus (scaphoid, lunate and triquetral, except pisiform). Anterior and posterior radiocarpal, radial and ulnar collateral ligaments.

Movements:
Flexion: Muscles: flexor carpi radialis, palmaris longus, and flexor carpi ulnaris
Extension: Muscles: extensor carpi radialis longus and brevis, and extensor carpi ulnaris
Adduction: Muscles: extensor carpi ulnaris and flexor carpi ulnaris
Abduction: Muscles: flexor carpi radialis, extensor carpi radialis longus, abductor pollicis longus, and extensor pollicis brevis.

### Carpal tunnel syndrome

Technique:
- Position: Patient to sit with the palm held upwads, make prominent palmaris longus tendon by flexing the wrist
- Toilet (sterilize) of the site with methyl alcohol (surgical spirit)
- Syringe: 2 ml with a 2.5 cm needle
- Ingredient: 1 ml steroid sol.
- Direction: Insert the needle slowly into the distal crease of the wrist on the radial side of the palmaris longus tendon, then distally, inject the steroid slowly.

### de Quervain's tenosynovitis

Technique:
- Position: Patient to sit with the thumb into the palm and make a fist, so as to make prominent borders of the snuffbox
- Toilet (sterilize) of the site with methyl alcohol (surgical spirit)

- Syringe: 2 ml with a 2.5 cm needle
- Ingredient: 1 ml steroid sol. mixed with 1 ml of 1% lignocaine plain
- Direction: Insert the needle slowly along the common synovial sheath of tendons (abductor policis longus and extensor pollicis brevis) forming the anterior border of the snuffbox, then proximally into the substance of tendon, inject the steroid sol. slowly.

### Trigger finger

Technique:
- Position: Patient to sit with the palm facing upwards, fingers fully extended
- Toilet (sterilize) of the site with methyl alcohol (surgical spirit)
- Syringe: 2 ml with a 2.5 cm needle
- Ingredient: 1 ml steroid sol. mixed with 1 ml of 1% lignocaine plain
- Direction: Insert the needle slowly over the crease of the MP joint of affected finger, then advance proximally into the flexor tendon, withdraw a little, and then inject the steroid sol.

### Knee

Clinical anatomy: It is a synovial joint of the hinge variety, formed by the distal end of femur, patella, and the proximal end of the tibia; largest and most complicated joint of the body, wherein all positions of the joint, the patella in contact with the femur and the femur with the tibia, while the bones do not interlock with one another; while its strength lies in the large areas of contact, and the surrounding strong ligaments and muscles (femoral condyles separated from the tibial condyles by the medial and lateral menisci or semilunal cartilages; anterior and posterior cruciate ligaments; medial and lateral collateral ligaments; quadriceps and popliteal ligaments; fascia lata and medial and lateral vasti; extensive synovial membrane and capsule.

Movements:
- Flexion (biceps femoris, popliteus, sartorius, gracilis, semitendinosus, semimembranous)
- Extension (quadriceps forceps)

Technique:
- Position: Patient lies on the bed or examination table, with the affected knee little flexed
- Toilet (sterilize) of the site with methyl alcohol (surgical spirit)
- Syringe: 2 ml with a 2.5 cm needle
- Ingredient: 1 ml steroid sol. mixed with 1 ml of 1% lignocaine plain
- Approach: Medial or lateral side of the patella
- Direction: Insert the needle slowly downward into the joint through the medial or lateral approach, aspirate the fluid using a 50 ml syringe with aspirating needle, then inject the steroid sol. slowly.

### Ankle

Clinical anatomy: It is a synovial joint of the hinge variety, formed by the talus and the distal ends of the tibia and fibula—that are firmly held together by the interosseous and other ligaments (allowing certain amount of laxity).

Ligaments: Joined together by their edges to form the fibrous capsule of the joint: Medial (deltoid), lateral, anterior and the posterior talo-fibular, calcaneofibular ligaments.

Movements: Dorsiflexion and plantar flexion (extension), and little side-to-side movement with joint plantar flexed.

Technique:
- Position: Patient lies on the bed or examination table
- Toilet (sterilize) of the site with methyl alcohol (surgical spirit)
- Syringe: 2 ml with a 2.5 cm needle
- Ingredient: 1 ml steroid sol. mixed with 1 ml of 1% lignocaine plain
- Approach: Anterior: space between the tibia and talus or between tendons of tibialis anterior and extensor hallucis longus
- Direction: Insert the needle slowly into the joint, then inject the steroid sol. slowly.

### Plantar fasciitis (syn, painful heel)
Technique:
- Position: Patient lies on the bed or examination table, prone
- Toilet (sterilize) of the site with methyl alcohol (surgical spirit)
- Syringe: 2 ml with a 2.5 cm needle
- Ingredient: 1 ml steroid sol mixed with 1 ml of 1% lignocaine plain
- Approach: Posterior or side of the heel
- Direction: Insert the needle slowly into the center of the heel, then advance down to the calcaneal spur, then inject the steroid sol.

| | |
|---|---|
| Postinjection care | Rest to the joint, to avoid lifting heavy weight for 2/56 |
| Complications | • Postinjection pain |
| | • Infection |
| | • Rupture: Tendons |
| | • Medicolegal issues: |
| | – Informed consent |
| | – Specific indication |
| | – Maintenance of records |
| | – Technique of procedure employed. |

## ASPIRATION AND DRAINAGE
### Lower Limb
### Hip

| | |
|---|---|
| Preface | Early diagnosis and prompt evacuation of the pus by aspiration or surgical drainage are mandatory. |
| Aspiration | Difficult to confirm diagnosis by aspiration in case the joint contains little fluid or the fluid highly purulent, whereby drainage is considered over aspiration |

Technique:

Approach: Anterior, posterior, and lateral.

Anterior:

- Direction: Insert the needle at right angle to the skin at a point 2.5 cm distal and lateral to the middle of inguinal ligament

Posterior:

- Direction: Insert the needle at the junction of middle and lateral 3rd of an imaginary line from center of greater trochanter to the postero-inferior iliac spine.

Lateral

- Direction: Insert the needle from the side, above the greater trochanter, then advance upwards and medially (at angle of 45 degree), parallel with the femoral neck for 5–10 cm, into the joint
- Insert the needle at right angle to the skin at a point 2.5 cm distal and lateral to the middle of inguinal ligament.

Drainage

Technique:

Approach: Posterior, anterior, medial or lateral

Posterior (Ober): To drain a fluctuating posterior abscess

- Incision parallel to femoral neck, from posterolateral border of greater trochanter, advanced upwards and medially towards posterosuperior iliac spine
- Divide gluteus maximus muscle in line of incision
- Isolate and ligate gluteal vessels
- Isolate sciatic nerve
- Isolate and divide muscles attached to greater trochanter
- Incise distended capsule to drain pus
- Insert rubber drain.

Anterior:

- Incision (vertical) from anterosuperior iliac spine, to expose and separate muscles (Sartorius, tensor fascia latae, vastus lateralis) to expose capsule
- Incise distended capsule to drain pus
- Insert rubber drain.

Lateral:

- Incision (vertical) parallel to anterior border of greater trochanter, to expose and separate vastus lateralis muscle from trochanter, then elevate periosteum from femoral neck to expose capsule
- Incise distended capsule to drain pus
- Insert rubber drain.

Medial (Ludolff):

- Incision (vertical) on the inner aspect of the hip and expose muscles (gracilis, adductor longus, pectineus and iliopsoas—behind that lies the hip joint)
- Incise distended capsule to drain pus
- Insert rubber drain.

Postoperative: Buck's traction.

## Knee

| | |
|---|---|
| Aspiration | Being a superficial joint, aspirated easily. |

Technique: Insert needle on the lateral or medial side at the level of proximal border of patella.

Drainage Technique:

Approach: Anterior, posterolateral, and posteromedial

Anterior:
- Incision: 5–10 cm long on each side of patella and patellar tendon
- Incise fasciae, capsule, and the synovium to drain pus
- Specimen for culture sensitivity and smears to identify the micro-organism
- Insert rubber drain.

Posterolateral:
- Incision 8 cm long on posterolateral aspect of flexed knee, anterior to fibular head and biceps tendon, avoids injury to common peroneal nerve, deepen incision through iliotibial band to expose the capsule
- Incise capsule to drain pus
- Insert rubber drain.

Posteromedial:
- Incision over joint, lateral to the semitendinosus tendon, isolate tendons of medial hamstrings, advance proximally along the gastrocnemius to expose the capsule
- Incise capsule to drain pus
- Insert rubber drain.

Postoperative: B/K cast or splint for 4–6/52.

## Ankle

Aspiration Difficult due to the swelling that hidden the malleoli and other landmarks, and because of swelling may be result of secondary effusion in tendon sheaths (acute suppurative arthritis)

Drainage Technique:

Approach: Anterolateral, posterolateral, anteromedial, and posteromedial

Anterolateral:
- Incision: Medial or lateral, 5–8 cm long parallel to long-axis of the foot
- Divide the superficial and deep fascia, open the capsule
- Drain the pus
- Specimen for culture sensitivity and smears to identify the micro-organism.

Postoperative: B/K cast or splint for 4–6/52.

## Tarsal Joints

Aspiration It is insufficient

Drainage Technique:
- Incision: Medial or lateral, 5–8 cm long parallel to long-axis of the foot

- Divide the superficial and deep fascia, open the capsule
- Drain the pus
- Specimen for culture sensitivity and smears to identify the micro-organism.

Postoperative: B/K cast or splint for 4–6/52.

## UPPER LIMB

### Shoulder

Aspiration     Aspirated easily as the fluctuant site palpable on the anterior aspect of the shoulder, usually needle inserted at this point.

Drainage     Technique:

Approach: Anterior and posterior.

Anterior:

- Incision from acromion, distally over center of humeral head, incise fasciae, deltoid fibers in line, to expose capsule
- Incise the capsule to drain pus
- Insert rubber drain.

Posterior:

- Incision from base of scapular spine, distally for 7.5 cm in line with deltoid fibers, divide deltoid to expose external rotators of the shoulder, deepen dissection between infraspinatus and teres minor, medial to greater tuberosity of humerus to expose capsule
- Incise the capsule to drain pus
- Insert rubber drain.

Postoperative: Abduction splint and as symptoms subside—exercises.

### Elbow

Aspiration     Position: Elbow held in acute flexion, the needle inserted on the posterior aspect lateral to the olecranon into the distended bursa, and the fluid aspirated.

Drainage     Technique:

Approach: Medial and lateral

Medial:

- Incision: 8 cm, centered over the medial humeral condyle, avoids injury to ulnar nerve that lies over posterior aspect of medial epicondyle
- Incise the superficial and deep fasciae, open space between triceps (posteriorly) and brachialis (anteriorly), incise periosteum to excise capsule
- Open the capsule to drain the pus
- Specimen for culture sensitivity and smears to identify the micro-organism.

Postoperative: A/E POP splint with elbow flexed at 90 degree for 4/52, followed by exercises.

## Wrist

**Aspiration**  Insert needle just below the radial or ulnar styloid process, advance in, perpendicular to the styloid process, into the joint and aspirate the fluid.

**Drainage**  Technique:

Approach: Medial, lateral, or posterior

Medial:
- Incision 5 cm centered over the head of the ulna, between tendons of flexor and extensor carpi ulnaris, expose end incise the ulnar collateral ligament and synovium.

Lateral:
- Incision 5 cm centered over snuffbox, between combined synovial sheath (tendons of abductor pollicis longus and extensor pollicis brevis) and extensor pollicis longus, deepen into snuffbox, isolate radial artery, incise the radial collateral ligament and synovium.

Posterior:
- Incision 5 cm centered over the medial aspect of the dorsum of the wrist, between extensor carpi ulnaris and extensor digiti minimi
- Drain the pus
- Specimen for culture sensitivity and smears to identify the micro-organism.

Postoperative:
- Cock up splint for 4/52
- Eexercises of fingers.

## SURGICAL APPROACHES TO JOINTS AND LONG BONES

**Preface**  Operative surgery is mainly the application of anatomical knowledge regarding surgical approaches to joints and bones:

Principles of surgical approach:
- To provide easy access to all required structures.
- To make the incision long enough so as not to hinder any part of the operation; to be placed parallel or follow the natural skin creases, to avoid undesirable scars.
- To avoid a longitudinal incision on the flexor surface of a joint, as that may result in a unsightly cosmetic lesion (scar or keloid); while a longitudinal midlateral incision esp. on a finger or thumb or on the inner border of the hand, that results in little scarring.
- To avoid approaching joints from their flexor surfaces, because of the presence of large vessels and nerves on the flexor aspects of joints.
- To establish properly the position of the patient prior to operation; the surgeon to be able to approach all parts of the surgical field easily.

Regional

## Shoulder Joint

### Anterior approach (Ollier):

Indication: It is the most commonly used approach that gives access to the joint, subdeltoid bursa, and the upper part of humerus.

Technique:
- Incision: 10 cm longitudinal, from coracoid process down the arm, over the sulcus separating deltoid from the pactralis major (in line of cephalic vein)
- Exposure of cephalic vein, and retracted medially with pectoralis major; deltoid retracted laterally
- Exposure of structures from above down: tip of coracoid process with origin of coracobrachialis; humeral toberosities; humeral surgical neck; tendon of pectoralis major; bicipital/or intertubercular sulcus lodging long tendon (head of) biceps
- Exposure of capsule by dividing the humeral tuberosities along with attached muscles (supraspinatus, Infraspinatus, and teres minor)
- Open: The joint.

### Posterior approach (Kocher):

Indication: It is used for the diseased glenoid cavity

Technique:
- Incision curved, beginning from acromioclavicular joint, extending back along inner border of acromion, then curved over junction of acromion with scapular spine, towards posterior axillary fold, ending 5 cm above it.
- Exposure of structures: from above down: acromioclavicular joint by dividing superior ligament of joint; trapezius divided from its acromial attachment; deltoid exposed below the scapular spine and divided from spine.
- Exposure of capsule: Supra and infraspinatus exposed and detached from acromion, that is divided and displaced laterally with deltoid, exposing the capsule of the joint
- Open: The joint.

### Superior approach:

Indication is used only in those cases of paralyzed deltoid; arthrodesis of joint; and for infantile paralysis.

Technique:
- Incision: Transverse centered over the top of the shoulder
- Exposure of structures: of deltoid muscle; divided and reflected down, exposing the humeral head and greater tuberosity with attached muscles
- Exposure of capsule by separating muscles attached to the greater tuberosity
- Isolate: Axillary nerve and the anterior and posterior circumflex humeral vessels
- Open: The joint.

## Elbow Joint

### Lateral J approach (Kocher):

Indication: Excision of the joint

Technique:
- Incision: Begin 5 cm proximal to the joint line, over the lateral epicondylar ridge of humerus, extends it down to radial head

- Exposure of lateral condyle and capsule by dissecting between triceps posteriorly and brachioradialis and extensor carpi radialis longus muscles anteriorly
- Exposure of posterior aspect of capsule by separating muscles (extensor carpi ulnaris and anconeus) around back and sides of joint; divide the distal fibers of anconeus in line with incision
- Reflect: Periosteum from anterior and posterior surfaces of distal humerus
- Reflect: Anteriorly common origin of extensor muscles from lateral epicondyle subperiosteally
- Incise: Capsule longitudinally
- Reflect: Anconeus subperiosteally from proximal ulna to dislocate the joint for examination.

### Medial approach (Campbell):

Indication: Fractured medial humeral epicondyle (fragment displaced distally and laterally into the joint cavity); to remove loose bone from the joint.

Technique:
- Incision: With elbow flexed right angled; make a 10 cm incision centered over the tip of medial epicondyle
- Isolate and retract posteriorly ulnar nerve from its groove posterior to the epicondyle
- Denude: Soft tissues from the epicondyle except common origin of flexor muscles
- Divide: The epicondyle with osteotome, and reflect it distally with its attached tendons
- Reflect: Muscles originating from medial epicondyle; protect median nerve branches entering these muscles
- Divide: Medial aspect of coronoid process
- Incise: Capsule, detach it subperiosteally from anterior and posterior aspects of humerus; avoid injuring median nerve crossing over front of joint.
- Dislocate the joint.

## Wrist Joint

Anatomically, incisions can be neither anterior (because of flexor sheaths and vessels and nerves), nor on the radial border (because of radial vessels); thus, the approach is dorsal or medial.

### Dorsal approach (Boyd)

Indication: Arthroplasty or arthrodesis of wrist joint.
Technique:
- Incision: Transverse curved, centered over medial aspect of ulnar head, extend it across dorsum of wrist to 1 cm proximal and posterior to radial styloid
- Exposure: Radial aspect of dorsum of wrist, by retracting skin, fasciae, and tendons
- Exposure: Ulnar aspect of dorsum of wrist, by incising through dorsal carpal ligament between extensor digiti minimi and common extensor tendons
- Exposure: Capsule by separating extensor digiti minimi and common extensor tendons
- Incise: Capsule transversely.
- Open: The joint.

### Medial approach (Sir Patrick Heron Watson):

Indication: Excision of joint and arthrodesis.

**Technique**
- Incision: 10 cm vertical incision on the ulnar border of the hand and forearm, centered over wrist joint (from 5 cm above ulnar styloid to middle of 5th metacarpal).
- Exposure and isolate the dorsal branch of ulnar nerve at proximal and of incision
- Deepen: Incision between extensor and flexor carpi ulnaris
- Exposure: Dorsal aspect of carpus by separating extensor tendons.

## Hip Joint

Anatomy: The hip joint is anatomically most stable joint of limbs; situated far away from the surface; femoral head and acetabulum form a very close articulation; approach is most difficult of limb joints (formidable undertaking)

### Anterior approach: Anterior iliofemoral (Smith-Peterson):
Indication: All surgical procedures of hip joint, i.e. osteotomy, dividing femoral neck, or internal fixation of fracture neck femur.

Technique:
- Incision: From middle of iliac crest to ASI spine, then distally 10 cm
- Divide: Superficial and deep fasciae and free attached gluteus medius and tensor fasciae latae muscles from iliac crest
- Strip: Subperiosteally attached gluteus medius and minimus from lateral surface of ilium; control nutrient bleeding by packing
- Divide: Deep fascia of thigh and deepen dissection between tensor fasciae latae laterally and sartorius and rectus femoris medially
- Ligate: Ascending branch of lateral femoral circumflex artery
- Retract: Medially, lateral femoral cutaneous nerve crossing sartorius
- Exposure and incise capsule transversely to expose femoral head and acetabular margin
- Divide: Ligamentum teres with curved scissors to dislocate femoral head.

### Lateral approach (Ollier):
Indication: Arthroplasty of hip joint.

Technique:
- Incision: From ASI spine distally to greater trochanter, then curve it posteriorly and proximally to end midway between trochanter and PSI spine
- Exposure of trochanter by separating gluteus medius posteriorly and tensor fasciae latae anteriorly; divide trochanter en bloc and reflect it proximally with attached piriformis, obturator, gemellio, and gluteal muscles
- Exposure: Capsule by separating fibers of gluteus maximus in line of incision
- Exposure: Femoral neck and hip joint by incising capsule vertically both anteriorly and posteriorly along superior surface of femoral neck; avoid injuring capsular branch of medial femoral circumflex artery.

### Posterior approach (Osborne):
Indication: Most popular approach for extensive operative procedures on the joint, e.g. excision of hip joint.

Technique:

- Incision: It is an angled one—angle at the tip of trochanter; upper limb extends towards PSI spine for 8 cm, lower limb extends vertically down limb axis for 8 cm
- Separate: Fibers of gluteus maximus parallel with line of incision; control bleeding by packing
- Divide: Insertion of gluteus maximus into fasciae latae for 5 cm
- Exposure of capsule by dividing insertion of tendons of piriformis and gamelli into trochanter
- Divide: Capsule longitudinally to expose femoral neck and acetabular margin.

## Knee Joint

### Anteromedial approach (Langenbeck):

Indication:

- Arthroplasty, e.g. TKR,
- IDK
- Excision osteophytes
- Removal of foreign body
- Arthrodesis
- Removal of tumors.

Technique:

- Incision: Beginning at the medial border of quadriceps tendon 10 cm. Proximal to patella, curve it around medial border of patella, then distally towards midline, ending at or distal to tibial tuberosity
- Divide and retract fascia
- Deepen: Dissection between vastus medialis and medial border of the quadriceps tendon, to expose capsule
- Incise: Capsule and synovium along medial borders of quadriceps tendon and patella, and patellar tendon
- Exposure of joint by retracting patella laterally and flexing the knee.

Split patella approach (Jones and Brackett):
Indication: Patellectomy.

Technique:

- Incision: Beginning 5 cm proximal to patella, extend it distally in the midline, ending at 2.5 cm distal to tibial tuberosity
- Exposure and divide quadriceps tendon, patella, and patellar tendon in the same plane; splitting patella with electric saw.

### Posteromedial and posterolateral approaches:

Anatomy: Sometimes a median septum separates posterior aspect of knee joint into two compartments; the posterior cruciate ligament is extrasynovial and projects anteriorly in the septum (shares partition); middle genicular artery runs anteriorly in the septum to supply tissues of femoral intercondylar notch; septum is important for tracing any foreign body or draining the joint.

Indication: To drain the suppurative arthritis and removal of foreign body.
Posteromedial approach (Henderson):

**Technique:**

- incision: Curved, 8 cm long distally from adductor tubercle, along the course of tibial collateral ligament, anterior to the relaxed tendons of semimembranosus, sartorius, gracilis, and semitendinosus muscles
- Exposure and incise oblique part of tibial collateral ligament
- Exposure of knee joint by incising capsule longitudinally.

## Posterolateral approach (Henderson)
**Technique:**

- Incision: Curved, on the lateral aspect of flexed knee, anterior to biceps femoris tendon and fibular head; avoid injuring common peroneal nerve, that crossover lateral aspect of fibular head
- Exposure: Lateral femoral condyle and origin of fibular collateral ligament; popliteus tendon lies between biceps tendon and fibular collateral ligament; retract it posteriorly to expose the capsule
- Exposure of joint by incising the capsule longitudinally.

Transverse approach (Charnley):

Indication: Meniscectomy (medial meniscus).

## Technique:
Medial meniscus:

- Incision: 5 cm long transverse, centered over tibial articular surface, extending laterally from the medial border of the patellar tendon to the anterior margin of tibial collateral ligament
- Incise: Capsule along the same line; then dissect proximal edge of divided capsule from synovium and retract it proximally
- Incise: Synovium along the proximal margin of medial meniscus
- Divide: Anterior attachment of meniscus, retract tibial collateral ligament and complete the excision of the meniscus.

Lateral meniscus:

- Incision: Hockey stick incision into capsule, that runs transversely along the joint line and then curves obliquely proximally along the anterior margin of the iliotibial band
- Incise: Synovium by retracting capsule.

## Ankle Joint

**Anterolateral approach:** Provides excellent exposure of ankle joint, talus, and most of the tarsal bones and joints; spares main vessels and nerves.

Indication: Called 'universal approach' for the ankle and foot (because most of reconstruction operations and procedures involving exposed structures); permits excision of whole talus; exception: cannot expose tarsal joints between navicular and the 1st and 2nd cuneiforms.

Technique:

- Incision: Beginning over the anterolateral aspect of leg, medial to fibula, and 5 cm proximal to ankle joint, extending distally over the joint, anterolateral aspect of talar body, and calcaneocuboid joint, ending at the base of 4th metatarsal
- Incise: Fascia and the transverse crural and cruciate crural ligaments to the tibial periosteum and capsule of ankle joint; avoid damaging malleolar and lateral tarsal arteries

- Isolate: Branches of superficial peroneal nerve
- Divide: Extensor digitorum brevis and reflect it distally
- Exposure: Expose the capsule by retracting extensor tendons, dorsalis pedis artery, and deep peroneal nerve medially; incise capsule
- Exposure: Talonavicular joint by incising capsule (deeper to tendons) transversely
- Incise: Capsule of calcaneocuboid joint
- Exposure: Subtalar joint by incising mass of fat lateral and inferior to talar neck
- Dissect: Extend distally dissection to the joints between cuboid and 4th and 5th metatarsals, and between navicular and 3rd cuneiform.

**Lateral approach (Kocher):**Provides excellent exposure of midtarsal, subtalar, and ankle joints.

Indication: Arthrodesis

Technique:
- Incision: Beginning just lateral and distal to the talar head, curve incision 2.5 cm below the tip of lateral malleolus, then posteriorly and proximally, ending 2.5 cm posterior to fibula and 5 cm proximal to tip of lateral malleolus
- Incise: Fascia down to peroneal tendons; retract them posteriorly, thereby saving the small saphenous vein and sural nerve
- Divide: Tendons by Z-plasty for wider operative field
- Exposure: Subtalar joint by dividing calcaneofibular ligament
- Exposure: Calcaneocuboid joint through distal part of incision
- Divide: Talofibular ligaments
- Dislocate: Ankle joint

Disadvantage: Skin may often slough about incision margins.

**Ollier approach:**Provides excellent approach for a triple arthrodesis; three joints exposed through a small opening.

Indication: Tripple arthrodesis.

Technique:
- Incision: Beginning over the dorsolateral aspect of talonavicular joint, extend it obliquely inferoposteriorly, ending 2.5 cm below the lateral malleolus
- Divide: Cruciate crural ligament in line of skin incision
- Exposure: Long extensor tendons to toes in the proximal part of the incision; retract them medially
- Exposure: Peroneal tendons in the distal part of the incision, retract them inferiorly
- Divide: Extensor digitorum brevis at its origin; retract it distally to expose sinus tarsi
- Exposure: Subtalar, calcaneocuboid, and talonavicular joints, by extending dissection.

**Posterolateral approach (Gatellier and Chastang)**

Indication:
- ORIF of fractures of ankle involving posterior tibial lip
- Osteochondritis dissecans of talus dome
- Osteochondromatosis of ankle.

Technique:
- Incision: Beginning 10 cm proximal to the tip of lateral malleolus; extend it distally to malleolar tip; then curve it anteriorly for 4 cm in line of peroneal tendons

- Exposure: Fibula including lateral malleolus subperiosteally
- Incise: Sheaths of peroneal tendons and retinacula—to allow tendons to be displaced anteriorly
- Divide: Fibula (nonfractured) 10 cm proximal to the lateral malleolus tip; then free the distal fragment by dividing interosseous membrane and the anterior and posterior malleolar ligaments; preserve the calcaneofibular and talofibular ligaments to maintain integrity of ankle postoperatively
- Exposure: Lateral and posterior aspects of distal tibia and lateral aspect of ankle joint.

## ARTHROPLASTY

Definition      Arthroplasty is defined as a reconstructive procedure to restore joint motion and function of the muscles, ligaments and other soft tissues controlling it or function of a joint. Over the years, many different types of hip arthroplasties have been described.

Types      Classification:
- Pseudarthrosis and resection arthroplasty
- Interposition arthroplasty
- Cup arthroplasties
- Double cup or surface replacement arthroplasty
- Femoral endoprostheses
- Bipolar endoprosthesis
- Total hip replacement (THR)
- Hybrid total hip replacement.

1. Pseudarthrosis and resection arthroplasty:

Example: Girdlestone Pseudarthrosis

Indication: Degenerative disease of the hip, tuberculous arthritis, and septic arthritis.

2. Interposition arthroplasty:

Indication: Interposition of soft tissues, e.g. muscle and fascia lata between articular surfaces.

3. Cup arthroplasties:

It is a unique type of interposition arthroplasty, which in large part was responsible for development of modern total hip replacement

Example: Vitallium cup arthroplasty

Indication: Painful hip, chronic arthritis.

4. Double cup or surface replacement arthroplasty:

Two metallic cups fixed with acrylic cement, one onto the femoral head and other into the acetabulum.

Hemiarthroplasty: Using a metallic cup mounted on a short curved intramedulary stem. The femoral head not resected but reamed to fit within the thin walled metal cup

Indication: Rarely used currently, due to unacceptable number of failures, although research and development are continuing with this device.

5. Femoral endoprostheses:

> Example: Moore (long stem) and Thompson (short stem) metallic prostheses
>
> Indication: Fracture neck femur, degenerative arthritis.

6. Bipolar endoprosthesis:

> Example: Metallic cups lined with high density polyethylene locked securely onto the head of the femoral component
>
> Indication: Fracture neck femur, degenerative arthritis.

7. Total hip replacement (THR):

> Indication: Fracture neck femur, AVN of femoral head, and degenerative arthritis (secondary osteoarthritis of hip).

8. Hybrid total hip replacement:

> It is a combination of cementless acetabular component and a cemented femoral component
>
> Indications:
> - Traumatic: To relieve pain
> - Infective: Infective arthritis, tubercular arthritis
> - Inflammatory: RA

C/I

> Tuberculosis: Causing ankylosis in a single joint
> Shortening: By growth impairment (due to injured epiphysis)
> Osteoporosis: Severe
> Osteomyelitis: Causing extensive sclerosis of bone
> Age: Young children
> Occupation: Workers doing strenuous work.

## Evolution of the Prosthesis Design

Preface

> Components of the prostheses used in total hip arthroplasty in current Orthopedic practice have evolved over the years and are discussed as follows:
>
> A. Acetabular components:
>   i. Cemented components:
>      - Charnley modified cup with a thin extended flange.
>      - Metal backed cemented acetabular components with screws
>   ii. Noncemented components
>
> Advantages: To increase longevity and to lessen incidence of aseptic loosening.
>
> Cups: Noncemented cups used with femoral components
>
> Types:
> - Press fit cups and no press fit cups available:
> - All have some form of additional fixation
> - All plastic: Hemispherical cup with two metal screws
> - Ingrowth cups: Porous surface to allow tissue ingrowth, and screws and spikes as additional fixation
> - Threaded cups, e.g. truncated cones, rings, hemispherical shells

B. Femoral components:
  i. Cemented Femoral Stems:
- Charnley femoral component:
  Head diameter 22–25 mm, standard stem
- Muller femoral component:
  Head diameter 32 mm, a collar and neck (3) lengths
  Curved saber neck
- Harris modular femoral component:
  3 cm of proximal stem precoated with methyl methacrylate for better bonding with stem.

  ii. Uncemented Femoral Stems:

    Types: Press fit femoral components:
- Moore and thompson, and Judet femoral prosthesis

Macrointerlock components: Press-fit supplemented by mechanical interlock such as steps, ribs, threads, flutes

Porous-coated metal stem components: Femoral stems have porous coating, with surface openings of 50–400 microns in diameter

Advantage: Uncemented femoral stems are widely used all over the world.

Disadvantage: Thigh pain, insufficient immediate fixation to enable bone ingrowth to take place, stress shielding of the proximal femur

Uncemented modular S-Rom prosthesis:

Composition: It is a proximally modular stem made of titanium alloy; distal part is cylindrical with flutes to improve rotational stability, and a coronal slot to reduce stem stiffness.

Types: Primary and revisions arthroplasty.

**Technique:**
Preoperative planning
- X-ray templating
- Neck resection: At predetermined level
- Femoral canal entry: Opening femoral canal at the piriformis fossa
- Reaming: Distal reaming with blunt nosed distal reamer
- Cone reaming: With assembled cone reamer
- Select the triangular reamer by noting the color-coded band of the cone reamer
- Calcar triangle milling: To prepare proximal femur for the calcar triangle portion of the final sleeve, to be placed in the medial proximal femur
- Trialing: Attach the trial to the stem body. Seat the trial sleeve; select and assemble stem trial with templated neck style; introduce the trial stem through the trial sleeve
- Confirm joint stability, and then extract the trials
- Implantation: Implant insertion through the sleeve using horseshoe stem inserter

## Hybrid Total Hip Replacement

| | |
|---|---|
| Definition | It is a combination of cementless acetabular component and a cemented femoral component |
| Concept | Clinical behavior and mechanism of loosening of femoral component differs from that of acetabular component |
| Cementing | Techniques: |
| | The handling of the cement and its application will determine the future performance of THR |
| | The cementing techniques have evolved through following stages: |
| First generation | Manual mixing and finger packing of bone cement into femoral canal |
| Disadvantages | Inclusion of air while mixing |
| | Interposition of blood and debris |
| Second generation | |
| | Use of a plug and cement gun with/without a proximal seal |
| Third generation | Use of high-pressure lavage, an intramedullary plug and brush, tamponade of the femoral canal, proximal pressurization and use of vacuum mixed cement. |

### Total hip replacement:

| | |
|---|---|
| Types | Cemented |
| | Uncemented |
| | Hybrid |

### Components of prostheses:

A. Acetabular components:

   i. Cemented components: Charnley modified cup with a thin extended flange

                               Metal backed cemented acetabular components with screws

   ii. Uncemented components:

      Advantages     To increase longevity

                       To lessen incidence of aseptic loosening

     Cups: Uncemented cups used with femoral components

     Types: Press fit cups:

     No pure press fit cups available.

     All have some form of additional fixation

     All plastic—hemispherical cup with two metal screws

     Ingrowth cups—porous surface to allow tissue ingrowth

     Spiked cups—screws/spikes as additional fixation

     Threaded cups, e.g. truncated cones, rings, hemispherical

B. Femoral components:

   i. Cemented femoral stems: Charnley femoral component:

                              Head diameter 22–25 mm standard stem

     Muller femoral component:

     Head diameter 32 mm   A collar and neck (3) lengths

     Curved saber neck

     Harris modular femoral component:

     3 cm of proximal stem precoated with methyl methacrylate for better bonding with stem.

ii. Uncemented femoral stems:

Types: Press fit femoral stems: Moore and Thompson, and Judet femoral prosthesis

Macrointerlock stem       : Press-fit supplemented by mechanical interlock such as steps, ribs, threads, flutes

Porous-coated metal stem  : Femoral stems have porous coating with surface openings

Uncemented femoral stems are widely used all over the world.

Disadvantages   Thigh pain

Insufficient immediate fixation to enable bone in growth to take place

Stress shielding of the proximal femur

Uncemented Modular S-Rom Prosthesis:

Composition     It is a proximally modular stem made of titanium alloy

Distal part is cylindrical with flutes to improve rotational stability, and a coronal slot to reduce stem stiffness

Indication      Primary and revisions arthroplasty

Method          Preoperative planning

X-ray templating

Neck resection—at predetermined level

Femoral canal entry—opening femoral canal at piriformis fossa

Reaming: Distal reaming—with blunt nosed distal reamer

Cone reaming—wirh assembled cone reamer

Select the triangular reamer by noting color-coded band of the cone reamer

Calcar triangle milling: To prepare proximal femur for the calcar triangle portion of the final sleeve—to be placed in the medial proximal femur

Trialing: Attach the trial to the stem body. Seat the trial sleeve

Select and assemble the stem trial with templated neck style

Introduce trial stem through the trial sleeve

Confirm joint stability, and then extract the trials.

Implantation    Implant insertion through the sleeve using horseshoe stem inserter

## C. Hybrid total hip replacement

Definition      It is a combination of uncemented acetabular component and a cemented femoral component

Concept         Clinical behavior and mechanism of loosening of femoral component differs from that of acetabular component

Cementing techniques:

Handling of cement and its application determines  the success of THR

Techniques      A. Manual mixing and finger packing of bone cement into femoral canal

Disadvantages:

• Inclusion of air while mixing

• Interposition of blood and debris

B. Use of a plug and cement gun with/without a proximal seal

C. Use of high-pressure lavage, an intramedullary plug and brush, tamponade of the femoral canal, proximal pressurization and use of vacuum mixed cement.

## ARTHRODESIS

| | |
|---|---|
| Indications | Pain—relief of pain |
| | Stability—to provide stability at the expense of movement |
| Types | Intra-articular arthrodesis |
| | Extra-articular arthrodesis |
| | Intra-articular and Extra-articular arthrodesis |
| Joints | Lower limb—Hip, knee, ankle, |
| | Upper limb—Shoulder |
| | Spine—anterior and posterior |

## OSTEOTOMY

| | |
|---|---|
| Indications | Deformity—Correction of deformity |
| | Pain—relief of pain |
| | Bone shape—alteration |
| | Lengthening—limb |
| | Traumatic—malunited fracture: Lateral tibial condyle, lateral femoral condyle, Pott's fracture of ankle |
| | Nonunited fracture: Neck of femur—esp. in younger age |
| | Slipped upper femoral epiphysis |
| | Osteoarthritis—Hip or knee |
| C/I | Acute arthritis (inflammatory) |
| Sites | Femur: Upper end: Displacement osteotomy—proximal to lesser trochanter, e.g. McMurray's osteotomy |
| | Angulation osteotomy—distal to lesser trochanter, e.g. Blount's osteotomy |
| | Lower end: Realignment osteotomy |
| | Tibia: |
| | Upper end: High tibial valgus osteotomy |
| | Lower end: Realignment osteotomy |
| | Humerus: Realignment osteotomy. |

## SYNOVECTOMY

| | |
|---|---|
| Indications | Rheumatoid arthritis: |
| | • Relief of pain |
| | • Restoration of joint function |
| | Traumatic synovitis |
| C/I | Polyarticular synovitis |

## ARTHROSCOPY (ENDOSCOPY) AND ARTHROSCOPIC SURGERY

It cannot be emphasized too strongly that arthroscopic surgery should only be attempted by surgeons who have total confidence in their arthroscopic technique

| | |
|---|---|
| Types | Diagnostic and operative (surgical) |
| Indications | Diagnostic: |
| | Preoperative assessment of internal derangement of knee |
| | Postoperative assessment of problems, e.g. persistent symptoms |
| | Operative: |
| | Synovial biopsy |
| | Synovectomy |
| | Adhesions and ankylosis—release |
| | Excision of fat-pad |
| | Removal of loose bodies, foreign bodies |
| | Trimming, shaving, drilling of articular cartilage of patella, femur, tibia |
| | Meniscectomy |
| | Prolapse intervertebral disk (PIVD) |
| Techniques | Single and double puncture techniques |
| Rules | Precise clinical diagnosis preoperatively |
| | Plan the approach preoperatively |
| Instruments | Arthroscope set includes: |

i. Arthroscope:
- Straight forward telescope 0 degree, enlarged view, diameter 4 mm, length 18 cm, autoclavable, fiber optic light transmission
- Operating tube, oval
- Obturator blunt, for use with operating tube
- Working insert, for use with operating tube, with working channel, diameter 8 mm and irrigation channel
- Localization device for fluoroscopic localization of point of incision, for insertion of operating tube

ii. Bone punch, 90 degree upbiting, 3 mm, working length 18 cm

iii. Bone punch, 45 degree upbiting, 3 mm, working length 18 cm

iv. Trephine, diameter 3.5 mm, working length 22 cm

v. Rongeur, oval jaws, 4 × 10 mm, working length 20 cm

vi. Bipolar coagulating forceps, with connector pin for bipolar coagulation, jaws 1 mm, diameter 3.5 mm, working length 20 cm

vii. Chisel, flat, 10 mm, with handle, length 15 cm

viii. Elevator, sharp, 5 mm, working length 18 cm

ix. Palpation hook, blunt, hook angled 90 degree

x. Suction tube, cut off hole, angled, working length 11 cm

xi. Fiberoptic light cable, size 3.5 mm, length 230 cm

xii. Surgical handle—Bard Parker

xiii. Surgical blades—sterile

| | |
|---|---|
| Method | Preoperative: |
| | General or local anesthesia |

Examination under anesthesia

A tourniquet applied—for knee procedures

Skin preparation and draping of the part

Distension of the joint—with irrigation fluid

Approaches: Anterolateral, central, anteromedial, posteromedial, insertion of the arthroscope:

- Knee flexed to 90 degree by surgeons who have total confidence in their arthroscopic technique

**Types** — Diagnostic and operative (surgical)

**Indications** — Diagnostic:

Preoperative assessment of internal derangement of knee

Postoperative assessment of problems, e.g. persistent symptoms

Operative:

Synovial biopsy

Synovectomy

Adhesions and ankylosis—release

Excision of fat-pad

Removal of loose bodies, foreign bodies

Trimming, shaving, drilling of articular cartilage of patella, femur, tibia

Meniscectomy

Prolapse intervertebral disk (PIVD)

**Techniques** — Single and double puncture techniques

**Rules** — Precise clinical diagnosis preoperatively

Plan the approach preoperatively

**Instruments** — Arthroscope set includes:

i. Arthroscope:
   - Straight forward telescope 0 degree, enlarged view, diameter 4 mm, length 18 cm, autoclavable, fiberoptic light transmission
   - Operating tube, oval
   - Obturator blunt, for use with operating tube
   - Working insert, for use with operating tube, with working channel, diameter 8 mm and irrigation channel
   - Localization device for fluoroscopic localization of point of incision, for insertion of operating tube

ii. Bone punch, 90 degree upbiting, 3 mm, working length 18 cm

iii. Bone punch, 45 degree upbiting, 3 mm, working length 18 cm

iv. Trephine, diameter 3.5 mm, working length 22 cm

v. Rongeur, oval jaws, 4 × 10 mm, working length 20 cm

vi. Bipolar coagulating forceps, with connector pin for bipolar coagulation, jaws 1 mm, diameter 3.5 mm, working length 20 cm

vii. Chisel, flat, 10 mm, with handle, length 15 cm

viii. Elevator, sharp, 5 mm, working length 18 cm

ix. Palpation hook, blunt, hook angled 90 degree

x. Suction tube, cut off hole, angled, working length 11 cm

xi. Fiberoptic light cable, size 3.5 mm, length 230 cm

                xii.  Surgical handle—Bard Parker

             xiii.  Surgical blades—sterile

**Method**         Preoperative:

General or local anesthesia

Examination under anesthesia

A tourniquet applied—for knee procedures

Skin preparation and draping of the part

Distension of the joint—with irrigation fluid

Approaches: Anterolateral, central, anteromedial, posteromedial, insertion of the arthroscope:

- Knee flexed to 90 degree
- A 5 mm incision made with blade at a point 2 mm above the anterior horn of lateral meniscus, close to patellar tendon
- A sharp trocar, locked into the arthroscope sheath, pushed upwards, medially and backwards towards intercondylar notch
- Patella lifted by the tip of the sheath, and the scope passed into the suprapatellar pouch, as the knee straightened
- Assembly of the scope—by insertion of the telescope and attachment of the light cable and irrigation tube

**Examination**     The examination made in chronological manner, e.g.

- Suprapatellar pouch
- Patellofemoral joint
- Medial compartment
- Intercondylar notch
- Lateral compartment
- Posteromedial compartment
- Posterolateral compartment
- Use of percutaneous needles and blunt hooks to manipulate structures.

**Post care**     A single stitch of monofilament nylon through skin and subcutaneous tissues and a sterile gauze dressing applied.

## AMPUTATIONS

**Indications**     Traumatic—Crush injury

Infective—Gangrene, severe burne

Vascular—Peripheral vascular disease

Neoplastic—malignant tumor

## Bibliography

1. Abbott LC, Carpenter WF. Surgical approaches to the knee joint, J. Bone Joint Surg. 27:277, 1945.
2. Abbott LC, et al. Surgical approaches to the shoulder joint, J. Bone and Joint Surg. 31-A:235, 1949
3. Apley AG, Solomon L. Orthopaedic procedures and appliances. Concise System of Orthopaedics and Fractures. Arnold London 2000.
4. Bell AD, Conaway D. Corticosteroid injections for painful shoulders. Int J Clin Prac. 59:1178–86, 2005.

5. Bost FC, et al. Surgical approaches to the elbow joint, American Academy of Orthopedics Instructional Course Lectures, vol. X, Ann Arbor, J.W. Edwards, p. 180, 1953.

6. Boyd HB. Surgical exposure of the ulna and proximal third of the radius through one incision, Surg., Gynec. and Obst. 71:86, 1940.

7. Campbell WC. Incision for exposure of the elbow joint, Am. J. Surg. 15:65, 1932.

8. Charnley J. Horizontal approach to the medial semilunar cartilage, J. Bone and Joint Surg. 30-B:659, 1948.

9. Charnley J. Total prosthetic replacement of the hip. Triangle 8: 211, 1968.

10. Clark JMP. Modern Trends in Orthopedics Fracture Treatment (1962) Butterworths, London.

11. Clark JMP. Modern Trends in Orthopedics Fracture Treatment, Butterworths, London, 1962.

12. Crenshaw AH, Milford l. Arthrodesis. Campbell's operative orthopaedics. Mosby Co. Tokyo 1963

13. Crenshaw AH, Milford L. Synovectomy for Rheumatoid arthritis of knee. Campbell's operative orthopaedics. Mosby Co. Tokyo 1963.

14. Dandy DJ, Jackson RW. Arthroscopic Surgery Knee. Churchill Livingstone 1981.

15. Gilltes H, Seligson D. Arthrograpgy and Arthroscopy: Precision in the Diagnosis of Meniscal Lesions: A Comparison of Clinical Evaluation, J. Bone and Joint Surg. 61-A: 343–346, 1979.

16. Henderson MS. Posterolateral incision for the removal of loose bodies from the posterior compartment of the knee joint, Surg., Gynec. and Obst. 33:698, 1921.

17. Jones A, et al. importance of placement of intra-articular steroid injections. BMJ. 307:1329–30, 1993.

18. Kapoor PS. Kapoor's Textbook of Accident and Emergency, 2nd ed, CBS, New Delhi, 2016.

19. Kocher T. Textbook of operative surgery, 3rd English ed (translated by H.J. stiles, and C.B. Paul), Adam and Charles Black, London, 1911.

20. Love M, et al. Bailey and Love's Short Practice of Surgery, ed. 13th, H.K. Lewis and Co., London, 1965.

21. Love M, Rains AJH, Capper WM. Bailey and Love's Short Practice of Surgery (1965) H.K. Lewis and Co., London.

22. Mc Rae R. Practical Fracture Treatment, ed. 1st, Churchill Livingstone, 1981.

23. McGinty JB, Matza RA. Arthroscopy of the Knee: Evaluation of an out-Patient Procedure under Local Anesthesia, J Bone and Joint Surg. 60-A: 787–9, 1978.

24. McGREGOR AL. A Synopsis of Surgical Anatomy, ed 9, John Wright and Sons Ltd., Bristol, 1963.

25. McGunty JB, Matza RA. Arthroscopy of the Knee. Evaluation of an Out-Patient Procedure under local Anaesthesia. Journal of Bone and Joint Surgery 60A: 787–9.

26. Oh I, Harris WH. A cement fixation system for total hip arthroplasty. Clin Orthop 164: 221–9, 1982.

27. Operative Principles of Ilizarov: Fracture Treatment—Nonunion, Osteomyelitis—Lengthening, Deformity correction, ASAMI Group, Williams and Wilkins, Milan, Italy, 1991.

28. Oretorp N, Gillquist J. Transcutaneous Meniscectomy under Arthroscopic Control. International Orthopaedics 3:19–25, 1979.

29. Silver T, Silver D. Joint and soft tissue injection. ed 4, Radcliffe Publishing LTYD., Oxford, UK, 2010.

30. Smith H. Surgical approaches: Campbell's Operative Orthopaedics, ed. 9th, vol I C.V. Mosby Co., Saint Louis, 1998.

31. Smith-Peterson MN. Approach to and exposure of the hip joint for mold arthroplasty, J. Bone and Joint Surg. 31-A:40 1949.

32. Watanabe M, Takeda S, Ikeuchi H. Atlas of Arthroscopy, 2nd Ed., Igaku Shoin Ltd., Tokyo, 1969.

33. Zaman M, Leonard MA. Meniscectomy in children: A study of fifty-nine knees. Journal of Bone and Joint Surgery 1978, 60-B: 436.

Part

# III

# ELECTIVE ORTHOPEDICS

# ORTHOPEDICS

| | |
|---|---|
| Definition | It is defined as the branch of surgery concerned with treating problems involving the musculoskeletal system. The musculoskeletal system includes bones, joints, ligaments, muscles, tendons, fascia and nerves. |
| History | The Greek word 'Ortho' means straight and 'pedics/paedics' derives from the Greek word 'Pais' meaning child. For many centuries orthopedic surgeons have been involved in the treatment of crippled children. Over the years, orthopedic field has expanded to encompass many sub-specialties and the treatment of a wide variety of musculoskeletal disorders in patients of all ages. Nowadays, the orthopedic surgeons specialize in the diagnosis and treatment of a wide range of problems of the musculoskeletal system, typically involving the upper limb (shoulder to hand), lower limb (hip to foot) and the spine. |

The commonest orthopedic problem is osteoarthritis ('wear and tear' arthritis affecting a joint). Other common problems include bone and joint deformities, overuse injuries (misuse), joint intability, bone and joint infection, arthritis and allied rheumatic diseases, and nerve compression.

| | |
|---|---|
| Types | Elective orthopedics: does not usually include the care of recent injuries, being covered under trauma, but may include the treatment of long-term problems caused by a previous injury. |

Trauma orthopedics: includes the care of recent injuries and may also of old injuries.

| | |
|---|---|
| Triage | Orthopedic patients are usually referred initially by the GPs and are seen as an outpatient in an Orthopedic Clinic. A patient may be seen initially by a musculoskeletal physiotherapy practitioner in a MCAS (Musculoskeletal Clinical Assessment Services) clinic. Further the case is seen by an orthopedic surgeon, whose task is diagnose a musculoskeletal problem and recommend appropriate treatment (include a range of options, including conservative measures as well as surgical procedures). The diagnosis may be confirmed by requesting special investigations, such as X-rays, ultrasound scans, MRI scans, CT scans, bone scans, and nerve conduction studies. The orthopedic surgeon may also arrange treatment with other medical professionals, such as physiotherapists, hand therapists, plaster technicians, orthotists, rheumatologists, or pain clinic specialists. |
| Management | The treatment of orthopedic problems may involve either conservative (nonsurgical) or surgical treatment. |

Conservative treatment: includes measures:

Pain relief medication

Weight loss

Exercise

Physiotherapy: Exercise (active/passive), heat/cold therapy, shortwave, infrared, ultrasound, magnetic, traction (cervical, lumbar, foot), orthotics (braces, belts, jackets, splints, or special footwear.

Surgical treatment: includes procedures:

Arthroscopy (keyhole surgery)

Osteotomy (realignment of a bone)

Arthroplasty

Arthrodesis (fusion of a joint)

Ligament reconstruction (e.g. ACL reconstruction)

Tendon repair (e.g. rotator cuff repair)

Excision of a bony/or soft tissue lump

Removal of metallic appliance

Nerve decompression (e.g. carpal tunnel decompression/or spinal decompression)

# Deformities

<table>
<tr><td>Definition</td><td>Deformity is defined as an abnormal shape of body part; it may be congenital or acquired (postural) in origin, and fixed or mobile in type; fixed deformities cannot be corrected by gentle manipulation exerted manually, whereas mobile deformities can be corrected as such.</td></tr>
<tr><td>Etiology</td><td>Based on pathological changes occurring in the anatomical structures skin and subcutaneous tissues: burns—common cause of fixed deformities by forming scars across the flexor aspects of joints, e.g. Dupuytren's contracture—a spontaneous contracture of the fibrous tissue of the palmar fascia.</td></tr>
</table>

Muscles and tendons: Ischemic contracture of muscle post-trauma or embolism resulting from contraction of scar tissue leftover necrosis of contractile mass of muscle belly.

Bones:
- Congenital deformities: Familial growth errors: fragilitas ossium, bones absence, achondroplasia
- Traumatic deformities: Malunited fractures
- Irregular epiphyseal growth: By trauma or disease
- Metabolic deformities: Rickets, renal rickets
- Fibrous dysplasias of bone: Paget's disease, osteitis fibrosa cystica

Joints:
- Congenital deformities: CDH, club foot, cleft foot, pseudarthrosis of tibia, Madelung's deformity
- Traumatic deformities: dislocation
- Arthritis and allied rheumatic deformities: rheumatoid arthritis, ankylosing spondylitis, Reiter's syndrome, systemic lupus erythematosus
- Hysterical deformities: Defined by the patient, holding the joint in an abnormal position for longer period
- Nervous lesions: Spastic deformities by Little's disease, hemiplegia flaccid deformities: poliomyelitis, peripheral nerve injury.

<table>
<tr><td>Prevention</td><td>Early diagnosis and management mostly rendered unnecessary need of surgical intervention, e.g. in the case of acute anterior poliomyelitis.</td></tr>
<tr><td>Management</td><td>Procedures for correction of deformities:<br>• Manipulation: Correction of club foot</td></tr>
</table>

- Surgery on soft structures: Fasciotomy, tenotomy, tendon transplantation/transfering
- Surgery on bones: Osteotomy, excision, amputation
- Surgery on joints: Arthrodesis of the tarsus for a flail ankle joint.

Criteria for intervention:

Age: Older the patient may not need correction, as may adept to the existing deformity, e.g. fixed equinus in paralytic lower limb due to poliomyelitis, may mechanically assist the weak quadriceps to hold the knee in extension, thus help in walk without help of a caliper. During childhood, usually the body comparatively not heavy, and the child moreover not adapted to strenuous physical activity, the postural affections that may begin during this period often unnoticed until adolescence; while during adolescence and adulthood, the body becomes heavier, and the person adopts an occupation that requires prolonged sitting and standing postures; thereby any postural affection that starts during childhood, tends to increase and become symptomatic; an early diagnosis and precise management, an affection may often be corrected, and the disability that might have ensued thus prevented.

Type: Most of the deformities that require surgical management are postural caused by unfair distribution of body weight while sitting, standing, or walking; while sitting or standing the body weight exerts a continuous downward pressure (by gravity) that is distributed evenly throughout spine and lower limbs; during body's motion, body weight constantly redistributed; postural deformities usually caused by:

- Normal body weight with abnormal supporting structures (spine and lower limbs)
- Normal supporting structures with abnormal havy body weight; the spine and lower limbs usually the only supporting structures for weight bearing, thereby are the structures usually subjected to postural affections.

Asymmetrical development: May be caused by atrophic or hypertrophic growth of one-half of body (hemiatrophy or hemihypertrophy) or of a limb or part of a limb.

## CONGENITAL DEFORMITIES OF BONES AND JOINTS

- Club foot
- Flat foot
- Cleft foot
- Congenital pseudarthrosis of tibia
- Congenital dislocation of hip
- Congenital coxa vara
- Osteogenesis imperfecta
- Vertebral anomalies:
  - Congenital spina bifida
  - Congenital scoliosis

- Spondylolisthesis
- Congenital torticollis
• Congenital elevation of scapula
• Made lungs deformity
• Congenital contracture of little finger
• Dupuytren's contracture
• Hereditary multiple exostosis
  (Diaphyseal aclasis (syn. multiple exostoses)
• Ollier's disease

## CLUB FOOT (TALIPES EQUINOVARUS FOOT)

Definition | It is defined as a group of foot deformities whereby the sole of the foot is no longer plantigrade. The deformity varies in severity, i.e. the entire foot in equines and varus, the forefoot in adduction, a cavus deformity to one much less severe in which the foot is in mild equines and varus. Mostly accompanied by internal tortion of tibia.

Etiology | Unknown.
Muscular imbalance: Calf muscles, tibialis anterior, and tibialis posterior rather than the peronei.

Pathogenesis | Contracture of medial plantar ligaments, deltoid ligament, posterior tibial tendon, abductor hallucis, tendocalcaneus capsules of tarsometatarsal and tarsal joints, posterior part of capsule of ankle joint, and the anterior tibial tendon. Talus deviated medially and plantarward, the head of talus—prominent subcutaneously on the dorsum of foot, navicular displaced medially and rotated, cuboid displaced medially on the calcaneus, the calcaneus displaced medially and in varus.

Diagnosis | Congenital type:
Deformity: Bilateral usually
Skin, subcutaneous tissues, muscles—appear normal
A transverse crease across medial sole
Callosities and bursae: In a walking child.

### Acquired type
Deformity: Unilateral usually
Skin: Cold, cyanotic, trophic changes, transverse crease absent
Muscles: Wasting, flaccid (infantile paralysis), spastic (upper motor neurone lesions).
Bones of the affected leg/s thin.

Investigation | X-ray feet, spine, pelvis
Management | Conservative treatment:
Should begin within first two weeks after birth, as with increasing age the deformity becomes more difficult to correct.

Manipulation: Into direction of over-correction: Steps:
• Adduction and varus of forefoot
• Varus of calcaneus

- Equinus of forefoot
- Equinus of ankle.

Postreduction X-ray: To confirm reduction, i.e.

- Adduction of forefoot: Axis of 1st metatarsal in line with body and neck of talus
- Varus: Distal ends of talus and calcaneus separated and long-axis of 5th metatarsal in line with that of calcaneus—equinus and cavus: normal height of longitudinal arch, no equinus of forefoot, body of talus centered under tibia.

Immobilization:

Plaster of Paris: Applied at regular intervals, to hold the correction

Denis Browne splints: Attached to the boots, later used as night splint, till walking established.

Shoe: Rigid shank and a low lateral wedge.

### Surgical treatment

Indication:

Failure of conservative treatment; interrupted or managed ineffectively, or resistant deformity, muscle imbalance in spina bifida, or persistence/ or recurrence of one or more elements of deformity, after one or more years of continuous and well managed conservative treatment, in older children whose deformity either has never been corrected or has recurred post correction.

Surgery: Depend upon patient's age and his deformity.

Children < 10 years: Operations confined mainly to the soft structures, as the bones of the foot have not ossified enough to permit procedures (arthrodesis) without loosing too much cartilage (unacceptable small foot)

Children 5–10 years: Procedures: tendon lengthening and osteotomy (Dwyer) :

Equinus: Tendocalcaneus lengthening + conservative treatment (corrective casts)

Congenital atresia of articulation for talus head: soft tissue releasing operations:

Brockman: Release plantar fascia and muscles from the calcaneus, lengthening of posterior tibial tendon

McCauley: Abductor hallucis displaced distally, sheaths of posterior tibial, flexor hallucis longus, flaxor digitorum longus excised, capsulotomies of joints, freeing plantar calcaneonavicular deltoid ligaments, lengthening of tendocalcaneus and posterior capsulotomy of ankle joint

Children > 10 years: Advanced ossification permits arthrodesis, and in severe cases operations on soft structures alone insufficient.

### Recurrent/residual cases:

Procedures:

- Equinus deformity: Lengthening of tendocalcaneus
- Varus deformity: Transposition of tibialis anterior tendon to the outer

border of foot, and division of all contracted ligaments around the tarsal joints on the inner side of foot.

Muscular imbalance: (Fried): Correction of deformity conservatively or surgically followed by transferring of tibialis posterior tendon anteriorly through the interosseous membrane to the dorsolateral aspect of the foot

Arthrodesis of midtarsal and subtalar joints:
Persistent varus of heel: (Dwyer) osteotomy of calcaneus
Deformity midtarsal joints: (Evans) resection and arthrodesis of calcaneocuboid joint
Tibial torsion: (Sell) derotation osteotomy of tibia
Persistent/untreated: Wedge resection of midtarsal joint
Postoperative: A long leg cast applied for 2/52.
Check up. If deformity persists—is corrected and POP cast applied for 8–12/52.

## Flat Foot (Pes Planus)

| | |
|---|---|
| Definition | It is defined as flattening of the longitudinal arch of the foot |
| Etiology | Congenital: Flexible type caused by postural factors |
| | Traumatic: Pott's fracture, fracture calcaneus, sprain |
| | Spastic: Peroneal spasm |
| Pathogenesis | Talus distorted plantarward and medially, calcaneus in quines, forefoot dorsiflexed at midtarsal joints, navicular on dorsal aspect of talar head, convex sole, deep creases on dorsolateral aspect of foot, contracted capsules, ligaments and tendons on dorsum of foot. |
| Diagnosis | Deformity: Flattening of medial arch of foot |
| | Rocker bottom flatfoot: Convex sole as both talus and calcaneus in equines and forefoot dorsiflexed at midtarsal joints |
| | Local tenderness |
| | Movements of tarsal joints restricted and painful |
| Investigation | X-ray feet, spine, pelvis |
| Management | Conservative treatment: |

Difficult to correct as tends to recur by conservative measures, e.g. moulding feet into inversion by the parents regularly, wedging casts, braces or modified shoes (inner borders raised with a crooked and extended heel, teaching child to practice walking on the outer borders of the feet with the toes turned in.

Surgical treatment: To be preferred:

Surgery: Release of contracted soft structures, placing displaced tarsals in normal positions, stabilizing tarsals by ORIF with Kirschner wires, or transferring peroneus brevis tendon to the talar neck (Osmond-Clarke).

Recurrence of deformity: (Grice) arthrodesis (extra-articular) of subtalar joint.

Adults: Tripple arthrodesis (subtalar and midtarsal joints).

Postoperatve: Apply POP cast with foot dorsiflexed.

## CLEFT FOOT (LOBSTER FOOT)

| | |
|---|---|
| Definition | It is defined as an abnormal foot whereby a single cleft extends proximally into the foot, in certain cases even up to tarsus, with absence of one or more toes and corresponding metatarsals (partially or complete). |
| Etiology | Unknown. |
| Pathogenesis | Deformity variable in degree and type, 1st and 5th rays usually present. |
| Diagnosis | Deformity: A single cleft extending proximally into foot |

- Toes: One or more missing
- Metatarsals: Partially, complete absent

Movements of tarsal joints restricted and painful

| | |
|---|---|
| Investigation | X-ray foot |
| Management | Surgical treatment: |

Aims: To improve function and appearance.

Surgery: (Joplin's): To correct splaying of forefoot, to narrow the distal part of forefoot:

- 1st and 5th rays present: Tendons available for the job.
- Cleft extending proximally between metatarsals: Skin
- Excision of opposing surfaces within cleft, closure of cleft by suturing dorsal and plantar flaps.
- Metatarsal without corresponding toe: Resecting of metatarsal.

## Congenital Pseudarthrosis of Tibia

| | |
|---|---|
| Definition | It is defined as a specific type of nonunion that may be present or incipient (starting to happen or exist) |

Types: three types:

i. Pseudarthrosis present at birth

ii. Post fracture: Through bone cyst

iii. Post fracture: Through bowed bone

| | |
|---|---|
| Etiology | Unknown |
| | Neurofibromatosis (closely related) |
| Predisposing | Congenital cyst and congenital bowing of bone |
| Pathogenesis | Bone bowed, narrow and sclerosed, medullary canal absent partially or complete |
| Diagnosis | Deformity: Bowed bone |
| | Pain |
| | Local tenderness |
| | Movements: May be painful and restricted |
| Investigation | X-ray leg: Bowed tibia and fibula (often), narrow and sclerosed, medullary canal partially or completely absent, bone cyst, fractured bone |
| Management | Conservative treatment: |
| | Rest |
| | Analgesics, NSAIDs |

**Surgical treatment**

Cyst without fracture:
- Curettage and bone grafting (dual cortical grafts)
- Amputation.

Complications:
- Age of the patient
- Union: Delayed or nonunion
- Shortening of leg.

Amputation: Indications:
- Shortening: > 8–10 cm
- Bowing of tibia: Severe
- Foot: Deformed severely
- Refracture of tibia.

Postoperative: Apply long leg POP cast or a spica cast (small fatty child) for 2/52, reapply casts till the bone unites.

## Congenital Dislocation of Hip

| | |
|---|---|
| Definition | It is defined as an abnormal development, usually of the acetabulum, the proximal femur, and the soft structures of hip joint. The condition is often familial or hereditary. Usually occurs during first two years after birth (rarely before birth). Common amongst girls. |

Types: Three types as per severity:
- Femoral head in normal position within abnormal acetabulum
- Subluxation of femoral head, lies partially beneath the acetabular roof
- Head fully dislocated from the acetabulum.

| | |
|---|---|
| Etiology | Unknown. |
| Pathogenesis | Shallow or flat acetabulum (mal developed roof), the femoral head and neck anteverted, the acetabulum and femoral head's contact missing, impaired capsule and acetabular labrum, contracted joint muscles. |
| Diagnosis | At birth: Clinical signs of dysplasia may be absent (periodic examination required to detect for dysplasia). |

No clinical sign diagnostic, finding any sign suggests dysplasia:
- Buttocks/or thighs: Asymmetry of the skin creases on the inner aspects of the thighs
- Shortening of leg
- Movements: Restricted abduction
- Ortolani sign (clicking on entry and exit of head into the acetabulum): +ve
- Telescoping of flexed and adducted thigh on the pelvis.

Late childhood:

Gait: Waddling (bilateral) and lurching (unilateral)
- Shortening: Above greater trochanter (as revealed by Nelaton's line)
- Greater trochanter: Prominent

- Spine: Lordosis
- Perineum: Widened (bilateral)
- Femoral pulsation:
  - ve due to absent femoral head behind it at the level of inguinal (Poupart's) ligament
  - Movements: Restricted abduction due to adductor's shortening

Trendelenburg's sign: +ve (standing on defective hip

**Investigation**

X-ray pelvis (at birth and during infancy)—ill defined.

Observation: Any one of following suggests dysplasia

- Acetabular index, horizontal reference line of

Hilgenreiner, the vertile reference line of Perkins, the arcuate lines of Shenton, and Y coordinate of Ponseti.

(Normal reference: Femoral head's epiphysis lies inferior to horizontal reference line and medial to the vertical line and low acetabular index).

Arthrography: Diagnostic:

- Presence of mild dysplasia
- Joint: Subluxated or dislocated
- Reduction by manipulation possible
- Acetabular labrum: Condition and position
- Development of acetabulum and femoral head: Normal/or abnormal.
  X-ray Pelvis (late childhood)—well defined
- Displaced (upward) femoral head (distorted Shenton line)
- Upper femoral epiphysis: Smaller (underdeveloped), lies above the horizontal line and lateral to vertical line
- Femoral neck: Anteverted

**Management**

Earlier diagnosis and earlier treatment yields better results.

Infancy: Conservative treatment:

Abduction of thighs: By using a pillow or folded diaper, later on an abduction splint used for this purpose

Children (1–2 years old):

Skeletal traction: For 2/52, prior to manipulation (closed reduction):
Aims:

- To loosen, relax, or stretch the contracted soft tissues, to allow the femoral head to the level of acetabulum, for easy reduction of dislocation
- To lessen the trauma of forced reduction
- To avoid chances of later development of coxa vara in children and OA in adults.

Closed reduction under anesthesia, followed by POP dual hip spica with hips placed in 90 degree flexion, fully abducted and externally rotated ("frog leg" plaster) for 8/52. The cast changed and checked by X-rays at intervals of 8/52, to know status of acetabulum.

Physiotherapy: After the cast discarded.

### Late childhood

Closed reduction (skeletal):
* Reduction satisfactory: no further treatment required.

Open reduction:
* Reduction unsatisfactory: Arthrography:
  - Skeletal traction followed by open reduction:
  Aims: To achieve anatomic and functional restoration.

Procedures:
* Open reduction and debridement of the acetabulum
* Acetabuloplasty or osteotomy of innominate bone for dysplastic acetabulum.

Postoperative: Apply POP double hip spica, (with the hip slightly abducted, flexed, and internally rotated) for 12/52, followed by a splint (Ponseti).
* Rotational osteotomy: anteversion > 35 degree.
  Postoperative: Apply a spica cast for 8/52, followed by non weight bearing exercises in bed for 3–4/52, then allowed up (usually 8–12/52.
* Arthrodesis: Late unreduced cases (> 12 years).

## Congenital Coxa Vara

| | |
|---|---|
| Definition | It is defined as a progressive decrease in the angle between the femoral neck and shaft, consequently by a progressive shortening of the limb and by the presence of a defect in the medial part of neck. |
| Etiology | Unknown |
| Pathogenesis | Abnormal epiphyseal plate, irregular columnar arranged cells in the defective cartilage, atypical ossification, adjacent metaphyseal bone osteoporotic, its trabeculae atrophic, lots of connective tissue in irregularly arranged cartilage and bone, delayed ossification. |
| Diagnosis | Overweight<br>Shortening of limb |
| Investigation | X-ray pelvis focusing affected hip/hips: Slipping of femoral epiphysis |
| Management | Conservative treatment: of little/or no value. As the child becomes older and heavier, the deformity increases till the greater trochanter lies superior to the femoral head, may develop pseudarthrosis of femoral neck. |

## Osteogenesis Imperfecta

| | |
|---|---|
| Definition | It is defined as a familial disorder due to certain congenital defect in the evolution of the connective tissue cells. |

Types:
* Prenatal: Incompatible with survival
* Postnatal: Tendency to fracture even as late as 5 years of age
* Infantile: Child born alive, the fragile limbs break
Easily
* Childhood/adolescence: Tendency to fracture

| | |
|---|---|
| Etiology | Unknown. |
| Pathogenesis | Developed fibrous tissue or bone forming cells, blue osteosclerosis. |
| Diagnosis | Fracture: Bones tendency to fractures, less painful |
| | Deformity: Diminished stature |
| | Appearance: Elf-like (flattened skull, pointed ears) |
| Investigation | X-ray bones, skull |
| Management | Preventive care: Protecting from risk of injury |
| | Specific treatment: |
| | Treatment of fracture |
| | Treatment of deformities: Multiple osteotomies. |

## VERTEBRAL ANOMALIES

### Congenital Spina Bifida

| | |
|---|---|
| Definition | It is defined as failure of fusion of vertebral arches, usually with associated maldevelopment of the spinal cord and membranes. |
| Types | • Spina bifida occulta: Commonest type; due to failure of fusion of neural arches, without protrusion of spinal cord of membranes, usually affecting a single vertebra in the lumbosacral region. |
| | • Meningocele: Protrusion of meninges through defective spino-laminar segment |
| | • Meningomyelocele: Normally developed spinal cord or cauda equina, may lie adherent to the posterior aspect of the sac |
| | • Syringomyelocele: Rarest type, characterized by dilated central canal of the spinal cord, and the sac contains spinal cord along with nerves originating from it. |
| | • Myelocele: Characterized by an elliptical raw surface (ununited groove), CSF discharging from central canal at its upper end. |
| | Commonest type of spina bifida second to spina bifida occulta. |
| Etiology | Unknown. |
| Pathogenesis | • Spina bifida occulta: A fibrous band—membrane reunions, connecting skin to the spina theca, growth of body yields pulling of spinal theca and nerve roots by the membrane. |
| | • Meningocele: Contains CSF only |
| | • Meningomyelocele: Spinal cord or cauda equine adherent to sac |
| | • Syringomyelocele: Dilated central canal of spinal cord |
| | • Myelocele: Discharging CSF from spinal central canal. |
| Diagnosis | Deformity: Swelling over lumbosacral reion, talipes |
| | Skin: Depression in the skin, patch of hair, trophic ulcers |
| | Discharging sinus: CSF discharge |
| | Muscular weakness, paralysis of legs (advance case) |
| | Incontinence of urine and feces. |
| Investigation | Transillumination test: Cord and nerves seen as dark shadows; to distinguish meningocele from meningomyelocele. |
| | X-ray lumbosacral spine: Reveals bony deficiency. |

| Management | Surgical treatment of choice; to be provided ASAP, by a team of neurosurgeon (for spina bifida repair) and the orthopedic surgeon (for lower limb deformities correction) |
| | Preoperative: Mandatory neurological examination to detect any area of anesthesis. |

## Congenital Scoliosis

| Definition | It is defined as a congenital disorder, characterized by lateral curved spine, caused by anomalies of one or more vertebrae. |
| Etiology | • Anomalies of one or more vertebrae: Hemivertebrae, failure of segmentation of posterior elements |
| | • Contractures: Muscular or ligamentous |
| Pathogenesis | • Primary curve: A single, sharp, lateral curve |
| | • Secondary curves develop with growth |
| Diagnosis | • Cervical: Short, thick neck, restricted movements |
| | • Dorsal: Deformity |
| | • Lumbar: Accompanying kyphosis |
| | • Shortening. |
| Investigation | X-ray spine |
| | MRI |
| | CT Scan |
| Management | Conservative treatment: |
| | Maintenace of posture |
| | Leg lengthening: By applying lift to the shoe |
| | Milwaukee brace: To control and correct rapidly increasing scoliosis |
| | Surgical treatment: |
| | Excision of hemivertebra |

## Spondylolisthesis

| Definition | It is defined as an anomaly characterized by slipping forward of a lower lumbar vertebra, usually the fifth one, through the plane of the intervertebral disk below it, thereby carrying with it the whole of the upper part of the spine. |
| | Grades: Four: |
| | Grade I: Displacement < 25% of anteroposterior diameter of first sacral segment |
| | Grade II: 25–50% |
| | Grade III: 50–75% |
| | Grade IV: > 75%. |
| Etiology | Unknown. |
| | Hereditary |
| | Incidence: 5% |
| | Sex: Equal in men and women. |
| Pathogenesis | The essential lesion is separation of the body of the vertebra from the posterior articulation, lamina, and spinous process due to defective pedicles, that hold together these two parts of the vertebra. |

| Diagnosis | Age: Rarely seen in children < 5 years old, increases until the late teens |
| | Pain: Aching round the loin, radiating into legs |
| | Weakness of lower limbs |
| | Deformity: The trunk appears usually short, a transverse furrow seen encircling the trunk, between ribs and iliac crests, thereby reducing the space, prominent upper edge of the sacrum with a depression above it. |
| Investigation | X-ray: Ap and Lateral views: confirms diagnosis: shows a congenital defect in the pedicles development. |
| Management | Conservative treatment: |
| | Rest |
| | Local heat, shortwave diathermy, infrared heat |
| | Lumbosacral belt or corset |
| | Analgesics |
| | Surgical treatment: Usually not required |
| | Indications: Younger patient with acute condition |
| | Persistent low backache, radiating pain in the buttocks and thighs to incapacitate a person for work |
| | Preoperative: Inspection of 5th lumbar and 1st sacral nerve roots for any protruding intervertebral disks and fibrocartilaginous tissue. |
| | Surgery: Arthrodesis of unstable spine by posterior fusion |

Note: Excision of protruding intervertebral disks and fibrocartilaginous tissue prior to posterior fusion, for symptoms of pressure on nerve roots (5th lumbar and 1st sacral) to avoid persisting radiating pain after fusion.

Postoperative:
- Rest on firm bed for 8/52
- Brace fitting and patient allowed up.

## Congenital Torticollis (syn. Wryneck)

| Definition | It is defined as a congenital anomaly characterized by tilting of head towards the affected side and the chin pointing to the opposite side. The lesion usually appears within two weeks post birth, may involve the sternocleidomastoid muscle diffusely or localized near its clavicular attachment, attains its size within 6–8/52, aggravated by growth. |
| Etiology | Unknown |
| Pathogenesis | Tumor, a fibromatosis within sternomastoid muscle |
| | Microscopically: Muscle fibers replaced by a diffuse infiltration of fibroblasts, arranged in organoid pattern, thickened acellular mass of disorganized fascial tissue consisting of small areas with multiple cells |
| Diagnosis | History of obstructed labor |
| | Deformity: Head tilted towards the affected side and the chin pointing to the opposite side, elevated shoulder, head shorter (anteroposterior). |
| | Sternomastoid muscle: Swollen entirely or partially |
| Investigation | X-ray neck, head |
| | Miroscopic examination of sternomastoid tumor |

| Management | Transient torticollis (20%): No treatment required |
| | Surgical treatment: |
| | Surgery: |

- Sternocleidomastoid release at clavicle
- Sternocleidomastoid release at mastoid
- Sternocleidomastoid tumor excision
- Tenotomy.

Postoperative:

- Physiotherapy including manipulation (stretching) of neck t.i.d. x couple of months.
- POP casts or braces: usually not effective.

## Congenital Elevation of Scapula (Sprengel's Deformity)

| Definition | It is defined as an elevation of the scapula, whereby the scapula lies more superiorly than normally in relation to the thoracic cage, and usually hypoplastic and misshapen. Other congenital anomalies, e.g. cervical rib, malformed ribs, cervical vertebrae, are usually present. |
| Etiology | Unknown. |
| Pathogenesis | Hypoplastic and misshaped scapula. |
| Diagnosis | Deformity: Elevated small scapula with restricted abduction movement, and very small and highly elevated (severe form); the inferior angle internally rotated |
| | Head: Tilted to the affected side |
| | Disability: Mild or severe. |
| Investigation | X-ray cervical and thoracic spine—AP and LAT views |
| | CXR |
| Management | Surgical treatment of choice. |
| | Indications: |

- Deformity and disability mild: No treatment required
- Deformity and disability severe: Surgical treatment.

Surgery:

- Release of muscles
- Excision scapula (cosmetic factor)

Physiotherapy: Regularly for couple of months.

## Madelung's Deformity (Syn. Manus Valga)

| Definition | It is defined as a congenital anomaly of the wrist characterized by posterior and lateral bowing of the distal radius, short radius, dorsal subluxation of the distal ulna, and secondary carpal deformities, triangular carpus wedged proximally between the deformed radius and the elongated ulna. There may be atrophic radial head and hypertrophic capitulum with wider space between them. |
| Etiology | Unknown. |
| Pathogenesis | A localized form of dyschondroplasia, fused ulnar half of distal radial epiphysis. |

| Diagnosis | Sex: More common in girls than in boys |
| | Age: Not present at birth, but develops in adolescence |
| | Mild: Asymptomatic |
| | Severe: Painful, weak, instable wrist |
| | Deformity: Bowed radius, subluxated ulnar head |
| Investigation | X-ray wrist: Shows deformity |
| Management | Mild: No treatment required |
| | Severe: Correction of deformity by surgical treatment |

Surgery:

Children: Ulnar shortening

Adults: Resection of lower end of ulna.

Postoperative: POP long arm cast, with wrist fully extended to engage the distal radial fragment and forearm in neutral position/rotation, applied for 6/52.

## Congenital Contracture of the Little Finger

| Definition | It is defined as a congenital anomaly of the little finger; characterized by hyperextended MCP joint and flexed PIP joint of the little finger; usually bilateral and symptomless, without any skin lesion, occurs in young persons. |
| Etiology | Unknown. |
| Pathogenesis | Contracted little finger, hyperflexed MCP and flexed PIP joint' |
| Diagnosis | Deformity: Hyperextended metacarpophalangeal joint, and flexed proximal interphalangeal joint of little finger |
| | Skin: Normal |
| Investigation | X-ray hand—AP and lateral views |
| D/d | Dupuytren's contracture: Rarely seen in younger age; usually inflammatory in origin; involves usually the metacarpophalangeal joint (flexed—draws that finger into palm) of little or ring finger. |
| Management | Treatment seldom required. |
| | Surgical treatment: Correction of the deformity. |
| | Postoperative: Physiotherapy: Exercises. |

## Dupuytren's Contracture

| Definition | It is defined as an affection of the palmar fascia, characterized by the localized thickening of the palmar aponeurosis that involves the overlying skin of the palm, resulting in tendency to contract which draws the affected fingers into fixed flexion. Mostly starts near the base of the ring or little finger, thereafter draws that finger into the palm of the hand. |
| Etiology | Unknown |
| | Hereditary: Familial |
| | Traumatic: Occupational hazzard |
| Pathogenesis | Primary disorder of the collagen substance of the fibrous tissue: lesion starts as a fibroblastic nodule in the subcutaneous palmar fascia, undergoes changes: proliferative, involutional, residual stage. |

| | |
|---|---|
| Diagnosis | Deformity: |
| | Age: Middle age |
| | Sex: in men > in women |
| | Deformity: Flexed proximal and middle phalanx, unaffected terminal phalanx. |
| | • In advanced case: Permanent changes in the affected joints render futile any attempts to straighten the fingers. |
| | Skin: Adherent skin of palm puckered |
| Investigation | X-ray hand: AP and Lateral views. |
| Management | Conservative treatment: |
| | Early case: Night splintage and active exercises: gentle stretching of fingers by the patient. |
| | Radiotherapy (RT): limited role in early phase. |
| | Surgical treatment: |
| | Aims: |
| | Surgery: Fasciotomy: |
| | Subcutaneous: Elderly, arthritic, or poor health |
| | Partial: Small affected area, immature nodule, early contracture produced by a fascial cord |
| | Complete: Younger patient with disabling contracture |
| | Postoperative: Immobilization by a splint for 1/52, followed by active exercises. |

## Hereditary Multiple Exostosis (Syn. Diaphyseal Aclasis)

| | |
|---|---|
| Definition | It is defined as a common hereditary anomaly characterized by the outgrowth of cancellous osteomata near the ends of long bones, occasionally all the long bones may be affected, with multiple growths. |
| Etiology | Unknown. |
| | Failure of tubulation |
| Pathogenesis | Distorted growth, outgrowth pedunculated with a cartilage cap on the tip from where it grows with an overlapping bursa, failed tubulation of growing bone (failure of periosteum to remodel external surface of new bone produced by epiphyseal growth. |
| Diagnosis | Deformities: Multiple growths near ends of long bones |
| | Pain: Due to pressure exerted by outgrowths |
| | Pressure symptoms: Numbness or pain (nerves) |
| | Muscular wasting |
| | Movements: Restricted and painful |
| Investigation | X-ray of long bones: Show multiple exostoses, deformities, blunt and widened metaphyses. |
| Management | Conservative treatment: |
| | • Analgesics |
| | Surgical treatment: Excision. |
| | Indications: |
| | • Pressure symptoms on surrounding structures—severe enough to justify surgery. |

- Childhood: unusual spurt of growth
- Adulthood: reactivation of growth

## Ollier's Disease (Syn. Enchondromatosis)

| | |
|---|---|
| Definition | It is defined as a chondrodysplasia characterized by the growing epiphysis leaving behind masses of cartilage in the center of the shaft of the bone. It is a developmental and not an hereditary disorder. |
| Etiology | Unknown.<br>Failure of tubulation |
| Pathogenesis | Impaired epiphyseal growth, broadened metaphyses, weakened and bowed long bones, malignant features in > half cases. |
| Diagnosis | Deformities: Dwarfed and bowed bones<br>Bones: Long bones (femur and tibia at the knee; humerus upper end, and lower end of radius), occasionally phalanges of hands and feet)<br>Pain: Due to pressure exerted by growths<br>Pressure symptoms: Numbness or pain (nerves)<br>Muscular wasting<br>Movements: Restricted and painful |
| Investigation | X-ray of long bones: Show cystic lesions in widened metaphyses. |
| D/d | Multiple exostoses: While Ollier's disease is endosteal and cartilaginous, the multiple exostoses is periosteal and cancellous bone. |
| Management | Aim: To prevent and correct deformities and to detect malignancy.<br>Conservative treatment: |

- Analgesics

Surgical treatment:
- Osteotomy: To correct deformity/s
- Amputation: For grossly deformed fingers.

## Bibliography

1. Barr JS. Spondylolisthesis (editorial). J. Bone and Joint Surg. 37-A:878, 1955.
2. Blount WP, et al. The Milwaukee brace in the operative treatment of scoliosis, J. Bone and Joint Surg. 40-A:511, 1958.
3. Blount WP. Congenital scoliosis: In Societe Internationale de Chirurgie Orthopedique etde Traumatologie, Huitieme Congres, New York, 1960, Brussels, 1961, Imprimerie des Scinces, p. 748.
4. Burrows HJ. An operation for the correction of Madelung's deformity and similar conditions, Proc. Roy. Soc. Med. 30:31, 1937.
5. Charnley J. Deformities: 333, 13th Ed. Bailey and Love's Short Practice of Surgery. Love M, Rains A.J. H., Capper W.M.; H.K. Lewis and Co., London, 1965.
6. Coventry MB, Harris L. Congenital muscular torticollis in infancy. Some observations regarding treatment, J. Bone and joint Surg. 41-A;815, 1959
7. Farmer AW. Congenital hallux varus, Am. J. Surg. 95:274, 1958.
8. Gill GG, Manning JG, White HL. Surgical treatment of spondylolisthesis without spine fusion, J. Bone and Joint Surg. 37-A: 493, 1955.
9. Goldner J Leonard. Surgical correction of foot deformities in children, spectator letter, 1959.
10. Green WT. The surgical correction of congenital elevation of the scapula (Sprengel's deformity), Proceedings of the American Orthopaedic Association, June 24–27, 1957, J. Bone and Joint Surg. 39-A:1439, 1957.

11. Gunn DR, Molesworth BD. The use of tibialis posterior as a dorsiflexor, J. Bone and Joint Surg. 39-B:674, 1957

12. Kandel B. Treatment of congenital clubfoot, Bull. Hosp. Joint Dis. 19:20, 1958.

13. Kapoor PS. Deformities, 2nd Ed. Accident and Emergency. Etiology, diagnosis, and management, CBS, New Delhi, 2016.

14. Massie WK, Howorth MB. Congenital dislocationof the hip. Part III. Pathogenesis, J. Bone and Joint Surg. 33-A:190,1951.

15. McCauley JC, Jr. Surgical treatment of club foot, S. Clin. North America 31:561, 1951.

16. McFarland B. Congenital deformities of the spine and limbs. In Platt, Sir Harry, editor: Modern Trends in Orthopedics, New York, 1950, Paul B. Holder, Inc.

17. McRae R. Fracture deformity: 10, 1st Ed.: Practical Fracture Treatment. Churchill Livingstone, 1984.

18. Scott JC. Volkmann's contracture, tibial fractures: 201:3. Modern Trends in Orthopedics Fracture Treatment. Clark JMP; Butterworths, London, 1962.

19. Somerville EW. Open reduction in congenital dislocation of the hip, J. Bone and Joint Surg. 35-B:363, 1953.

20. Trevor D. Treatment of congenital hip dysplasia in older children. President's address, Proc. Roy. Soc. Med. 53:481, 1960.

21. Wilkinson J, Carter C. Congenital dislocation of the hip. The results of conservative treatment, J. Bone and Joint Surg. 42-B:669, 1960.

## POSTURAL DEFORMITIES OF BONES AND JOINTS

- Pes planus (syn. Flat Foot)
- Hallux valgus (syn. Bunion)
- Hallux varus
- Hallux rigidus
- Bunionette (syn. Tailor's Bunion)
- Clavus durum (Hard Corn)
- Clavus mollum (syn. Soft Corn)
- Morton's toe (syn. Metatarsalgia)
- Hammer toe
- Kohler's disease (syn. Freiberg's Disease)
- Plantar callosities
- Ingrown toenail
- Calcaneal spur
- Scoliosis:
  - Idiopathic scoliosis

### Pes Planus (Syn. Flat Foot)

Definition   It is defined as deformity of the foot characterized by depressed longitudinal arch, clinically classified by whether the arch being relatively too flexible or too rigid, and whether the peroneal muscles spastic or normal.

Types: Four principal types:
i. Flexible with normal peroneals
ii. Rigid with normal peroneals
iii. Rigid with spastic peroneals

iv. Rocker bottom (vertical): Position of talus distorted obliquely downward (congenital deformity).

| | |
|---|---|
| Etiology | Congenital |
| | Traumatic: Fractures of the os calcis, malunited Pott's fracture |
| | Inflammatory: Strain foot—common in waitresses, policemen, watchmen |
| | Spastic: Peroneal spasm |
| Pathogenesis | Flexible: Longitudinal arch disappears only on weight bearing, joints of foot hypermobile, short tendocalcaneus rigid with normal peronei: fibrous or bony ankylosis rigid with spastic peronei: ankylosis (fibrous, osseous, or cartilaginous) |
| Diagnosis | Deformity: Longitudinal arch: depressed |
| | Pain: Disabling |
| | Local tenderness |
| | Movements of tarsal joints: Painful and restricted |
| Investigation | X-ray feet: AP and Latera and oblique views to rule out an accessory navicular |
| Management | Conservative treatment: |
| | Children: Manipulation of feet under anesthesia followed by walking POP cast for 24/52, may be relapse in certain cases. |
| | Adults: Treatment more difficult because of obscure pathology. |
| | Surgical treatment of choice. |
| | Preoperative: Criteria of surgery: |

- Amount of disability
- Functional basis
- Occupation of the patient

Indications:

- Tripple arthrodesis: Flexible pes planus so severe that heel in valgus position and sagged talonavicular joint
- Kidner, Miller, Young, or Hoke procedures: Flexible pes planus whereby the tarsal bones distorted and undergo few adaptive changes in the soft tissues.
- Lowman or Young: Sagging at talonavicular joint
  Procedures: Lengthening of tendocalcaneus may be indicated (with caution) with anyone of following procedures:
  - Excision of accessory navicular bone and transplanting posterior tibial tendon to the inferior surface of the navicular, with or without lengthening of tendocalcaneous (Kidner)
- Transferring insertion of the anterior tibial tendon with (Lowman) or without (Young) arthrodesis of the talonavicular joint
- Transferring distal attachment of calcaneonavicular ligament and the insertion of the posterior tibial tendon with arthrodesis of the joints between navicular and first cuneiform and between first cuneiform and first metatarsal with or without lengthening of tendocalcaneous (Miller)
- Arthrodesis of joints between navicular and 1st, and 2nd cuneiform joints (Hoke)

- Arthrodesis of talonavicular and subtalar joints (Harris and Beath)
- Tripple arthrodesis of the midtarsal and subtalar joints with or without lengthening of tendocalcaneous.

Postoperative:
- Check X-ray
- POP cast with the foot in equines and the heel in varus position, the cast extended with the ankle in dorsiflexion. Removal of cast and sutures after 2/52, then a plaster boot (walking) applied for 4/52, followed by modified shoes (fitted with arch supports) to be worn.

## Hallux Valgus (Syn. Bunion)

| | |
|---|---|
| Definition | It is defined as a deformity of the foot characterized by valgus of the phalanges of the greater toe with angulated metatarsophalangeal joint, medially prominent first metatarsal head so called Bunion, and varus of first metatarsal. |
| Etiology | Traumatic<br>Inflammatory |
| Pathogenesis | Adherent capsule of the first metatarsophalangeal joint, subchondral cystic lesions in the metatarsal head |
| Diagnosis | Deformity: Abducted big toe, associated hammer toe (2nd toe)<br>Pain; agonizing<br>Swelling (Bunion) over first matatarsophalangeal joint<br>Local tenderness |
| Investigation | X-ray: Shows osteophytic outgrowths, malalignment of the bones |
| Management | Conservative treatment: Unsatisfactory.<br>Shoes: Low heels, wide fronts, straight inner borders<br>Surgical treatment of choice<br>Indication: Marked discomfort and gross deformity. |

Surgery:

Keller operation: Excision of the base of the proximal phalanx, augmented by an osteotomy of the base of the first metatarsal and closure of the enlarged gap between and the second metatarsal (Stamm). The corrected position held by inserting excised bone to hold the osteotomy open on the medial aspect.

Postoperative: After 2/52 the Kirschner wire or the cast, looped wire, and rubber bands and sutures removed.

Partial walking allowed, increased gradually, in a modified shoe (fitted with arch support) for 6/12.

McBride operation: Indicated in middle age and in younger patients (modified)

Aim: Deals primarily with the soft tissues correction, when the deformity is moderate.

Procedure: Freeing adductor hallucis tendon from the proximal phalanx, and attached it the first metatarsal.

Postoperative: After 2/52 allowed walk with partial weight bearing on the heel, followed by wearing modified shoe

Lapidus operation: Correction of the varus of the first metatarsal and resection of the bone/or revision of soft structures or both.

Aim: To narrow the wide angle at the bases of the first and second metatarsals, and to remove any exostotic bone from the head of the first metatarsal

Procedure: Correction of the varus of the first metatarsal at the first metatarsocuneiform joint, and correction of deformity of first metatarsophalangeal joint by revision of the soft tissues.

Postoperative: A wide steel corset stay used for holding the great toe in 10 degree of varus and externally rotated, for 4/52, then wide shoes fitted for 6/52.

Duncan McKeever operation: Arthrodesis of the first metatarsophalangeal joint.

Procedure: Correction of the deformity of first metatarsophalangeal joint, and decreasing the varus of the first metatarsal.

Postoperative: Permitted weight bearing in a shoe after 1/52.

## Hallux Varus

| | |
|---|---|
| Definition | It is defined as a deformity of the foot characterized by medial angulation of the greater toe at the level of metatarsophalangeal joint, usually associated with an equinovarus deformity of the foot, infrequent, and difficult to correct. |
| Etiology | Congenital |
| | Traumatic |
| | Infective |
| | Muscular imbalance: Weak adductors vs abductors |
| | Postoperative: Operative hallux valgus |
| Pathogenesis | Muscular imbalance |
| Diagnosis | Deformity: Medial angulation of the greater toe at level of metatarsophalangeal joint |
| | Pain |
| | Local tenderness (traumatic, infective) |
| | Movements of metatarsophalangeal joint of greater toe painful (traumatic, infective) |
| Investigation | X-ray foot |
| D/d | Metatarsus primus varus: Angle between bases of first and second metatarsal greater than normal, with the normal metatarsophalangeal joint. |
| Management | Surgical treatment of choice. |
| | Deformity: Soft tissue correction and tendon transplantation |
| | Recurrence of deformity: Arthrodesis of the first metatarsophalangeal joint, and a syndactylism created. |
| | Postoperative: Spica cast applied to the foot for 2/52 |
| | After 2/52 the Kirschner wire, the cast, and sutures removed. |
| | Partial walking allowed, increased gradually, in a modified shoe (fitted with arch support) for 6/12. |

## Hallux Rigidus

| | |
|---|---|
| Definition | It is defined as a postural anomaly of greater toe characterized by painful, restricted dorsiflexion with ankylosed plantar flexion. |

Types: Two distinct types:

- Adolescent type: As a result of traumatic synovitis of the first metatarsophalangeal joint, associated wityh muscular spasm
- Adult type: Non-articular osteoarthritis, precipitated by trauma. The restricted movement, on account of interlocked osteophytes and flattened metatarsal head.

| | |
|---|---|
| Etiology | Traumatic: Synovitis, muscular spasm |
| | Degenerative: Non-articular osteoarthritis |
| Pathogenesis | Degenerative changes, osteophytes |
| Diagnosis | Pain |
| | Disability |
| | Movements: Plantar flexion and dorsiflexion—painful and restricted |
| Investigation | X-ray foot |
| Management | Surgical treatment of choice. |

Keller operation: The painful rigid toe replaced by a pseudarthrosis at the metatarsophalangeal joint.

Procedure: Resection of the proximal half of the proximal phalanx, and resection of any osteophytes

Postoperative: Spica cast applied to the foot for 2/52

After 2/52 the Kirschner wire, the cast, and sutures removed.

Partial walking allowed, increased gradually, in a modified shoe (fitted with arch support) for 6/12.

Arthrodesis: An alternative procedure.

## Bunionette (Syn. Tailor's Bunion)

| | |
|---|---|
| Definition | It is defined as a deformity of the foot characterized by varus angulation of fifth toe at metatarsophalangeal joint, usually associated with hallux valgus in the same foot—relaxed or splayed. |
| Etiology | Inflammatory |
| Pathogenesis | An adventitious bursa on the outer aspect of fifth metatarsal head and hard corn on the dorsolateral aspect of the proximal interphalangeal joint of fifth toe. |
| Diagnosis | Pain |
| | Deformity: Varus angulation of fifth toe MTP joint |
| | Local tenderness |
| | Movements: Painful and restricted |
| Investigation | CBC, ESR |
| | X-ray foot |
| Management | Conservative treatment: |
| | Rest, fomentation |
| | Analgesics, NSAIDs |
| | Surgical treatment of choice. |

Procedures:
- Resection of the lateral third of the fifth metatarsal head
- Resection of the entire head of the fifth metatarsal.

Indication: Recurrence (relaxed and splayed)

Postoperative: Weight bearing resumed after 2/52,

Wide shoes with low heels to be worn for couple of months.

## Clavus Durum (Hard Corn)

| | |
|---|---|
| Definition | It is defined as a deformity of the foot characterized by thickening of the soft tissue (hard corn) usually on the dorsolateral aspect of the fifth toe |
| Etiology | Traumatic: Pressure of the shoe on the prominent outer part of head of proximal phalanx |
| Pathogenesis | Local cornification of skin |
| Diagnosis | Pain |
| | Local tenderness |
| | Deformity: Flexion-adduction of the toe |
| Investigation | X-ray foot |
| Management | Conservative treatment: |
| | Analgesics: Paracetamol, NSAIDs |
| | Surgical treatment of choice. |

Procedures:
- Excision of the proximal interphalangeal joint
- Excision of the entire proximal phalanx (may cause flail toe)
- Shortening of the fifth toe and removal of osseous

Prominence.

## Clavus Mollum (Syn. Soft Corn)

| | |
|---|---|
| Definition | It is defined as a deformity of the foot characterized by painful and often disabling soft swellings, developed frequently between the toes, and on the lateral aspect of the base of the fourth toe between fourth and fifth toes, usually macerated by the moisture. |
| Etiology | Traumatic: By pressure of the base of the proximal phalanx of the fourth toe against the fifth toe. |
| Pathogenesis | Macerated soft corn |
| Diagnosis | Pain |
| | Disability |
| Investigation | CBC, ESR, blood sugar |
| Management | Conservative treatment: |

- Toilet of the lesion with liquid betadine (Piodine), dusting powder application
- Analgesics: Paracetamol, NSAIDs
- Antibiotics: For infective lesions.

Surgical treatment:

Surgery: Excision of lateral half of the base of the proximal phalanx of the fourth toe

Complications: Subluxation or dislocation.

Postoperative:
- Pressure sterile dressing of the forefoot
- Walking permitted after 1/52.

## Morton's Toe (Syn. Metatarsalgia)

| | |
|---|---|
| Definition | It is defined as a deformity of the foot characterized by the development of a neuroma, usually of the most lateral branch of the medial plantar nerve, between the third and fourth, or less frequently between any two of the metatarsal heads. |
| Etiology | Traumatic: Neuroma pressing on the lateral most branch of the medial plantar nerve |
| Pathogenesis | Neuroma |
| Diagnosis | Pain: Excruciating while walking |
| | Disability |
| | Movements of toes painfull and restricted |
| Investigation | X-ray foot |
| Management | Conservative treatment: |
| | Analgesics: Paracetamol, NSAIDs |
| | To avoid narrow toe shoes |
| | Surgical treatment of choice |
| | Surgery: Excision of the neuroma. |
| | Postoperative: Weight bearing after 1/52. |

## Hammertoe

| | |
|---|---|
| Definition | It is defined as a deformity of the foot characterized by hyperextension of the metatarsophalangeal joint, flexed proximal interphalangeal joint, flexed or extended distal interphalangeal joint, depressed and prominent metatarsal head, callosities formed over the bony prominences |
| Etiology | Congenital |
| | Traumatic: Wearing of tight fitted shoes |
| Pathogenesis | Corn or adventitious bursa on the dorsum of first |
| | Interphalangeal joint, contracted fascia and ligaments |
| Diagnosis | Pain |
| | Disability |
| | Deformity: Hyperextended metatarsophalangeal, hyperflexed first interphalangeal, and hyperextended terminal joint. |
| | Movements: Walking painful and restricted. |
| Investigation | X-ray foot |
| Management | Conservative treatment: |
| | Wearing of wide shoes |
| | Analgesics, NSAIDs |
| | Surgical treatment: |
| | Surgery: Resection of the proximal interphalangeal joint (Sir Robert Jones). |
| | Postoperative: Weight bearing after 1/52. |

## Kohler's Disease (Syn. Freiberg's Disease)

| | |
|---|---|
| Definition | It is defined as a deformity of the foot characterized by degenerative changes occurring in the head of the second or third metatarsal. |
| Etiology | Unknown |
| Pathogenesis | Degenerative changes in the metatarsal head |
| Diagnosis | Pain: Excruciating while walking |
| | Disability |
| | Swelling |
| | Local tenderness |
| | Movements of toes painfull and restricted |
| Investigation | X-ray foot; shows flattening of the articular surface and irregular sclerosis of the metatarsal head, loose bodies within the joint |
| Management | Conservative treatment: |
| | Analgesics: Paracetamol, NSAIDs |
| | To avoid narrow toe shoes |
| | Surgical treatment of choice |
| | Surgery: |

- Excision of metatarsal head
- Remodeling the head and excising the proximal half of the proximal phalanx.

Postoperative: Weight bearing after 1/52.

## Plantar Callosities and Metatarsalgia

| | |
|---|---|
| Definition | It is defined as a deformity of the foot characterized by presence of hypertrophic callosities, mostly under the heads of the 2nd and 3rd metatarsals. |
| Etiology | • Disturbed functioning of the toes, secondary either to deformed toes, such as claw toes or hammertoes |
| | • Static disorder of the metatarsal bones |
| Pathogenesis | Hypertrophic callosities, cone shaped extensions like plantar warts |
| Diagnosis | Pain |
| | Local tenderness |
| | Deformity: Deformed toes (hammertoes, claw toes) |
| | Disability: In walking |
| | Skin: Hard, rough |
| Investigation | X-ray foot: AP and Lateral views |
| Management | Conservative treatment: |
| | Analgesics, NSAIDs |
| | Anti-inflammatory ointment |
| | Shoes: Properly fitted substantial shoes, with metatarsal bars or leather-cork arch supports with metatarsal pads |
| | Surgical treatment: |
| | Indications: Conservative treatment failure and severe pain |

Surgery: Procedures:
- Trimming of the callosities
- Resecting metatarsal head
- Shortening of metatarsal (McKeever)
- Modified shortening of metatarsal (Giannestras)

Postoperative: POP walking cast for 4/52

Complications: Ulceration of plantar callosity

Management: Excision of entire ray (Dickson).

## Ingrown Toenail

**Definition**

The word ingrown toenail is misnomer. It is defined as a deformity of the foot characterized by overgrowth of the soft tissues that obliterate medial or lateral groove for the nail.

**Etiology**
- Improper trimming (pairing) of the nail
- Overcrowding of the toes in the shoes (narrow pointed).

**Pathogenesis**

Improperly trimmed nail grows, its corner penetrating the tissue—inflamed, infective (suppurated).

**Diagnosis**

Pain: Mostly severe

Local tenderness

Movements of greater toe painful and restricted

Deformity: Imbedded nail, swollen toe, obliterated medial or lateral grove for the nail.

**Investigation**

CBC, ESR, blood sugar

X-ray foot focusing greater toe

**Management**

Conservative treatment:

Rest

Fomentation: Wet packs

Analgesics, NSAIDs

Antibiotics

Trimming of protruding nail's edge

Surgical treatment:
- Excision of the nail (partly): (Heifetz)
- Excision of the whole nail (Zadic)
- Excision of the inflammed/septic soft tissue (Vandenbos and Bowers)
- Excision of entire nail bed and tuft of distal phalanx (Thompson and Terwillinger)

Postoperative: ASD, elastic crepe bandage, foot elevation.

## Calcaneal Spur

**Definition**

It is defined as a deformity of the foot characterized by a transverse ridge or bar of bone at the anterior plantar edge of the calcaneal tuberosity, mostly its sharpe free edge pointing towards the toes. It develops at the attachment of the plantar fascia, extending into the fascia itself.

| | |
|---|---|
| Types | • Large but painless |
| | • Large and painful |
| | • Rudimentary |
| Etiology | Unknown |
| Pathogenesis | Plantar fasciitis developing into spur |
| Diagnosis | Pain |
| | Swelling |
| | Deformity: |
| | Disability: Painful walking |
| Investigation | X-ray foot: Ap and Lateral views: seen as a transverse ridge or bar of bone at the anterior plantar edge of the tuberosity of the calcaneus |
| Management | Conservative treatment: |
| | Painless: No treatment required |
| | Painful: |

• Hot wet packs, infrared therapy, short-wave therapy
• Analgesics, NSAIDs, corticosteroids PO
• Shoe: Sponge in the heel

Surgical treatment:

Indication: Pain disabling and persistent despite conservative measures

Surgery: Excision of the spur

Postoperative: Weight bearing after 2/52, using a sponge in the heel of the shoe.

## Scoliosis

**Definition**    It is defined as a deformity of the spine (lateral curve/s), characterized by deviation of several or all vertebrae from their normal positions in the midline of the body. The deformity is considered pathological, whereby the patient himself/herself either cannot correct it, or can but unable to maintain it corrected, and the involved vertebrae rotated abnormally.

Curves: Primary and secondary: criteria:
• Vertebrae in primary curve mostly displaced from midline to the side of convexity of the primary curve, whereas in secondary curve they are mostly displaced to the side of the concavity of the secondary curve
• In case of three curves, the middle one is mostly primary
• In case of four curves, two middle ones are mostly primary
• In case of greater curve, or one towards which trunk shifted is the primary curve
• In case of the curve that is least flexible and least correctible is primary curve—confirmed by Schmidt's lateral bending test.

**Etiology**    Primary (Idiopathic): (80%): cause unknown
Secondary: (20%): cause known:
• Congenital anomalies of the spine
• Traumatic

- Inflammatory: poliomyelitis
- Infective: empyema
- Neurofibromatosis
- Muscular dystrophy
- Friedreich's ataxia
- Cereabral palsy.

## Idiopathic Scoliosis

**Pathogenesis**

Primary curves: Deform and develop structural changes (wedging, angulation, rotation) simultaneously and do not tend to correct themselves spontaneously

Secondary curves: Develop structural changes (wedging, angulation, rotation) more slowly, tend to retain much longer the ability to correct themselves spontaneously.

**Diagnosis**

History: In idiopathic scoliosis majority of characteristic features of primary curve/s present at onset of deformity and rarely change GPE

Neurological signs:

Deformity:
- In high dorsal curves: Elevated shoulder, prominent scapula, projected ribs (razorback)
- In lumbar scoliosis: Less deformity

Height (standing and sitting): Increased or decreased

**Investigation**

X-ray spine AP view: To show severity of structural change in each curve (to show how much primary and secondary curves can be passively corrected prior to spinal arthrodesis).

Lateral view: To rule out anomalies: epiphysitis, infective.

### Measurement of curves

Cobb's method: Steps:
- Locate the top vertebra of the curve, its superior surface tilts towards side of concavity of curve to be measured, the intervertebral space above this top vertebra is mostly wider on concave side of curve, while one below it narrower on this side. These may findings be variable in case of the vertebral wedging.
- Locate the bottom vertebra of the curve, its inferior surface tilts towards side of concavity of curve to be measured, the intervertebral space below this bottom vertebra is mostly wider on concave side of curve, while one above it narrower on this side. These findings may be variable in case of the vertebral wedging.
- Draw intersecting perpendiculars from superior surface of top vertebra and inferior surface of bottom vertebra.

Angle of curve: Angle of deviation of these perpendiculars from a straight line.

Ferguson method: Steps:
- Locate the top and bottom vertebrae as per Cobb's method

Draw lines from centre of body of top and bottom vertebrae to the center of body of vertebra at the apex of curve.

Angle of curve: Angle of deviation of these two lines from a straight line.

Management    Conservative treatment:
- Symptomatic
- Brace: Milwaukee brace in growing children
- Turnbuckle cast
- Localizer cast

**Surgical treatment**
Idiopathic scoliosis:
Aims:
- To correct the deformity
- To maintain the correction.

Indications:
Growing child: Increasing curve
Adolescent: Severe deformity with asymmetry of trunk
Older patients: Pain uncontrollable by conservative measures

Surgery:
Correction of curves:
Aim: To restore the symmetry of the trunk by centering the first dorsal vertebra above the sacrum
Preoperative: Turnbuckle cast application (Risser)
Surgery: Arthrodesis of spine

Methods:
- Hibbs technique for extra-articular fusion
- Goldstein technique for extra-articular fusion
- Moe technique for intra-articular fusion
- Risser technique for intra-articular fusion
- Harrington technique (instrumentation and fusion)

Postoperative: The cast changed at intervals of 2–3 months until the fusion is mature.

**Complications**
Occurring during correction of curves:
- Pressure sores over bony prominences: Due to improper padded cast
  Treatment: Proper padding prior to cast application
- Burning pain: Due to pressure on the skin
  Treatment: Release the pressure
- Brachial palsy: Due to traction on the cervical nerve roots or pressure by improper padded cast.

Treatment: Avoided by bending patient's head toward concavity of primary curve prior to applying cast.

Occuring during spinal fusion:
Shock: Avoided by blood transfusion coverage during operation and gentle manipulation of spine
Hyperpyrexia: Avoided by proper sterile technique

Respiratory distress: Avoided by using endotrachial anesthesia

Occuring postoperatively:

Pneumonia: Due to patient's low vital capacity

Wound infection: Antibiotic coverage, incision and drainage of pus

Recurrence of scoliosis: Due to faulty surgical technique, inadequate bone graft, inadequate immobilization.

### Paralytic scoliosis

Aims of surgery:

Correction of curves

Prevention of recurrence

Stabilization of weakened trunk

Indications: For fusion and determination of fusion area are different from those in idiopathic scoliosis.

Surgery:

Preoperative: Milwaukee brace, Risser localizer cast

Harrington instrumentation

Fusion of spine from D-1 to L-3 or L-4 in 2–3 stages (Blount): For paralytic scoliosis associated with extensive weak trunk and respiratory distress.

### Neurofibromatosis scoliosis:

Types:

- Long gentle curve: Due to involvement of soft tissues outside the spine

Treatment: Conservative measures: exercises

Sharp localized curve: Due to a neurofibromatosis

Treatment: Fusion of spine.

## Bibliography

1. Baker LD, Kuhn HH. Morton's metatarsalgia, South. M.J. 37:123, 1944.
2. Biickel WH, Dockerty MB. Plantar neuromas, Mortan's toe, Surg., Gynec., and Obst. 84:111, 1947.
3. Blount WP, Schmidt AC, et el. The Milwaulkee brace in the operative treatment of scoliosis, J. Bone and Joint Surg. 40-A:511, 1958.
4. Charnley J. Deformities: 333, 13th Ed. Bailey and Love's Short Practice of Surgery. Love M, Rains A.J. H., Capper W.M.; H.K. Lewis and Co., London, 1965
5. Cobb JR. Spine arthrodesis in the treatment of scoliosis, Bull. Hosp. Joint Dis. 19:187, 1958.
6. Cobb JR. Technique, after-treatment, and results of spine fusion for scoliosis, American Academy of Orthopedic Surgeons. Instructional Course Lectures, Vol. IX, Ann Arbor, 1952, J. W. Edwards, p. 261.
7. Cobb JR. The treatment of scoliosis, M.J. 7:467, Connecticut, 1943.
8. Ferguson AB. The study and treatment of scoliosis, South. M.J. 23:116, 1930.
9. Harrington Paul R. Treatment of scoliosis. Correction and internal fixation by spine instrumentation, J. Bone and Joint Surg. 44-A:591, 1962.
10. Harris RI. Rigidvalgus foot due to talocalcaneal bridge, J. Bone and Joint Surg.
11. Heifetz CJ. Operative management of ingrown toenail, J. Missouri M.A. 42:213, 1945.
12. Jordan HH, Brodsky AE. Keller operation for hallux valgus and hallux rigidus, an end result study, A,M.A. Arch. Surg. 62:586, 1951.
13. Kapoor PS. Fracture deformity: 404, 2nd Ed. Accident and Emergency: Etiology, Diagnosis and Management, CBS, New Delhi, 2016.

14. Kleinberg S. Scoliosis: Pathology, etiology, and treatment. Williams and Wilkins Co., Baltimore, 1951

15. McBride ED. Hallux valgus, bunion deformity: its treatment in mild, moderate, and severe stages, J. Internat. Coll. Surgeons 21:99, 1954.

16. McRae R. Fracture deformity: 10, 1st Ed.: Practical Fracture Treatment. Churchill Livingstone, 1984.

17. Mercer W. Orthopedic surgery, Ed. 4. Williams and Wilkins Co., Baltimore, 1950.

18. Risser JC. Modern trends in scoliosis, Bull. Hosp. Joint Dis. 19:166, 1958.

19. Risser JC. Plaster bodt-jacket, Am. J. Orthop. 3:19, 1961.

20. Scott JC. Volkmann's contracture, supracondylar fractures of the elbow: 201:3. Modern Trends in Orthopedics Fracture Treatment. Clark J.M.P.; Butterworths, London, 1962.

21. Scott JC. Volkmann's contracture, tibial fractures: 201:3. Modern Trends in Orthopedics Fracture Treatment. Clark J.M.P.; Butterworths, London, 1962.

22. Simmonds FA, Menelaus MB. Hallux valgus in adolescents, J. Bone and Joint Surg. 42-B: 761, 1960.

23. Smith NR. Hallux valgus and rigidus treated byarthrodesis of the metatarsophalangeal joint, Brit. M.J. 2:1385, 1952.

24. Vandenbos Kermit Q, Bowers Warner F. Ingrown toenail: a result of weight bearing on soft tissue, U.S. Armed Forces M.J. 10:1168, 1959.

25. Zadic FR. Obliteration of the nail bed of the great toe without shortening the terminal phalanx, J. Bone and Joint Surg. 32-B:66, 1950.

# 14

# Affections of Muscles, Tendons, and Tendon Sheaths

Traumatic:
- Contusion
- Rupture muscles and tendons:
  - Shoulder cuff injuries:
  - Ruptured supraspinatous tendon
- Biceps muscle, tendons injuries:
  - Ruptured muscle
  - Tendon (long head)
  - Tendon (distal end)
- Ruptured ulnar collateral ligament
- Ruptured extensor tendon (Mallet finger)
- Ruptured flexor tendons (Trigger finger)
- Ruptured tendocalcaneus/achilles
- Ruptured patellar tendon
- Ruptured quadriceps femoris tendon

Inflammatory:
- Tennis elbow (lateral epicondylitis)

Vascular:
- Volkmann's ischemic contracture:
  - Upper limb
  - Lower limb
- Anterior tibial compartment syndrome (March gangrene)

Muscular:
- Muscle hernia
- Displaced muscles, tendons:
  - Biceps brachii tendon
  - Peroneal tendons

## Contusion

| | |
|---|---|
| MOI | Direct trauma |
| | RSA |
| | Sports injury |
| Pathogenesis | Extravasation of blood within muscle sheath (at site of injury or at a distance from actual site of injury) |
| Diagnosis | Pain |
| | Swelling |

| | |
|---|---|
| | Local tenderness |
| | Movements: Painful and restricted |
| Investigation | X-ray AP and LAT views: To rule out any bony injury. |
| Management | Conservative treatment: |
| | Rest |
| | Pressure dressings |
| | Analgesics, NSAIDs |
| | Antibiotics. |
| | Surgical treatment: |
| | Surgery: Needle aspiration of blood/pus. |

## Rupture of Muscles and Tendons

| | |
|---|---|
| Preface | Rupture of a muscle mostly occurs at the junction of tendon and muscle itself (quadriceps extensor ruptures just above the patella); rupture of the muscle belly of rectus femoris occurs at mid thigh level. A tendon may rupture during normal activity or during unusual physical activity/stress (weight lifting or avulsion of a finger extensor tendon at its insertion by traumatic injury). |
| MOI | Direct trauma: Violence |
| | Indirect trauma: Sudden quadriceps contraction |
| | RSA |
| | Sports injury: Weight lifting, jumps, martial arts |
| | Degenerative: In elderly (trivial injury, i.e. stumbling) |
| Pathogenesis | Torn muscle fibers/tendon; extravasation of blood; hematoma |
| Incidence | Muscles and tendons that rupture most often are: |
| | • Muscles: Rectus femoris, biceps brachii |
| | • Tendons: Quadriceps femoris tendon, supraspinatus tendon, patellar tendon, biceps brachii, tendocalcaneus, extensor pollicis longus, extensor digitorum communis. |
| Diagnosis | Pain |
| | Gap: Visible and palpable on contracting the affected muscle |
| | Local tenderness |
| | Movements: Painful and restricted. |
| Investigation | X-ray—AP and LAT views: To rule out any bony injury. |
| Management | Conservative treatment: |
| | Rest |
| | Pressure dressings |
| | Analgesics; NSAIDs |
| | Antibiotics |
| | Surgical treatment: ASAP esp. in a young person/laborer |
| | Surgery: |
| | • Muscle: Repair with interrupted silk mattress sutures |
| | • Tendon: Apposition of ruptured ends without tension; lacerated parts of tendon to be excised; ruptured large tendon to be repaired by suturing of strips of fascia lata across line of repair; followed by support with a cast or splint. |

## Shoulder Cuff Injuries

| | |
|---|---|
| Anatomy | Shoulder cuff comprises—tendons of supraspinatus, teres minor, and infraspinatus. |
| MOI | A little trauma may cause tears (lesions) in the degenerated shoulder cuff. These lesions are: |

- Supraspinatus tendonitis
- Rupture of supraspinatus tendon
- Calcification of supraspinatus tendon
- Subdeltoid bursitis.

Diagnosis    Supraspinatus tendonitis (Painful Arc Syndrome):

- Pain appears in the shoulder over an arc—60 to 120 degree of abduction, with freedom from pain on movement outside limits of that range.
- Tenderness over greater tuberosity, i.e. insertion of supraspinatus.

Rupture of supraspinatus tendon:

- Pain and tenderness over greater tuberosity
- Abduction painful at 90 degree.

Calcification of Supraspinatus tendon:

- Pain in the shoulder
- Stiffness
- X-ray shows calcified deposit above head.

Subdeltoid or subacromial bursitis:

- Pain in the shoulder
- Tenderness over greater tuberosity
- Painful restricted abduction.

Management    Conservative treatment:

Short-wave diathermy or Infrared fomentation plus analgesics

Intra-articular inj. Hydrocortisone with lignocain 2%, plus exercises.

Surgical treatment:

Surgery: Repair of the lesion – esp. in the young patient.

**Refer:** To the next fracture clinic.

## Ruptured Supraspinatus Tendon

| | |
|---|---|
| Preface | Rupture of the supraspinatus tendon usually affects the middle-aged persons, that may occur post a trivial trauma; rupture may be complete or incomplete; majority of patients with complete rupture of supraspinatus do not require surgerical repair. |
| Anatomy | Supraspinatus muscle originates from 2/3rd of the floor of supraspinous fossa; fibers pass laterally under acromion; end in a short, stout tendon that is inserted to the top of greater tubercle of the humerus; the tendon is closely adherent to the capsule of the shoulder joint. |
| MOI | Direct trauma |
| | RSA |
| | Sports injury |

| | |
|---|---|
| Pathogenesis | Extravasation of blood within muscle sheath (at site of injury or at a distance from actual site of injury); inflamed subacromial bursa |
| Diagnosis | Pain |
| | Gap: Visible and palpable at site of rupture |
| | Local tenderness |
| | Movements: Painful and restricted |
| Investigation | X-ray shoulder—AP and LAT views: To rule out any bony injury. |
| Management | Conservative treatment: Symptomatic: |
| | Rest |
| | Analgesics, NSAIDs |
| | Antibiotics |
| | Physiotherapy: IR, SWD, massage, exercises |
| | Immobilization: By an arm pouch |

Intra-articular injection of steroid (hydrocortisone/triamcinolone) + lignocaine plain 1%

Technique:
- Position: Patient placed supine on examination table; or sitting on a stool
- Toilet/sterile skin with spirit/alcohol, and drape shoulder
- Insert a sterile aspiration needle into the deposit; aspirate; inject steroid + lignocaine slowly
- Seal the area.

Surgical treatment:
Indication: Failure of conservative treatment (persisting pain and disability)
Surgery: Repair of complete/incomplete tears.

Technique:
- Incision: Along the coracohumeral or coracoscapular ligament
- Exposure of ruptured part of the tendon
- Detach: Supraspinatus tendon by a transverse incision along the greater tuberosity
- Bury supraspinatus flap into a trench made into the bone at level of anatomical neck
- Fixation of the flap with silk sutures passed through the tendon and through holes drilled in the bone
- Suturing: Side to side of the supraspinatus to the infraspinatus and subscapularis tendons
- Wound closure.

After care: Physiotherapy: exercises.

## Rupturted Biceps Muscle

| | |
|---|---|
| Definition | |
| MOI | Direct violence |
| | RSA |

|  | Fall from a height |
|---|---|
|  | Neoplastic. |
| Diagnosis | Pain |
|  | Swelling: Becomes prominent on flexion elbow against resistance |
|  | Local tenderness |
|  | Movements of shoulder and elbow and restricted |
| Investigation | X-ray of arm—AP and LAT views. |
| Management | Conservative treatment: |
|  | Indication: Incomplete tear |
|  | Immobilization: With an arm sling/pouch |
|  | Analgesics and NSAIDs |
|  | SWD or IR heat therapy |
|  | Surgical treatment: |
|  | Indication: Complete tear or an old tear |
|  | Surgery: Repair of torn muscle |
|  | Technique: |

- Incision: Anterolateral, parallel with outer border of the beceps close to sulcus
- Suturing of ruptured muscle, by apposing the ends with interrupted mattress sutures of silk; extensive tears sutured with fascia lata across the lesion; old neglected tears (fibrosed) are to be debrided prior to suturing.

Postoperatively: Rest in an arm sling/pouch, with elbow flexed for 3/52.

After care: Exercises: Active and passive.

**Refer:** The patient to next fracture clinic.

## Ruptured Biceps Tendon (Long Head)

| Preface | Rupture of the tendon of long head of biceps may occur while fraying in the bicipital grove usually in elderly (osteoarthritis of shoulder joint); hypertrophic short head may partially compensate for the resulting disability. |
|---|---|
| Anatomy | It is a vital factor in the mechanism of the shoulder joint; enters the shoulder joint through an opening between the two tubercles of humerus; by its position within the capsule and in the sulcus between the tubercles of the humerus, it keeps head of the humerus in place, and to steady it in shoulder movements. |
| MOI | Direct trauma |
|  | RSA |
|  | Sports injury: Weight lifting |
| Pathogenesis | Extravasation of blood within muscle sheath (at site of injury or at a distance from actual site of injury); rupture usually transverse, occurring within shoulder joint or within intertubercular sulcus, or may occur at the musculotendinous junction or at its glenoid attachment; tendon flattened, frayed, and ruptured. |

| | |
|---|---|
| Diagnosis | Pain |
| | Bunching of the muscle nearer the elbow than normal; displaced downwards on flexing the elbow |
| | Local tenderness |
| | Movements of shoulder and elbow weakened. |
| Investigation | X-ray arm—AP and LAT views: to rule out any bony injury. |
| Management | Conservative treatment: |
| | Rest |
| | Analgesics, NSAIDs |
| | Antibiotics. |
| | Surgical treatment: End to end suturing is impractical until and unless the rupture occurs at or near the musculocutaneous junction |
| | Surgery: Repair of ruptured tendon: |
| | Indications: Shoulder exploration for: |

- Rupture of rotator cuff or any pathology
- Excision of ruptured intra-articular portion of tendon
- Fixation of distal ruptured end of tendon into the bicipital sulcus or into the coracoids process
- Excision of proximal segment of bicipital tendon and tenodesis of distal segment.

Technique:
- Incision: 10 cm anterior longitudinal
- Exposure of ruptured part of the tendon
- Reinforce the sutures, with strips of fascia lata
- Fixation: With interrupted.

## Ruptured Biceps Tendon (Distal End)

| | |
|---|---|
| Preface | Rupture of the distal end of biceps tendon may occur due to fraying of the tendon against radial tuberosity by supination and pronation of the forearm usually in elderly, or avulsion of the tendon from its insertion at the tuberosity by lifting heavy weights, or from sudden violent muscle contraction. |
| MOI | Direct trauma |
| | RSA |
| | Sports injury: Weight lifting |
| Pathogenesis | Extravasation of blood within tendon sheath (at site of injury or at a distance from actual site of injury); rupture usually transverse, occurring within elbow joint or at the musculotendinous junction, or at tuberosity attachment; tendon flattened, frayed, and ruptured. |
| Diagnosis | Pain |
| | Swelling |
| | Local tenderness |
| | Movements of supination painful and restricted. |
| Investigation | X-ray elbow—AP and LAT views: To rule out any bony injury. |

Management    Conservative treatment:
Rest
Analgesics, NSAIDs
Antibiotics.

Surgical treatment:
Indication: To restore biceps power of supination.

Surgery:
- Repair of ruptured tendon: End to end suturing is impractical until and unless the rupture occurs at or near the musculocutaneous junction
- Reinserting the tendon into radial tuberosity: Method of choice
Technique:
- Incision: Curvilinear, centered over the anterior aspect of the elbow
- Exposure: Distal tendon of biceps; pass silk suture through it
- Exposure: Radioulnar tunnel through which tendon passed prior to

Injury:
- Incision: 2nd incision on the posterolateral aspect of flexed elbow
- Exposure: Radial head and neck by detaching muscles from lateral aspect of olecranon and retracting them laterally, thus saving the deep branch of radial nerve as it enters supinator
- Exposure: Radial tuberosity by pronating forearm
- Drill holes: Into tuberosity; pass the ends of the silk suture in the biceps tendon into the tunnel and bring out through 2nd incision; pull the tendon through; tie the suture.

Postoperatively: Immobilization: by a posterior POP splint applied to the forearm with flexed elbow for 2/52; removal of stitches, and change of splint post for another 3–4/52.

After care: Exercises.

## Ruptured Ulnar Collateral Ligament (Gamekeeper's Thumb)

MOI    Direct violence: Forced abduction.
Diagnosis    Deformity—persistent flexion of terminal phalanx
Pain
Local tenderness
Movements of thumb painful and restricted esp. grasping.
Investigation    X-ray of thumb—AP and LAT views.
Management    Conservative treatment:
Indication: Incomplete tear or undisplaced avulsion fracture
Method: Plaster fixation (Scaphoid type cast) for 6/52.
Surgical treatment:
Indication: Complete tear or rotated fracture
Surgery: Repair of torn ligament and open reduction of fracture.
Postoperative: Followed by plaster fixation (Scaphoid type cast) for 6/52.
After care: Physiotherapy—active exercises.

**Refer:** The patient to next fracture clinic.

## Ruptured Extensor Tendon (Mallet Finger)

| | |
|---|---|
| MOI | Forced flexion of finger from extension position. The extensor tendon tears its attachment to the phalanx (avulsion injury). |
| Diagnosis | Deformity: Persistent flexion of terminal phalanx |
| | Pain |
| | Swelling |
| | Local tenderness |
| | Movement: Loss of extension of terminal phalanx. |
| Investigation | X-ray hand—AP and LAT views. |
| Management | Conservative treatment: |
| | Apply splint in hyperextension (DIP joint) for 5/52. |
| | Surgical treatment: |
| | Indication: Failure of conservative treatment |
| | Surgery: Arthrodesis in extreme cases of failure. |

**Refer:** The patient to next fracture clinic.

## Ruptured Flexor Tendons (Trigger Finger)

| | |
|---|---|
| Definition | It is a condition affecting the flexor tendons of the finger or thumb. |
| Etiology | Thickening of flexor tendon or constriction in the tendon sheath |
| Diagnosis | Disability: Difficulty in flexing or extending the affected finger |
| | Little force: Suddenly releases the finger with a click |
| | Palpation: A nodule palpated opposite MP joint of the affected finger. |
| Investigation | X-ray hand—AP and LAT views. |
| Management | Conservative treatment: |
| | Splintage. |
| | Surgical treatment of choice. |
| | Indication: Failure of conservative treatment. |
| | Surgery: Slitting the fibro-osseous tunnel at the level of the constriction. |
| | After care: Active exercises. |

## Ruptured Tendocalcaneus/Achilles

| | |
|---|---|
| MOI | Direct trauma |
| | RSA |
| | Sports injury |
| Pathogenesis | Extravasation of blood within muscle sheath (at site of injury or at a distance from actual site of injury) |
| Diagnosis | Pain |
| | Gap: Visible and palpable at site of rupture |
| | Local tenderness |
| | Movements: Painful and restricted |
| D/d | Rupture of plantaris tendon (younger age) |
| Investigation | X-ray AP and LAT views: To rule out any bony injury. |
| Management | Conservative treatment: |
| | Rest |
| | Pressure dressings |

Analgesics, NSAIDs
Antibiotics.

Surgical treatment:
Surgery: Suturing of tendon.

Technique:
- Incision: 10 cm posterior longitudinal
- Exposure of ruptured part of the tendon
- Pullout suturing: Modified Bunnel pullout suturing technique used
- Reinforce the sutures, with strips of fascia lata, or by using a tongue or strip of tendon, turned distally from proximal to the rupture tendon
- Fixation: With interrupted silk sutures
- Wound closure.

Postoperative: Apply a long leg cast with knee flexed and foot in an equines position; wire sutures protruding through the cast.
After care: Removal of cast and wires post 4/52; then apply walking cast for 4/52.

## Ruptured Patellar Tendon

| | |
|---|---|
| Preface | Rupture of the patellar tendon mostly occurs at the lower border of the patella; patella is a part of the proximal segment of the tendon and usually retracted 2 to 5 cm proximally due to contraction of the quadriceps muscle. |
| Anatomy | It is a broad, thick tendon that connects the patella with tibial tuberosity, and via that the quadriceps is attached to the tibia. |
| MOI | Direct trauma |
| | RSA |
| | Sports injury. |
| Pathogenesis | Torn tendon; extravasation of blood within tendon sheath. |
| Diagnosis | Pain |
| | Gap: Visible and palpable at site of rupture |
| | Local tenderness |
| | Movements of knee painful and restricted. |
| Investigation | X-ray AP and LAT views: To rule out any bony injury. |
| Management | Conservative treatment: |
| | Rest |
| | Pressure dressings |
| | Analgesics, NSAIDs |
| | Antibiotics. |
| | Surgical treatment: |
| | Surgery: Repair of tendon. |
| | Technique: |

- Incision: 20 cm long midline anterior longitudinal
- Exposure of ruptured part of the tendon
- Drain the hematoma, and debride the ruptured ends of tendon

- Drill a transverse hole through middle of patella
  Pass a strip of fascia lata through the patellar hole
- Appose the ruptured tendon ends by extending the knee, and pulling down the proximal part of the tendon distally with a clamp
- Suturing of tendon ends with silk or chromic catgut
- Reinforce the sutures, with strips of fascia lata, or by using a tongue or strip of tendon, turned distally from proximal to the rupture tendon
- Fixation with interrupted silk sutures
- Wound closure.

Postoperative: Apply a long leg cast with knee flexed and foot in an equines position; wire sutures protruding through the cast.

After care: Removal of cast and wires post 4/52; then apply walking cast for 4/52.

## Ruptured Quadriceps Femoris Tendon

| | |
|---|---|
| Preface | Rupture of the quadriceps tendon mostly occurs just above the patella; usually occurs in elderly, through a zone of degeneration; supplement of the sutures with fascial strips is beneficial. |
| Anatomy | It is a broad, thick tendon that is attached to the upper border of patella, while some of its fibers continue distally, across front of patella, into the ligamentum patellae. |
| MOI | Direct trauma<br>RSA<br>Sports injury. |
| Pathogenesis | Torn tendon; extravasation of blood within tendon sheath. |
| Diagnosis | Pain<br>Gap: Visible and palpable at site of rupture<br>Local tenderness<br>Movements of knee painful and restricted. |
| Investigation | X-ray AP and LAT views: To rule out any bony injury. |
| Management | Conservative treatment:<br>Rest<br>Pressure dressings<br>Analgesics, NSAIDs<br>Antibiotics.<br>Surgical treatment:<br>Surgery: Repair of tendon.<br>Technique: |

- Incision: 20 cm long midline anterior longitudinal
- Exposure of ruptured part of the tendon
- Drain the hematoma, and debride the ruptured ends of tendon
- Appose the ruptured tendon ends by extending the knee, and pulling down the proximal part of the tendon distally with a clamp
- Suturing of tendon ends with silk or chromic catgut

- Reinforce the sutures, with strips of fascia lata, or by using a tongue or strip of tendon, turned distally from proximal to the rupture tendon
- Fixation: With interrupted silk sutures
- Wound closure

Postoperative: Apply a long leg cast with knee flexed and foot in an equines position; wire sutures protruding through the cast.

After care: Removal of cast and wires post 4/52; then apply walking cast for 4/52.

## Aspiration and Needling of Calcified Deposits

| | |
|---|---|
| Indication | Calcification of short rotator muscles |
| | Technique: |

- Position: Patient placed supine on examination table; or sitting on a stool
- Toilet/sterile skin with spirit/alcohol, and drape shoulder
- Anesthesia: Local (lignocaine/xylocaine 1%) infiltration of skin and deeper tissue
- Insert a sterile aspiration needle into the deposit; aspirate deposit withdraw the needle, and seal the area.

## Lateral Epicondylitis (Tennis Elbow)

| | |
|---|---|
| Definition | It is a very common disorder of unknown pathogenesis. |
| Etiology | Traumatic: RSA, sports injury, direct violence. |
| MOI | Abrupt pronation of the forearm, causing strain on the extensor aponeurotic fibers. |
| Diagnosis | Pain—over the outer aspect of the elbow |
| | Local tenderness—over lateral epicondyle |
| | Movements—passive pronation to the full extent exaggerate pain. |
| Investigation | X-ray elbow—AP and LAT views. |
| Management | Conservative treatment: |
| | Heat—IR or SWD |
| | Elbow support |
| | Local—inj. hydrocortisone 25–50 mg + Inj. lignocain 2%. |
| | Surgical treatment: |
| | Surgery: Release of extensor aponeurosis. |

**Refer:** To the next fracture clinic.

## Volkmann's Ischemic Contracture (VIC)

| | |
|---|---|
| Definition | It is defined as a progressive degeneration of muscle, resulting from impaired vasculature of a limb (partial or complete). |
| Etiology | • Direct trauma: Causing arterial or venous (rare) obstruction |
| | • Immobilization: Tight splints or casts |
| | • Spasmodic: Local arterial spasm with an associated reflex spasm of the collateral vascular supply, due to arterial trauma (obstruction). |

| Pathogenesis | Impaired vasculature by obstruction (swelling); muscle ischemia; muscle tissue necrosis and degeneration; muscle tissue replaced by fibrous tissue; resulting contracture, deformity, or paralysis due to ischemic nerves (irreparable ischemia). |

### VIC of Upper Limb

| Incidence | Upper limb: Most often occurs post supracondylar fracture of humerus; and occasionally post fractures both bones of forearm (radius and ulna). Muscles: Commonly forearm flexors (esp. flexur digitorum profundus and flexur pollicis longus) severely involved; flexor digitorum sublimis less affected. |
| Diagnosis | Impending S/S: Severe pain in flexor muscles of forearm post fracture |

Confirmed signs:
- Deformity: Claw hand (flexed all phalanges with flexed wrist); unable to extend the fingers
- Sensations: Impaired
- Skin: Pallor or cyanosis of fingers
- Pulse: Impaired radial pulse

| Management | First aid treatment: ASAP: |

- Reduction: Failure to reduce fracture is unimportant, vide severe disability of an established VIC
- Removal of pressure from front of elbow; bivalve or remove the cast/splint; cutting of dressings up to skin
- Joint: To be partly extended
- Sympathetic nerve block (inj. Papaverine): To relieve vascular spasm

Surgical treatment:

Indications:
- Impending VIC (to cover risk)
- Established VIC

Surgery:
- Fasciotomy + arteriectomy
- Sympathectomy

Technique:
- Incision: Curved incision centered over the elbow medial to the biceps tendon
- Divide the deep fascia; drain any hematoma—relieves the vascular obstruction; if not then:
- Exposure of brachial artery:
  - For lacerated: Ligate it above and below
  - For spasmodic: Incise the arterial wall; remove the thrombus if present; repair the arterial incision
  - Arteriectomy: Segmental excision of 5 cm long + end to end ligation
  - Sympathectomy of choice vide arteriectomy
- Exposure of flexor muscle bellies: divide intermuscular septa

- Exposure of median nerve: Suturing of laceated nerve
- Skin suturing only.

Postoperative: Immobilization of arm in cast in extended position.

## *VIC of Lower Limb*

| | |
|---|---|
| Incidence | Lower limb: Most often occurs post supracondylar fracture of femur; displaced fractures of upper part of tibia; and occasionally post-fractures both bones of leg (tibia and fibula). |
| | Muscles: Commonly calf muscles involved. |
| Diagnosis | Impending S/S: Severe pain in the calf muscles post fracture, aggravated by passive dorsiflexion of ankle |
| | Local tenderness: Over calf |

Confirmed signs:
- Deformity: Equinovarus of foot and ankle; unable to correct the foot
- Sensations: Impaired
- Skin: Pallor or cyanosis of toes
- Pulse: Impaired dorsalis pedis pulse.

Management  First aid treatment: ASAP:
- Reduction: Failure to reduce fracture is unimportant, vide severe disability of an established VIC
- Removal of pressure: Bivalve or remove the cast/splint; cutting of dressings up to skin
- Joint: Release elbow flexion and allow it to be partly extended
- Blockage of stellate ganglion with lignocain/xylocain
- Sympathetic nerve block (inj. Papaverine): To relieve vascular spasm.

Surgical treatment:

Indications:
- Impending VIC (to cover risk)
- Established VIC.

Surgery:
- Fasciotomy + arteriectomy
- Sympathectomy
- Reconstruction: TA lengthening + wedge osteotomy of tarsus
- Tendo-achilles (TA) lengthening (Z-plastic tenotomy of TA).

Technique:
- Position: Patient placed on unaffected side or prone
- Incision: 10 cm long longitudinal incision medial to the tendo-achilles
- Incise tendon sheath to expose the tendon
- Divide the tendon from side to side, leaving the posterior flap attached to calcaneus and an anterior flap attached to the gastrocnemius and soleus muscles
- Dorsiflex fully the foot; appose and suture the raw surfaces of tendon flaps
- Posterior capsulectomy: For contracted posterior part of ankle capsule
- Skin suturing only.

Postoperative: Immobilization: apply a long leg cast from midthigh to toes with knee flexed to 20 degree, for 6/52, followed by active and passive exercises.

Osteotomy (wedge) of tarsus

Indication: Deformity: Established equines by ankylosis.

Technique:
- Incision: 10 cm longitudinal incision over the anterolateral aspect of ankle and foot
- Exposure of joint by subperiosteal dissection; avoiding injury to the dorsalis pedis artery and the extensor tendons
- Osteotomy: Removing a cuneiform wedge of bone with its anterior base
- TA lengthening + posterior capsulectomy: If required
- Manipulation: Dorsiflex the foot forcibly
- Skin sutures

Postoperative: Apply a below knee cast for 4/52, followed by a walking boot cast.

## Anterior Tibial Compartment Syndrome (March Gangrene)

| | |
|---|---|
| Definition | It is defined as a syndrome that occurs in army/police personnels/athletes due to long marches/races; resulting in ischemic myositis of muscles of the anterior compartment of the leg. |
| Etiology | Direct trauma |
| | Vascular: Embolism |
| Pathogenesis | Strenuous exercise resulting in edema and micro-hemorrhages in the muscles; muscle ischemia due to pressure from edema; muscle necrosis; fibrosis; contractures; paresis; deformities; |
| Diagnosis | Age: Common in younger persons |
| | Sex: In male > in female |
| | Pain: Acute post strenuous march/or exercise |
| | Swelling |
| | Skin: Localized erythema |
| | Muscle power: Loss of functioning (anterior tibial, extensor digitorum longus, and extensor hallucis longus) |
| | Sensation: Paresis between 1st and 2nd toes (peroneal nerve) |
| | Deformity: Develops in late case due to fibrous contractures. |
| Management | Surgical treatment of choice: |
| | Surgery: |
| | • Fasciotomy of crural fascia |
| | • Arteriectomy |
| | • Sympathectomy |
| | Technique: |
| | • Incision: 15 cm longitudinal anteromedial along the anterior border |
| | • Divide the deep fascia; drain any hematoma—relieves the vascular obstruction; if not then |

- Exposure of posterior tibial artery:
  - For lacerated: Ligate it above and below
  - For spasmodic: Incise the arterial wall; remove the thrombus if present; repair the arterial incision
- Arteriectomy: Segmental excision of 5 cm long + end to end ligation
- Sympathectomy of choice vide arteriectomy
- Exposure of flexor muscle bellies: Divide intermuscular septa
- Exposure of posterior tibial nerve: Suturing of laceated nerve
- Skin suturing only.

Postoperative: Immobilization of leg in cast in extended position.

## Muscle Hernia

| | |
|---|---|
| Preface | Herniation of a muscle through a tear in the muscle sheath is rare; Examples: Usually occurs in the lower limb below the knee, and in the upper limb (adductors and biceps brachii); variable in size (large to less than 1 cm). |
| Etiology | Direct trauma: Violence (blow) |
| | Sports injury: Common amongst mountain climbers, skiers, marchers, Athletes |
| | Surgical removal: |
| Pathogenesis | On contraction, muscle fibers protrude through the torn muscle sheath; hypertrophic muscles; distended fascial compartment; weak fascial sheath splits; herniation occurs through these weak areas; fascial defect— oval, with sharp well defined edges; underlying muscle not thickened. |
| Diagnosis | Swelling: Over the belly of the muscle, reducible, decrease in size or disappear on muscle contraction |
| | Site: Commonly seen in thighs (large hernias) anterolaterally; in legs over the anterior tibial muscle, and over the peroneal muscles. |
| | Size: Large or small |
| | Pain: On exertion |
| | Fatigue |
| | Disability |
| D/d | Torn muscle: A gap appears between the two torn segments, on muscle Contraction |
| | Varicose veins |
| | Angiomas |
| Management | Required only when the symptoms are severe and disabling: Conservative treatment: |

- To avoid strenuous physical activity/exertion
- Analgesics/NSAIDs
- Elastic support.

Surgical treatment:

### Technique

Large symptomatic hernia:
- Repair of hernia with a peace of fascia or mesh.

Small hernias:
- Repair by undermining the fascia and closure of the tear with the interrupted nonabsorbable mattress sutures; Alt:
- Closure with a fascial graft, Alt:
- Enlarging the hernia orifice in both directions.

## DISPLACEMENT OF TENDONS

### Displacement of Biceps Brachii Tendon

| | |
|---|---|
| Definition | Displacement of biceps brachii tendon is defined as a symptom complex  caused by dislocation of the tendon from the intertubercular groove. |
| Etiology | Direct trauma: Violence (blow) |
| | Sports injury: Common amongst mountain climbers, skiers, marchers, athletes |
| | RSA |
| Pathogenesis | On contraction, the tendon dislocates through the intertubercular groove hypertrophic muscles; distended fascial compartment; weak fascial sheath splits. |
| Diagnosis | Swelling: Over the belly of the muscle, reducible, decrease in size or disappear on muscle contraction |
| | Site: Commonly seen in arms over the intertubercular groove |
| | Size: Large or small |
| | Pain: On exertion |
| | Fatigue |
| | Disability |
| D/d | Torn muscle: A gap appears between the two torn segments, on muscle contraction |
| | Varicose veins |
| | Angiomas |
| Management | Required only when the symptoms are severe and disabling: |
| | Conservative treatment: |
| | • To avoid strenuous physical activity/exertion |
| | • Analgesics/NSAIDs |
| | • Elastic support |
| | Surgical treatment of choice. |
| | Surgery: Fixation of tendon in the intertubercular groove. |
| | Technique: |
| | • Incision: Anterior longitudinal centered over the deltopectoral groove |
| | • Exposure: Tendon of long head of biceps |
| | • Replace: The tendon in the intertubercular groove |
| | • Suture: Transverse humeral ligament across the groove to secure the tendon in the groove. |
| | Postoperatively: Immobilization: By an arm pouch or sling for 2/52 |
| | After care: Exercises. |

## Displacement of Peroneal Tendons

| | |
|---|---|
| Definition | Displacement of peroneal tendons is defined as a common entity due to a congenitally shallow groove of the lateral malleolus or total absence of the groove. |
| Etiology | Congenital |
| | Direct trauma: Violence (blow) |
| | Sports injury: Common amongst mountain climbers, skiers, marchers, athletes |
| | RSA |
| Pathogenesis | Mechanical impairment: Loss of fulcrum pull: on contraction, the tendons muscle fibers disllocate from their normal position on the posterior aspect of the lateral malleolus, to lie over the lateral aspect of the distal third of the fibula. |
| Diagnosis | Swelling of ankle (lateral aspect) |
| | Site: Over the outer side of ankle |
| | Size: Large or small |
| | Pain: On exertion |
| | Fatigue |
| | Disability |
| D/d | Torn muscle: A gap appears between the two torn segments, on muscle contraction |
| | Varicose veins |
| | Angiomas |
| Management | Required only when the symptoms are severe and disabling: |
| | Conservative treatment: |

Management (continued):

- To avoid strenuous physical activity/exertion
- Analgesics/NSAIDs
- Elastic support

Surgical treatment of choice.

Surgery: Reconstruction

Technique:

- Incision: Posterior longitudinal centered over the posterior aspect of the distal 1/3rd of the fibula, extend over the lateral border of the foot up to the cuboid
- Exposure: Deep fascia by lifting the posterior skin flap
- Formation of an ample flap with its base attached to tip of the lateral malleolus
- Replace: The tendons
- Suture: Fascial flap to the soft tissues on the lateral border of the calcaneus, to secure the tendons in the groove
- Skin: Closure.

Postoperatively: Immobilization—with a POP cast A/A with ankle at 90 degree for 1/12

After care: Walking allowed post 1/12.

## Bibliography

1. Anderson LD. Affections of muscles tendons, and tendon sheaths: Campbell's Operative Orthopaedics, ed. 9th, Vol I-IV. C.V. Mosby Co., Saint Louis, 1998.
2. Campbell's Operative Orthopaedics (1998) 9th Ed. Vol I-IV. Canale S. Terry, Daugherty K, and Jones Linda. Mosby.
3. Canale ST, et al. Campbell's Operative Orthopaedics, ed. 9th, Vol I-IV. C.V. Mosby Co., Saint Louis, 1998.
4. Clark JMP. Modern Trends in Orthopedics Fracture Treatment, Butterworths, London, 1962.
5. Clark JMP. Modern Trends in Orthopedics Fracture Treatment. Butterworths, London, 1962.
6. Kapoor PS. Accident and Emergency, ed. 2nd, Part I, CBS, New Delhi, 2016.
7. Kapoor PS. Accident and Emergency: Etiology, Diagnosis and Management, 2nd Ed., CBS, New Delhi, 2016.
8. Love M, et al. Bailey and Love's Short Practice of Surgery, ed. 13th, H.K. Lewis and Co., London, 1965.
9. Mc Rae R. Practical Fracture Treatment, ed. 1st, Churchill Livingstone, 1981.
10. Mercer W. Orthopaedic Surgery, 4th Ed., Williams and Wilkins Co., Baltimore, 1950.
11. Practical Fracture Treatment (1981) 1st Ed. Mc Rae R, Churchill Livingstone.
12. Scott JC. Volkmann's contracture, supracondylar fractures of the elbow: 201:3. Modern Trends in Orthopedics Fracture Treatment. Clark JMP; Butterworths, London, 1962.
13. Scott JC. Volkmann's contracture, tibial fractures: 201:3. Modern Trends in Orthopedics Fracture Treatment. Clark JMP; Butterworths, London, 1962.

# 15

# Affections of Fascia and Bursae

**Fascial affections**
- Palmar fibromatosis (Dupuytren's contracture)
- Plantar fibromatosis (Plantar fasciitis)
- Snapping (clicking) joints:
  - Snapping hip
  - Snapping knee
  - Snapping shoulder
  - Snapping scapula

**Bursae affections**
- Bursitis of shoulder:
  - Subdeltoid and/or subacromial bursitis
  - Subscapularis bursitis
- Bursitis of elbow:
  - Olecranon bursitis (Student's elbow)
- Bursitis of hip:
  - Trochanteric bursitis
  - Ischiogluteal bursitis (Weaver's bottom)
- Bursitis of knee:
  - Prepatellar bursitis (Housemaid's Knee)
  - Popliteal cyst (Baker's cyst)
- Bursitis of foot and ankle:
  - Tendo-achilles (retrocalcaneal) bursitis

## FASCIAL AFFECTIONS

Preface

Affections of fascia and the bursae are common disorders in office practice, mostly managed by the conservative measures (respond favorably to such treatment, e.g. rest, heat, elevation, massage, and local or systemic medication); hardly few require surgery in case of failure of conservative measures or is not indicated.

### Palmar Fibromatosis (Syn. Palmar Fasciitis; Dupuytren's Contracture)

Definition

It is defined as an affection of the palmar fascia, characterized by the localized thickening of the palmar aponeurosis that involves the overlying skin of the palm, resulting in tendency to contract which draws the affected fingers into fixed flexion. Mostly starts near the base of the ring or little finger, thereafter draws that finger into the palm of the hand; similar in histology and pathogenesis to that of the plantar fascia, with some variation peculiar to the anatomy of the part.

| | |
|---|---|
| Anatomy | Palmar fascia (deep) consists of three portions (medial and lateral, that are thin and weak; and intermediate, that is thick and strong); covers the vessels, nerves, muscles, and tendons. |

Medial portion: Covers the hypothenar eminence in the hand.

Lateral portion: Covers the thenar eminence in the hand.

Intermediate portion (palmar aponeurosis): Related to inner four digits vide five toes in the foot.

Arrangement: Fascia triangular in shape; apex attached to transverse carpal ligament and the palmaris longus tendon; base divides opposite metacarpal heads int four processes, one going to each of four fingers, site of division held by transverse fibers; neurovascular bundle and lumbrical muscles pass between these slips.

**Etiology**

Unknown

Hereditary: Familial

Traumatic: Occupational hazard

Inflammatory

Metabolic

**Pathogenesis**

Primary disorder of the collagen substance of the fibrous tissue: Lesion starts as a fibroblastic nodule in the subcutaneous palmar fascia, undergoes changes: proliferative, involutional, residual stage.

**Diagnosis**

Deformity:

Age: Middle age

Sex: In men > in women

Deformity: Flexed proximal and middle phalanx, unaffected terminal phalanx.

- In advanced case: Permanent changes in the affected joints render futile any attempts to straighten the fingers.
   Skin: Adherent skin of palm puckered

**Investigation**

X-ray hand: AP and Lateral views.

**D/d**

Fibrosarcoma: Difficult to differentiate histologically

Synovial sarcoma

**Management**

Conservative treatment:

Early case: Night splintage and active exercises: gentle stretching of fingers by the patient.

Radiotherapy (RT): limited role in early phase.

Surgical treatment:

Aims:

Surgery: Fasciotomy:

- Subcutaneous: Elderly, arthritic, or poor health
- Partial: Small affected area, immature nodule, early contracture produced by a fascial cord
- Complete: Younger patient with disabling contracture.

Technique:

Subcutaneous fasciotomy:

- Puncture wounds: With a pointed scalpel, on the medial side of palmar fascia, at the levels (apex of palmar fascia; at the proximal palmar crease; at the distal palmar crease)
- Insert: A fasciatome through each of punctured wounds; pass it across palm, between skin and fascia
- Divide: Facial cords
- Skin: Free skin from underneath adherent palmar fascia.

Partial fasciectomy:

- Incision/s: Transverse across contracture
- Excision of involved palmar fascia
- Suture: Skin.

Complete fasciectomy:

- Incision: Parallel to the distal palmar crease
- Separate: Skin from adherent palmar fascia by sharp dissection
- Exposure of affected palmar fascia; avoid injury to neurovascular bundle
- Excision of entire deep fascia from the palm
- Suture: Incisions closure with interrupted mattress sutures.

Postoperative: Immobilization by a splint for 1/52, followed by active exercises.

## Plantar Fibromatosis (Plantar Fasciitis)

| | |
|---|---|
| Definition | Plantar fasciitis is defined as the inflammation of the plantar fascia; similar in histology and pathogenesis to that of the palmar fascia, with some variation peculiar to the anatomy of the part. |
| Anatomy | Plantar fascia (deep) consists of three portions (medial and lateral, that are thin and weak; and intermediate, that is thick and strong); covers the vessels, nerves, muscles, and tendons.<br>Medial portion: Covers the abductor hallucis of great toe<br>Lateral portion: Covers the abductor digiti minimi; stronger than medial portion<br>Intermediate portion (plantar aponeurosis): Covers flexor digitorum Brevis; posterior end narrow, attached to medial tubercle of calcaneus anteriorly splits into five processes that proceed towards toes; bound together by transverse fibers. |
| Etiology | Traumatic<br>Inflammatory<br>Infective<br>Metabolic |
| Pathogenesis | Most often affects the medial part of plantar fascia; proliferated fibroblasts, that blend with fascia, beneath the tarsal bones; nodular thickening of the plantar fascia |
| Diagnosis | Pain<br>Swelling<br>Local tenderness |

| | |
|---|---|
| Investigation | CBC, ESR, blood sugar |
| D/d | Fibrosarcoma: Difficult to differentiate histologically |
| | Synovial sarcoma |
| Management | Surgical treatment of choice to avoid recurrences. |

Surgery: Block resection of plantar fascia.

Technique:

- Apply a tourniquet
- Incision: A long longitudinal, along medial border of the plantar fascia
- Exposure of the affected area
- Resect: Block of plantar fascia (includes full width and lesion)
- Protect medial neurovascular structures
- Remove: Tourniquet prior to wound closure.

After care: Bedrest with elevated leg for several days, followed by full weight bearing.

## Snapping (Syn. Clicking) Joints

| | |
|---|---|
| Preface | Defined as an ability to produce sounds (loud clicks) from what would appear to be otherwise normal joints. |

Sources: Two main sources of these sounds/clicks (intra-articular menisci of joints, and the sliding of tendons over bony anatomical prominences near the joints); may be habitual (obsessive neurotics–finding solace in a trivial intolerable discomfort).

Intra-articular menisci: Occur in jaw and the knee

Snapping tendons: Occur in hip, shoulder, and peroneal tendons.

| | |
|---|---|
| D/d | Stenosing tenosynovitis: Characterized by trigger phenomenon |
| Pathogenesis | Deranged articular menisci and tendons. |

## Regional

### Snapping Hip

| | |
|---|---|
| Definition | It is defined as an audible, palpable, or visible snap; usually produced by a tense fascial band catches while sliding over the superior margin of the greater trochanter, when the hip is flexed, adducted, or internal rotated; usually the band is the thickened posterior border of the iliotibial band, or the anterior border of the gluteus maximus muscle near its insertion. |
| Etiology | Voluntarily: Painless |
| | Involuntarily: Painful and habitual |
| | Traumatic: Subluxation of hip |
| | Inflammatory: Osteochondritis |
| | Bursitis: Trochanteric |
| | Loose bodies |
| Pathogenesis | Thickened posterior border of the iliotibial band; thickened anterior border of the gluteus maximus muscle; iliotibial band (tendon of tensor fasciae) sliding forwards and backwards over the greater trochanter's prominence (obsessive neurosis). |

| | |
|---|---|
| Diagnosis | Painless: Occasionally painful and habitual |
| | Snap/click: Voluntarily produced. |
| Management | Rarely rquires surgery as it is usually painless, and the patient usually prefer no treatment after being explained about its cause (mostly neurosis). |
| | Surgical treatment: |
| | Indication: Very severe snapping/clicking |
| | Surgery: Excision of fascia at the level of greater trochanter |
| | Technique: |
| | Anesthesia: Local preferred. |

- Incision: 2.5 cm posterior and 5 cm distal to the anterosuperior iliac spine; continue incision distally to the posterior border of greater trochanter and further distally for 10 cm over the thigh
- Incise: Fascia lata longitudinally just posterior to the iliotibial band
- Divide: Transversally posterior half of iliotibial band
- Flap formation: Form a flap of the posterior half of iliotibial band
- Transferring: Anteriorly distal end of the band
- Suturing of flap on the anterolateral surface of the thigh with the interrupted sutures.

After care: Active exercises post healing of the wound.

## Snapping Knee

| | |
|---|---|
| Etiology | Congenital: Discoid cartilage (solid disk, thicker in the center than at the periphery, that slips to produce a snap/click (no neurotic element) |
| Pathogenesis | Solid disk, thicker in the center than at the periphery; slippery |
| Diagnosis | Age: Common amongst adolescents |
| | Snap/click: Loudly audible even at a distance |
| | Knee: Hyperactive though dislocating |
| Investigation | X-rays knee AP and LAT views |
| Management | Surgical treatment of choice |
| | Indication: Very severe snapping/clicking |
| Surgery | Excision of disk. |

## Snapping Shoulder

| | |
|---|---|
| Etiology | |

- Supraspinatus sliding over greater trochanteric prominence (obsessive neurosis)
- Short head of biceps tendon sliding over lesser trochanter
- Long head of biceps displaced from bicipital groove
- Supraspinatus syndrome (lesions) of rotator cuff of shoulder.

| | |
|---|---|
| Pathogenesis | Supraspinatus tendon sliding over the greater trochanter's prominence; muscle fibers originating from outer border of the short head of biceps passed distally and laterally toward the long head, passing over the lesser trochanter, as the shoulder abducted and rotated. |
| Diagnosis | Pain |
| | Muscle spasm |
| | Local tenderness |

Snap/click: Less audible

Movements of shoulder painful and restricted (obsessive neurosis)

Muscle atrophy

**Investigation**    X-rays shoulder: May show calcified spots

**Management**    Rarely rquires surgery as it is usually painless, and the patient usually prefer no treatment after being explained about its cause (mostly neurosis).

Conservative treatment: Symptomatic:

- Rest
- Physiotherapy: Heat, massage, exercises
- Analgesics/NSAIDs
- Immobilization: By a sling/or an arm pouch
- Aspiration and needling of the calcified mass.

Surgical treatment:

Indication: Very severe snapping/clicking

Surgery: Fixation of tendon of long head in the bicipital groove

Technique:

- Incision: Anterior incision over the deltopectoral border
- Exposure of intertubercular groove by deepening the incision
- Isolate: Tendon of long head of biceps; replace it in the groove
- Suture: Transverse humeral ligament over the tendon.

Postoperative: Immobilization: arm support for 2/52

After care: Exercises.

## Snapping Scapula

**Preface**    Snapping or clicking beneath the scapula occurs more often; annoying; occasionally painful or disabling; variable—from a fine clicking/grating to a coarse audible popping or thumping.

**Etiology**    Traumatic

Lesions of scapula:

- Increased anterior curve of the superior angle of the scapula
- Osseous/or fibrocartilaginous nodule on the anterior aspect of superior angle of the scapula
- Tumors: Osteochondromas of anterior surface of the body of scapula

**Diagnosis**    Pain

Muscle spasm

Local tenderness

Snap/click: Less audible

Movements of shoulder painful and restricted (obsessive neurosis).

Muscle atrophy

**Investigation**    X-rays scapula: AP and oblique views: to rule out tumor.

**Management**    Rarely rquires surgery as it is usually painless, and the patient usually prefer no treatment after being explained about its cause (mostly neurosis).

Conservative treatment: symptomatic:
- Rest
- Physiotherapy: Heat, massage, exercises
- Analgesics/NSAIDs
- Immobilization: By a sling/or an arm pouch

Surgical treatment:

Indication: Disability—very severe snapping/clicking; persisting pain

Surgery: Exploration of the scapula.

Technique:
- Incision: Longitudinal along the vertebral border of the scapula from its superior to inferior angle
- Mobilize: Skin flaps; then divide the trapezius in line with the incision to expose vertebral border of scapula
- Exposure of subscapularis by freeing rhomboids from the scapula
- Removal of the causative lesion (resection of medial 2.5 cm. of body of scapula).

## BURSAE AFFECTIONS

### Bursitis

| | |
|---|---|
| Definition | It is defined as an acute or chronic inflammation of the bursal sac/s; usual sites are the subdeltoid, olecranon (student's elbow), ischial (Weaver's bottom), trochanteric, and prepatellar (Housemaid's knee) areas. |
| Anatomy | Bursae are closed sacs lined with a cellular membrane that resemble synovium; are usually situated about joints, or adjoining structures (skin, tendon, or muscle) moving over a bony prominence; may or may not communicate with the joint; anatomically and physiologically, the bursae are similar to tendon sheaths and synovial membranes of joints. |
| | Function: To reduce friction and to protect sensitive structures from pressure; to facilitate mobility of tendons and muscles over the bony prominences. |
| Etiology | Traumatic: Anatomical bursae<br>Prolonged pressure: Adventitious bursae<br>Inflammatory<br>Infective: Pyogenic, tuberculous, syphilitic<br>Rheumatic diseases: RA, gout |
| Pathogenesis | Inflamed; infective; periarticular calcific deposits, fibrosed, ankylosed |
| Diagnosis | Pain<br>Swelling<br>Local tenderness<br>Movements: Painful and restricted |
| Investigation | CBC, ESR, blood uric acid, blood sugar<br>X-ray |
| Management | Conservative treatment:<br>Rest |

Immobilization

Diathermy

Analgesics/NSAIDs

Injection: I/A corticosteroid + local:
- Hydrocortisone acetate 25 mg/ml + lignocaine 0.5%
- Triamcinolone acetonide 40 mg/ml + lignocaine 0.5%

Antibiotics

Surgical treatment:

Indication: Not required in most of cases

Procedures:
- Aspiration and injection of an appropriate drug
- Incision and drainage
- Excision of bursae.

After care:

Physiotherapy: exercises.

Regional

## Bursitis of Shoulder

### Subdeltoid and/or Subacromial Bursitis

| | |
|---|---|
| Anatomy | Subdeltoid and subacromial bursae form one large sac that separates the deltoid muscle from the upper part of the humeral shaft below and intervenes between under surface of the acromion and the humeral tuberosities above; disappears entirely under the acromion while in the right angled abduction—fact utilized in isolating the subdeltoid bursitis from other lesions around the shoulder joint. |
| Preface | Subacromial bursitis occurs more often than any other regional bursitis, the inflammation in the bursa being rarely primary; rather results from tendinitis of the rotator cuff of the shoulder, either with/or without calcification. |
| Etiology | Traumatic or frictional |
| | Inflammatory: Pyogenic, tuberculous |
| | Rheumatic: RA, gout, rheumatic fever |
| Pathogenesis | Periarticular calcific deposits |
| Diagnosis | Pain |
| | Swelling |
| | Local tenderness |
| | Movements: Painful and restricted |
| Investigation | CBC, ESR, blood sugar, blood uric acid |
| | X-ray: May show calcific deposits |
| Management | Conservative treatment: |
| | Rest |
| | Immobilization |
| | Diathermy |

Analgesics/NSAIDs

Injection: I/A corticosteroid + local:

- Hydrocortisone acetate 25 mg/ml + lignocaine 0.5%, Alt:
- Triamcinolone acetonide 40 mg/ml + lignocaine 0.5%

Antibiotics

Surgical treatment:

Indication: Not required in most of cases

Procedures:

- Aspiration and injection of an appropriate drug
- Incision and drainage
- Excision of bursae.

## Subscapularis Bursitis

| | |
|---|---|
| Anatomy | Subscapular bursa forms a sac between the subscapularis and the front of the scapular's neck and the coracoids's base. |
| Definition | It is defined as an inflammation of the subacromial bursa; results from tendinitis of the rotator cuff of the shoulder, either with/or without calcification. |
| Etiology | Traumatic or frictional |
| | Inflammatory: Pyogenic, tuberculous |
| | Rheumatic: RA, gout, rheumatic fever |
| Pathogenesis | Periarticular calcific deposits |
| Diagnosis | Pain |
| | Swelling |
| | Local tenderness |
| | Movements: Painful and restricted |
| Investigation | CBC, ESR, blood sugar, blood uric acid |
| | X-ray shoulder: May show calcific deposits |
| Management | Conservative treatment: |
| | Rest |
| | Immobilization |
| | Diathermy |
| | Analgesics/NSAIDs |

Injection: I/A corticosteroid + local:

- Hydrocortisone acetate 25 mg/ml + lignocaine 0.5%, Alt:
- Triamcinolone acetonide 40 mg/ml + lignocaine 0.5%

Antibiotics

Surgical treatment:

Indication: Not required in most of cases

Procedures:

- Aspiration and injection of an appropriate drug
- Incision and drainage

## Bursitis of Elbow

### Olecranon Bursitis (Student's Elbow)

| | |
|---|---|
| Anatomy | Olecranon bursa forms one large sac that separates the triceps expansion and subcutaneous triangular area on the olecranon's dorsal surface; large and very important bursa; acute inflammation of this bursa causes a widespread sympathetic inflammation of the adjoining soft structures. |
| Preface | Olecranon bursitis occurs more often; the inflammation in the bursa being rarely primary; rather results from tendinitis of the triceps. |
| Etiology | Traumatic: Fresh trauma or recurrent traumas (frictional) <br> Inflammatory: Pyogenic, tuberculous <br> Rheumatic: RA, gout, rheumatic fever |
| Pathogenesis | Repeated friction/pressure; inflammation; effusion; periarticular calcific deposits |
| Diagnosis | Pain <br> Swelling <br> Local tenderness <br> Movements of elbow painful and restricted |
| Investigation | CBC, ESR, blood sugar, blood uric acid <br> X-ray elbow AP and LAT views: May show calcific deposits |
| Management | Conservative treatment: <br> Rest <br> Immobilization: Splints, cuff and collar sling <br> Diathermy <br> Analgesics/NSAIDs <br> Injection: I/A corticosteroid + local: |

- Hydrocortisone acetate 25 mg/ml + lignocaine 0.5%, Alt:
- Triamcinolone acetonide 40 mg/ml + lignocaine 0.5%

Antibiotics

Surgical treatment:

Indication: Not required in most of cases

Procedures:

- Aspiration and injection of an appropriate drug
- Incision and drainage
- Excision of entire bursa.

## Bursitis of Hip

### Trochanteric Bursitis

| | |
|---|---|
| Anatomy | The trochanteric bursa is a large synovial sac that separates the aponeurotic part of gluteus maximus from the lower part of the outer aspect of the greater trochanter of the femur. |
| Preface | The trochanteric bursitis occurs more often than any other regional bursitis, the inflammation in the bursa being rarely primary; rather results from the tendinitis of the glutei tendons of the hip, mainly due to recurrent friction. |

| Etiology | Traumatic or frictional |
| --- | --- |
| | Inflammatory: Pyogenic, tuberculous |
| | Rheumatic: RA, gout, rheumatic fever. |
| Pathogenesis | Inflamed synovial; effusion, fibrosed; ankylosed. |
| Diagnosis | Pain |
| | Swelling |
| | Local tenderness |
| | Limp |
| | Movements of hip painful and restricted |
| Investigation | CBC, ESR, blood sugar, blood uric acid |
| | X-ray hip: May show synovitis; calcific deposits |
| Management | Conservative treatment: |
| | Rest |
| | Immobilization: traction |
| | Diathermy |
| | Analgesics/NSAIDs |
| | Injection: I/A corticosteroid + local: |

- Hydrocortisone acetate 25 mg/ml + lignocaine 0.5%, Alt:
- Triamcinolone acetonide 40 mg/ml + lignocaine 0.5%

Antibiotics

Surgical treatment:
Indication: Not required in most of cases

Procedures:
- Aspiration and injection of an appropriate drug
- Incision and drainage
- Excision of the entire bursa.

Technique of drainage:
- Incision: A longitudinal incision centered over the posterolateral aspect of the greater trochanter; deepen incision through deep fascia
- Divide: Fascia lata posterior and distal to the fibers of tensor fascia latae muscle
- Exposure of bursa by opening space between the vastus lateralis and gluteus maximus tendon
- Drainage of acute pyogenic bursitis.

## Ischiogluteal Bursitis (Weaver's Bottom)

| Anatomy | The ischiogluteal bursa separates the gluteus maximus muscle from the ischial tuberosity. |
| --- | --- |
| Preface | The ischiogluteal bursitis is usually caused by constant irritation/friction that occurs most often in persons with sedentary occupation (weaver); the inflammation in the bursa being rarely primary; rather results from tendinitis of the glutei of the hip. |
| Etiology | Traumatic or frictional |
| | Inflammatory: Pyogenic, tuberculous |
| | Rheumatic: RA, gout, rheumatic fever |

| | |
|---|---|
| Pathogenesis | Inflamed synovial, effusion, fibrosed, ankylosed. |
| Diagnosis | Pain |
| | Swelling |
| | Local tenderness |
| | Limp |
| | Movements of hip painful and restricted |
| Investigation | CBC, ESR, blood sugar, blood uric acid |
| | X-ray: May show synoivial effusion calcific deposits |
| Management | Conservative treatment: |
| | Rest |
| | Immobilization |
| | Diathermy |
| | Analgesics/NSAIDs |

Injection: I/A corticosteroid + local:
- Hydrocortisone acetate 25 mg/ml + lignocaine 0.5%, Alt:
- Triamcinolone acetonide 40 mg/ml + lignocaine 0.5%

Antibiotics

Surgical treatment:
Indication: Not required in most of cases

Procedures:
- Aspiration and injection of an appropriate drug
- Incision and drainage
- Excision of the entire bursa

Technique:
- Incision: 8 cm long, centered over prominence of ischial tuberosity, in line of distal fibers of gluteus maximus muscle
- Exposure of bursa by dividing the muscle by blunt dissection
- Isolate: The sciatic nerve lying just lateral to the tuberosity
- Incision and drainage: For acute pyogenic bursitis
- Excision of bursa for chronic bursitis.

## Bursitis of Knee

### Prepatellar Bursitis (Housemaid's Knee)

| | |
|---|---|
| Anatomy | The prepatellar bursa (Housemaid's bursa) forms one large sac that separates the front of the lower half of the patella and the upper half of the patellar ligament from the skin; patellar nerve plexus lying between bursa and the skin; often causes inflammation (bursitis). |
| Preface | Prepatellar bursitis occurs more often than any other regional bursitis, the inflammation in the bursa being rarely primary; rather results from tendinitis of the quadriceps of the knee; chronic enlargement of this bursa from friction/pressure is called the Housemaid's knee, as during scrubbing, the hands rest on the floor, the bursa brought into contact with the ground. |
| Etiology | Traumatic: Recurrent injuries |
| | Inflammatory: Pyogenic, tuberculous |

|                 | Rheumatic: RA, gout, rheumatic fever |
|-----------------|--------------------------------------|
| Pathogenesis    | Inflamed synovial; effusion; fibrosed; ankylosed. |
| Diagnosis       | Pain |
|                 | Swelling |
|                 | Local tenderness |
|                 | Limp |
|                 | Movements: Painful and restricted |
| Investigation   | CBC, ESR, blood sugar, blood uric acid |
|                 | X-ray: May show calcific deposits |
| Management      | Conservative treatment: |
|                 | Rest |
|                 | Immobilization |
|                 | Diathermy |
|                 | Analgesics/NSAIDs |

Injection: I/A corticosteroid + local:
- Hydrocortisone acetate 25 mg/ml + lignocaine 0.5%, Alt:
- Triamcinolone acetonide 40 mg/ml + lignocaine 0.5%

Antibiotics

Surgical treatment:
Indication: Not required in most of cases

Procedures:
- Aspiration and injection of an appropriate drug
- Incision and drainage
- Excision of bursa.

Technique of incision and drainage:
- Incision: Two longitudinal incisions (medial and lateral
- Exposure of bursa
- Incision and drainage of bursa.

Technique of excision of bursa:
- Incision: A transverse incision centered over the bursa
- Separate: Bursa from the overlying skin and subcutaneous tissue, and the deeper patellar aponeurosis
- Excision of the entire bursa
- Closure of wound: Skin edges apposed with interrupted mattress sutures.

Postoperative complication:
- Hematoma formation:
  Treatment: Obliteration of dead space by inserting mattress sutures through skin and deeper tissues on each side of the incision; post apposition of skin edges with interrupted sutures, the mattress sutures tied over large buttons.
  After care: Exercises.

## Popliteal Cyst (Baker's Cyst)

| | |
|---|---|
| Anatomy | Semimembranosus bursa form one large sac that separates the tendon and the medial head of the gastrocnemius muscle; often curves round the medial side of the gastrocnemius to communicate with a bursa that separates the medial head of gastrocnemius from the back of the knee joint. |
| Preface | Semimembranosus bursitis occurs more often than any other regional bursitis, the inflammation in the bursa being rarely primary; rather results from tendinitis of the gastrocnemious of the knee joint. |
| Etiology | Traumatic or frictional |
| | Inflammatory: Pyogenic, tuberculous, syphilitic |
| | Rheumatic: RA, gout, rheumatic fever |
| | Degenerative: Osteoarthritis |
| Pathogenesis | Herniation of the synovial membrane through the posterior part of the capsule of the knee; or overflow of synovial fluid through the communication of semimembranosus bursa with the knee. |
| Diagnosis | Common in children |
| | Pain |
| | Swelling |
| | Local tenderness |
| | Limp |
| | Movements of knee painful and restricted |
| | Muscular: Weakness |
| Investigation | CBC, ESR, blood sugar, blood uric acid |
| | Serological test |
| | Aspirated fluid analysis, culture |
| | X-ray: May show |
| D/d | Lipomas |
| | Xanthomas |
| | Fibrosarcoma |
| Management | Conservative treatment: |
| | Rest |
| | Immobilization |
| | Diathermy |
| | Analgesics/NSAIDs |
| | Injection: I/A corticosteroid + local: |
| | • Hydrocortisone acetate 25 mg/ml + lignocaine 0.5%, Alt: |
| | • Triamcinolone acetonide 40 mg/ml + lignocaine 0.5% |
| | Antibiotics |
| | Surgical treatment: |
| | Indication: Not required in most of cases |
| | Procedures: |
| | • Aspiration and injection of an appropriate drug |
| | • Incision and drainage |
| | • Excision of cyst |

Technique:
- Incision: 8 cm long curved longitudinal incision over the medial aspect of the popliteal space
- Develop: Plane of cleavage between the semimembranosus and the medial head of the gastrocnemius; separate the cyst wall from these muscles
- Separate: The cyst from adjoining structures by sharp dissection
- Excision of the cyst in toto.
- Closure of wound: Skin edges apposed with interrupted mattress sutures.

Postoperative: Immobilization of the knee by a posterior splint for 2/52.

After care: Quadriceps exercises.

## Bursitis of Foot and Ankle

### Tendo-Achilles (Retrocalcaneal) Bursitis

| | |
|---|---|
| Anatomy | Tendo-achilles (calcaneus) is the strongest tendon in the body; a small bursa separates the tendon from the upper part of the posterior surface of the calcaneus; the bursa may extend beyond the tendo-achilles (calcaneus) tendon, medially and laterally. |
| Preface | Tendo-achilles (calcaneus) bursitis occurs more often than any other regional bursitis, the inflammation in the bursa being rarely primary; rather results from tendinitis of the tendo-achilles. |
| Etiology | Traumatic or frictional<br>Sports injury<br>Inflammatory: Pyogenic, tuberculous<br>Rheumatic: RA, gout, rheumatic fever |
| Pathogenesis | Periarticular calcific deposits |
| Diagnosis | Pain<br>Swelling<br>Local tenderness<br>Limp<br>Movements of ankle painful and restricted |
| Investigation | CBC, ESR, blood sugar, blood uric acid<br>X-ray ankle AP and LAT views |
| Management | Conservative treatment:<br>Rest<br>Warm fomentation/diathermy<br>Elevation of foot<br>Immobilization of the affected part<br>Analgesics/NSAIDs<br>Injection: I/A corticosteroid + local:<br>• Hydrocortisone acetate 25 mg/ml + lignocaine 0.5%, Alt:<br>• Triamcinolone acetonide 40 mg/ml + lignocaine 0.5%<br>Antibiotics |

Surgical treatment:

Indication: Not required in most of cases

Procedures:

- Aspiration and injection of an appropriate drug
- Incision and drainage
- Excision of the bursa in toto.

Technique:

- Incision: A curved longitudinal incision along the lateral side of the tendocalcaneus and the proximal part of its inserted portion to the calcaneus
- Exposure of the bursa and the calcaneus' posterosuperior angle
- Excision of the entire bursa
- Resection of the angle of the calcaneus (if required)
- Closure of wound: Skin edges apposed with interrupted mattress sutures.

Postoperative: Immobilization of the foot by a posterior splint for 2/52.

After care: Exercises.

## Bibliography

1. Allen RA, et al. Soft-tissue tumors of the sole. With special reference to plantar fibromatosis, J. Bone and Joint Surg. 37-A:14, 1955.
2. Bailey and Love's Short Practice of Surgery. Love M, Rains A.J. H., Capper W.M.; H.K. Lewis and Co., London, 1965.
3. Burleson RJ, Bichel WH, Dahlin DC. Popliteal cyst. A clinicopathological survey, J. Bone and Joint Surg. 38-A: 1265, 1956.
4. Canale ST, et al. Campbell's Operative Orthopaedics, ed. 9th, Vol I-IV. C.V. Mosby Co., Saint Louis, 1998.
5. Childress HM. Popliteal cysts and posterior lesions of the medial meniscus. In DePalma A.F., editor: Clinical orthopedics, Vol. 18, J.B. Lippincott Co. p. 136, Philadelphia, 1960
6. Clarekson P. Dupuytren's contracture, Proc. Roy. Soc. Med. 47;365, 1954
7. Clark JMP. Modern Trends in Orthopedics Fracture Treatment, Butterworths, London, 196
8. Clark JMP. Modern Trends in Orthopedics Fracture Treatment. Butterworths, London, 1962.
9. Hendryson IE. Bursitis in the region of the fibular collateral ligament, J. Bone & Joint Surg. 28:446, 1946.
10. Kapoor PS. Accident and Emergency: Etiology, Diagnosis and Management 2nd Ed. CBS, New Delhi, 2016.
11. Kuhns JG. Adventitious bursas, Arch. Surg. 46:687, 1943
12. Love M, et al. Bailey and Love's Short Practice of Surgery, ed. 13th, H.K. Lewis and Co., London, 1965.
13. Mc Rae R. Practical Fracture Treatment 1st Ed. Churchill Livingstone, 1981.
14. Mc Rae R. Practical Fracture Treatment, ed. 1st, Churchill Livingstone, 1981.
15. Milch H. Partial scapulectomy for snapping of the scapula, J. Bone and Joint Surg. 32-A: 561, 1950.
16. Speed JS. Affections of fascia and bursae: Campbell's Operative Orthopaedics 9th Ed. Vol I-IV, Mosby, 1998.
17. Steffensen JCA, Evensen A. Bursitis retrocalcanea achili. Acta orthop. Scandinav. 27: 228, 1957–8.

# 16

# Affections of Bones and Joints

### Inflammatory
- Acute osteomyelitis
- Chronic osteomyelitis
- Acute suppurative arthritis
- Chronic suppurative arthritis
- Tuberculosis of bones and joints
- Periosteal tuberculosis
- Tuberculous spondylitis
- Syphilis of bones and joints
- Gonorrheal arthritis
- Mycotic infections

### Cervicobrachial pain syndrome
- Cervical spondylosis
- Thoracic outlet syndrome
- Periarthritis shoulder (Frozen shoulder)
- Scapulohumeral calcareous tendinitis
- Scapulocostal syndrome
- Shoulder hand syndrome
- Causalgia
- Epicondylitis (Tennis elbow)
- Carpal tunnel syndrome
- Acute suppurative tendosynovitis
- Acute stenosing tenosynovitis (de Quervain's disease)
- Trigger finger and thumb

## INFLAMMATORY

### Acute Osteomyel tis (Acute Pyogenic Infection of Bone/Acute Osteitis)

| | |
|---|---|
| Definition | It is defined as an acute inflammation of the bone due to infection. |
| Etiology | Direct: Compound fractures, penetrating wounds, operations, diagnostic procedures, e.g. intramedullary aspiration, injection. |
| | Indirect: Hematogenous (bacteremia or septicemia secondary to infective skin, upper respiratory tract (URC), genitorurinary tract. |
| Transmission | Primary: Direct intrusion of microorganisms in the bone |
| | Secondary: Hematogenous—through bloodstream (mostly through arteries). |

459

| | |
|---|---|
| Organisms | Bacteria: Staphylococcus, streptococcus, pneumococcus, gonococcus meningococcus, *haemophilus influenzae*, gram-negative bacilli, mycobacterium tuberculosis or bovis. |
| | Sceondary: Hematogenous—through bloodstream (mostly through arteries. |
| | Viruses: Smallpox, measles, mumps |
| | Fungi: Actinomyces, blastomyces, coccidioides |
| | Parasites: Echinococcus granulosus. |
| Pathogenesis | Variable with the age of the patient due to differences in the structure and blood supply at different ages. |
| | Infants and children: Metaphyseal abscess formed on the mataphyseal side of the epiphyseal plate (epiphysis mostly saved due to firm attachment of periosteum to the epiphyseal plate) ruptures the elevated periosteum to form subperiostea abscess, usually ruptures the periosteum and form the soft tissue abscess. Stripping of periosteum from the diaphyseal bone causes impaired blood supply of the bone, resulting in bone necrosis (sequestrum formation), periosteum becomes thickened (involucrum formation) perforated by cloacae, through that pus escapes and bursts through the skin, forming sinus leading down to the bone. |
| | Adults: Rare except in the spine. Spreading of subperiosteal abscess is slow because of dense bone, the spread of an abscess is usually towards the medullary canal. Sinuses formed in the cortex, resulting in formation of extraperiosteal abscess. |
| | Pathological fracture may occur due to local absorption of the cortex. |
| Diagnosis | Age—common in children |
| | Bone—tibia, femur, humerus are commonly affected |
| | Site—bone ends (metaphysis) |
| | Onset—sudden |
| | Pain—severe |
| | Fever with chills, prostration |
| | Swelling |
| | Skin—hot, red |
| | Local tenderness—over the bone |
| | Swelling of joint—absent initially, may present later on |
| | Movements—free initially, and later on may be painful and restricted |
| Investigation | CBC, hematocrit |
| | TLC and DLC—leukocytosis |
| | ESR—raised |
| | Blood culture |
| | Aspiration of lesion and smear and culture sensitivity of the aspirate |
| | Urinalysis |
| | X-ray: Normal in early cases. Later on there occurs rarefaction of the metaphysis, and subperiosteal bone formation. |
| D/d | • Suppurative arthritis |
| | • Cellulitis |

- Rheumatic fever
- Acute poliomyelitis Deormity or shortening
- Ewing's sarcoma

Complications
- Chronic osteomyelitis: Due to delayed diagnosis, waiting for manifest X-ray evidence, or inadequate early treatment
- Suppurative arthritis: Due to extension into joints
- Soft tissue abscess formation
- Pathological fracture: At the site of extensive bone necrosis
- Deformity: Due to impaired epiphysis, e.g. manus valgus
- Brodie's abscess.

Management
Principles: The possibility of acute osteomyelitis always to be kept in mind, and necessary treatment for it should start ASAP, once the provisional/clinical diagnosis is made.

General measures:

Bedrest

Immobilization—by splint, traction

Elevation of the part

Warm fomentation

Antibiotics: Bactericidal agents to be preferred

Analgesics

Fluids—orally or IV

Blood transfusion: If necessary

Surgical measures: To be avoided during first 2–3 days post onset of acute infection, esp. in infants and young children.

Procedure: Incision and drainage of abscess under general anesthesia

Indications:
- Swelling (overlying)
- Acute local tenderness: Persisting for > than 24 hours
- Fever: Persisting for > than 24 hours

Procedure: Decompression of medullary canal by bur holes

Indications: Drainage of abscess in the medullary canal

Postoperative: Immobilization by POP cast or splint, with ankle in neutral position and knee in 20 degree flexion.

## Chronic Osteomyelitis (Chronic Pyogenic Infection of Bone)

Definition
It is defined as chronic inflammation of the bone that may occur as a result of missed diagnosis or inadequate treatment of acute infection, or may occur without preceding acute infection as an indolent, slowly progressive process without any specific symptoms. It may remain quiescent for months or years, but from time to time, acute or subacute exacerbations occur.

Etiology
Chronic osteomyelitis is the reparative stage of acute Osteomyelitis, due to missed diagnosis or inadequate Treatment.

Risk factors
Anxiety, overwork, or other debilitating conditions.

| | |
|---|---|
| Diagnosis | History of trauma |
| | Symptoms and Signs: Mild and insidious: |
| | Pain: Unremitting |
| | Fever: Recurrent |
| | Swelling |
| | Skin: Redness of overlying skin |
| | Discharging sinuses: Periodic or constant discharge of pus |
| | Movements—free initially, and later on may be painful and restricted. |
| Investigation | Hemogram—anemia |
| | TLC and DLC—leukocytosis |
| | ESR—raised |
| | Blood culture |

X-ray: May show:

- A sequestrum, separated from the surface of the bone or may lie in a cavity
- Increased bone density: Due to absorption of calcium from surrounding vascularized bone
- Involucrum and new bone formation: Subperiosteal or within bone
- Resorption of sclerosed bone: healing in cancellous bone.
- CT Scan: To localize an occult infection

**D/d**
- Pathological fracture: Fatigue
- Specific infections: Tuberculosis, syphilis, mycotic
- Tumors: Benign and malignant

**Complications**
- Septic arthritis
- Amyloidosis
- Pathological fracture
- Deformity/or shortening.

**Management**
Conservative: General measures:
Bedrest
Immobilization—by splint, traction
Elevation of the part
Warm fomentation
Antibiotics
Analgesics
Fluids—orally or IV.

Surgical procedures:
- Incision and drainage of abscess.

Indications: Soft tissue abscesses.
- Sequestrectomy and curettage
- Saucerization
- Amputation: To forestall the onset of amyloid disease.

Postoperative: POP cast applied, and a window is cut over the wound for dressings.

## Acute Suppurative Arthritis

| | |
|---|---|
| Definition | It is defined as an acute inflammation of the joint due to infection. It is a serious crippling disorder, usually monoarticular and in case of polyarticular, is acute in one or more joints, while subacute or mild in others. |
| Etiology | Direct: Compound fractures involving the joint, penetrating wounds, operations, diagnostic procedures, e.g. intra-articular aspiration or injection. |
| | Local: Extension from a neighboring focus, e.g. acute arthritis of the hip joint (intra-articular) from osteomyelitis of femoral neck. |
| | Indirect: Hematogenous (bacteremia or septicemia secondary to infective skin, upper respiratory tract (URC), genitourinary tract. |
| Transmission | Primary: Direct intrusion of microorganisms into the joint |
| | Sceondary: Hematogenous—through bloodstream (mostly through arteries. |
| Organisms | • Bacteria: Staphylococcus, streptococcus, pneumococcus, gonococcus meningococcus, *haemophilus influenzae*, gram-negative bacilli, mycobacterium tuberculosis or bovis. |
| | • Viruses: Smallpox, measles, mumps |
| | • Fungi: Actinomyces, blastomyces, coccidioides |
| | • Parasites: Echinococcus granulosus. |
| Pathogenesis | Variable with the age of the patient due to differences in the structure and blood supply at different ages. |
| | Infants and children: Metaphyseal abscess formed, enters the joint (intra-articular), resulting in suppurative arthritis, articular cartilage destruction (partially or completely). Pus may spread into the muscular plane or s/c tissue. |
| Diagnosis | Age: Common in children |
| | Joint: Knee and hip are commonly affected |
| | Site: Bone ends (intra-articular) |
| | Onset: Sudden |
| | Pain: Severe |
| | Fever with chills, prostration |
| | Swelling |
| | Skin: Hot, red |
| | Local tenderness |
| Movements | Painful and restricted. |
| Investigation | CBC |
| | TLC and DLC—leukocytosis |
| | ESR—raised |
| | Blood culture |
| | Synovial fluid analysis: leukocytosis |
| | Smear and culture study of causative organism |
| | X-Ray: Normal in early cases, but later on shows the demineralization, bony erosion, narrowing of joint space, followed by osteomyelitis and periostitis |

| | |
|---|---|
| D/d | • Pneumococcal arthritis |
| | • Tuberculous arthritis |
| | • Syphilitic arthritis |
| | • Gonococcal arthritis |
| | • Rheumatoid arthritis |
| | • Hemophilic joints |
| | • Rheumatic fever |
| | • Gout |
| | • Reiter's syndrome |
| | • Traumatic synovitis |
| Complications | • Chronic arthritis due to delayed diagnosis, waiting for manifest X-ray evidence, or inadequate early treatment |
| | • Soft tissue abscess formation: pelvic abscess |
| | • Persistent infection |
| | • Pathological fracture: at the site of extensive bone necrosis |
| | • Pathological dislocation of hip |
| | • Deformity: Ankylosis (fibrous or bony), due to partial or complete destruction of articular cartilage. |
| Management | Conservative treatment: |
| | General measures: |
| | Bedrest |
| | Immobilization of joint by traction or splint |
| | Elevation of the part |
| | Warm fomentation |
| | Antibiotics |
| | Analgesics fluids: Orally or IV |
| | Surgical treatment: |
| | Aspiration of joint |
| | Incision and drainage |
| | Tarsal joints: |
| | • Aspiration: Insufficient |
| | • Drainage of choice (medial or lateral approach) |
| | Ankle: |
| | • Aspiration: Insufficient |
| | • Drainage of choice (posterolateral approach) |
| | Knee: |
| | • Aspiration: Easily aspirated (lateral side of the suprapatellar pouch) |
| | • Drainage: Anterior, posteromedial, and posteolateral approaches |
| | Hip: |
| | • Aspiration: Anterior, posterior, or lateral approaches |
| | • Drainage: Anterior, lateral, and posterior approaches |
| | Shoulder: |
| | • Aspiration: Anterior, posterior, or lateral approaches |
| | • Drainage: Anterior (preffered) or posterior approach. |

Elbow:
* Aspiration: Posterolateral approach (flexed elbow)
* Drainage: Medial or lateral approach

Wrist:
* Aspiration: Dorsal aspect (medial to snuffbox)
* Drainage: Medial, lateral, or posterior approach.

## Amputation

Indications:
* Patient's life-threatened
* Amyloidosis due to prolonged suppuration
* Painful deformity.

## Chronic Suppurative Arthritis

| | |
|---|---|
| Definition | It is defined as a polyarticular infection, characterized by slight effusion in the joints; considerable edema of the synovial membrane and the periarticular structures, and formation of adhesions and stiffness. |
| Preface | Chronic infective arthritis usually follows untreated or unsuccessfully managed acute primary or secondary infective arthritis; inadequate management is manifested by persisting infection, but the course is either intermittent or continuous one at a slow rate; may remain quiescent for months or years, but from time to time acute or subacute exacerbations recur. |
| Etiology | Untreated or unsuccessfully managed acute primary or secondary infective arthritis. |
| | Direct: Compound fractures involving the joint, penetrating wounds, operations, diagnostic procedures, e.g. intra-articular aspiration or injection. |
| | Local: Extension from a neighboring focus, e.g. acute arthritis of the hip joint (intra-articular) from osteomyelitis of femoral neck; septic wound. |
| | Indirect: Hematogenous (bacteremia or septicemia secondary to infective skin, upper respiratory tract (URC), genitourinary tract. |
| Transmission | Primary: Direct intrusion of microorganisms into the joint |
| | Sceondary: Hematogenous—through bloodstream (mostly through arteries. |
| Organisms | • Bacteria: Staphylococcus, streptococcus, pneumococcus, gonococcus meningococcus, *haemophilus influenzae*, gram-negative bacilli, mycobacterium tuberculosis or bovis. |
| | • Viruses: Smallpox, measles, mumps |
| | • Fungi: Actinomyces, blastomyces, coccidioides |
| | • Parasites: Echinococcus granulosus. |
| Pathogenesis | Pathogen/s induce a purulent inflammatory response within a joint; superinfection may occur post open surgical trauma and antibiotics; discharging sinuses |
| Diagnosis | Age: Common in adults |
| | Joint: Knee and hip are commonly affected |

|  | Site: Bone ends (intra-articular) |
|--|--|
|  | Onset: Slow |
|  | Pain: Mild to moderate, continuous |
|  | Fever: May or may not be present |
|  | Swelling |
|  | Skin: Red, grey, or pale |
|  | Local tenderness |
|  | Deformity: Increasing |
|  | Sinus/s |
|  | Movements: Painful and restricted. |
| Investigation | CBC |
|  | TLC and DLC—leukocytosis |
|  | ESR—raised |
|  | Blood culture |
|  | Synovial fluid analysis: Leukocytosis |
|  | Smear and culture study of causative organism |
|  | X-Ray: Shows demineralization; bony erosion, narrowing of joint space (progressive cartilage destruction); infarction or cavitation. |

**D/d**
- Pneumococcal arthritis
- Tuberculous arthritis
- Syphilitic arthritis
- Gonococcal arthritis
- Rheumatoid arthritis
- Hemophilic joints
- Rheumatic fever
- Gout
- Reiter's syndrome
- Traumatic synovitis

**Complications**
- Soft tissue abscess formation: pelvic abscess
- Persistent infection
- Pathological fracture: At the site of extensive bone necrosis
- Pathological dislocation of hip
- Deformity: Ankylosis (fibrous or bony), due to partial or complete destruction of articular cartilage.

**Management**

Aims:
- To eradicate infection
- To restore maximum joint function

**Conservative treatment**

General measures:

Bedrest

Immobilization of joint by traction or splint

Elevation of the part

Warm fomentation

Antibiotics

Analgesics fluids: Orally or IV

**Surgical treatment**

Aspiration of joint

Incision and drainage

Tarsal joints:
- Aspiration: Insufficient
- Drainage of choice (medial or lateral approach)

Ankle:
- Aspiration: Insufficient
- Drainage of choice (posterolateral approach)

Knee:
- Aspiration: Easily aspirated (lateral side of the suprapatellar pouch)
- Drainage: Anterior, posteromedial, and posteolateral approaches

Hip:
- Aspiration: Anterior, posterior, or lateral approaches
- Drainage: Anterior, lateral, and posterior approaches

Shoulder:
- Aspiration: Anterior, posterior, or lateral approaches
- Drainage: Anterior (preffered) or posterior approach.

Elbow:
- Aspiration: Posterolateral approach (flexed elbow)
- Drainage: Medial or lateral approach

Wrist:
- Aspiration: Dorsal aspect (medial to snuffbox)
- Drainage: Medial, lateral, or posterior approach.

Debridement of the wounds

Saucerization of the bone

Arthrodesis:

Amputation: Resection of the bone

Indications:
- Patient's life-threatened
- Amyloidosis due to prolonged suppuration
- Painful deformity.

## Tuberculosis of Bones and Joints

Definition     It is defined as an inflammation of bones and joints due to the bacterial infection (Mycobacterium tuberculosis); bone and joint tuberculosis is a slow unrelenting manifestation of a systemic disease; mostly secondary to a primary focus in the respiratory or the gastrointestinal tract.

Etiology       Mycobacterium tuberculosis (acid-fast)

Transmission   Hematogenous spread from a primary focus

Pathogenesis   Tuberculous-osteitis originates in the cancellous bone by the lodging blood borne bacilli, mostly at the ends of long bones (intra-articular); resulting in tuberculous arthritis (exception: Pott's disease of the spine), and the subperiosteal abscess formed; discharging sinuses are formed.

| | |
|---|---|
| Diagnosis | Tuberculous osteitis is insidious in its onset and course |

Site: Ends of long bones and short bones of hand and feet

Pain: Dull aching

Swelling of the bone

Weakness

Skin: Shiny, pale

Periosteum: Thickened due to edema; subperiosteal abscess may form

Sinuses: Pathognomonic

**Investigations**  CBC, ESR

Sputum tests for active tuberculosis:

- Smear microscopy for acid and alcohol, fast bacilli (AAFB)
- Nucleic acid amplification test (NAAT)
- Culture

Montoux test

Heaf test: Tuberculin injected by multiple punctures:

Report:

- A +ve reaction (induration > 10 mm) post 3/7, indicates past or current infection; but a +ve test always not confirmatory for the presence of disease and at best can be only supportive
- A-ve reaction rules out tuberculosis
- Rapid culture method like: BACTEC and mycobacterial growth indicator
- Tube (MGIT) method, continue to be costly and mostly nonavailable
- Sputum culture: Methods remain a limited option for majority of patients.
- Molecular biology techniques like: Polymerase chain reaction (PCR)
- Synovial fluid/tissue exudates analysis: Recovery of acid-fast bacilli
- Biopsy of lesion or regional lymph node: Acid-fast bacilli.

X-ray shows bone destruction (caries) seen as rarefaction of bone (thinning and erosion of bony lamellae, with a cavity containg small sequestrae); recalcification occurs at the healing stage; new bone formation and bone sclerosis are not characteristic of a tuberculous lesion, but may be seen with subsequent secondary infection.

**D/d**  Chronic osteomyelitis

Chronic pyogenic arthritis

Syphilis of bones and joints

Rheumatoid arthritis

Gouty arthritis

**Complications**
- Cold abscess
- Sinus formation
- Paraplegia (spinal tuberculosis).

**Management**  Conservative treatment:

General measures:
- Hygienic atmosphere, fresh air
- Bedrest

- Immobilization: By splint or plaster
- Diet: Balanced, nutritious
- Appropriate treatment of associated lesions (pulmonary, genito-urinary, gastrointestinal)
- Chemotherapy: Systemic administration of antitubercular agents (in combinations):

Antitubercular (AT) agents/drugs:

Primary: Isoniazid, streptomycin, PAS, ethambutol, rifampicin:

- Isoniazid (INH): Most effective drug, when used in combination with other (AT) drugs

    Dose: Adult dose: 0.60 g PO, t.i.w.

    Child dose: 10–15 mg/kg PO, t.i.w.

- Streptomycin: Less effective than isoniazid; is not used currently; except for resistant organisms

    Dose: Adult dose: 0.75–1 g (0.5 g for pts. > 50 years or < 30 kg) IM t.i.w.

    Child dose: 15 mg/kg IM, t.i.w.

    Toxicity: May cause injury to 8th cranial nerve (vertigo, deafness)

- PAS (paras-aminosalicylic acid): Less effective, but when used in combination with other (AT) drugs, it delays resistant organisms-emergence.

    Dose: 4–5 g PO, t.i.w.

- Ethambutol: Relatively safer drug; currently used as a substitute for PAS

    Dose: Adult dose: 1.20 g PO, t.i.w.

    Child dose: 30 mg/kg PO, t.i.w.

    Toxicity:

    – Affects visual activity

    – To be avoided in infants and young children.

    – Rifampin is one of the latest available (AT) drug; cost is main disadvantage

    Dose: Adult dose: 0.45–0.60 g PO, t.i.w.

    Child dose: 10–20 mg/kg PO, t.i.w.

- Pyrazinamide (PZA): Less effective than abovesaid primary (AT) drugs

    Dose: Adult dose: 1.50 g PO, t.i.w.

    Child dose: 35 mg/kg PO, t.i.w.

    Toxicity: Toxic hepatitis.

Surgical treatment: Many types of surgical treatment are required for chronic or advanced tuberculosis of bones and joints based upon the site of the lesion and the age and general condition of the patient; availability of the effective antitubercular drugs for systemic use has widened indications for synovectomy and debridement; conversely, the indication for more radical surgical procedures, e.g. arthrodesis and amputation has decreased; the supplementary chemotherapy allows healing to proceed; usually arthrodesis of the weight bearing joints is preferred in case the beneficial function cannot be salvaged.

Surgery: Various surgical measures applicable to the tuberculosis of the bones and joints are:
- Aspiration of joint:
  Indication: Synovitis in early stage
- Arthrostomy (biopsy, synovectomy, debridement, and bone grafting):
  Indication: Subacute hypertrophic lesions, involving tendon sheaths, bursae, or joints.
- Curettage or bone grafting:
  Indication: Evacuation of extra-articular bone lesions
- Excision of bones and joints:
  Indication: Extensive sinuses and secondary infection
- Arthrodesis:
  Indication: Extensive destruction of bone and cartilage
- Amputation:
  Indication: Extensive destruction of bone and cartilage.

## Regional Surgical Measures

Foot

Tuberculosis of bones of the foot may occur at any age; chronic infection is widespread in neglected cases; incidence—in descending order: calcaneus, talus, 1st metatarsal, navicular, and cuneiforms.

Curettage or bone grafting:
Indication: Evacuation of extra-articular bone lesions

Technique:
- Incision: Centered over the focus or directly through the abscess or sinus
- Curettage: Removal of devitalized tissue, esp. sequestra; avoid curetting soft bone that surrounds the cavity as it may revascularize and recalcify
- Bone grafting: Packing of cavity with cancellous bone; avoid bone grafting in case of secondary infection
- Closure of wound in absence of secondary infection; otherwise close the wound around a catheter/drain.

Excision of bones:
Indication: Extensive sinuses and secondary infection
Bones: Metatarsal, cuneiforms, navicular, cuboid, calcaneus, and talus.
Principle: Reconstructive measures combined with excision of a tarsal bone to restore normal mechanics and to provide a stable, painless weight bearing foot, e.g. when a midtarsal bone excised, then a proportionate amount of normal bone removed from the opposite side of the foot, so as to alloy proper alignment.

Excision of metatarsal:
Technique:
In presence of secondary infection:
- Incision: Longitudinal, centered over the affected bone, from the distal row of tarsal bones to the middle of proximal phalanx

- Incise: Superficial and deep fasciae between tendons, without opening their sheaths
- Exposure: Tarsometatarsal and metatarsophalangeal joints, by dividing periosteum
- Excision: The bone with intact periosteum
- Closure: Wound in layers/or pack it open with sterile gauze.

In absence of secondary infection:

- Incision: Longitudinal incision extended distally around base of the corresponding toe
- Excision: The entire ray, by dissecting metatarsal from adjoining tissues
- Divide: Nerves and tendons of toe as far as possible; and ligate vessels
- Divide: Adjacent metatarsals, for excised 2nd, 3rd, or 4th ray
- Shifting: Each bone medially or laterally to block the intervening space
- Closure: Wound in layers.

After care: Immobilize foot in a cast from toes to proximal third of leg for 3/52; walking cast with provision for weight bearing up to 8/52; walking to continue in an orthopedic shoe fitted with a steel arch support.

Excision of cuneiform bones:

Anterior tarsectomy for multi bones involvement

Technique:

- Incision: 5 cm lateral incision in the longitudinal axis of foot
- Exposure of joint between cuboid and 5th metatarsal
- Exposure of 1st cuneiform and base of 1st metatarsal through a similar medial incision
- Exposure of 2nd and 3rd cuneiforms subperiosteally
- Excision of anterior half of cuboid and three cuneiforms
- Resect: Articular cartilage from anterior surface of navicular and bases of all five matatarsals; approximate roughened cancellous surfaces of metatarsals to the navicular and cuboid
- Closure of incisional wounds.

After care: Same as for excision of navicular bone described.

## Excision of navicular:

Arthrodesis: Postnavicular excision, a midtarsal arthrodesis may be performed, so as to stabilize the foot in alignment.

Technique:

- Incision: Anterolateral, centered over the midtarsus
- Exposure: Talonavicular and naviculocuneiform joints, by dividing the capsules
- Excision of navicular bone by denuding all ligamentous attachments
- Exposure of calcaneocuboid joint by inferior and lateral dissections

- Excise: Articular cartilage and superficial bone from anterior end of calcaneus and posterior 2/3rd of cuboid
- Removal of articular cartilage of talar head and posterior surfaces of 1st and 2nd cuneiforms
- Approximate: Raw surfaces of cuboid to the calcaneus and cuneiforms to talus, obliterating space—position to be maintained by crossed threaded wires.
- Closure: Wound in layers.

After care: Immobilize foot in a cast from toes to proximal third of leg for 3/52; walking cast with provision for weight bearing up to 8/52; walking to continue in an orthopedic shoe fitted with an ankle brace for 6/12.

### Excision of cuboid:

Technique:
- Incision: Anterolateral, centered over the affected bone
- Excision: The bone, by denuding ligamentous attachments
- Resect: Articular surfaces and adjacent superficial bone from posterior aspect of cuneiforms and 5th metatarsal, and anterior surface of the calcaneus
- Excise: Navicular and articular cartilage and superficial bone from head of talus
- Approximate: Bony surfaces of cuneiforms and 5th metatarsal to talus and calcaneus
- Fixation: With crossed threaded wires to maintain position.
- Closure: Wound in layers.

After care: Immobilize foot in a cast from toes to proximal third of leg for 3/52; walking cast with provision for weight bearing up to 8/52; walking to continue in an orthopedic shoe fitted with an ankle brace for 6/12.

Excision of calcaneus:
Disability post excision of calcaneus severe, but the result preferable to that offered by amputation through leg and use of an artificial limb.

Technique:
- Incision: Kocher incision, 10 cm proximal to lateral malleolus; extend it along lateral border of tendocalcaneus to superior surface of the calcaneus; continue to inferior to the lateral malleolus, ending 2.5 cm anterior to calcaneocuboid joint.
- Incise: Fibular collateral ligament of ankle joint and displace peroneal tendons superiorly and anteriorly.
- Incise: Capsule of the calcaneocuboid joint and denude the ligamentous
- Exposure: Ligaments of sinus tarsi and other ligaments between talus and calcaneus
- Dislocate: Calcaneus at the subtalar joint; denude its attachments
- Removal of calcaneus by denuding attached soft tissue includes tendocalcaneus from it.

- Isolate: Tibial nerve and vessels on the medial side while separating ligaments
- Suture: Tendocalcaneus to the inferior surface of talus and the short muscles of foot.

After care: Immobilize foot in equines in a cast from toes to proximal third of thigh, with knee at 30 degree of flexion for 2/52; cast changed extending to knee with foot in equines for 8/52; followed by a walking boot cast, with partial weight bearing for 4/12; then a heel brace may be used for 6/12; thereafter support is discarded.

### Excision of talus:

Talus affected more often by tuberculosis (2nd to calcaneus) than any other bone of foot.

Technique:

- Incision: Kocher or anterolateral approach
- Exposure: Ankle, subtalar, and talonavicular joints; severe the capsule, and ligamentous attachments of talonavicular joint on the dorsolateral and inferior surfaces
- Divide: Fibular collateral ligament attached to lateral malleolus
- Dislocate: Ankle joint and displace medially the talus with entire foot
- Excision of the talus by denuding attached soft tissues and ligaments
- Displace: Entire foot posteriorly and insert anterior part of calcaneus between the malleoli
- Closure: Wound in layers, with foot in equines.

After care: Immobilize foot in equines in a cast from toes to proximal third of thigh, with knee at 30 degree of flexion for 2/52; cast changed extending to knee with foot in equines for 8/52; followed by a walking boot cast, with partial weight bearing for 4/12; then a heel brace may be used for 6/12; thereafter support is discarded.

Ankle

Measures/procedures:

- Immobilization + antibacterial therapy: For tuberculosis confined primarily to the synovial membrane
- Incision drainage: For abscess/s
- Curettage: For localized bone lesion
- Arthrodesis of ankle joint: For extensive destruction of bone and cartilage.

Knee

Measures/procedures:

- Immobilization + antibacterial therapy: For tuberculosis confined primarily to the synovial membrane
- Incision drainage: For extra-articular abscess/s
- Curettage: For localized bone lesion
- Synovectomy: For involved sunovium
- Arthrodesis of knee joint: For extensive destruction of bone and cartilage.

### Arthrotomy of knee

Technique:

- Incision: That opens the knee joint by the most direct approach to the bone lesion

- Evacuate: Necrotic, caseous, and purulent matter and loose bony fragments (caution: avoid curetting soft bone that adjoins the area of destruction, as it may revascularize and recalcify)
- Packing: Lesion with sterile gauze.

After care: Immobilize limb in a splint for 2/52; gauze packing removed; active exercises; weight bearing allowed as per progress.

**Hip**

Measures/procedures:

- Arthrotomy: For tuberculosis confined primarily to the synovial membrane
- Incision drainage: For abscess/s
- Synovectomy and curettage: For localized bone lesion
- Arthrodesis of hip joint: For extensive destruction of bone and cartilage (of choice).

## Arthrotomy of hip:

Technique:

- Incision: Anterolateral incision; open capsule and synovial membrane
- Excision: Portion of thickened capsule and synovial membrane
- Curettage: Foci in the femoral head, neck, or acetabulum
- Suture: Wound in layers.

After care:

- Immobilization: By traction to prevent rotation and adduction
- Exercises: Active exercises after disappearance of muscle spasm
- Weight bearing: Permitted only post radiological evidence of healing.

## Extra-articular lesions of hip:

Tuberculous foci in the os ilium above the acetabulum, may be curetted without arthrostomy of normal (spared from spread) hip

Technique:

- Incision: Anterolateral
- Dissection (under C-arm scanning): Extra-articular (outside capsule
- Curettage of lesion (cavity)
- Bone grafting: For clean case (without secondary infection): packing with cancellous bone chips
- Wound closed in layers.

After care:

- Immobilization: By traction to prevent rotation and adduction
- Exercises: Active exercises after disappearance of muscle spasm
- Weight bearing: Permitted only post radiological evidence of healing.

## Femoral neck's lesion:

To be evacuated, thus preventing spread into the hip joint

Technique:

- Incision: Lateral incision over greater trochanter and femoral shaft
- Exposure of greater trochanter and 5 cm of femoral shaft
- Window: Removed from the cortex in the subtrochanter area

- Locate: Lesion radiologically
- Curettage: Focus with a curet (protect epiphyseal plate)
- Bone grafting: Packing cavity with cancellous bone chips
- Wound closure in layers.

After care:

- Immobilization: By traction to prevent rotation and adduction
- Exercises: Active exercises after disappearance of muscle spasm
- Weight bearing: Permitted only post radiological evidence of healing.

**Arthrodesis of hip:**

Indication:

- Tuberculosis of hip joint in adults (of choice)
- Gross destruction of hip joint in children.

Surgery: Intra-articular arthrodesis

Technique:

- Incision: Anterior iliofemoral or lateral U incision
- Exposure and dislocation of hip joint
- Excise: Cartilage from the femoral head and acetabulum
- Reduction of joint to approximate osseous surfaces
- Synovectomy: For tuberculous synovium
- Resection of head and neck and a large part of acetabulum
- Denude: Trochanter and approximate it to the raw surface of the acetabulum.

Postoperative:

Fixation:

- Adults: Hip held at 20 degree of flexion
- Children: Hip held in full extension

Hip spica: Plaster cast applied from nipple line to the toes on the affected side, while above knee on the normal side; cast changed post 8/52 intervals, as per radiological findings (usually 4/12).

After care: Observation for development of deformities: for one year in case of adults, while in children to be observed for many years.

**Abscesses of hip:**

May develop during nonoperative management of tuberculosis of hip joint or postoperatively; with ruptured capsule, the abscess may be located subcutaneously: in the adductor region, anterior surface of thigh—distally to anterosuperior iliac spine, laterally over the trochanter, or in the gluteal region.

Surgery: Incision and drainage of abscess.

Technique:

- Incision: Centered over the abscess
- Drainage: And thorough irrigation of the cavity
- Closure of the wound primarily.

### Excision of hip:

Indication: In adults only for extensive destruction of femoral head and neck, and the ilium, complicated by secondary infection.

Technique:
- Incision: Ollier's lateral U incision, or Gibson's posterolateral incision
- Incise: Capsule, to excise femoral head and neck
- Removal of pathological tissue from acetabulum
- Removal portion of ilium with the acetabulum
- Reduction of trochanter into the acetabulum
- Closure of the wound around a gauze drain (to be removed post 2/52.

Postoperatively:
Immobilization: A double hip spica with the hip held in 40 degree abduction

**Note:** The results of excision of hip are far from gratifying; residual instability corrected by the Schanz osteotomy or by the arthrodesis; Girdlestone described a more extensive procedure instead of excision.

**Sacroiliac**
Tuberculosis of sacroiliac joint occurs infrequently; post antibacterial era, currently treated surgically.

Measures/procedures:
- Debridement and open drainage, Alt:
  - Dèbridement and arthrodesis

Postoperatively: Immobilization in double spica cast from nipple line to the knees for 3/12.

**Spine**
Measures/procedures:
- Drainage of abscess
- Arthrodesis.

### Tuberculous abscesses of spine:

May be palpable externally, as per their size, involved vertebrae, the adjoining fascial planes and musculature, or pressure symptoms exerted on the organs, e.g. spinal cord or pharynx.

Regional spine's abscesses:

### Tuberculous abscess/s of lumbar spine:

Lumbar/or paravertebral abscess:
Surgery: Drainage of abscess

Technique:
- Incision: 10 cm longitudinal incision, 5 cm lateral to midline and parallel to the spinous processes
- Divide: Dorsolumbar fascia in line with the incision
- Puncture: Dorsolumbar fascia with a curved hemostat; then force the hemostat along the anterior border of transverse process to encounter the abscess; evacuate the abscess thoroughly
- Closure of wound in layers.

Psoas abscess:

Surgery: Drainage of abscess

Technique:

Through Petit's triangle:

- Incision: 7.5 cm incision, 2.5 cm proximal to and parallel with the posterior crest of ilium, starting lateral to the erector spinae group of muscles, to expose the Petit's triangle
- Incise: Through the internal oblique muscle directly into the abscess; evacuate the abscess thoroughly
- Closure of wound in layers.
  Through lateral incision
- Incision: 10 cm incision along the middle 1/3rd of the iliac crest
- Releae: Attachments of internal and external oblique muscles
- Puncture: The abscess with a curved hemostat;

Caution: Avoid peritoneal rupture.

Through anterior incision

- Incision: Longitudinal, from ASIS distally for 5 cm over front of thigh
- Deepen dissection: To inner border of Sartorius muscle, to level of AIIS
- Isolate: Femoral nerve
- Puncture: The abscess with a curved hemostat, under the inguinal lig.
- Closure: Wound in layers.

Pelvic abscess

Source: In tuberculosis of lower lumbar and lumbosacral vertebrae, the abscess formed may gravitate into the pelvis, forming an abscess anterior to sacrum

Surgery: Drainage of abscess.

Technique:

- Incision: 15 cm elliptical, centered over the coccyx
- Disarticulate: Coccyx from the sacrum, by denuding its soft tissue attachments
- Puncture: The abscess with a curved hemostat, through pyramidal tunnel of sacrum
- Packing of wound with sterile gauze (changed frequently), until the wound healed up by granulation tissue from within.

## Tuberculous abscess/s of dorsal spine:

Surgery: Drainage of abscess

Technique: Costotransversectomy.

- Incision: Midline, centered over three spinous processes
- Reflect: Periosteum and soft tissue from spinous processes and laminae
- Exposure of middle transverse process and resect it at the base
- Resect: Subperiosteally medial end of rib, 5 cm from the tip of the transverse process; bevel rib's end (avoid puncturing pleura)

- Puncture: The abscess with a curved hemostat, close to vertebral body
- Closure of wound in layers.

## Tuberculous abscess/s of cervical spine:

The abscess usually presents retropharyngeally in the posterior triangle of neck, or supraclavicular region, or may gravitate to form the mediastinal abscess under the prevertebral fascia.

Surgery: Drainage of retropharyngeal abscess.

Technique:

- Incision: 7.5 cm along posterior border of sternocleidomastoid muscle at junction of its middle and upper thirds
- Incise: Superficial layer of cervical fascia; protect spinal accessory nerve
- Exposure: Levator scapulae and splenius muscles; displace internal jugular vein to expose the abscess in front of transverse process and bodies of vertebrae
- Puncture: The abscess with a curved hemostat; evacuate thoroughly
- Closure of wound in layers.

Debridement and anterior arthrodesis:

Indication: Tuberculosis of spine at any level: to evacuate pus, removal of sequestra and necrotic matter

## Technique

Cervical spine:

- Incision: Anterior approach, or Alt: 10 cm oblique incision centered over level of lesion across left sternocleidomastoid muscle
- Divide: Sternocleidomastoid muscle transversely; save accessory nerve
- Divide or denude muscles enveloping vertebrae; save vertebral artery
- Removal of pus, granulation tissue, and necrotic matter, anterior to the vertebral bodies
- Debridement of lesion
- Grafting: Packing of cavity with bony chips; Alt:
- Roughen: Lateral and anterolateral surfaces of diseased vertebral bodies; cut a groove in the vertebrae (includes healthy vertebra above and below)
- Wedging of graft: Full-thickness rib graft into the groove made.
- Closure of wound in layers.
  Postoperative:
- Immobilization: In an anterior or posterior plaster shell for 3/12; followed by ambulation in a Minerva jacket.

Dorsal spine:

- Incision: Anterolateral approach
- Exposure of ribs and transverse processes
- Resection of ribs and transverse processes
- Exposure of abscess

- Divide or denude muscles enveloping vertebrae
- Removal of pus, granulation tissue, and necrotic matter, anterior to the vertebral bodies
- Debridement of lesion
- Grafting: Packing of cavity with bony chips; Alt:
- Roughen: Lateral and anterolateral surfaces of diseased vertebral bodies; cut a groove in the vertebrae (includes healthy vertebra above and below)
- Wedging of graft: Full-thickness rib graft into the groove made.
- Closure of wound in layers.

Postoperative:
- Immobilization in an anterior or posterior plaster shell for 3/12; followed by ambulation in a Minerva jacket.

Lumbar spine:
- Incision: Left oblique abdominal incision with patient placed on the right side on a kidney rest; beginning proximally at the lateral border of the quadrates lumborum, extend it anteriorly and distally to the lateral border of rectus abdominis
- Divide or denude muscles enveloping vertebrae
- Removal of pus, granulation tissue, and necrotic matter, anterior to the vertebral bodies
- Debridement of lesion
- Grafting: Packing of cavity with bony chips; Alt:
- Roughen: Lateral and anterolateral surfaces of diseased vertebral bodies; cut a groove in the vertebrae (includes healthy vertebra above and below)
- Wedging of graft: Full-thickness rib graft into the groove made.
- Closure of wound in layers.

Postoperative:
- Immobilization: In an anterior or posterior plaster shell for 3/12; followed by ambulation in a plaster body jacket.

## Periosteal Tuberculosis

Preface  Mostly affects the flat bones (skull, sternum, and ribs); infection originates in the deeper layers of the periosteum, that becomes edematous; and then gets separated from the underlying bone by the granulation tissue; caseation and cold abscess formation may follow; superficial structures becoming progressively adherent and invaded, while the bone itself gets eroded; in case of a rib, the abscess extends along the bone to discharge at a distance from the site of origin; finally, the skin gets involved and the abscess discharges on the surface; and secondary infection may follow.

Etiology  Mycobacterium tuberculosis (acid-fast)

Transmission  Hematogenous spread from a primary focus

| | |
|---|---|
| Pathogenesis | Infection originates in the deeper layers of the periosteum, that becomes edematous; and then gets separated from the underlying bone by the granulation tissue; caseation and cold abscess formation may follow; superficial structures becoming progressively adherent and invaded, while the bone itself gets eroded; in case of a rib, the abscess extends along the bone to discharge at a distance from the site of origin; finally, the skin gets involved and the abscess discharges on the surface; and secondary infection may follow. |
| Diagnosis | Onset and course: Insidious |
| | Site: Ends of long bones and short bones of hand and feet |
| | Pain: Dull aching |
| | Swelling of the bone |
| | Weakness |
| | Skin: Shiny, pale |
| | Periosteum: Thickened due to edema; subperiosteal abscess may form |
| | Sinuses: Pathognomonic |
| Investigation | CBC, ESR |
| | Montoux-test |
| | Synovial fluid/tissue exudates analysis: Recovery of acid-fast bacilli |
| | Biopsy of lesion or regional lymph node: acid-fast bacilli X-ray shows bone destruction (caries) seen as rarefaction of bone (thinning and erosion of bony lamellae, with a cavity containg small sequestrae); recalcification occurs at the healing stage; new bone formation and bone sclerosis are not characteristic of a tuberculous lesion, but may be seen with subsequent secondary infection. |
| Management | For treating localized tuberculous lesions in a bone or joint, the orthopedic surgeon must never forget that the patient is a tuberculous one and that the systemic approach to the disease is essential; once the systemic element appears to be under control, only then local surgery to be considered; often spontaneous healing takes place post improved general physique of the patient. |

Conservative treatment:

General measures:

- Bedrest
- Immobilization: By splint or plaster
- Diet: Nutritious
- Appropriate treatment of associated lesions (pulmonary, genito-urinary, gastrointestinal)
- Chemotherapy: Systemic administration of antitubercular agents (in combinations).

Surgical treatment:

Indication: With the antibiotic coverage, surgery is indicated much earlier, and spontaneous discharging sinuses and secondary infection avoided; also the inevitable amputation may be much less so since the advent of chemotherapy (CT).

Surgerry:
- Incision and drainage of the abscess/s
- Curettage of the underlying diseased bone.

## Tuberculous Spondylitis (Syn. Pott's Disease)

| | |
|---|---|
| Definition | It is defined as the tuberculous disease of the spine, affecting any age. |
| Etiology | Infection: Mycobacterium tuberculosis |
| Pathogenesis | Originates as an osteitis in the cancellous bone of a vertebral body adjoining an intervertebral disk—that is destroyed at an early stage by extending abscess, followed by rarefaction of adjacent bone surface, vertebral bodies collapse producing kyphosis, the perispinal abscess travels along muscle planes and forms a subcutaneous cold abscess, far away from its source, abscess bursts forming a discharging sinus, resulting paraplegia due to pressure on the spinal cord by the abscess, loose fragments of dead bone or disk. |
| Investigations | X-ray spine: AP and LAT views shows: |

- Narrowing of intervertebral space
- Erosion of adjacent vertebral body: earliest definite sign
- Perispinal abscess
- Collapsed vertebrae
- Wedging of vertebrae.

| | |
|---|---|
| Management | Post diagnosis, treatment should start immediately, and status of spinal cord function to be observed carefully. |

Conservative treatment:

General measures:

Bedrest

Immobilization: On a spinal frame or in a plaster bed

Ambulation: In a brace, in late stage

Diet: Nutritious

Appropriate treatment of associated lesions (pulmonary, genitourinary, gastrointestinal)

Chemotherapy: Systemic administration of antitubercular agents (in combinations)

Surgical treatment:

Aspiration of abscess at intervals:

Indication: In early stage

Arthrodesis:

Indication: No evidence of spontaneous fusion

Technique: Posterior spinal fusion

Pott's Paraplegia: Management:

Surgery: Procedures:

- Mechanical decompression of the spinal cord
- Laminectomy
- Laminectomy with arthrodesis of spine.

Indications:
- Mechanical causes pressing cord
- Paraplegia getting worse
- Severe paraplegia of rapid onset
- Painful paraplegia
- Onset in old age.

Prognosis:
Poor: In case of flaccid paralysis or with extreme flexion contractions, with urinary retention, sensory loss in legs.

## Syphilis of Bones and Joints

| | |
|---|---|
| Preface | Syphilitis of bones and joints is defined as an inflammation of the bones and joints caused by the spirochaetal infection (Treponema pallidum), that may occur during any stage of the congenital or acquired systemic disease; tertiary lesions of syphilis that affect the joints, are seen rarely as the disease being detected early and treated effectively; syphilitic lesions of joints usually respond well to adequate chemotherapy. |
| Epidemiology | Continue to be significant problems (venereal) in certain regions of Africa and south-east Asia. |
| Etiology | Treponema pallidun (syn. Spirochaeta pallid). |
| Transmission | Hematogenous spread from a primary focus. |
| Pathogenesis | Infants: Typical manifestation of congenital syphilis is metaphysitis and epiphysitis, focal perosteal thickening about the anterior fontanel forms |

Parrot's nodes.

Childhood and adolescence: Manifestations of congenital syphilis are periostitis and osteoperiostitis, symmetrical bone involvement, and periosteal proliferation along the tibial crest forms Saber shin, painless bilateral effusion of the knees (Clutton's joints)—is a rare congenital manifestation.

Adulthood: Tertiary manifestation of congenital or acquired syphilis is Gumma formation—characterized by localized bone destruction with surrounding areas of sclerosis (periostitis, osteitis, and arthritis); the periosteal nodes; transitory and symmetrical effusions in larger joints; pathological fractures occurring due to the structural weakening caused by destruction and rarefaction.

Diagnosis    Congenital syphilis:
- Clutton's joints: Bilateral, painless hydrops of knee in a child.

Acquired syphilis:
- Secondary stage: Arthralgia and hydrarthrosis (fleeting bone pains due to periostitis)
- Tertiary stage: Diffuse periosteal gumma, usually form in the tibia, clavicle, and manubrium.

Lesion: Painless, symmetrical hydrops with free and painless mobility (pathognomonic).

| | |
|---|---|
| Investigation | X-ray: Syphilitic osteitis not diagnostic, while bone production is more pronounced than bone destruction<br>CBC: Leukocytosis<br>Serological test: Wassermann's reaction+ve. |
| Management | The only local treatment that is mandatory for the skeletal lesion is immobilization to provide comfort or protection from fracture of weak osteoporotic bone; lesions of bones and joints respond markedly and promptly to adequate chemotherapy of the systemic disease. |

### Conservative treatment
Preventive measures:
- To avoid sex with an unknown person
- To use condom prior to sexual act
- To maintain good hygiene
- Antibiotic: Procain penicillin 2.4 million units IM in each buttock od.

Systemic measures:
- Antibiotic: Benzyl penicillin (penicillin G)

### Surgical treatment:
Indications:
- Residual disability of joints due to destruction

Surgery: Procedures:
- Synovectomy for thickened synovial membrane
- Arthrodesis for destroyed articular surfaces of the joint.

## Gonorrheal Arthritis

| | |
|---|---|
| Preface | Gonorrheal arthritis (syn. gonococcal arthritis; and gonorrheal rheumatism), is defined as an acute inflammatory disorder caused by *Neisseria gonorrhoeae*, that is secondary to genitourinary infection; encountered more commonly in women having occult genitourinary infections, and occasionally in children; symptoms pertaining to the musculoskeletal system usually occur post 3/52 of primary infection; manifested in various forms ranging from arthralgia to acute arthritis; suppuration not a common feature; may be monoarticular (knee or elbow), or polyarticular (small/or large). |
| Etiology | Infective: Secondary to genitourinary infection.<br>Bacteriology: *Neisseria gonorrhoeae* (Gram – ve diplococci) |
| Pathogenesis | Joint infection via bloodstream; synovitis with effusion; purulent exudate; destroyed cartilage; fibrous/or bony ankylosis; tenosynovitis of wrist. |
| Diagnosis | Male: (2/52 post sexual intercourse with an infected partner): |

- Itching, burning sensation
- Polyuria: Frequency/or urgency
- External urethral meatus: Balanitis (reddish, sticky lips)
- Discharge: Purulent per urethrum, dysuria
- Prostatitis, proctitis
- Joint/s: Arthralgia, swelling, tendered, ankylosed, movements painful and restricted.

Female: (Early symptoms less pronounced than in the male):
- Discomfort of the vulva (burning sensation)
- Urethritis
- Dysuria
- Cervicitis
- Vaginitis, bartholinitis, salpingitis, proctitis
- Discharge: Blood stained discharge P/v
- Backache
- Joint/s: Arthralgia, swelling, tendered, ankylosed, movements painful and restricted.

| | |
|---|---|
| Investigation | CBC, ESR |
| | Blood culture |
| | Synovial fluid analysis: Culture, complement fixation test |
| D/d | Nongonococcal urethritis (chlamydiae, mycoplasmas) |
| | RA |
| | Suppurative arthritis |
| | Reiter's disease |
| | Gout |
| Management | Preventive treatment: |
| | Sexual abstinence |
| | Condom: To be used properly |
| | Drugs: To be taken within 24 hours. |
| | Systemic treatment: |

- Procaine penicillin G 4.8 million units IM into each buttock od; Alt:
- Ampicillin 3.5 g PO + probenecid 1 g PO, Alt:
- Tetracycline 1.5 g PO stat, then 0.5 g PO qds

Local treatment:
- Immobilization of joint by splintage
- Diathermy: SWD or IR

Surgical treatment:
Aspiration of joints
After care: Physiotherapy: exercises.

## Mycotic infections of Bones and Joints

| | |
|---|---|
| Preface | Fungus infections of bones and joints are usually secondary to a primary infection I another organ system, mostly the lower pulmonary tract; although bones and joints have a predilection for the cancellous ends of long bones and the vertebral bodies, the main lesion—a granuloma with varying degrees of necrosis and abscess formation—does not form a characteristic clinical picture. |

### Coccidioidomycosis

| | |
|---|---|
| Preface | It is defined as a fungal infection of bones and joints; usually secondary to the primary (pulmonary infection); initial phase of pulmonary infection is characterized by arthralgia, periarticular swelling (esp. of |

knees and ankles); osseous lesions usually occur in the cancellous bone of the vertebrae or adjoining ends of long bones

| | |
|---|---|
| Etiology | Mycotic infection (coccidioidomycosis) |
| Pathogenesis | Villonodular synovitis; granulomatous lesions in cancellous bone of vertebrae or near ends of long bones; local bone atrophy; focal destruction (cystic); abscess formation; sinus formation. |
| Diagnosis | Pain |
| | Swelling |
| | Local tenderness |
| | Skin: Reddish |
| | Arthritis septic arthritis |
| | Abscess |
| | Sinus formation |
| Investigation | CBC, ESR |
| | Complement fixation test |
| | Microscopic appearance: Spherules containing endospores |
| | Culture of synovial fluid for detection of coccidioides immitis |
| | X-rays of bone: Rarefaction simulate those of tuberculosis. |
| Management | Conservative treatment: |
| | Immobilization of joints by splint/plaster cast |
| | Avoid weight bearing |
| | Antibiotics: Amphotericin B |
| | Surgical treatment: Procedures: |

- Surgery: Curettage or saucerization
  Indication: Chronic infection of bone
- Surgery: Amputation
  Indication: Progressive stubborn bone infection
- Surgery: Synovectomy
  Indication: More advanced joint infections

Surgery: Debridement of the local lesion.
Indication: More advanced joint infection
Afer care: Physiotherapy: execises.

## Histoplasmosis

| | |
|---|---|
| Preface | It is defined as a fungal infection of the bones and joints; is rare; usually secondary to the primary (pulmonary infection); skeletal lesions may be single or multiple; initial phase of pulmonary infection is characterized by arthralgia, periarticular swelling (esp. of knees and ankles); osseous lesions usually occur in the cancellous bone of the vertebrae or adjoining ends of the long bones; the granulomatous lesions are not characteristic. |
| Etiology | Mycotic infection (histoplasmosis) |
| Pathogenesis | Villonodular synovitis; granulomatous lesions in cancellous bone of vertebrae or near ends of the long bones are not characteristic; local one atrophy; focal destruction (cystic); abscess formation; sinus formation. |

| | |
|---|---|
| Diagnosis | Pain |
| | Swelling |
| | Local tenderness |
| | Skin: Reddish |
| | Arthritis septic arthritis |
| | Abscess |
| | Sinus formation |
| Investigation | CBC, ESR |
| | Complement fixation test |
| | Microscopic appearance: Spherules containing endospores |
| | Culture of synovial fluid for detection of coccidioides immitis |
| | X-rays of bone: Rarefaction simulate those of tuberculosis |
| Management | Conservative treatment: |
| | Immobilization of joints by splint/plaster cast |
| | Avoid weight bearing |
| | Analgesics/NSAIDs |
| | Antibiotics: Amphotericin B |
| | Surgical treatment: Procedures: |

- Surgery: Curettage/or saucerization
  Indication: Chronic infection of bone
- Surgery: Amputation
  Indication: Progressive stubborn bone infection
- Surgery: Synovectomy
  Indication: More advanced joint infections

Surgery: Debridement of the focal lesion.
Indication: More advanced joint infection
Afer care: Physiotherapy: Execises.

## CERVICOBRACHIAL PAIN SYNDROMES

| | |
|---|---|
| Preface | Cervicobrachial pain syndromes include a large number of articular and extra-articular disorders; characterized by the pain that may involve simultaneously the neck, shoulder girdle, and upper limb; diagnostic differentiation is usually difficult; while some of these disorders and clinical syndromes represent primary disorders of the cervicobrachial region, others are local manifestations of systemic diseases; the clinical picture becomes further complicated when two or more of these disorders occur coincidentally. |
| Classification | Some of the more common disorders are: |

- Cervical spondylosis (syn. Degenerative arthritis)
- Periarthritis shoulder (syn. Scapulohumeral, Frozen shoulder)
- Scapulohumeral calcareous tendinitis
- Scapulocostal syndrome
- Shoulder-hand syndrome
- Causalgia (syn. Reflex sympathetic dystrophy)
- Epicondylitis (syn. Tennis elbow)
- Carpal tunnel syndrome.

## Cervical Spondylosis (Syn. Degenerative Arthritis)

| | |
|---|---|
| Definition | It is defined as a degenerative condition characterized by degeneration of the intervertebral disks with the formation of bony ridges running across the anterior surface of the neural canal, and the formation of ostyeophytes from the neurocentral joints of Luschka that project backwards into the intervertebral foramen; condition may be symptomless or may cause neurological symptoms. |
| Etiology | Direct trauma: Violence |
| | RSA |
| | Fall from a height |
| | Degenerative: Osteoarthritis |
| Pathogenesis | Progressive thinning of articular cartilage; subchondral osteosclerosis; osteophytic proliferation around the joint margins of cervical spine. |
| Diagnosis | Initially spinal pain may have specific and nonspecific features, including fever, night sweats, weight loss, progressive pain; chronic spondylotic symptoms due to whiplash injuries; later on radicular symptoms and signs develop due to progressive degenerative process (Table 16.1). |
| | Age: Common in persons above 35 years. |
| | Pain: Referred in the occipital or post-auricular areas and between the shoulder blades |
| | Swelling: Over nape of neck |
| | Numbness of arms and fingers |
| | Movements of neck and shoulder painful and restricted. |
| Investigation | X-rays cervical spine—AP and LAT views: shows: |
| | • Straightening of spine (an early finding is loss of normal anterior convexity of the cervical curve; reduced disk space |
| | • Reduced disk space/s |
| | • Osteophyte formation (a late finding). |
| | MRI: To demonstrate nerve root or spinal cord compression. |
| D/d | Cervicobrachial pain syndromes |
| | RA |
| | AS |
| | Cervical sprains (whiplash injuries) |
| | Bone tumors (Primary and Secondary) |

**Table 16.1:** Radicular symptoms and signs of progressive spondylosis

| Level | Pain radiation | Sensory loss | Motor loss | Reflex loss |
|---|---|---|---|---|
| C4 | Neck to outer shoulder, arm | Shoulder | Deltoid | N/A |
| C5,6 | Outer arm to thumb, Index finger | Index finger, thumb | Biceps, wrist externsors | Biceps, triceps, supinator |
| C7 | Outer arm to middle Finger | Index, middle finger | Triceps | Triceps |
| C8 | Inner arm to ring, little finger | Ring, little finger | Hand muscles | Finger jerks may be brisk |

| Management | Patient's education: Key to treating cervical spondylotic symptoms, i.e. to know that pain does not signify ongoing tissue inflammation or damage |
|---|---|

Conservative treatment:

Ice packs or warm fomentation, SWD, or IR therapy

Cervical collar: For short (2/52) period to avoid muscle trophy

Cervical brace

Cervical traction: Continuous or periodic

Analgesics + NSAIDs

Physiotherapy and exercises: Isometric and other exercises to maintain muscle power and flexibility of neck muscles.

### Surgical treatment

Indication:

- Persistent pain in the occipital and posterior auricular areas surgery: Excision of involved nerves
- Persistent pain in the lower cervical region

  Surgery: Arthrodesis (bone grafting—paraspinal inlay) to immobilize joints
- Bony ridges (on the anterior surface of cord) to cause neurological symptoms and spasticity (disk lesion)

  Surgery: Division of dentate ligaments
- Intraforaminal compression by osteophytes to cause compression of multiple nerve roots

  Surgery: Nerve roots decompression by hemifacetectomy.

  After care:
  - To wear collar for 1/12
  - Exercises of neck to be started ASAP.

## Thoracic Outlet Syndrome

| Definition | It is defined as a syndrome that includes disorders characterized by varied manifestations that are caused by compression of the neurovascular structures supplying the upper limb: |
|---|---|

- Cervical rib syndrome
- Costoclavicular syndrome
- Scalenus anticus and medius syndromes
- Pectoralis minor syndrome
- Wright's syndrome

| Etiology | Congenital |
|---|---|

Traumatic

Inflammatory

Degenerative

Neoplastic

Predisposing factors:

Age: Elderly

Faulty posture

|                  | Occupational |
|                  | Chronic illness |
| Pathogenesis     | |
| Diagnosis        | Pain: Radiate to the nape of neck, axilla, shoulder girdle, arm, forearm and hand |
|                  | Paresthesia: Volar aspect of 4th and 5th digits; sensory symptoms may be aggravated at night or by strenuous exercises |
|                  | Muscular weakness and atrophy |
|                  | Vascular: Pallor of fingers on elevation of the arm, cold sensitivity; digits gangrene. |
|                  | Reflexes: Deep reflexes unaffected. |
| Investigation    | X-rays: Most helpful in differential diagnosis |
|                  | Color Doppler: Arterial and venous: to locate site of obstruction |
|                  | Nerve conduction: To localize the site of nerve compression. |
| D/d              | Osteoarthritis of cervical spine |
|                  | Periarthritis of shoulder |
|                  | Cervicobrachial pain syndromes. |
| Management       | Conservative treatment: |
|                  | Rest |
|                  | To avoid strenuous exercises aggravating the condition |
|                  | To improve posture |
|                  | Analgesics/NSAIDs |
|                  | Surgical treatment: More likely to relieve neurological rather than the vascular component causing symptoms. |
|                  | Indication: Failure of conservative measures |
|                  | Surgery: Decompression of nerves. |

## Periarthritis Shoulder (Syn. Scapulohumeral, Frozen Shoulder)

| Definition    | It is defined as an inflammatory disorder of multiple etiology involving primarily the soft tissue |
| Etiology      | Primary: Idiopathic |
|               | Secondary: |
|               | • Traumatic: Fracture or dislocation |
|               | • Inflammatory: RA |
|               | • Degenerative: OA |
|               | • Pulmonary tuberculosis |
|               | • Cervical radiculopathy |
|               | • Apical lung tumors. |
| Pathogenesis  | Synovitis; tendinitis; inflamed ligaments, capsule, bursae, and the bicipital tendon sheath; calcareous tendinitis; rotator cuff attrition. |
| Diagnosis     | Age and sex: Common in women post 5th decade |
|               | Pain: Acute or insidious; worst at night; aggravated by joint motion. |
|               | Local tenderness: +ve over greater trochanter or bicipital groove |
|               | Movements of shoulder joint painful and restricted. |

| | |
|---|---|
| Investigation | X-rays of shoulder—AP and LAT views |
| Management | Aims: Pain relief, restoration of movement, and treatment of underlying cause. |

Conservative treatment:
- Rest
- To avoid strenuous exercises aggravating the condition
- To improve posture
- Analgesics/NSAIDs

Surgical treatment: More likely to relieve neurological rather than the vascular component causing symptoms.

Indication: Failure of conservative measures

Surgery: Exploration.

## Scapulohumeral Calcareous Tendinitis

| | |
|---|---|
| Definition | It is defined as acute or chronic inflammatory disorder of the rotator cuff (capsule-tendinous—esp. supraspinatous part); characterized by the deposit of calcium salts (usually hydroxyapatite) in the tendon fibers; the calcium deposit may be restricted to the tendon substance, or may rupture into the overlying subacromial bursa. |
| Etiology | Traumatic |
| | Inflammatory |
| | Degenerative |
| Pathogenesis | Calcium salts deposits in the rotator cuff (capsule-tendinous. |
| Diagnosis | Age and sex: Common in females above the age of 30 years. |
| | Pain: Severe or subacute onset with progressive worsening at night; diffuse or localized over the humeral head; may radiate to nape of neck and deltoid area |
| | Local tenderness |
| | Movements of shoulder painful and restricted. |
| Inveatigation | X-rays shoulder—AP and LAT views: may show calcified deposits in the shoulder cuff. |
| Management | Depends on the clinical presentation; also influenced by the presence of impingement. |

Conservative treatment:

Warm fomentation

Occupational: To avoid strenuous exercises

Analgesics + NSAIDs

Local corticosteroids

Surgical treatment:

Indication: Failure of conservative measures

Surgery: Removal of calcific deposits by open or arthroscopic surgery.

## Scapulocostal Syndrome

| | |
|---|---|
| Definition | It is defined as acute or chronic inflammatory disorder characterized by fatigue associated with habitually faulty posture that exerts tension |

on the deep cervical fascia and adjoining muscles, causing pain in the posterior cervical region.

| | |
|---|---|
| Etiology | Traumatic |
| | Inflammatory |
| | Degenerative |
| Pathogenesis | Spasmodic muscles attached to the vertebral border of scapula. |
| Diagnosis | Age and sex: Common in females above the age of 30 years. |
| | Pain: Severe or subacute onset with progressive worsening at night; diffuse or localized; may radiate to occiput, vertebral border of the scapula, and down the arm and forearm to the ulnar side of the hand, or to the region of 4th and 5th ribs posteriorly. |
| | Local tenderness |
| | Movements of shoulder painful and restricted. |
| Investigation | X-rays shoulder—AP and LAT views: may show degenerative changes; soft tissue calcification calcified deposits in the shoulder cuff. |
| Management | Depends on the clinical presentation; also influenced by the presence of impingement. |

Conservative treatment:
Warm fomentation
Occupational: To avoid strenuous exercises
Analgesics + NSAIDs
Local corticosteroids

Surgical treatment:
Indication: Failure of conservative measures

Surgery:
- Exploration
- Removal of underlying cause.

## Shoulder Hand Syndrome

| | |
|---|---|
| Definition | It is defined as a variable complex of symptoms and signs occurring from various painful disorders of the shoulder joint and hand of the same limb; is a manifestation of reflex neurovascular dystrophy; is essentially a combination of scapulohumeral periarthritis and Sudeck's atrophy of the hand and wrist. |
| Etiology | Traumatic |
| | Inflammatory |
| | Degenerative |
| Pathogenesis | Reflex neurovascular dystrophy; scapulohumeral periarthritis. |
| Diagnosis | Age: Common in middle age group. |
| | Pain: Severe or subacute onset with progressive worsening at night; diffuse or localized; may radiate to arm, forearm, and hand |
| | Local tenderness |
| | Movements of shoulder painful and restricted. |
| Investigation | X-rays shoulder—AP and LAT views: may show calcified deposits in the shoulder cuff. |

| Management | Depends on the clinical presentation; also influenced by the presence of impingement. |
|---|---|
| | Conservative treatment: |
| | Warm fomentation |
| | Occupational: To avoid strenuous exercises |
| | Analgesics + NSAIDs |
| | Local corticosteroids |
| | Surgical treatment: |
| | Indication: Failure of conservative measures |
| | Surgery: |
| | • Exploration |
| | • Removal of calcific deposits by open or arthroscopic surgery. |

## Causalgia (Syn. Post-traumatic/Reflex Sympathetic Dystrophy)

| Definition | It is defined as an uncommon pain syndrome that affects either the lower or upper limb. |
|---|---|
| Etiology | Unknown |
| Predisposing factors: | • Traumatic: In upper limb: Usually due to the complete/or incomplete laceration of the median nerve or brachial plexus |
| Pathogenesis | Calcified deposits into the subacromial bursa |
| Diagnosis | Pain: Severe, burning, often paroxysmally precipitated by friction, worse at night |
| | Local tenderness |
| | Hyperesthesia |
| | Vasomotor: Skin warm, dry, swollen, and red or cyanotic, nails ridged |
| | Spasm: Affected limb held in position by spasmodic muscles |
| | Joints: Held in deformed position |
| | Movements of shoulder joint painful and restricted. |
| Investigation | X-ray shows: Calcified deposits |
| Management | Conservative treatment: |
| | Warm fomentation |
| | Physiotherapy: Active and passive exercises |
| | Analgesics + NSAIDs |
| | Local corticosteroids |
| | Surgical treatment: |
| | Indication: Failure of conservative measures |
| | Surgery: |
| | • Sympathetic blocks (Stellate ganglion or lumbar), Alt: |
| | • Sympathectomy |
| | • Exploration; removal of calcified deposits. |

## Epicondylitis (Syn. Tennis Elbow)

### Tennis Elbow (Lateral Epicondylitis)

| Definition | It is defined as a single or multiple clinical disorders; some defined and some vague, that cause pain and local tenderness in the lateral epicondyle of the elbow. |
|---|---|

| Etiology | Traumatic: Direct violence |
| | RSA |
| | Occupational: Strain |
| | Inflammatory |
| MOI | Abrupt pronation of the forearm, causing strain on the extensor aponeurotic fibers. |
| Pathogenesis | Periostitis due to repeated strains; small tears (single or multiple) in the conjoined tendon of origin of extensor muscles of forearm |
| Diagnosis | Pain: Over the outer aspect of the elbow |
| | Local tenderness—over lateral epicondyle |
| | Movements: Passive pronation to the full extent exaggerate pain. |
| Investigation | X-ray elbow—AP and LAT views. |
| Management | Conservative treatment: |
| | Rest |
| | Diathermy: SWD or IR |
| | Elbow support |
| | Local: Inj. Hydrocortisone 25–50 mg + Inj. Lignocain 2%. |

Surgical treatment:
Surgery: Release of extensor aponeurosis.

Technique:
- Incision: 8 cm posterolateral centered over the lateral; epicondyle, extending distally along the extensor aponeurosis
- Release: The fibrous part of the aponeurosis from its lateral epicondyle origin, and retract it distally; free it from underlying joint capsule and the lateral collateral and annular ligaments
- Exposure: Radial head and the radiohumeral joint by pronating and supinating the forearm
- Release: Insertion of annular ligament from ulna
- Divide: 0.5 cm of the lateral epicondyle, and bevel the surface by rasp
- Reattach: Extensor aponeurosis to the soft tissue of lateral epicondyle
- Closure of the wound.

Postoperatively: immobilization: by a posterior POP splint for 2/52.
After care: Exercises.

**Refer:** To the next fracture clinic.

## Acute Carpal Tunnel Syndrome (Syn. Tardy Median Nerve Palsy)

| Definition | It is defined as a space occupying lesion due to the median nerve compression in the wrist at the level of carpal tunnel; any condition that reduces the space of the carpal canal may initiate the symptoms. |
| Etiology | Traumatic: |
| | RSA |
| | Sports injury |
| | Falls from a height |
| | Occupational: Lifting heavy weight |

| | Inflammatory: Tenosynovitis |
|---|---|
| | Degenerative: Osteoarthritis. |
| Diagnosis | Usually a middle aged female |
| | Pain—severe, burning or severe pins and needles in the hand and fingers |
| | Paresthesiae in the median nerve distribution—may be chief symptom |
| | Morning stiffness of fingers |
| | Tinel's sign +ve. |
| Investigation | X-ray of hand—AP and LAT views. |
| Management | Conservative treatment: |
| | Indication: Mild S/S present for < 2/12 |
| | Treatment: Inj. Hydrocortisone 25–50 mg weekly into the carpal tunnel |
| | Surgical treatment: |
| | Indication: Severe and progressive S/S |
| | Procedure: Decompression of the tunnel by a longitudinal ventral incision (division of the deep transverse carpal ligament). |

## Acute Suppurative Tendosynovitis

| Definition | It is definerd as an acute inflammation of a tendon sheath, following suppuration from wounds (extension from whitlows, or systemic); severe pain resulting from a movement that causes the tendon to glide in its sheath; suppuration caused by a virulent organism may rapidly extends along the tendon sheath; may result in sloughing of tendons if not adequately treated. |
|---|---|
| Etiology | Traumatic |
| | RSA |
| | Sports injury |
| | Fall from a height |
| | Inflammatory: Wounds, bursitis, tuberculosis. |
| Diagnosis | Pain: Severe |
| | Swelling |
| | Local tenderness |
| | Movements: Painfull |
| | Sloughing of tendons. |
| Investigation | CBC, ESR |
| | X-ray of hand—AP and LAT views |
| | Culture of aspirated fluid/pus |
| Management | Conservative treatment: |
| | Antibiotics |
| | Analgesics and NSAIDs |
| | Immobilization: Splintage of the affected part. |
| | Surgical treatment: |
| | Surgery: Incision drainage of the affected tendon sheath. |

## Acute Stenosing Tenosynovitis (De Quervain's Disease)

| Definition | It is defined as a fibrous thickening of a tendon sheath, mostly the tendon sheaths of abductor policis longus and extensor pollicis brevis, |
|---|---|

|               |                                                                                  |
|---------------|----------------------------------------------------------------------------------|
|               | at the level of outer aspect of the radial styloid (esp. those who use their thumbs excessively, e.g. washerwomen/men wringing clothes) |
| Etiology      | Traumatic: RSA, sports injury, falls, lifting heavy weight                       |
|               | Inflammatory: Bursitis                                                            |
|               | Degenerative: Osteoarthritis.                                                     |
| Investigation | X-ray of hand—AP and LAT views.                                                  |
| Management    | Conservative treatment:                                                          |
|               | Shortwave, infrared therapy                                                      |
|               | Analgesics, NSAIDs                                                               |
|               | Exercises                                                                        |
|               | Surgical treatment:                                                              |
|               | Surgery: Incision of the thickened tendon sheath.                                |

## Trigger Finger and Thumb

|               |                                                                                  |
|---------------|----------------------------------------------------------------------------------|
| Definition    | It is defined as a clinical condition characterized by difficulty in flexing or extending the affected finger or thumb beyond a certain position, due to involvement of the flexor tendons of the finger or thumb. |
| Etiology      | Traumatic: violence                                                              |
|               | RSA                                                                              |
|               | Sports injury                                                                    |
|               | Inflammatory                                                                     |
| Pathogenesis  | Thickening of flexor tendon or a constriction in the tendon sheath, while entering the fibro-osseous tunnel at the level of the MCP (metacarpophalangeal) joint. |
| Diagnosis     | Age: infants—often affects several fingers of both hands; adults—usually affects a single finger or thumb |
|               | Deformity: Difficulty in flexing/or extending the affected finger; snapping/or triggering of distal joint (little force-suddenly releases the finger with a click |
|               | A nodule: Palpated opposite the MP joint of the affected finger.                 |
| Investigation | X-ray hand—AP and LAT views.                                                     |
| Management    | Conservative treatment:                                                          |
|               | Active exercises                                                                 |
|               | Analgesics and NSAIDs                                                            |
|               | Surgical treatment:                                                              |
|               | Surgery: Slitting the fibro-osseous tunnel at the level of constriction.         |
|               | Postoperative: Active exercises.                                                 |

## Bibliography

1. Aegerter E. Kirkpatrick JA. Orthopedic diseases, W.B. Saunders Co., Philadelphia, 1958.

2. Anderson LD. Miscellaneous affections of joints: Campbell's Operative Orthopaedics, ed. 9th, Vol I-IV, C. V. Mosby Co., Saint Louis, 1998.

3. Bailey and Love's Short Practice of Surgery (1965) Love M, Rains A.J. H., Capper W.M.; H.K. Lewis and Co., London.

4. Basom WC. Tuberculous osteomyelitis of the shafts of the long bones, Proc. Staff Meet. Mayo Clin. 16:397, 1941.

5. Bickel WH, Bateman JG, Johnson WE. Treatment of chronic hematogenous osteomyelitis by means of saucerization and bone grafting, Surg., Gynec. and Obst. 96:265, 1953.

6. Blanche DW. Osteomyelitis in infants, J. Bone and Joint Surg. 34-A:71, 1952.

7. Buchman J. Osteomyelitis, American Academy of Orthopaedic Surgeons Instructional Course Lectures, vol. XVI, C.V. Mosby Co., St Louis, 1959.

8. Calandruccio A. Miscellaneous affections of bones: Campbell's Operative Orthopaedics, ed. 9th, Vol I-IV, C. V. Mosby Co., Saint Louis, 1998.

9. Campbell's Operative Orthopaedics (1998) 9th Ed. Vol I-IV. Canale S. Terry, Daugherty K, and Jones Linda. Mosby.

10. Canale ST, et al. Campbell's Operative Orthopaedics, ed. 9th, Vol I-IV. C.V. Mosby Co., Saint Louis, 1998.

11. Clark JMP. Modern Trends in Orthopedics Fracture Treatment (1962); Butterworths, London.

12. Clark JMP. Modern Trends in Orthopedics Fracture Treatment, Butterworths, London, 1962.

13. Conner CL. Monilia from osteomyelitis, J.Infect. Dis. 43:108, 1928.

14. Crenshaw AH. Tuberculosis. Campbell's Operative Orthopaedics, ed. 4th, Vol II, C.V. Mosby Co., Saint Louis, 1998 p 942.

15. Crooks F, Birkett AN. Fractures and Fracture-dislocations of the Cervical Spine. Brit. J. Surg 1944: 31: 252.

16. Dykes J, Segesman JK, Birsner JW. Coccidioidomycosis of bone in children, A.M.A. Am. J. Dis. Child. 85:34, 1953.

17. Garcia A, et al. Hematogenous pyogenic vertebral osteomyelitis, J. Bone and Joint Surg. 42-A:429, 1960.

18. Kapoor PS. Accident and Emergency: Etiology, Diagnosis and Management (2016) 2nd Ed. CBS, New Delhi.

19. Kapoor PS. Osteoarthritis. Accident and Emergency, ed. 2nd, Part I, CBS, New Delhi, 2016.

20. Key JA. Amputation for chronic osteomyelitis, J. Bone and Joint Surg. 26: 350, 1944.

21. Love M, et al. Bailey and Love's Short Practice of Surgery, ed. 13th, H.K. Lewis and Co., London, 1965.

22. Mc Rae R. Practical Fracture Treatment (1981) 1st Ed. Churchill Livingstone.

23. Mc Rae R. Practical Fracture Treatment, ed. 1st, Churchill Livingstone, 1981.

24. Mercer W. Orthopaedic Surgery, 4th Ed., Williams and Wilkins Co., Baltimore, 1950.

25. Morse TS, Pryles CV. Infections of the bones and joints in children, New England J. Med. 262:846, 1960.

26. Murray DuBose, Young Bennett H. Osteogenesis imperfect treated by fixation with intramedullary rod, South. M. J. 53:1142, 1960.

27. Shannon JG, Woolhouse FM. Treatment of chronic bone infection, J. Bone and Joint Surg. 36-A, 841, 1954.

28. Speed JS, Boyd HB. Bone syphilis, South. M. J. 29:371, 1936.

29. Wishner JG. Chronic sclerosing osteomyelitis (Garr'e), J. Bone and Joint Surg. 15:723, 1933.

# 17

# Arthritis and Allied Rheumatic Diseases

- Rheumatoid arthritis
- Ankylosing spondylitis (AS)
- Acute gout
- Acute low backache
- Acute sciatica
- Prolapse intervertebral disk (PIVD)
- Reiter's syndrome
- Rheumatic fever
- Systemic lupus erythematosus (SLE)
- Raynaud's disease
- Progressive systemic sclerosis (Scleroderma)
- Sjogren's (Sicca) syndrome
- Wegener's syndrome

## Rheumatoid (Syn. Atrophic) Arthritis

| | |
|---|---|
| Definition | It is a chronic inflammatory disease, characterized by symmetric polyarthritis often leading to serious morbidity. |
| | Incidence: 1 to 3% in general population |
| | Sex : Female : Male 3:1 |
| | Age : 20–40 |
| Etiology | Unknown. |
| Possibility | May be due to autoimmunity, or infection |
| Diagnosis | Diagnostic criteria of Rheumatoid Arthritis, based on American Rheumatology Association: At least 4 of 7 criteria are required to diagnose a patient as having rheumatoid arthritis. Failure to meet these criteria esp. during early phases of the disease does not rule out the diagnosis. |
| Criteria | 1. Morning stiffness |
| | 2. Symmetric joint swelling |
| | 3. Arthritis of hand joints, e.g. PIP, MCP, wrist |
| | 4. Arthritis of toes, ankles, knees |
| | 5. Subcutaneous nodule over bony extensor aspects |
| | 6. Rheumatoid factor—Positive |
| | 7. Radiologic changes |

Other Sign/Symptoms:
- Warmth
- Local tenderness
- Fever, malaise, loss of weight
- Sweating
- Paresthesia
- Scleritis, iritis.

**Investigation**    CBC, ESR
- Rheumatoid factor (Latex Particle Agglutination)
- Immunoglobulin (Quantitative)—IgA, IgM, IgG
- X-Ray wrists and hands: Early changes seen are osteoporosis around the affected joint and erosion of cartilage at the periphery of the joint surface.

**Management**    The treatment is unsatisfactory. Till date any specific treatment of Rheumatoid arthritis not available.

Conservative measures:

Rest: Complete bedrest indicated in patients with profound systemic and articular involvement, while in mild cases: few hours rest may suffice, allowing patient to continue his routine work, while avoiding strenuous activities.

Heat and cold: Used for their muscle relaxant and analgesic effect.
- Infrared and short-wave therapy—very effective
- Even cold application helps in relief of pain.

Drugs:

1. Nonsteroidal anti-inflammatory drugs (NSAID) with or without analgesics form the mainstay of therapy of RA.

   Action: By inhibiting cyclooxygenase (COX) these NSAID reduce the synthesis of prostaglandins (main mediators of inflammation). But these NSAID provide only symptomatic relief and do not cure or alter the disease process.

   Variety of NSAID: Almost equally effective and is advisable not to change NSAID frequently, as response may take sometime to be seen

   Combinations of NSAID—may better be avoided

   Elderly patients—more prone to side effects

   Side effects—GI tract disturbances. Can be minimized by use of antacids

2. Analgesics—Paracetamol or dextropropoxyphene

3. Corticosteroiods:
   - Cortisone, hydrocortisone
   - Prednisone, prednisolone
   - Triamcinolone
   - Dexamethasone, betamethasone

   May be of great help, but underuse or overuse may be harmful.

Intra-articular steroids: Helpful particularly in the inflammation of selective joints

4. Disease modifying antirheumatics drugs (DMARDs): Although unable to cure RA, has the potential to modify the disease process favorably and thereby reduce the chances of joint destruction. These agents should start at earliest.

DMARDs:
- Antimalarial agents—Chloroquin
- Sulfasalazine
- Methotraxate
- Cyclosporin.

5. Gold: Lysosomal stabilizer, although exact mode of action unknown
Side effects: Monitor carefully for side effects of these DMARDs.

6. Newer therapy: Anti TNF therapy—very expensive, and under study
Physiotherapy and rehabilitation: It is an integral part of management of RA.

It helps in:
- Controlling pain
- Preventing deformity
- Improving joint function
- Maintaining muscle strength

**Refer:** The patient to medical outpatients or the GP

Surgery: Has an important role to play in very early disease when significant synovitis is present in one or few joints and in advanced (late) disease. Though surgery cannot cure arthritis, it plays an important role esp. in rehabilitating the patient

Surgical options: Available are:

In early stages:
- Arthroscopy and arthroscopic debridement
- Synovectomy
- Tendon reconstruction

In later stages:
- Excision arthroplasty
- Arthrodesis
- Osteotomy
- Joint replacement:
  - Unicompartmental joint replacement
  - Hemiarthroplasty
- Total joint replacement:
  - Total Hip Replacement (THR)
  - Total Knee Replacement (TKR).

## Regional Arthritis

Hip

Surgery:
- Mold arthroplasty of choice for RA of the hip; in case of bilateral ankylosed hips, arthroplasty of one is imperative (revised later on).

Technique:
- Mold arthroplasty (Smith-Petersen) + capsulectomy + synovectomy
- Revised arthroplasty: Prosthetic replacement.
- Prosthetic replacement: Indicated in short, osteoporotic femoral neck; may be reserved for failed mold arthroplasty.
- Arthrodesis: Indicated in case of unilateral ankylosed hip, esp. for the prolonged standing or walking requirement.

**Knee**

Surgery:
- Synovectomy: Indicated usually in monarticular ankylosed knee
- Synovectomy + patellectomy: Indicated for pain underneath patella due to irregular surface
- Arthroplasty and reconstruction: Indicated in severe ankylosed knee
- Arthrodesis: Indicated in painful and disabled knee, when arthroplasty contraindicated
- Arthrodesis + arthroplasty: Indicated in bilateral RA knees (arthrodesis of one knee and arthroplasty of other one).

**Ankle**

Surgery:
- Tendo-achilles lengthening + posterior capsullectomy: Indicated in the fixed equines deformity
- Osteotomy + TA lengthening + Arthrodesis: Indicated in the ankylosed ankle joint.

**Feet**

Surgery:

Procedures: Surgical procedures for managing the various deformities of the feet mentioned in Table 17.1. As no two rheumatoid feet are alike, uniform suggestions for surgery are difficult to make; usually multiple procedures indicated upon the two feet.

| Table 17.1: Surgical management of deformities in RA feet | |
|---|---|
| *Deformity* | *Surgery* |
| Hallux valgus | Bunionectomy |
| Hallux rigidus | Excision of proximal 2/3rd of proximal phalanx + excision of metatarsal head |
| Bunionette | Excision lateral 1/3rd of 5th metatarsal head/or excision of whole metatarsal head |
| Hammertoe | Excision of PIP joint + dorsal MTP capsulotomy |
| Hammertoe + deformed distal IP joint (corn) | Excision of PIP joint/amputation distal ½ of toe |
| Claw toe: | |
| • Mild/moderate | Excision of proximal phalanx |
| • Severe/multiple | Excision of metatarsal heads |
| • Rigid/severe + metatarsalgia | Amputation at metatarsal necks |
| Hypertrophied toe nail (onychogryposis) | Greater toe: excision nail + amputation tuft; other toes: amputation distal phalanx |
| Rheumatoid sc nodules (tarsus and metatarsals bases) | Excision |

Technique:
Bunionectomy

Excision:
- Metatarsal heads, phalanx, PIP joint, MTP capsulotomy, sc nodules Amputation.

Spine    Surgery:
- Osteotomy: Indicated in the flexion deformity; usually made at the upper lumbar level as anatomically the spinal canal here is large, and the osteotomy is distal to the spinal cord's end; a compensatory lumbar lordosis developed for thoracic kyphosis; spine mobility not increased.

Shoulder    Surgery:
- Acromioplasty: Indicated in the subacromial bursitis to relieve pain
- Acromionectomy of choice; indicated in the RA involvement of the acromioclavicular joint

Elbow    Surgery:
- Synovectomy: Indicated in the restricted mobility (flexion, extension, pronation, and supination) in RA of elbow joint
- Excision of radial head: Indicated in diaplaced radiohumeral joint (impaired relationship between radial head and capitulum).

## Ankylosing Spondylitis

Definition    It is a crippling disease that affects mostly young men (20–40 years). It is a chronic inflammatory disease that affects mainly the spine and sacroiliac joints, peripheral joints and extra-articular structures

Etiology    Unknown

Diagnosis    Low backache—pain may radiate down the thighs and legs
Morning stiffness
Chest expansion—restricted
Difficulty in breathing
Movements of spine—painful and restricted

Investigation    CBC
ESR
Rheumatoid factor
Antinuclear antibodies
C-Reactive Protein
Uric acid
Bone densitometry
X-Ray chest shows: Fuzziness or erosion of sacroiliac joints, narrowing of intervertebral spaces, ossification of ligaments, osteophytes formation, deformed joints in advanced cases.

Management    No specific treatments known for this distressing condition.
Conservative treatment:
General measures:
Bedrest

Warm fomentation
Deep breath exercises
Drugs: Analgesic
   NSAID
   Corticosteroids
Physiotherapy:
Exercises: Active—patient puts joints through range of motion
- Passive—someone puts joints through range of motion
- Isometric—muscle is contracted, but not shortened
- Isotonic—muscle is contracted and shortened

Heat therapy: Infrared, shortwave diathermy
Radiotherapy: Symptomatic relief
Side effects: High incidence of leukemia
Surgical treatment: Indicated in severe flexion deformity of the spine.
Surgery: Osteotomy (wedge) of the spine.

## Acute Gout

| | |
|---|---|
| Definition | It is a metabolic disease of heterogeneous nature, associated with hyperuricaemia, resulting from a disturbed purine metabolism or from abnormal excretion of uric acid. Any abrupt change in the serum uric acid concentration may provoke an acute attack of gout. |
| Risk factors | Alcohol consumption<br>Fasting<br>Diet—purine rich foods, e.g. bacon, salmon, sweetbreads<br>Obesity<br>Hypertension<br>Lead exposure—occupational and environmental |
| Diagnosis | Pain—agonizing pain accompanied by signs of inflammation: Swelling, redness, warmth and tenderness<br>Fever—low grade<br>More than one attack of arthritis<br>Maximum inflammation develops within 1 day<br>Monoarthritis attack<br>Attack usually start during night, and is moderate initially.<br>Pain becomes persistently worse, continuous gnawing type.<br>First (great toe) metatarsophalangeal joint painful and swollen<br>Tophi—nodular masses of urate crystals deposited in soft tissues |
| Investigation | Complete blood cell count<br>Serum uric acid<br>Serum creatinine<br>BUN<br>Synovial fluid examination—urate crystals and leukocytes<br>Aspiration of tophus—for study of urate crystals<br>X-ray shows: Asymmetrical swelling around a joint |

Subcortical cysts without erosions
MRI

## Management

| | |
|---|---|
| General measures | Control of body weight |
| | Control over alcohol intake |
| | Diet—Purine restricted diet, e.g. red meat, pulses, cheese |
| | Plenty of fluids orally |
| | Control of hypertension and hyperlipidemia |
| Drugs | NSAIDs: Indomethacin may be preferred 25–50 mg t.d.s. |
| | Naproxen 250–500 mg b.d. |
| | Diclofenac 50 mg b.d. or t.d.s. |
| | Colchicine 0.5 mg tablets given orally. Repeat hourly till depending upon patient's response |
| | IV colchicine—given rarely Dose 2 mg IV in 20 ml saline |
| | Side effects: Nausea, vomiting, diarrhea |
| | Allopurinol: 300 mg/day, avoided during an acute attack of gout |
| | Side effects: Nausea, vomiting, diarrhea, skin rash |
| | Probenecid: Used as a uricosuric agent. Dose 0.5 g b.d. |
| | C/I: Urine output < 1 ml/mt, renal calculi |
| | Corticosteroids: Used only when NSAIDs and colchicine noneffective |
| | • Prednisone 20–30 mg/day |
| | • Intra-articular injection—indicated in monarthric gout |

**Refer:** The patient to the orthopedic team

## Acute Low Backache

| | |
|---|---|
| Definition | One of the penalities that mankind pays for having adopted an upright posture during the course of evolution, instead of going on all four limbs, is that human beings are prone to backache. The prevalence of backache and difficulty of exact diagnosis, have made management of this disorder challenging to some and frustrating to most. Most people are affected by backache at one or other time. |
| Etiology | Traumatic: RSA, sports injury, falls, lifting heavy weight |
| | Inflammatory: Osteomyelitis (bacterial, tubercular) discitis, sacrolitis, ankylosing spondylitis, spondyloarthropathies, prostatitis, endometritis, appendicitis, cholecystitis |
| | Endocrinal and Metabolic: Diabetes, thyroid disorders, osteoporosis |
| | Degenerative: Spondylosis, spondylolisthesis, prolapsed disk |
| | Postural: Habitual, spinal deformity, e.g. kyphosis, scoliosis |
| | Neoplastic: Carcinoma colon |
| | Miscellaneous: Paget's disease, fluorosis. |
| Diagnosis | Pain: |
| | • Lumbar or dorsal pain during the night |
| | • Buttock pain if affecting right or left |
| | • Heel pain |

Pain:
- May worsen on activity (mechanical)
- May aggravates on coughing, sneezing
- May or may not radiate to the thigh, legs depending on whether there is compression of nerve roots

Muscle spasm

Deformity—kyphosis or scoliosis may be present

Local tenderness

Movements painful and restricted

Neurological deficit—may or may not be present depending on whether there is compression of nerve roots

Straight leg raising (SLR) test, and forward bending test

| | |
|---|---|
| Investigation | Hemogram, ESR, TLC and DLC, RA factor |
| | X-ray lumbosacral spine—AP and LAT views |
| | MRI |
| | Myelogram |
| | CT scan |
| Management | Conservative treatment: |
| | General measures: |
| | Bedrest |
| | Heat therapy—Infrared, short wave diathermy |
| | Traction, lumbar belt |
| | Analgesics, NSAIDs |
| | Antibiotic—to control infection if present |
| | Specific treatment: |
| | Epidural block |
| | Treatment of underlying cause. |

**Refer:** The patient to the orthopedic team

## Acute Sciatica

| | |
|---|---|
| Definition | Few diseases cause more suffering and economic loss than sciatica. It is most resistant to treatment and is often difficult to treat satisfactorily, because its etiology may remain obscure even after careful physical and radiological examinations. |
| Etiology | Traumatic: RSA, sports injury, lifting heavy weight |
| | Inflammatory: Tuberculosis, spondylitis |
| | Infection of genitourinary, gastrointestinal, nervous system |
| | Endocrinal: Diabetes |
| | Neoplastic: Vertebral or pelvic tumors |
| | Degenerative: PIVD, spondylosis, spondylolisthesis |
| Diagnosis | Pain down thigh and leg |
| | SLR test |
| | Forward bending test |
| Investigation | Hemogram, TLC and DLC, ESR |
| | X-ray lumbosacral spine |

| | |
|---|---|
| | Myelography |
| | CT scan |
| Management | Conservative treatment: |
| | General measures: |
| | Bedrest |
| | Heat therapy—Infrared, short wave diathermy |
| | Traction |
| | Lumbar belt |
| | Analgesics |
| | NSAIDs |

Specific treatment:
Treatment of underlying cause

Surgical treatment:
Surgery indicated only in limited cases:
- PIVD
- Spinal tumors

Refer: The patient to the orthopedic team.

## Prolapse Intervertebral Disk (PIVD)

| | |
|---|---|
| Anatomy | The intervertebral disks are a series of white fibrocartilage, interposed between the bodies of two adjacent vertebrae; disks are thicker behind than in front (in thoracic region); peripheral part of each disk (annulus fibrosus) is fibrous and firm; central part (nucleus pulposus) is soft and pulpy (contains 80% of water: subjected to dehydration and growing age) being held under pressure by the surrounding strong part; these disks increase the elasticity of the vertebral column; the intervertebral disks are the main union between the vertebral bodies, that unite each of the vertebra to the succeeding one from the 2nd cervical to the lumbosacral junction; contribute much to the length of the vertebral column above the sacrum, and also contribute to a variable extent to the curvature of the vertebral column; relationship of the nerve roots and nerves to the itervertebral disks and intervertebral foramina is of special interest because of increasing frequency of nerves injury at these levels. Remarkable mobility of the vertebral column results primarily from the elasticity and compressibility of the intervertebral disks, that allow movement of the vertebral bodies upon each other. Movements: of the vertebral column largely depend upon the ratio between the height of the disks and the height of the bony column. |
| Function | - To give shape to the vertebral column |
| | - To act as a remarkable series of shock absorbers or buffers (exposed to jars and strains constantly, even during sleep acted upon by column movements). |
| Definition | It is the main cause of low backache and pain down thigh, legs, or arms. It commonly affects adults from 30 to 50, most often males. It results from compression upon nerve root or cord, by the backward protrusion of nucleus pulposus, due to weakning of posterior longitudinal |

ligament and the annulus fibrosus as a result of trauma. The vast majority affect the disk between the L5 and S1 vertebrae. Disk between L4 and L5 is the next most vulnerable. The root of 5th lumbar or 1st sacral is commonly affected.

| | |
|---|---|
| Etiology | Direct traumatic—violence |
| | RSA |
| | Sports injury |
| | Fall from height |
| | Lifting heavy weight |
| | Injury by a lumbar puncture needle |
| | Degenerative |
| Risk factors | Postural |
| | Deformity, e.g. kyphosis, scoliosis |
| | Spondylitis |
| | Vertebral osteophytes |
| | Violent actions—sneezing, coughing, lurching |

Pathogenesis　　Each disk likened to a coiled up spring—spring bulge at the weak area due to damaged confining walls, resulting in:

- Nuclear expansion: Nucleus bulges into the vertebral body because of loss of support given by vertebral cancellous bone to the cartilage plates.
- Nuclear retropulsion PIVD: Damaged posterior longitudinal ligament and the annulus fibrosus; backward protrusion of the nucleus pulposus, covered by the weakened ligaments.

Diagnosis　　Symptoms are those of sciatica in most cases, depending on type of lesion (nerve root compression):

Cervical　　Ruptured disk between C5 and C6 (compression of C6 nerve root):

Pain: In the neck, shoulder, vertebral border of scapula, lateral aspect of arm, and posterior aspect of forearm

Numbness: Thumb and index finger

Weakness: Biceps

Reflexes: Biceps jerk: Decreased or absent

Ruptured disk between C6 and C7 (compression of C7 nerve root)

Pain: In the neck, shoulder, vertebral border of scapula, lateral aspect of arm, and posterior aspect of forearm

Numbness: Index and middle fingers

Weakness: Triceps

Reflexes: Triceps jerk: Reduced or absent

Ruptured disk between C7 and T1 (compression of C8 nerve root)

Pain: Neck, vertebral border of scapula, front of chest, inner aspect of upper arm and forearm

Numbness: Little and ring fingers

Weakness: Massive

Reflexes: Triceps jerk: Reduced or absent

L5 lesions　　Pain: In the hip, groin, thigh (posterolateral) outer calf, lateral malleolus, foot (dorsum), toes (1, 2, 3rd)

| | |
|---|---|
| | Numbness: In the area of affected nerve, e.g. more medial over tibial region—extending over big toe, medial malleolus, and related part of sole |
| | Local tenderness: Outer gluteal region and near fibular's head |
| | Weakness: Extensor of greater toe and foot |
| | Ankle jerk: Depressed |
| SLR | Positive |
| S1 lesions | Pain: In the sacroiliac joint, thigh (back), calf (back) to heel, sole (plantar surface) and toes (4th and 5th) |
| | Numbness: In the area of affected nerve, e.g. outer side of leg, foot, outer two toes and sole |
| | Local tenderness: Over sacroiliac joint, back of thigh and leg |
| | Weakness: Hamstrings, flexor of foot, flexor and abductors of toes |
| | Ankle jerk: Diminished or absent |
| | SLR: Positive |
| | Lumbar curve: May be diminished or lost |
| | Prominent spinous processes (L3, 4, 5) |
| Investigation | CBC, ESR |
| | Serum proteins |
| | CSF examination |
| | X-ray lumbar spine—AP and LAT views: may produce "false" alarms as signs of disk degeneration present in a very high percentage of the healthy persons having no problem at all |
| | Bone scans |
| | MRI: Many imaging-based degenerative features, likely part of normal aging, not associated with pain |
| | CT Scan |
| Management | Conservative treatment: symptomatic. Most slipped disk cases self-heal within 4–6/52, but chances of recurrence, in case the underlying cause remains untreated. |

Measures:

- Bedrest
- Physiotherapy: Heat therapy, massage, supervised exercises of the back and leg, as soon as the acute backache and sciatica subside
- Traction: For muscle spasm
- Support: Lumbar belt/back brace
- Analgesics, NSAIDs.

Surgical treatment:

Indication: May be indicated in 10% of cases, when compression of nerve roots or spinal cord causes neurologic deficit. Surgery is advised only in those severe cases where their bowel or bladder is to be compromised. Even in such cases conservative treatment must be attempted prior to recommended surgery. Surgery may not be fastest route, can take from 3–12/12, for complete recovery.

Procedures: Microsurgical arthroscopic lateral-approach laser-assisted fluoroscopic discectomy—gold standard for treating disk prolapse, as it can be performed as a day care procedure, and has proven to be a safe and least traumatic procedure

Alternative surgical procedures:
- Laminectomy with or without arthrodesis spine
- Percutaneous lumbar discectomy—automated
- Percutaneous lumbar discectomy—endoscopic
- Percutaneous laser discectomy
- Microdiscectomy—transforaminal endoscopic
- Microdiscectomy—stereostactic lumbar
- Artificial disk replacement or intervertebral disk transfer—future holds (procedures) in store.

**Refer:** The patient to the next orthopedic clinic.

## Reiter's Syndrome

| | |
|---|---|
| Definition | It is defined as a clinical tetrad of unknown etiology, consisting of polyarthritis, urethritis, conjunctivitis/or uveitis and mucocutaneous manifestations; occurs commonly in young men; venereal in origin; may occur within 4/52 post sexual intercourse with infected partener |
| Etiology | Unknown |
| Predisposing factors | Venereal contact (unprotected sexual intercourse) or diarrhea. |
| Pathogenesis | Incubation period: 1–4/52; systemic reaction including fever. |
| Diagnosis | Arthritis: Asymmetrical, usually large weight bearing joints (knee, ankle), sacroiliitis, ankylosing sponylitis; onset insidious; articular stiffness; movements painful (relieved by rest) and restricted; valgus or varus deformity of the knee common; joint effusion |
| | Eyes: Conjunctivitis, uveitis |
| | Mucocutaneous lesions: Stomatitis, keratoderma, balanitis, uethritis |
| | CVS: Carditis, AR |
| | Fever, malaise, loss of weight |
| Investigation | CBC—anemia |
| | ESR: Elevated |
| | WR: +ve |
| | Autoantibody screen |
| | RA factor: + ve |
| | X-ray joints: Knees, ankle, spine, chest |
| D/d | Gonococcal arthritis |
| | RA |
| | Ankylosing spondylitis |
| | Psoriatic arthritis |
| Management | Conservative treatment: symptomatic: |
| | Analgesics and NSAIDs: Paracetamol, diclofenac, aceclofenac, ibuprofen, naproxen, piroxicam |
| | Antibiotics |
| Prognosis | Most signs of disease disappear within days/weeks, the arthritis may continue for couple of months/years. |

## Rheumatic Fever

| | |
|---|---|
| Definition | It is defined as a subacute or chronic systemic disease of unknown etiology; may either be self-limiting or may be a slowly progressive valvular deformity; rarely acute or fulminating; commonest amongst persons under fifty years of age; ranks third behind hypertension and atherosclerotic coronary disease. |
| Etiology | Unknown |
| | Infective: Post URC (tonsillitis, nasopharyngitis, otitis media), caused by streptococci hemolytic A |
| Pathogenesis | Acute lesion: perivascular granulomatous reaction with vasculitis; pink granulations on the surface of edematous valves, endocarditis, myocarditis, percarditis; pleuritis, synovitis chronic: complete healing or progressive scarring over months/years. |
| Diagnosis | Age: Common under fifty years of age (commonest 5–15 years of age) |
| | Sex: Common in males; while corea seen more in females |

Major criterias:

- Carditis: Endocarditis; myocarditis; pericarditis, CHF
- Skin: Erythema
- Subcutaneous nodules: Common in children; nodules few or many
- Chorea (Sydenham): Occurs suddenly or during course of overt fever
- Polyarthritis: Migratory polyarthritis of sudden or gradual onset; may involve large joints sequentially; inflamed (red, hot, swollen, and tender); synovitis; arthralgia and arthritis are common in children and young adults.

Minor criterias:

- Fever: In association with arthritis and carditis; low grade; continuous or intermittent type; may be normal in certain cases
- Arthralgia: Poly
- Malaise, anorexia, loss of weight
- Pain abdomen: Variable in site and intensity (may from hepatomegaly, peritonitis, or rheumatic arteritis)
- Arthralgia.

| | |
|---|---|
| Investigation | CBC (WBC and ESR—raised) |
| | C-reactive protein: Increased |
| | Urine: Proteinurea, hematurea |
| | Throat culture: For beta-hemolytic streptococci |
| | ECG: Prolonged P-R interval |
| | X-rays joint/s |
| D/d | RA |
| | Traumatic arthritis |
| | Osteomyelitis |
| | SBE |
| | Pulmonary tuberculosis |
| | DLE |

| | |
|---|---|
| | Serum sickness |
| | Leukemia. |
| Complications | CHF |
| | Cardiac arrhythmias |
| | Pericarditis with effusion |
| | Pulmonary embolism |
| | Heart: Valvular defects |
| Management | Preventive treatment: |

Aim: To avoid URC (beta-hemolytic streptococcal infections) and to treat

Infections with appropriate antibiotics.

General measures:
- Bedrest
- To avoid contact with persons having bad cold includes URC
- To use antibiotics (benzyle penicillin G 1.2 million units IN every 4/52
- Warm saline/listerine gargles.

**Medical treatment**

Drugs:
- Salicylates: As analgesics, antipyretics, anti-inflammatory agents
  Sod. Salicylate 1–2 g every 4 hourly PO, for fever and pain
- Aspirin: As an alternative to sod. salicylate (same dosages).
- Antibiotics: Penicillin
- Corticosteroids: Prompt relief; use with caution

Prednisone 5–10 mg PO q.i.d. for 3/52

| | |
|---|---|
| Prognosis | Recurrences are common in children, while uncommon after the age of 20 years; immediate mortality is 2%; poor prognosis in cases of persistent rheumatic activity with CHF (30% of children die within ten years of initial attack); 80% of children attain adult life with little restriction of activity; in adults residual heart damage occurs in < 20%; 20% of those having chorea may develop valvular deformity. |

## Systemic Lupus Erythematosus (SLE)

| | |
|---|---|
| Definition | It is defined as an inflammatory syndrome, that involves primarily the vascular and connective tissues of multiple organs, resulting in multiple local and systemic manifestations. |
| Etiology | • Viral (myxoviruses – measles and parainfluenza type I, and Epstein-Barr) infection (demonstrated in capillary endothelial cells. <br> • Heredity |
| Pathogenesis | Exact mechanisms unknown. May be altered immune mechanism. <br> Necrotized vasculitis (cellular infiltras to fibrinoid necrosis. |
| Diagnosis | Systemic: Fever, sweating, weight loss, weakness, malaise, fatigue <br> Skin: Erythematous rash on face (butterfly) or other areas (forehead, neck, arms, legs, back or abdomen exposed to sunlight <br> Eyes: Corneal opacity and retinopathy (exudative) <br> Lungs: Pulmonary dysfunction with basilar atelectatic pneumonitis, pleural effusion |

|  | |
|---|---|
|  | CVS: Pericarditis, pericardial effusion, myocarditis, endocarditis, tachycardia, gallop rhythm, heart failure, hypertension |
|  | Hematopoietic: Hemolytic anemia, thrombocytopenic purpura, hypersplenism |
|  | GI tract: Nausea, vomiting, diarrhea, dysphagia, stomatitis, pain abdomen, ileitis, peritonitis, bleeding per rectum |
|  | Liver: Hepatomegaly, hepatic failure |
|  | Kidneys: Nephritis (proteinuria, hematuria, nephrotic syndrome), renal failure |
|  | Musculoskeletal: Myalgia, arthralgia, myositis, polyarthritis, synovial nodules and cysts |
|  | CNS: Psychosis, peripheral neuritis, convulsions, hemiplegia, coma |
|  | Lymhatic system: Lymphadenopathy, splenomegaly |
| Investigation | CBC: Anemia (normochromic, normocytic or hemolytic), Coombs test + ve |
|  | Leukopenia: Mild with lymphopenia |
|  | ESR raised |
|  | Serology: Serum globulin IgG increased, antinuclear antibodies present, serum complement levels low; RA factor + ve; LE cells in blood and tissues (diagnostic) due to anti-IgG |
|  | LFT: Usually abnormal |
|  | Biological: False positive STS |
|  | Urine: Proteinuria, hematuria, casts |
|  | Biopsy: Skin and kidney: detects antibody fluorescence. |
| D/d | Collagen disorders |
|  | Musculoskeletal disorders |
|  | Hematological disorders |
|  | Dermatological disorders (scleroderma, dermatositis) |
|  | Chronic infections: Syphilis |
|  | Drugs: Anticonvulsants, hydralazine, isoniazid, quinidine, sulfas, thiouracils, phenothiazines |
| Management | Symptomatic and supportive. |
|  | Diet: High caloric, high vitamin, iron supplements |
|  | Avoid exposure to sunlight/ultraviolet radiation |
|  | Avoid exposure to cold for Raynaud's phenomenon |
|  | Drug abuse: Avoid drugs causing SLE |

Medical:
Blood transfusion and iron supplements for anemia

Drugs:
- Corticosteroids: Prednisone 10–70 mg od PO

Caution: Reduction of daily dose on improvement
- Antimalarials: Chloroquine—caution: toxic retinopathy
- Antibiotics: To control infections, pneumonia
- Analgesics: Salicylates or anti-inflammatory drugs

- Immunosuppressives agents:
  - Alkylating agents (cyclophosphamide)
  - Purine antagonists (mercaptopurine)

| | |
|---|---|
| Prognosis | Mild: Improvement with corticosteroid therapy |
| | Fulminant: Death may occur within few weeks despite treatment. |

## Raynaud's Disease

| | |
|---|---|
| Definition | It is defined as a spasmodic condition commonly occurring in the young women, that affects the upper limbs more than the lower one; the peripheral pulses remain normal; attributable to abnormal sensitivity in the direct response of the arterioles to cold. |
| Etiology | Cold exposure |
| Pathogenesis | Attack: Cold exposure yields abrupt spasm of arterioles; metabolites accumulation in the capillary circulation; dilated capillaries filled with slowly flowing deoxygenated blood; part swollen and dusky, obliterative changes in peripheral vessels, necrosis, dry gangrene. |
| | Post-attack: Relaxed arterioles, dilated capillaries filled with oxygenated blood, hands become reddish. |
| Diagnosis | Incidence: Young women |
| | Limbs: Symmetrically upper limbs esp. fingers |
| | Skin: Paroxysmal bilateral symmetrical pallor and cyanosis followed by bright redness of skin of fingers, rarely of toes, sparing thumbs |
| | Attacks of numbness, tingling and blanching (syncope) followed or preceded by pain and cyanosis (asphyxia), terminate spontaneously or by warmth. May progress to atrophy of digital skin and fat pads, gangrene, ulcers. |
| | Recovery: Intense redness, throbbing, paresthesia, swelling. |
| Investigation | CBC, ESR, WR |
| | Oscillometry: To detect pulsations at different levels |
| | X-ray: For cervical rib, gas bubbles (gas gangrene) |
| | Arteriography: Color doppler for artery status |
| | Plethysmography: To estimate vasodilatation and increased blood flow rate |

D/d

- Thromboangitis oblitrans: common in men, absent/diminished peripheral pulses
- Arteriosclerosis oblitrans
- Thoracic outlet syndromes and cervical rib: Symptoms unilateral
- Scleroderma: Skin of face, neck, chest involved.

Management

Conservative treatment:

Measures:

- To protect from cold: wear gloves
- To keep body warm
- To avoid pulp and nail bed infections
- To avoid smoking

Drugs: Vasodilators: Reserpine, methyldopa, papaverine

**Surgical treatment**

Measures:

- Sympathectomy (preganglionic section of thoracic sympathetic chain)

Indication: Indicated for severe attacks.

Prognosis          Mild discomfort on exposure to cold.

Gangrene: Disability by severe pain, restricted movements and ankylosis of distal joints.

## Progressive Systemic Sclerosis (Scleroderma)

Definition          It is defined as a chronic disorder of unknown cause characterized by insidious onset of connective tissue proliferation in the dermis and in multiple internal organs, an early and progressive small arterial involvement disproportionate to the fibrosis.

Etiology          Unknown

Pathogenesis:

Diagnosis          Incidence: Middle aged women

Forms: Localized and systemic

Hands and feet: Stiffness, sweating of hands and feet, ulceration of fingers and toes

Raynaud's phenomenon + ve

Skin: Hard, thick, parched, glossy, pigmented, calcified around joints

Joints: Arthritis

GI tract: Dysphagia, nausea, vomiting, diarrhea

Chest: Constriction of thorax, pulmonary fibrosis, pneumonia

CVS: Pericarditis, myocarditis, CHF

CNS: Peripheral neuritis

Renal: Nephritis progressive causing death.

Investigation          ESR raised

Serum globulin elevated

LE phenomenon or increased antinuclear antibodies

Urine: Proteinuria, casts

X-ray: Subcutaneous calcification, osteoporosis, bone distruction

Plane X-ray abdomen: Peristalsis loss

Management          Symtomatic and supportive.

**Conservative treatment**

Measures:

- To avoid cold exposure
- Drugs: Vasodilators, corticosteroids

Prognosis          Better in young women.

Survival rate: Seven years, death occurs due to renal, cardiac failure or infection.

## Sjogren's (Sicca) Syndrome

Definition          It is defined as a generalized connective tissue disorder of unknown etiology that occurs usually in women over fifty years of age.

| | |
|---|---|
| Etiology | Unknown |
| | Faulty secretion by the lacrimal and salivary glands |
| Pathogenesis | Sicca complex due to faulty secretion by the lacrimal and salivary glands resulting in the kerato-conjunctivitis sicca and xerostomia; corneal ulceration; enlarged salivary (parotid) glands; arthritic joints; vasculitis. |
| Diagnosis | Incidence: Common in women > 50 years of age |
| | Eyes: Dryness (keratoconjunctivitis sicca) |
| | Mouth: Dryness (xerostomia) |
| | Nose: Dryness, rhinitis, epistaxis |
| | Respiratory: Dyspnea, bronchitis |
| | Joints: Arthritic changes similar to RA |
| | Vasculitis |
| | Splenomegaly |
| | Vagina: Dryness |
| | Peripheral neuritis |
| | Raynaud's phenomenon |
| | Hepatomegaly |
| | Thyroiditis |
| Investigation | CBC, ESR |
| | RA factor |
| | Antinuclear antibodies |
| | LE cells |
| | Fundoscopy |
| | P/V examination |
| Management | Conservative treatment: |
| | Local treatment: |

- Eyes: For dryness use irrigating sol. or artificial tears; corticosteroids to be used with caution
- Mouth: Listerine gargles
- Joints: Rest, physiotherapy; I/A injections of corticosteroids with caution.

General treatment: Symptomatic:
- Rest
- Analgesics/NSAIDs
- Corticosteroids systemic: With caution
- Physiotherapy.

| | |
|---|---|
| Prognosis | Subjected to remissions and exacerbations; usually not progressive. Prognosis depends upon the associated systemic diseases or connective tissue disorders. |

### Wegener's Syndrome

| | |
|---|---|
| Definition | It is defined as a syndrome characterized by a generalized connective tissue disorder of unknown cause, occurring usually in the middle aged (above 50 years) women, having dryness of eyes, nose, mouth, trachea, bronchi, vagina, and skin, with hypofunction of the lacrimal and parotid glands. |

| | |
|---|---|
| Etiology | Unknown |
| Pathogenesis | Hypofunction of lacrimal and parotid glands, xerostomia and keratoconjunctivitis sicca, corneal ulceration, swollen salivary glands, secretory insufficient nasopharynx, larynx, trachea, vagina. |
| Diagnosis | URC: Hypersecretion, dryness of eyes, nose, mouth, trachea, bronchii, ulceration, inability to swallow and chew foods |
| | Salivary glands: Swollen |
| | Vagina: Discharge, dryness |
| | Joints: Arthritis |
| | Vasculitis |
| | Peripheral neuritis |
| | Raynaud's phenomenon |
| | Purpura |
| | Thyroiditis |
| | GI tract: Achlorhydria, pancreatitis |
| | Hepatomegaly |
| | Splenomegaly |
| | Renal: Acidosis |
| Investigation | CBC: Anemia |
| | Rheumatoid factor |
| | Antinuclear antibodies |
| | LE cells |
| | X-ray joints, CXR |
| | Ophthalmologic examination |
| | Biopsy: Salivary glands of lower lip |
| Management | Unsatisfactory. |
| | Conservative treatment: |
| | Local treatment: |
| | Eyes: |

- Polyethylene glycol 400 and Propylene glycol sol. q.i.d. for the keratoconjunctivitis and corneal ulcers
- Corticosteroids: Fluorometholone suspension q.i.d.

Mouth: Oral gargles for dryness of mouth
Nose: Nasal drops (Otrivin/nasivion) for dryness of nose
Trachea, bronchi: Steam inhalation
Vagina: Vaginal lubricant cremes

| | |
|---|---|
| Complications | Increased incidence of lymphomas and reticulum cell sarcoma |
| Prognosis | Subject to remissions and exacerbations, depending upon the associated systemic and connective tissue involvement. |

## Bibliography

1. Apostolides PJ, Jackobowitz R, Sonntag VK. Lumbar discectomy microdiscectomy: The gold standard. Clin Neurosurg 43: 228–38, 1996.
2. Bell GR, Parkman RH. The conservative treatment of sciatica. Spine 9:54, 1984.
3. Brunch TW, et al. Synovial fluid complement: Usefulness in diagnosis and classification of rheumatoid arthritis. Ann Int Med 81:32, 1974.

4. Calabro JJ, Maltz BA. Ankylosing spondylitis, New England J Med 282:606, 1970.

5. Campbell's Operative Orthopaedics (1998) 9th Ed. Vol I-IV. Canale S. Terry, Daugherty K, and Jones Linda. Mosby.

6. Charnley J. Raynaud's disease. Bailey and Love's Short Practice of Surgery. 13th Ed., H.K. Lewis and Co. Ltd., 1965.

7. Chaturvedi V. Ankylosing Spondylitis: A Radical Shift In Management. Orthopaedics Today VI:42, 2004.

8. Cummings NA, et al. Sjogren's syndrome: Newer aspects of research, diagnosis, and therapy. Ann Int Med 75:937, 1971.

9. Cummings NA, et al. Sjogren's syndrome: Newer aspects of research, diagnosis, and therapy. Ann Int Med 75:937, 1971

10. Das K. Raynaud's disease. Clinical Methods in Surgery. 6th Ed. Imperial Art Cottage, Calcutta, 1962.

11. Dubois EL (Editor). Lupus Erythematosus, 2nd ed. Univ. of Southern California Press, 1974.

12. Engleman EP, Chatton MJ. Arthritis and Allied Rheumatic Disorders. Current Medical Diagnosis and Treatment, 474–98, 1975.

13. Engleman EP, Weber HM. Reiter's syndrome: Rheumatic manifestations of systemic disease, Clin Orthop 57:19, 1968

14. Ephraim P Engleman, Milton JC. SJogren's (sicca) Syndrome. Arthritis and Allied Rheumatic Disorders. Current Medical Diagnosis and Treatment, Maruzen, 1975.

15. Ephraim P, Chatton MJ. SLE, Arthritis and Allied Rheumatic Disorders, 480–482, 1975.

16. Ephraim P, Engleman, Milton JC. Diffuse Scleroderma (progressive Systemic Sclerosis). Arthritis and Allied Rheumatic Disorders. Current Medical Diagnosis and Treatment, Maruzen, 1975.

17. Feinstein AR, Stern EK. Clincal effects ofrecuirrent attacks of acute rheumatic fever: A prospective epidemiologic study of 105 episodes. J Chronic Dis 20:13, 1967.

18. Frymoyer JW. Back pain and sciatica. N Engl J Med 318:291, 1998.

19. Gifford RW Jr. The clinical significance of Raynaud's phenomenon and Raynaud's disease. M Clin North America 42:963, 1958.

20. Gokhale T, Hedge U, Jyotish CJ. Classification and diagnostic Criteria for Rheumatic Diseases. Journal of General Medicine 14:7–14, 2002.

21. Gulati Y. Lumbar microdiscectomy. Apollo Medicine 1; 34–37, Sept 2004.

22. Johnson JS, et al. Rheumatoid arthritis, 1970-72. Ann Int Med 78:937, 1773.

23. Joshi VR. ACR criteria for classification of acute gouty arthritis. Journal of General Medicine 14, 2002.

24. Kapoor PS. Accident and Emergency: Etiology, Diagnosis and Management. 2nd Ed. CBS, New Delhi, 2016.

25. Kapoor PS. Ankylosing Spondylitis. The Indian Express 4 June, 200.

26. Kapoor PS. Backache. The Indian Express 11 September, 2002.

27. Kapoor PS. Prolapse intervertebral disc management. Accident and Emergency 2nd Ed., CBS, New Delhi, 2016.

28. Kapoor PS. Prolapse intervertebral disc. Accident and Emergency 2nd Ed., CBS, New Delhi, 2016.

29. Kapoor PS. Rheumatoid arthritis. The Indian Express 18 September, 2003.

30. Kapoor PS. The truth about Sciatica. The Indian Express 30 October, 2002.

31. Kelley JH, et al. Multiple operations for protruded lumbar intervertebral disk, Proc. Staff Meet. Mayo Clin. 29:546, 1954.

32. Love M, Rains AJH, Capper WM. Bailey and Love's Short Practice of Surgery (1965). H.K. Lewis and Co., London.

33. Mathews HH. Transforaminal endoscopic microdiscectomy. Neurosurg Clin N Am 7(1): 59–63, Jan 1996.

34. Mc Rae R. Practical Fracture Treatment (1981) 1st Ed. Churchill Livingstone.

35. Morris R, et al. HL-A W27: A clue to the diagnosis and pathogenesis of Reiter's syndrome. New England J Med 290:554, 1974.

36. Muller R. Protrusion of thoracic intervertebral disks with compression of the Spinal cord, Acta med. Scandinav. 139:99, 1950.

37. Regan JJ, Guyer RD. Endoscopic techniques in spinal surgery. Clinical Orthopaedics, 335, 1.

38. Rothman RC, Simeone F. Lumbar Disc Disease. Philadelphia. Saunders, 1975. pp 443–58.

39. Russel ASA, Ansel BM. Septic arthritis. Ann Rheumat Dis 31:40, 1972 spati PK: Acute Gout. Journal of General Medicine 14, 2002.

40. Russel ASA, Ansel BM. Septic arthritis. Ann Rheumat Dis 31:40, 1972.

41. Shearn MA. Sjogren's Syndrome. Saunders, 1971.

42. Siegel RC. Progressive systemic sclerosis. California Med 119:35, Aug 1973.

43. Silvers HR. Microsurgical versus standard lumbar discectomy, Neurosurgery 22(5): 837–41, May 1988.

44. Sledge CB. Surgery for rheumatoid arthritis. Current Orthopaedics, 3,1. 1989.

45. Spati PK. Acute Gout. Journal of General Medicine 14, 2002.

46. Wilson DH, Harbaugh R. Microsurgical and standard removal of the protruded lumbar disc: A comparative study. Neurosurgery 8: 422–27, 1981.

# 18

# Infective Arthritis and Wounds of Joints

- **Acute suppurative arthritis**
- **Wounds of Joints**

## ACUTE SUPPURATIVE ARTHRITIS

| | |
|---|---|
| Definition | It is defined as an acute inflammation of the joint due to infection. It is a serious crippling disorder, usually monoarticular and in case of polyarticular, is acute in one or more joints, while subacute or mild in others. |
| Etiology | Direct: Compound fractures involving the joint, penetrating wounds, operations, diagnostic procedures, e.g. intra-articular aspiration or injection. |
| | Local: Extension from a neighboring focus, e.g. acute arthritis of the hip joint (intra-articular) from osteomyelitis of femoral neck |
| | Indirect: Hematogenous (bacteremia or septicemia secondary to infective skin, upper respiratory tract (URC), genitourinary tract. |
| Transmission | Primary: Direct intrusion of microorganisms into the joint |
| | Sceondary: Hematogenous—through bloodstream (mostly through arteries. |
| Organisms | • Bacteria: Staphylococcus, streptococcus, pneumococcus, gonococcus meningococcus, *haemophilus influenzae*, gram-negative bacilli, mycobacterium tuberculosis or bovis. |
| | • Viruses: Smallpox, measles, mumps |
| | • Fungi: Actinomyces, blastomyces, coccidioides |
| | • Parasites: Echinococcus granulosus. |
| Pathogenesis | Variable with the age of the patient due to differences in the structure and blood supply at different ages. |
| | Infants and children: Metaphyseal abscess formed, enters the joint (intra-articular), resulting in suppurative arthritis, articular cartilage destruction (partially or completely). Pus may spread into the muscular plane or sc tissue. |
| Diagnosis | Age: Common in children |
| | Joint: Knee and hip are commonly affected |
| | Site: Bone ends (intra-articular) |
| | Onset: Sudden |

|                 | Pain: Severe |
|-----------------|--------------|
|                 | Fever with chills, prostration |
|                 | Swelling |
|                 | Skin: Hot, red |
|                 | Local tenderness |
|                 | Movements: Painful and restricted. |
| Investigation   | CBC |
|                 | TLC and DLC—leukocytosis |
|                 | ESR—raised |
|                 | Blood culture |
|                 | Synovial fluid analysis: leukocytosis |
|                 | Smear and culture study of causative organism |

**Investigation** (continued)

X-Ray: Normal in early cases, but later on shows the demineralization, bony erosion, narrowing of joint space, followed by osteomyelitis and periostitis

**D/d**

- Pneumococcal arthritis
- Tuberculous arthritis
- Syphilitic arthritis
- Gonococcal arthritis
- Rheumatoid arthritis
- Hemophilic joints
- Rheumatic fever
- Gout
- Reiter's syndrome
- Traumatic synovitis.

**Complications**

- Chronic arthritis due to delayed diagnosis, waiting for manifest X-ray evidence, or inadequate early treatment
- Soft tissue abscess formation: Pelvic abscess
- Persistent infection
- Pathological fracture: At the site of extensive bone necrosis
- Pathological dislocation of hip
- Deformity: Ankylosis (fibrous or bony), due to partial or complete destruction of articular cartilage.

**Management**

Conservative treatment:

General measures:

Bedrest

Immobilization of joint by traction or splint

Elevation of the part

Warm fomentation

Antibiotics

Analgesics Fluids: Orally or IV

Surgical treatment:

Aspiration of joint

Incision and drainage

## Aspiration and Drainage

### Lower limb

Hip

| | |
|---|---|
| Preface | Early diagnosis and prompt evacuation of the pus by aspiration or surgical drainage are mandatory. |
| Aspiration | Difficult to confirm diagnosis by aspiration in case the joint contains little fluid or the fluid highly purulent, whereby drainage is considered over aspiration. |

Technique:

Approach: Anterior, posterior, and lateral.

Anterior:

- Direction: Insert the needle at right angle to the skin at a point 2.5 cm distal and lateral to the middle of inguinal ligament

Posterior:

- Direction: Insert the needle at the junction of middle and lateral 3rd of an imaginary line from center of greater trochanter to the postero-inferior iliac spine.

Lateral

- Direction: Insert the needle from the side, above the greater trochanter, then advance upwards and medially (at angle of 45 degree), parallel with the femoral neck for 5–10 cm, into the joint
- Insert the needle at right angle to the skin at a point 2.5 cm distal and lateral to the middle of inguinal ligament.

Drainage

Technique:

Approach: Posterior, anterior, medial or lateral

Posterior (Ober): To drain a fluctuating posterior abscess

- Incision parallel to femoral neck, from posterolateral border of greater trochanter, advanced upwards and medially towards posterosuperior iliac spine
- Divide gluteus maximus muscle in line of incision
- Isolate and ligate gluteal vessels
- Isolate sciatic nerve
- Isolate and divide muscles attached to greater trochanter
- Incise distended capsule to drain pus
- Insert rubber drain.

Anterior:

- Incision (vertical) from anterosuperior iliac spine, to expose and separate muscles (Sartorius, tensor fascia latae, vastus lateralis) to expose capsule
- Incise distended capsule to drain pus
- Insert rubber drain.

Lateral:

- Incision (vertical) parallel to anterior border of greater trochanter, to expose and separate vastus lateralis muscle from trochanter, then elevate periosteum from femoral neck to expose capsule

- Incise distended capsule to drain pus
- Insert rubber drain.

Medial (Ludolff):
- Incision (vertical) on the inner aspect of the hip and expose muscles (gracilis, adductor longus, pectineus and iliopsoas—behind that lies the hip joint)
- Incise distended capsule to drain pus
- insert rubber drain.

Postoperative: Buck's traction.

## Knee

| | |
|---|---|
| Aspiration | Being a superficial joint, aspirated easily. |
| | Technique: Insert needle on the lateral or medial side at the level of proximal border of patella. |
| Drainage | Technique: |

Approach: Anterior, posterolateral, and posteromedial

Anterior:
- Incision: 5–10 cm long on each side of patella and patellar tendon
- Incise fasciae, capsule, and the synovium to drain pus
- Specimen for culture sensitivity and smears to identify the micro-organism
- Insert rubber drain.

Posterolateral:
- Incision 8 cm long on posterolateral aspect of flexed knee, anterior to fibular head and biceps tendon, avoids injury to common peroneal nerve, deepen incision through iliotibial band to expose the capsule
- Incise capsule to drain pus
- Insert rubber drain.

Posteromedial:
- Incision over joint, lateral to the semitendinosus tendon, isolate tendons of medial hamstrings, advance proximally along the gastrocnemius to expose the capsule
- Incise capsule to drain pus
- Insert rubber drain.

Postoperative: B/K cast or splint for 4–6/52.

## Ankle

| | |
|---|---|
| Aspiration | Difficult due to the swelling that hidden the malleoli and other landmarks, and because of swelling may be result of secondary effusion in tendon sheaths (acute suppurative arthritis). |
| Drainage | Technique: |

Approach: Anterolateral, posterolateral, anteromedial, and posteromedial

Anterolateral:
- Incision: Medial or lateral, 5–8 cm long parallel to long-axis of the foot

- Divide the superficial and deep fascia, open the capsule
- Drain the pus
- Specimen for culture sensitivity and smears to identify the microorganism.

Postoperative: B/K cast or splint for 4–6/52.

## Tarsal Joints

| | |
|---|---|
| Aspiration | It is insufficient |
| Drainage | Technique: |

- Incision: Medial or lateral, 5–8 cm long parallel to long-axis of the foot
- Divide the superficial and deep fascia, open the capsule
- Drain the pus
- Specimen for culture sensitivity and smears to identify the microorganism.

Postoperative: B/K cast or splint for 4–6/52.

## Upper Limb

### Shoulder

Aspiration   Aspirated easily as the fluctuant site palpable on the anterior aspect of the shoulder, usually needle inserted at this point.

Drainage   Technique:

Approach: Anterior and posterior.

Anterior:

- Incision from acromion, distally over center of humeral head, incise fasciae, deltoid fibers in line, to expose capsule
- Incise the capsule to drain pus
- Insert rubber drain.

Poaterior:

- Incision from base of scapular spine, distally for 7.5 cm in line with deltoid fibers, divide deltoid to expose external rotators of the shoulder, deepen dissection between infraspinatus and teres minor, medial to greater tuberosity of humerus to expose capsule
- Incise the capsule to drain pus
- Insert rubber drain.

Postoperative: Abduction splint and as symptoms subside—exercises.

### Elbow

Aspiration   Position: Elbow held in acute flexion, the needle inserted on the posterior aspect lateral to the olecranon into the distended bursa, and the fluid aspirated.

Drainage   Technique:

Approach: Medial and lateral

Medial:

- Incision: 8 cm, centered over the medial humeral condyle, avoids injury to ulnar nerve that lies over posterior aspect of medial epicondyle

- Incise the superficial and deep fasciae, open space between triceps (posteriorly) and brachialis (anteriorly), incise periosteum to excise capsule
- Open the capsule to drain the pus
- Specimen for culture sensitivity and smears to identify the micro-organism.

Postoperative: A/E POP splint with elbow flexed at 90 degree for 4/52, followed by exercises.

## Wrist

| | |
|---|---|
| Aspiration | Insert needle just below the radial or ulnar styloid process, advance in, perpendicular to the styloid process, into the joint and aspirate the fluid. |
| Drainage | Technique: |

Approach: Medial, lateral, or posterior

Medial:
- Incision 5 cm centered over the head of the ulna, between tendons of flexor and extensor carpi ulnaris, expose and incise the ulnar collateral ligament and synovium

Lateral:
- Incision 5 cm centered over snuffbox, between combined synovial sheath (tendons of abductor pollicis longus and extensor pollicis brevis) and extensor pollicis longus, deepen into snuffbox, isolate radial artery, incise the radial collateral ligament and synovium

Posterior:
- Incision 5 cm centered over the medial aspect of the dorsum of the wrist, between extensor carpi ulnaris and extensor digiti minimi
- Drain the pus
- Specimen for culture sensitivity and smears to identify the micro-organism.

Postoperative:
- Cock up splint for 4/52
- Eexercises of fingers.

Tarsal joints:
- Aspiration: Insufficient
- Drainage of choice (medial or lateral approach)

Ankle:
- Aspiration: Insufficient (anterolateral, posterolateral, anteromedial, and posteromedial approach)
- Drainage of choice (posterolateral approach)

Knee:
- Aspiration: Easily aspirated (lateral side of the suprapatellar pouch)
- Drainage: Anterior, posteromedial, and posterolateral approaches

Hip:
- Aspiration: Anterior, posterior, or lateral approaches
- Drainage: Anterior, lateral, and posterior approaches.

Shoulder:
- Aspiration: Anterior, posterior, or lateral approaches
- Drainage: Anterior (preffered) or posterior approach.

Elbow:
- Aspiration: Posterolateral approach (flexed elbow)
- Drainage: Medial or lateral approach.

Wrist:
- Aspiration: Dorsal aspect (medial to snuffbox)
- Drainage: Medial, lateral, or posterior approach.

### Amputation

Indications:
- Patient's life-threatened
- Amyloidosis due to prolonged suppuration
- Painful deformity.

## WOUNDS OF JOINTS

| | |
|---|---|
| Preface | Suppurative arthritis resulting from wounds of joints is more difficult to manage than the hematogenous type, and the prognosis is less favorable; infection may not be confined to the joint but may have transmitted from the original wound through fascial planes and may have caused diffuse cellulitis or abscess/s; reactivation of the infection or scar contracture is more likely postsurgical or manipulation; every effort to be made to prevent serious infections, while treating original wound; great improvements in managing contaminated or septic wounds of joints have been developed. |
| Etiology | Direct trauma: Violence (blow, stab, gunshot) <br> RSA <br> Sports injuries <br> Fall from a height <br> Gunshot injuries |
| Pathogenesis | Torn tissues; contused adjoining structures; extravasation of blood; hematoma (localized hemorrhage); infected wound; diffuse ellulitis; abscess/s formed; reactivated infection; scarring; contracture of soft tissues; usually the knee joint with its extensive synovium, is more immune to infection than the bones, the tendons, or periarticular structures; wounds of knee may occur in cases where synovium, the capsule, and skin closed surgically—that later on resulted in an extra-articular infection, not an intra-articular one. |
| Transmission | Self infection or cross infection from other persons. |
| Organisms | Bacterial infections: <br> Gram +ve cocci: *Staphylococcus aureus, staphylococcus albus* <br> Gram +ve sporing bacilli: *Clostridia welchii, clostridia tetani* |

| | Gram –ve bacilli: *Escherichia coli and Klebsiella, Proteus, Pseudomonas pyocyanea, bacteroids* |
|---|---|
| Investigation | CBC, ESR |
| | Blood culture |
| | Culture of aspirated fluid/pus |
| | X-rays of the affected joint—AP and LAT views |
| Management | Conservative treatment: |

Aim: Choice of treatment depends upon two factors:

1. The time since injury: Much less important in wounds of joints than in others; for anticipated motion preservation, the synovium to be closed, as the exposed joints usually develop mixed infections, and the exposed cartilage degenerates rapidly.

2. The type of wound: May be classified as types 1, 2, and 3:

   Type 1: Soft tissue injury is slight, while the osseous and cartilaginous structures are usually uninjured, e.g. punctured wound of the knee inflicted by a nail, sharpened pen/pencil/hair pin/needle.

   Type 2: Soft tissue injury may be relatively extensive, while maceration and necrosis are usually slight, with little foreign matter may be found within the joint or soft tissues; injury to osseous and cartilaginous structures may be severe, e.g. compound fracture of the patella, and a gunshot wound of a joint (bone moderately or severely damaged, while the bullet is lodged in or near the joint.

   Type 3: Soft tissue injury is severe; foreign body present in the wound; tissue necrosis marked; and the synovium and capsule lacerated; injury to osseous and cartilaginous structures may be severe, e.g. gunshot wound caused by at close range.

Management of type 1 wounds:

Conservative treatment of choice:

- Toilet of the wound
- ASD
- Antibiotics
- Analgesics and NSAIDs
- Immobilization of the affected joint.

### Surgical treatment

Indication:

- Synovitis
- Remnant foreign body in the wound/adjoining soft tissues.

Surgery:

- Aspiration of joint: Diagnostic and therapeutic.
- Exploration of wound/soft tissue.

After care:

- Immobilize the joint with Buck's traction
- Exercises: Active and passive, to be started once the acute symptoms subsided; restoring function to be induced slowly; otherwise a

reaction may develop in the joint that may cause residual synovitis, or may even reactivate an infection; special exercises required to restore quadriceps power at the earliest possible

- Walking: Allowed with the aid of a long leg brace; the brace not to be discarded until a satisfactory range of motion esp. extension, restored.

Management of type 2 wounds:

Surgery: Debridement of wound and exploration of joint.

Technique:

- Debridement: External wound prepared and debrided
- Excision of damaged tissues

  Trimming: Sparingly of contused edges of synovium and capsule
- Exploration of joint thoroughly; removal of the blood clots, loose fragments of the bone or cartilage and foreign bodies; metallic bodies embedded in the bones (femoral or tibial condyles) away from the joint not to be disturbed (to avoid surgical trauma and flaring up of infection in the joint); edges of bones smoothed; vessels encountered to be ligated.
- Suturing of synovial membrane with catgut sutures
- Instill: Antibiotics into joint through closed synovium with a needle
- Flap of skin or fascia to close the wound, when loss of tissue prevents closure of synovium or capsule.

  After care:
  - Immobilize the joint with Buck's traction
  - Exercises: Active and passive, to be started once the acute symptoms subsided; restoring function to be induced slowly; otherwise a reaction may develop in the joint that may cause residual synovitis, or may even reactivate an infection; special exercises required to restore quadriceps power at the earliest possible
  - Walking: Allowed with the aid of a long leg brace; the brace not to be discarded until a satisfactory range of motion esp. extension, restored.

Management of type 3 wounds

**Note:** In most of type 3 wounds, infection is possible or probable, and the chances of restoring a mobile joint are remote.

Surgery:

- Debridement of wound and exploration of joint.

  Same as for a type 2 wound up to the point of closure.
- Arthrodesis: For a fresh wound (joint surfaces severely destroyed), may be considered.
- Alternatives: Based less upon the time since injury than upon the type of wound and the status of surgery, e.g. wound caused by a shotgun blast at close range may be so severe that thorough debridement impossible/or impracticable (inevitable infection).

Three alternatives:

A. Synovium closure: With left open skin and subcutaneous tissues

B. Drainage of wound: And dressed; closed secondarily on 5th day

C. • Drainage of wound: Through parallel incisions (posteromedial, posterolateral, and anterior); all wounds kept open.

 • Removal of metallic parts imbedded in bone near the joint, failing that may cause continuous irritation of tissues and result in sinuses formation.

After care:

- Immobilize the joint with Buck's traction
- Exercises: Active and passive, to be started once the acute symptoms subsided; restoring function to be induced slowly; otherwise a reaction may develop in the joint that may cause residual synovitis, or may even reactivate an infection; special exercises required to restore quadriceps power at the earliest possible
- Walking: Allowed with the aid of a long leg brace; the brace not to be discarded until a satisfactory range of motion esp. extension, restored.

## Bibliography

1. Bailey and Love's Short Practice of Surgery (1965) Love M, Rains A.J. H., Capper W.M.; H.K. Lewis and Co., London.
2. Blount WP. Unequal leg length, American Academy of Orthopedic Surgeons Instructional Course.
3. Campbell's Operative Orthopaedics (1998) 9th Ed. Vol I-IV. Canale S. Terry, Daugherty K, and Jones Linda. Mosby.
4. Canale ST, et al. Campbell's Operative Orthopaedics, ed. 9th, Vol I-IV. C.V. Mosby Co., Saint Louis, 1998.
5. Clark JMP. Modern Trends in Orthopedics Fracture Treatment, Butterworths, London, 1962.
6. Engleman EP. Chatton MJ. Acute infectious (septic) arthritis. Current Medical Diagnosis & Treatment, Maruzen, 1975.
7. Kapoor PS. Accident and Emergency: Etiology, Diagnosis and Management (2016) 2nd Ed. CBS, New Delhi.
8. Love M, et al. Bailey and Love's Short Practice of Surgery, ed. 13th, H.K. Lewis and Co., London, 1965.
9. Mc Rae R. Practical Fracture Treatment, ed. 1st, Churchill Livingstone, 1981.

# 19

# Endocrinal Affections of Bones and Joints

**Endocrinal affections**
- Pituitary gland:
  - Simmonds' disease (panhypopituitarism)
  - Gigantism and acromegaly
- Thyroid gland:
  - Cretinism and juvenile hypothyroidism
    Myxedema (adult hypothyroidism)
- Parathyroid gland:
  - Hypoparathyroidism (tetany)
  - Hyperparathyroidism

**Metabolic affections**
- Osteoporosis
- Rickets and osteomalacia
- Gouty arthritis
- Scurvy
- Marfan's syndrome
- Amyloidosis

**Nonmetabolic affections**
- Paget's disease
- Polyostotic fibrous displasia (osteitis fibrosa cystica)

## ENDOCRINAL AFFECTIONS

### Pituitary Gland (Syn. Hypophysis Cerebri)

| | |
|---|---|
| Anatomy | It is suspended from the bse of the brain by a projecting stalk so-called (infundibulum); lies in the pituitary fossa of the sella turcica of sphenoid bone in the middle fossa of the skull; covered by the sella diaphragm (dura)—pierced by the infundibulum; has two lobes (large anterior and small posterior); optic chiasma lies above the pituitary gland. |
| Physiology | Anterior pituitary functions: Controlled by regulating hormones (factors) generated by the hypothalamus: |

- Controls growth, esp. of bones, muscles, and viscera
- Regulates metabolism of carbohydrate, fat, and protein
- Controls growth, development, structural integrity, and activity of the thyroid, adrenal cortex, ovary, testis, and breast.

Hormones: Secreted are:
- Growth hormone
- Thyroid stimulating hormone (TSH)
- Corticotrophin hormone (ACTH)
- Follicle stimulating hormone (FSH)
- Luteinizing hormone (LH)
- Lactogenic hormone (Prolactin)
  Posterior pituitary functions;
- Controls secretion of urine by the kidney, thereby regulates water and electrolyte balance of the body fluids
- Stimulates release of lactogenic and galactopoietics factors from the anterior pituitary, thereby causes ejection of milk from the lactating breast; also have a physiological role in parturition.

Hormones secreted are:
- Antidiuretic hormone (ADH)
- Oxytocin hormone.

| | |
|---|---|
| Pathogenesis | Enlarged anterior pituitary (by tumors) leads to dyspituitarism: |

- Hyperpituitarism: Excessive skeletal growth:
  - Gigantism: Hyperpituitarism occurring prior to closure of epiphyses of long bones
  - Acromegaly: Hyperpituitarism occurring post closure of epiphyses.
- Hypopituitarism: Retarded skeletal growth:
  - Dwarfism: Stunted skeletal development in young persons; delayed genital maturity with delayed appearance of secondary sexual features.

## Disorders of Hypothalamus and Pituitary Gland

### Simmonds' Disease (Syn. Panhypopituitarism)

| | |
|---|---|
| Definition | It is defined as a disorder characterized by the inactivity of the pituitary gland, resulting in insufficiency of the target organs; all or many of the tropic hormones may get involved; isolated disorders, e.g. of the gonadotropins may not be rare; true pituitary cachexia is quite rare. |
| Etiology | Pituitary disorders: |

- Pituitary necrosis in post delivery circulatory collapse due to the hemorrhage (PPH)
- Granulomas
- Hemochromatosis
- Cysts (Rathke's pouch)
- Tumors: Cause hyper or hypopituitarism

Functional: In starvation, anemia

| | |
|---|---|
| Pathogenesis | hypothalamic lesions; destroyed/necrosed pituitary gland |
| Diagnosis | Weakness |
| | Fatigue |
| | Lack of resistance to stress, cold, and fasting |

Hair loss: Axillary and pubic

Skin: Dry, pallor, loss of pigmentation

Face: Sleepy appearance

Hypotension

Sexual dysfunction

Lactation: Abnormal

Visual field defects

| | |
|---|---|
| Investigation | CBC, ESR |

Blood sugar: Fasting low; flat glucose tolerance curve; insulin tolerance test shows insulin sensitivity

TFT: Low level of T4

Low levels of ACTH, TSH, LH, and FSH

X-rays skull may show a lesion in or above the sella; delayed bone age in children

Eye examination: Visual field defects may be present

**D/d**       Anorexia nervosa: May simulate hypopituitarism

Addison's disease

Myxedema.

**Complications**       As a result of patient's inability to cope with the minor stressful situations: Leading to:

- High fever
- Shock
- Coma
- Death.

**Management**       **Conservative treatment:**

Replacement therapy:

- Corticosteroids:
  - Hydrocortisone 20–30 mg PO od, Alt:
  - Prednisolone 5 mg PO od, Alt:
  - Dexamethasone 1 mg PO od
- Thyroid:
  - Thyroid extract 15–30 mg PO od, Alt:
  - Thyroxine 0.1 mg PO od
- Sex hormones:
  - Testosterone: Both for male and females: methyltestosterone (male 20 mg; female 10 mg) PO od
  - Anabolics: Estrogens for females: estradiol 0.5 mg PO od
  - Gonadotrophic hormone: APL + pituitary FSH or postmenopausal urinary gonadotrophin (to initiate fertility)
- Human growth hormone: Most effective agent for increasing height (Human placental lactogen).

Radiotherapy:

Indications: Spontaneous cystic involution; abnormal optic chiasma

Surgical treatment:

Indication: Tumor

Surgery: Removal of tumor.

## *Gigantism and Acromegaly*

| | |
|---|---|
| Definition | It is defined as hyperpituitarism that may occur pre (gigantism) or post closure (acromegaly) of the epiphyses of the long bones, due to (excessive growth hormone) overactivity of the anterior pituitary lobe, formed by a benign adenoma. |
| Etiology | • Tumors of the anterior pituitary lobe: benign adenoma; carcinomas<br>• Transient: Fugitive acromegaly |
| Pathogenesis | Hyperactive eosinophilic portion of anterior pituitary lobe; onset may be pre or post closure of epiphyses of long bones |
| Diagnosis | • Growth: Excessive growth of the hands (increased glove size), feet (increased shoe size), jaw (protruded lower jaw), malar bones (prominent lower half of face), separation of teeth, chest (increased AP diameter of chest); and internal organs<br>• Deformity: Kyphosis, big hands reaching down to knees, protruded lower jaw (Gorilla type)<br>• Amenorrhea<br>• Headache<br>• Sweating, weakness<br>• Bone and Joint: Aches and pains in the limbs; backache<br>• Hypotension<br>• Visual field: Loss |
| Investigation | • CBC, ESR<br>• Serum inorganic phosphorus: Elevated<br>• BMR: Elevated<br>• FSH: Low level<br>• Glycosuria<br>• Hyperglycemia<br>• Hypercalciuria<br>• T4 and PBI: Normal<br>• Eye examination: Visual field study may show bitemporal hemianopsia<br>• X-rays skull: May show large sella with destroyed clinoids; large frontal sinuses; thickened skull and long bones; dorsal kyphosis. |
| D/d | • Amenorrhea: Unexplained<br>• Diabetes mellitus: Insulin resistant (Type II)<br>• Goiter: With increased BMR<br>• Occupational. |
| Complications | • Pressure: On adjoining structures<br>• Carpal tunnel syndrome<br>• Cord compression: Due to large disks<br>• Rupture of tumor into brain or sinuses<br>• Heart failure. |

| Management | Conservative treatment: |
|---|---|

Conservative treatment:
- Hormonal therapy (HT):
  - Progesterone, growth hormone (somatostatin).
- Radiotherapy (RT): Treatment of choice for sensitive tumor, without visual field loss.

Surgical treatment (ST): Rarely required as per the patient's are poor risk, on account of heart and chest problems, and difficult surgical approach.

Indication: Radiotherapy hazardous; visual fields markedly reduced.

Surgery: Cryohypophysectomy.

## THYROID GLAND

**Anatomy**

The thyroid gland is composed of two lateral lobes connected by an isthmus; each lobe extends vertically from middle of thyroid cartilage's side, to the 6th tracheal ring; isthmus covers 2nd, 3rd, and 4th tracheal rings; external and recurrent laryngeal nerves are in intimate relationship with the gland (surgeon's main concern to protect these, in thyroid surgery).

**Physiology**

Secretes thyroxine and triiodothyronine (hormone iodine) present only in plasma (4–8 μg/dl.; regulated by the TSH of the anterior pituitary

Functions of thyroxine:
- Metabolism:
  - To stimulate metabolism in the tissues
  - To increase oxygen consumption (by catalyzing enzyme systems that are meant for oxidation processes)
  - To promote growth and development of internal organs
  - To promote absorption of glucose from small intestine
  - To stimulate conversion of glycogen into glucose in the liver.
- Bone:
  - To modify the calcium metabolism (removal of calcium and phosphorus from bones, causing rarefaction (osteoporosis); does not raise serum calcium (due to loss in feces and urine).
- Heart:
  - To accelerate normal and denervated heart
- Kidney:
  - To increase urine flow
  - To regulate fluid distribution in the body
- Breast:
  - To promote milk secretion

**Assaying thyroid function**

Thyroid function tests:
- Basal metabolic rate (BMR): Best index of the severity of thyroid Dysfunction: Elevated in hyperthyroidism, polycythemia, leukemia; low in myxedema, Simmond's disease
- Plasma protein bound iodine (PBI): Most useful test for suspected mild myxedema; high in hyperthyroidism, thyroiditis, ingestion of iodides, thyroxine, desiccated thyroid; low in hypothyroidism, ingestion of mercurial diuretics, nephrosis

- CBC, ESR
- Serum cholesterol: Elevated in hypothyroidism, myxedema; low in thyrotoxicosis
- Thyroid stimulating hormone (TSH): By immunohistochemistry
- Triiodothyronine (T3): By serum chemilumiescence
- Thyroxine (T4): By radio immunoassay/by serum chemiluminescence
- Thyroglobulin: By chemiluminescence.

**Pathogenesis**   Thyroid disorders leads to:

- Hypothyroidism: Retarded skeletal growth:
- Myxedema: In adults
- Cretinism and Juvenile hypothyroidism in children
- Hyperthyroidism: Retarded skeletal growth:
- Dwarfism: Stunted skeletal development in young persons; delayed genital maturity with delayed appearance of secondary sexual features.

## Disorders of Thyroid Gland

### Cretinism (Syn. Juvenile Hypothyroidism)

**Definition**   It is defined as a type of dwarfism, with marked mental retardation, resulting from congenital absence or maldevelopment of the thyroid gland

**Etiology**   Causes of cretinism and juvenile hypothyroidism (Wilkins)

Congenital (Cretinism):

- Thyroid gland: Absent or rudimentary
- Thyroid gland: Present but defective in hormone secretion, goitrous, or atrophied
- Extrinsic factor: Deficient iodine

Acquired (Juvenile Hypothyroidism):

- Thyroid gland: Atrophic, defective in function, thyroiditis,
- Operative: Thyroidectomy (lingual thyroid or toxic goiter)

**Pathogenesis**   Delayed skeletal maturartion; stippled epiphyses.

**Diagnosis**   Dwarfism: Delayed skeletal maturation

Long bones: Thickened

Apathy, listless

Mental retardation

Face: Pale, puffy, wrinkled

Skin: Dry and cold

Hair: Coarse, dry, brittle

Anorexia

Dentition: Delayed

GI tract: Constipation, large protruding tongue, pot belly, umbilical hernia

Limbs: Cold, hands thick and short

Sexual maturity: Retarded, sexual precocity

Amenorrhea or menometrorrhagia

| Investigation | • CBC, ESR |
|---|---|
| | • Serum cholesterol: Elevated |
| | • BMR: |
| |     – Thyroid stimulating hormone (TSH): By immunohistochemistry: high |
| | • Triiodothyronine (T3): By serum chemiluminescence |
| | • Thyroxine (T4): By radioimmunoassay / by serum chemiluminescence: low |
| | • Thyroglobulin: By chemiluminescence. |
| | X-rays: Shows delayed skeletal maturation, often with stippling of the epiphyses (e.g. of femoral head) with flattening; thickened cortices of long bones; absent cranial sinuses; delayed dentition |
| D/d | Hypopituitarism |
| | Down's syndrome: Retarded skeletal development rare |
| Management | Specific: Thyroid or a synthetic preparation used: |
| | Desiccated thyroid: |
| | • Initial dose: 60–120 mg PO od until age of 12 years. |
| | • Maintenance dose: 120–180 mg PO od for life |
| | Thyroxine sod: |
| | • Initial dose: 50–100 µg PO od, increased by 25 µg every 2/12 |
| | • Maintenance dose: 100–200 µg. PO od |

### Myxedema (Syn. Adult Hypothyroidism)

| Definition | It is defined as a disease caused by the inability of the thyroid gland to secrete a sufficient amount of the thyroxine hormone; usually affects middle aged women. |
|---|---|
| Etiology | Idiopathic |
| | Thyroidectomy: Total |
| | Thyrotoxic patients: Treated with radioiodine |
| | Antithyroid drugs: Overtreatment/overdosage |
| Pathogenesis | Atrophic thyroid gland; reduced iodide capacity; reduced formation of thyroxine and triiodothyronine |
| Diagnosis | Mental retardation; amnesia; slow speech, nervousness |
| | Muscular weakness, fatigue, lethargy, headache, bodyache |
| | Sexual functions impaired: menorrhagia, amenorrhea |
| | Face: Puffy |
| | Skin: Dry and coarse |
| | Hair: Thin, coarse, dry |
| | Nails: Brittle |
| | Weight gain: Due to reduced metabolism and edematous skin and organs |
| | Speech: Slow |
| | CVS: Pericardial effusion, heart enlargement |
| | Deep tendon reflexes: Delayed return. |
| Investigation | • CBC, ESR |
| | • Serum cholesterol: Elevated |

- BMR:
- Thyroid stimulating hormone (TSH): By immunohistochemistry: high
- Triiodothyronine (T3): By serum chemiluminescence
- Thyroxine (T4): By radio immunoassay/by serum chemiluminescence: low
- Thyroglobulin: By chemiluminescence.

X-rays: Shows flattening; thickened cortices of the long bones

D/d      Hypopituitarism

Down's syndrome: Retarded skeletal development rare

Management      Specific: Thyroid or a synthetic preparation used:

Desiccated thyroid:

- Initial dose: 60–120 µg PO od until age of 12 years.
- Maintenance dose: 120–180 µg PO od for life

Thyroxine sod.:

- Initial dose: 50–100 µg PO od, increased by 25 µg. Every 2/12
- Maintenance dose: 100–200 µg. PO od

## PARATHYROID GLAND

Anatomy      A small gland embedded in the thyroid gland in the neck, or located near it; usually there are two pairs of parathyroid glands; size of a split pea; related to the inferior laryngeal vessels and recurrent laryngeal nerves (surgeon's main concern to protect these, in thyroid surgery).

Physiology      Parathyroids secretes parathyroid hormone (active principles are parathormone and calcitonin) that regulates the calcium and phosphorus metabolism in the body; the production of parathyroid hormone depends directly on the level of calcium in the blood passing through the glands; any lowering of the blood's calcium level results in secretion of more parathyroid hormone; bone and kidney are the main target organs.

Functions of parathormone:

- To regulate excretion of inorganic phosphate in the urine: increased phosphate excretion in the urine results in hypophosphatemia, leads to reciprocal hypercalcemia (flow of calcium from bones into blood); hypercalcemia leads to increased calcium excretion by the kidney; causing rarefaction of bones, hypercalcemia, elimination of bone calcium in the urine
- To act directly on bone, by stimulating osteoclastic activity; leading to flow of calcium from bones into blood—hypercalcemia
- To act on the kidney, electrolyte equilibria, and the bones.

Functions of calcitonin:

- To lower the serum calcium and effects calcium storage in the bone; quite the opposite action to parathormone.

Pathogenesis      Hypoparathyroidism leads to decreased phosphate urinary excretion; hyperphosphatemia; reciprocal hypocalcemia (fall affects diffusible—ionized calcium); muscular spasms (tetany).

## Disorders of Parathyroid gland

### Hypoparathyroidism (Tetany)

| | |
|---|---|
| Definition | Hypoparathyroidism is usually seen following thyroidectomy or, post-operative removal of parathyroid tumor; characterized by muscular spasms (Tetany) due to hypocalcemia and alkalemia. |
| Etiology | Direct trauma: Violence (neck injury) |
| | Surgical: Post-thyroidectomy; post parathyroid surgery (tumor removal) |
| | Irradiation: Radiotherapy (RT) |
| | Neonatal: Underactivity of parathyroid |
| | Idiopathic: Associated with candidiasis, familial, Addison's disease |
| | Renal failure with phosphate retention |
| Pathogenesis | Hypoparathyroidism leads to decreased phosphate urinary excretion; hyperphosphatemia; reciprocal hypocalcemia (fall affects diffusible—ionized calcium); muscular spasms (tetany) |
| Diagnosis | Tetany, with muscle (hands, feet, and abdominal) cramps, stridor and wheezing, irritability, carpopedal spasms (adducted thumbs with the plantar-flexion of feet), and convulsions |
| | Personality changes, anxiety state |
| | Dyspnea: Due to spasm of respiratory muscles |
| | Face: Tingling and numbness of lips, nose, and limbs |
| | Eyes: Diplopia, photophobia, blurring of vision, late cataracts |
| | Nails: Thin, brittle |
| | Skin: Dry, scaly, candidiasis |
| | Eyebrows: Loss of hair |
| | Urinary: Frequency |
| | Chvostek's sign (facial contraction on tapping facial nerve near angle of jaw): +ve |
| | Trousseau's phenomenon (carpopedal spasm post application of a cuff) +ve |
| | Deep reflexes: Hyperactive |
| Investigation | Serum calcium: Low |
| | Serum phosphate: High |
| | Urinary phosphate: Low |
| | Urinary calcium: Low |
| | Alkaline phosphatase: Normal |
| | Creatinine clearance: Normal |
| | Radioimmunoassayable parathormone level: Low |
| | X-rays skull: May show calcified basal ganglia; denser bones |
| D/d | Metabolic or respiratory alkalosis |
| | GI tract: Pyloric stenosis, vomiting, diarrhea |
| | Primary hyperaldosteronism |
| | Brain tumor. |
| Complications | Respiratory obstruction |
| | Cardiac failure |
| | Growth: Stunting |
| | Brain damage |

| Management | Preventive treatment: |
|---|---|

- To isolate and embed parathyroid in the sternomastoid muscle, during subtotal thyroidectomy for a benign disorder
  Specific treatment of parathyroid tetany:
- Calcium gluconate (10% sol.) 10–20 ml IV slowly; rept. as per condion.
  Maintenance treatment:
- Parathyroid extract (parathormone) 30 IU IM bid
- Diet: Rich in calcium; or calcium lactate 8 G added to the diet.
  Avoid meat, fish, cereals, and dairy products (rich in phosphorus).
- Vitamin D2 (Calciferol) 50–200 K IU + calcium lactate 5–15 G od PO; to be given throughout life.

## Hyperparathyroidism

| Preface | Hyperparathyroidism may result from diffuse hyperplasia of all the parathyroids or from a localized tumor (adenoma, or rarely carcinoma) in one of them; characterized by rise of serum calcium, reciprocally fall of serum phosphate; withdrawal of calcium from bones; increased urinary excretion of calcium; decreased urinary excretion of phosphate |
|---|---|
| Etiology | Diffuse hyperplasia of all the parathyroids |
| | Localized tumor: Adenoma or carcinoma |
| Pathogenesis | Rise of the serum calcium; reciprocally fall of the serum phosphate; withdrawal of calcium from bones; increased urinary excretion of the calcium; decreased urinary excretion of phosphate; rarefaction of bones (osteoporosis); bone cysts formed (osteitis fibrosa cystica); pathological fractures; renal calculi formed due to calciurea. |
| Diagnosis | Skeletal manifestations: |

- Body aches, joint pains, backache
- Pathological fractures of spine, ribs, or long bones

Urinary tract manifestations:
- Renal calculi
- Polyuria, polydipsia, uremia

GI tract manifestations:
- Constipation, peptic ulcer

Hypercalcemia manifestations:
- Nausea, vomiting, anorexia, restlessness, prostration, and tachycardia

CVS manifestations:
- Hypertension

| Investigation | Serum calcium: Increased |
|---|---|
| | Serum phosphorus: Decreased |
| | Serum alkaline phosphatase: Increased |
| | Urine calcium: Increased |
| | Urine phosphate: High |
| | Slitlamp examination of eye: Band keratoplasty |
| | X-ray: Shows subperiosteal resorption; loss of lamina dura of teeth; renal parenchymal calcification or stones, bone cysts. |

| D/d | Multiple myeloma |
| | Metastatic (kidney, bladder, thyroid) |
| | Hyperthyroidism |
| | Sarcoidosis |
| | Bone disorders: Osteoporosis, cancer |
| | Vitamin D intoxication |
| | Drugs: Corticosteroids, chlorthiazides |
| Management | Conservative treatment: |

Fluids: IV fluids to minimize formation of calcium phosphate renal Stones.

Diuretics: Furosemide

Hemodialysis: May be life-saving

Calcitonin: Lowers serum calcium

Surgical treatment: Only curative treatment.

Surgery: Parathyroidectomy

Indication: Adenoma of parathyroid and hyperplasia of parathyroids

Preoperatively: 4 g of calcium lactate and 1 K units of calciferol, with 1 L of milk PO od for 3/7

Technique:

- Incision: Transverse incision following a crease of neck; flap dissected up to level of pomum adami
- Exposure of thyroid gland through a vertical median incision made into fasciomuscular planes from the hyoid bone to the suprasternal space of burns; parathyroid tumor is sought by sight and touch
- Excision of parathyroid tumor; Alt.
- Excision: 3/4th of hyperplastic parathyroid

Postoperatively:

Calcium + Vitamin D (calciferol):

- 4 g of calcium lactate and 1 K units of calciferol, with 1 L of milk PO od for 3/7 for 6/12.

## METABOLIC BONE DISEASES/DISORDERS/AFFECTIONS

### Osteoporosis

Osteoporosis is a world wide phenomenon, being considered now as a common geriatric disorder. No race or sex has been spared.

| Definition | It is defined as a progressive systemic disease characterized by reduced bone mass and deteriorating bone tissue (matrix), thereby resulting in increased bone fragility and subsecuently a fracture may occur with a minor injury, when the bone loss > 30%. |
| Etiology | Primary: Unknown |
| Secondary | Traumatic: Prolonged immobilization |
| | Inflammatory: Rheumatoid arthritis, tuberculous, syphilitic |
| | Endocrinal: Lack of androgens: senile osteoporosis |

|  | Lack of estrogens: Postmenopausal osteoporosis |
|---|---|
|  | Hypopituitarism: Hypogonadism |
|  | Hyperthyroidism: Thyrotoxicosis |
|  | Hyperparathyroidism |
|  | Excessive ACTH or corticosteroids: Cushing's syndrome |
|  | Diabetes mellitus |
|  | Pregnancy |
|  | Metabolic: Calcium deficiency |
|  | Neoplastic: Multiple myeloma. |
| **Risk factors** | Age:  > 60 years |
|  | Sex: F : M ratio 6 : 2 |
|  | Race: Asian |
|  | Built: Thin |
|  | Menopause: Early |
|  | Alcohol abuse: Excess intake |
|  | Smoking: Cigarettes |
|  | Diet: Poor diet |
|  | Lifestyle: Sedentary |
|  | Activity: Lack of physical activity (exercise) |
|  | Drugs: Heparin and corticosteroids—prolonged use. |
| **Diagnosis** | Asymptomatic to severe backache |
|  | May be found accidently on X-ray examination for a fracture |
|  | Fracture: Occurrence of a fracture is the most common finding, e.g. |

Sites:

- Fracture neck of femur
- Fracture vertebral body (crush)
- Colles' fracture

Pain: Low backache—localized or radiating

Deformity

Height: Loss of height.

| **Investigation** | Serum calcium, phosphate and alkaline phosphatase are normal |
|---|---|
|  | X-ray shows: Areas of demineralization of spine, pelvis, limbs |

Fracture:
- Compression fracture of vertebral body
- Fracture neck of femur
- Colles' fracture

Bone densitometry (BMD) measurement (Table 19.1): May be an important test in early diagnosis of bone mineral loss.

Technique: Ultrasound (US) of the os calcis.

Other sites: Lumbar spine, neck of femur and distal end of radius.

The BMD measurement is recorded as a T score:

(Patient's BMD compared  to BMD of a healthy young adult)

And a Z score:

(Patient's BMD compared to BMD of same sex and age person)

**Table 19.1:** T Score Interpretation

| T Score | Interpretation |
| --- | --- |
| 0 to –1 | Normal |
| 1 to –2.5 | Osteopenia |
| < –2.5 | Osteoporosis |
| < –2.5 with fracture | Frank osteoporosis |

(*Source*: World Health Organisation)

Interpretation: Depending on the T score the patient's fracture risk can be calculated and treated accordingly (Table 19.1).

CT scan  : Quantitative CT scan

MRI       : Quantitative MRI

DEXA     : (Dual Energy X-ray Absorptiometry)—is a valuable test. Disadvantage is an expensive procedure

Bone Biopsy: Rarely done—being an invasive and time consuming procedure.

**Management**  Aims: To prevent or reduce the level of osteoporosis.

General measures:

Diet: High protein diet and adequate in calcium (milk and milk products)

Exercise: Regular exercise esp. weight bearing

Stop smoking

Reduce alcohol intake

Calcium and vitamin D:

- Calcium (carbonate or lactate) 1–2 g od.
- Vitamin D: Alfacalcidol and calcitriol
- Alfacalcidol 0.25 µg-1.0 µg od.
- Calcitriol 0.25–0.5 µg od.

Analgesics and NSAIDs.

Specific measures:

I. Antiresorptives:

   A. Hormone replacement therapy (HRT):

   Indication: Postmenopausal osteoporosis

Drugs:

1. Estrogens:

   Indication: Postmenopausal osteoporosis

   Intact uterus: Estrogen along with progesterone given to reduce chances of malignancy

   Hysterectomised: Estrogen given alone

   Agents:

- Natural estrogens: Estradiol, estrone, conjugated estrogens
- Synthetic estrogens: Ethinyl estradiol, mestranol, stilbestrol

   Dose:

- Ethinyl estradiol 0.05 mg t.d.s. maintenance 0.025 mg/day,

- Eonjugated estrogen 0.625 mg/day,
- Estriol 4 mg/day for 2/52 Maintenance 1–2 mg/day

2. Combined Estrogen + Testosterone:

   Indication: postmenopausal osteoporosis

   Agents: Mixogen (ethinylestradiol + methyltestosterone)

   Dose: 1–2 mg/day PO or 1 mL IM every 3–4 weeks.

   C/I: Breast cancer, vaginal bleeding, pregnancy, liver disease

3. Progestogens:

   Indication: Adjunt to estrogen replacement therapy (HRT) in menopausal women with an intact uterus

   Agents: Norethindrone acetate

   Dose: 5–10 mg/day from 14th to 28th day of each cycle

4. Androgens:

   Indication: Hypogonadic androgen deficiency osteoporosis

   Agents: Testosterone 25–50 mg IM twice weekly for 4–6 weeks.

   C/I: Suspected cases of breast or prostate carcinoma

   B. Bisphosphonates:

   Indication: Postmenopausal, steroid induced and senile osteoporosis

   Agents:
   - Alendronate 10 mg/day or 70 mg/week
   - Etidronate 400 mg/day for 2/52 followed by 11/52, repeat 4 cycles/year.
   - Other newer drugs: Ibandronate, risodronate and tiludronate

   S/E: Esophagitis, gastritis and disturbance of bone mineralization

   C. Calcitonin:

   Indication: Postmenopausal osteoporosis and osteogenesis imperfecta

   Dose: 100 units/day IM or sc.

   S/E: Flushing, local irritation, diarrhea

   D. Thiazides:

   Indication: Hypercalciuria

   Dose: Hydrochlorothiazide 25–50 mg/day 5.

II. Mineral supplements:

- Calcium supplementation:

  Indication: Postmenopausal and senile osteoporosis

  Dose: Calcium (carbonate or lactate) 1000–2000 mg/day

- Fluoride supplementation:

  Indication: Enhances bone formation

  Dose: 20–50 mg od.

- Anabolic steroids:

  Indication: As an adjunctive therapy in the treatment of osteoporosis

  Agents:
  - Nandrolone decanoate (Metadec) 25–100 mg every 3rd week IM
  - Nandrolone phenylpropionate (Durabolin, Metabol) 25–50 mg/week IM

| D/d | Osteomalacia and Rickets: |
|---|---|
| | In osteoporosis there is a reduction in the bone mass and the mineral—matrix ratio is maintained, in contrast to osteomalacia and rickets—in which mineral—matrix ratio is disturbed due to reduced mineralization. |

## Rickets and Osteomalacia

| Preface | Characterized by disturbed mineral-matrix ratio due to reduced mineralization; rickets is a deficiency disease due to lack of vitamin D (component of natural fats and oils); osteomalacia is the adult form of rickets—common in females; tetany may occur in advanced cases.<br>Epidemiology: Prevalent in African, Asean, North China. |
|---|---|
| Etiology | Deficiency of calcium and phosphorus in the bone; may be caused by:<br>• Inadequate absorption from the intestine, either due to the lack of calcium alone, or lack of/or resistance to the action of vitamin D. Osteomalacia in adults may be found in association with:<br>  – Disorders of fat absorption (diarrhea, gastrectomy, pancreatitis, and sprue)<br>  – Renal calcium or phosphorus losses (vitamin D resistant rickets)<br>  – Fanconi's syndrome<br>  – Mesenchymal tumor. |
| Risk factors | Lack of sunshine<br>Diet: Poor in natural fats and oils<br>Sedentary: Immobilization, lack of exercises/yoga<br>Neoplastic |
| Pathogenesis | Epiphysitis; epiphyseal cartilages enlarged (longitudinally and laterally); histologically zone of provisional calcification either absent or present (irregular patches); thereby no specific line of demarcation exists between the proliferating cartilage and the medullary spaces; newly formed bone trabeculae are of osteoid tissue, that lack calcium salts, while medullary spaces filled up with vascular fibrocellular tissue instead of normal bone marrow; result in deformed bones. |
| Diagnosis | Flabby child with pot belly, sweating of head<br><br>Deformities:<br>• Stature: Diminished due to retarted bony growth (esp. femur and tibia); bending of leg bones, and spinal deformities<br>• Increased width of shaft due to increased epiphyses<br>• Ribs: Rickety rosary due to beading of costochondral junctions<br>• Long bones: Deformed legs (bowing) due to weight bearing:<br>• Femur: Natural curves increased, e.g. increased anterior curve of the femur; coxa vara<br>• Tibia: Abrupt curvature in the lower third of tibia (buttress formation)<br>• Skull: Craniotabs occurs due to severe constitutional disturbances; delayed closure of fontanelles and dentition; skull becomes broader and flatter (increased width between eyes—broadening of base) |

- Spine: kyphosis, followed by scoliosis due to the faulty posture or inequality of legs
- Pelvis

Pain: Bones aching esp. of long bones and ribs

Respiratory: Distress

GI tract: Disturbances

Hepatomegaly

Splenomegaly

Renal functions: Disorders

Umbilical hernia: Due to prolonged distension

Muscular weakness, paralysis.

|  |  |
|---|---|
| Investigation | CBC, ESR, blood urea |
|  | Serum calcium: Low |
|  | Serum phosphate: Low |
|  | Alkaline phosphatase: Elevated |
|  | Urinary calcium and phosphate: Low |
|  | Bone densitometer test: +ve |
|  | X-ray: Shows cupping of epiphyseal line; epiphyseal line blurred and concave towards the epiphysis; demineralization and bowing. |
| D/d | Osteoporosis |
|  | Hyperparathyroidism |
|  | Hyperthroidism |
|  | Osteogenesis imperfecta |
| Management | ASAP: Yields good results |

Conservative treatment:

Diet: High calcium diet, milk, cod liver oil, meat extracts

Calcium: Gluconate or lactate 5–20 g/day

Vitamin D: Metabolites of calciferol for osteomalacia resistant to vitamin D

Sunlight exposure (coverts ergosterol in the skin to vitamin D)

Deformities: Corrected by splinting

Osteoclasis: By manipulation.

Specific measures:

- Rickets: Vitamin D 2–5 K units/day
- Osteomalacia and renal rickets: Vitamin D 25–100 K units/day
- Pancreatic insufficiency: Pancreatic enzyme; high calcium intake
- Fanconi's syndrome: (Disturbed calcium and phosphorus metabolism; glycosuria, albuminuria, and cystinuria); rachitic changes in epiphysis in children while osteoporosis in adults: managed by calcium, vitamin D, and phosphorus intake.

Surgical treatment:

Indication: To correct deformities.

Surgery: Osteotomy in older children and adults

**Gouty Arthritis** Described in chapter on Arthritis and Allied Rheumatic Diseases

## Scurvy

| | |
|---|---|
| Definition | It is defined as a disease caused by a severe lack of vitamin C (ascorbic acid); may occur in infants who have been fed exclusively on sterilized food, the vitamin C content of that has thus been destroyed and not replaced by fruit juice; breastfed babies usually obtain enough vitamin C from the mother's milk; may also occur in adults (diet lacks fresh fruit and vegetables, that are rich in vitamin C), and in the old people living alone, or occasionally in those dieting 'on medical advice'. |
| Etiology | Deficiency of vitamin C due to:<br>Dietary:<br>• Infants: Fed exclusively on sterilized food (minus breastfeeding)<br>• Adults: Dietary: lacking fresh fruit and vegetables<br>• Elderly: Living alone or dieting on medical advice.<br>Metabolic: Increased metabolic needs |
| Physiology | Vitamin C (ascorbic acid) available in plant and animal kingdoms:<br>• Fresh juice (blackcurrant, strawberry, orange, lemon, grapefruit, etc.)<br>• Fresh vegetables: Sprouts, cauliflower, cabbage, tomato, potatoes, etc.<br>• Milk: Vitamin C content of human milk > that of cow's milk; Pasteurization: Destroys vitamin C of cow's milk (although counts for little vs benefits of pasteurization)<br>• Foods devoid of vitamin C: Meat, fish, eggs, fats and oils, cereal products includes Bread and nuts. |
| Requirement | Adults: 30–45 mg od<br>Pregnant and lactating mothers: 60 mg od |
| Pathogenesis | Bruises on limbs; extravasation of blood into the tissues; hemorrhagic gums; loosening of teeth; poor wound healing; epiphyseal changes. |
| Diagnosis | Gums: Edema and bleeding of gums<br>Dentine: Porosity<br>Hair follicles: Hyperkeratotic<br>Muscular weakness<br>Joints: Swollen<br>Bones: Rarefaction<br>Skin: Bruises<br>Lethargy<br>Breathing disorder |
| Investigation | CBC, ESR<br>Reduced capillary resistance<br>Serum ascorbic acid levels: Decreased<br>X-rays of long bones: May show typical changes; epiphyseal changes in children—pathognomic. |
| Management | Easy to treat:<br>Diet: Fresh fruit and leafy green vegetables<br>Vitamin C tablets 100 mg od PO as long as deficiency persists<br>Injection sodium ascorbate 100–500 mg IM. |

## Marfan's Syndrome

Definition       It is defined as an autosomal dominant hereditary of connective tissue; basic metabolic defect of that remains unknown; may be quite similar to that seen in patients with homocystinuria; disease involves primarily the skeletal system, CVS, and the eyes, besides many other clinical manifestations; mild, incomplete (atypical) forms of the disease may exist.

Etiology         Unknown.

Pathogenesis     Connective tissue disorder: Arachnodactyly; thin, tapered webbed fingers, pes planus, pes cavus, hammer toes, tower skull, high palatal arch, winged scapulae; lens dislocation; detached retinas; and CVS deformities.

Diagnosis        Build: Tall and thin
                 Deformity:
                 - Limbs: Long vs trunk
                 - Hands: Spider-like (arachnodactyly) with thin, tapered, webbed fingers
                 - Feet: Pes planus, pes cavus, and hammer toe may be present
                 - Skull: 'Tower skull' (long, narrow, and pointed head), and high palatal arch
                 - Chest: Pigeon or funnel shaped
                 - Scapula: Winging of scapulas.
                 - Eyes: Myopia, dislocation of lens (ectopia lentis), retinal detachment
                 CVS: Aortic dilatation; pulmonary dilatation, valvular insufficiency, ASD, and dissecting aneurysm.

Investigation    CBC< ESR
                 Serum mucoprotein: Low
                 Urinary hydroxyproline: High
                 X-rays: Skull, chest, affected limb/s, scapulae

Complications    Cardiovascular complications:
                 - ASD
                 - Disecting aneurysm

Management       Symptomatic and supportive
                 Treatment: Confined toward CV disorders

Prognosis        Mortality rate high during infancy.
                 Death: Occurs usually due to cardiac complications.

## Amyloidosis

Definition       It is defined as a poorly understood disorder of the protein metabolism that usually occurs secondary to chronic suppurative disease, but that may also occur as the primary type in patients without the apparent pre-existing disease; the onset insidious; clinical manifestations may vary as per organs/or tissues in which the peculiar homogeneous, filamentous glycoprotein (amyloid) substance that is deposited extra-cellularly; may be associated with the abnormalities of the serum globulins, e.g. multiple myeloma.

| Pathogenesis | **Types:** |
|---|---|

- **Primary (hereditary) systemic amyloidosis:** Rarely, occurs in patients without any pre-existing disease; usually transmitted as an autosomal dominant trait; amyloid deposited mainly in mesenchymal tissues, with resultant involvement of many organs.
- **Primary localized (tumor forming) amyloidosis:** Rarely, occurs in patients with involvement of upper respiratory tract (larynx); in the absence of pre-existing disease; and without evidence of amyloidosis in other tissues.
- **Amyloidosis associated with multiple myeloma:** May be variation of the primary systemic type, while the relationship is uncertain.
- **Secondary amyloidosis:** Commonest type; associated with chronic debilitating and suppurative disorders; amyloid deposited widely in parenchymatous organs (liver, spleen, kidneys, and adrenal glands); predisposing factors (tuberculosis, RA, ulcerative colitis, chronic osteomyelitis, and other chronic wasting and suppurative disorders.

| Diagnosis | Highly variable and atypical |
|---|---|
| | Hereditary |
| | Fever |
| | Weakness |
| | Weight loss |
| | Purpura |
| | Lymph adenopathy |
| | Pain abdomen |
| | Hepatosplenomegaly |
| | CHF |
| | Nephropathy. |
| Investigation | Microscopic examination of biopsy or surgical specimens post staining procedures: Diagnostic |
| | Fin needle biopsy of subcutaneous abdominal fat: diagnostic |
| | X-rays of affected parts. |
| D/d | Chronic osteomyelitis |
| | Chronic suppurative disorders |
| | Multiple myeloma. |

| Management | |
|---|---|

- No effective treatment of systemic amyloidosis.
- Surgical excision of localized amyloid tumors.
- Treatment of the predisposing disease may cause a temporary remission or slowdown the progress of the disease, but is unlikely that the established metabolic process is altered.
- An early adequate treatment of pyogenic infections (antibiotics and corticosteroids) may prevent much secondary amyloidosis.

| Prognosis | Poor esp. in systemic amyloidosis. |
|---|---|
| | Death usually occurs within 1–3 years. |

# NONMETABOLIC BONE DISEASES/DISORDERS/AFFECTIONS

## Paget's Disease (Osteitis Deformans)

| | |
|---|---|
| Definition | It is defined as a nonsystemic localized skeletal affection, in contrast to Hyperparathyroidism; may affect single or multiple bones, often involving only a part of a single bone; affects the spine (usually lumbar region), skull, sternum, ribs, clavicle, humerus, innominate, femur, and tibia, in descending order; spares the small bones. |
| Etiology | Unknown. |
| Pathogenesis | Increased blood flow to the affected bone; marked osteoclastic activity, abruptly followed by marked osteoblastic activity, forming irregular tortuous cemented lines in the bone; intertrabeculae marrow spaces filled with fibrous tissue (mosaic pattern), dense regular cortex replaced by spongy tissue—2 to 3 times thicker than normal cortex, subperiosteal bone formation, narrow/absent medullary canal. |
| Diagnosis | Symptomless (25%)<br>Pain: Prominent symptom of longer duration, intermittent in nature<br>Stature: Diminished due to kyphosis and scoliosis of spine, and bowing of long bones of legs<br>Head: Enlarged, forehead veins dilated<br>Face: Thickened facial bones<br>Chest: AP diameter increased<br>Backache, weakness, fatigue, tendered heels<br>Eyes and Ears: Impaired vision and hearing<br>Gait: Waddling due to coxa vara. |
| Investigation | X-rays: Diagnostic—appearance as per disease's stage:<br>• Normal bone destroyed<br>• Paget bone formed<br>• Paget bone destroyed<br>• Paget becomes healed or quiescent<br>• Areas of excessive new bone formation seen with alternate areas of lysis or cyst formation<br>• New bone: Coarsely trabeculated and honeycombed<br>• Long bones: Paget begins at one end, advancing toward other end<br>• Cortex of long bone: Thickened, irregular surfaces (Fuzzy)<br>• Skull: Thickened, wooly in appearance<br>• Vertebrae: Decreased height, increased width, wedging of vertebral bodies; vertebral collapse to compress the spinal cord. |
| Complications | • Pathological fracture: Spontaneous fracture common, transverse character (often revealed by X-ray).<br>• Osteoarthritis: Due to altered mechanics of the joint<br>• Paraplegia: Due to involved vertebrae (collapse)<br>• Bone sarcoma: May develop in 5% cases of Paget (osteoblastic or osteoclastic type)<br>• Death: Due to pulmonary distress. |

| | |
|---|---|
| Management | No specific treatment to control progress of Paget's disease. |
| | Medical treatment: Symptomatic: |
| | Pain: Anti-inflammatory drugs |
| | Radiotherapy: To relieve bone pain |

Surgical treatment:
Osteotomy: To relieve pain due to faulty mechanics.

### Treatment of complications
Pathological fracture:
- Close reduction and immobilization
- ORIF: To avoid prolonged immobilization.

Paraplegia: Due to collapsed vertebral compression:
- Laminectomy to decompress the spinal cord.

## Polyostotic Fibrous Dysplasia (Osteitis Fibrosa Cystica)

| | |
|---|---|
| Definition | Is defined as a rare fibrocystic disease of bone that manifests itself by softening, bending, and often fracture; that is usually mistaken for osteitis fibrosa generalized due to the hyperparathyroidism, as both disorders are manifested by bone cysts and fractures; polyostotic fibrous dysplasia not a metabolic disorder of the bone, but a congenital dysplasia being characterized by nonformation of bone and cartilage while remaining as fibrous tissue; polyostotic fibrous dysplasia with "brown spots" with ragged margins and true precocious puberty—is known as Albright's syndrome; may be associated with hyperthyroidism and acromegaly. |
| Etiology | Unknown. |
| Pathogenesis | Generalized bone resorption resulting in diffuse cystic changes that are widely scattered throughout the skeleton, affecting mostly the long bones and skull; bone cysts and pathological fractures; in congenital |
| | Type: Bone and cartilage are formed and replaced by fibrous tissue. |
| Diagnosis | Age: Usually in the 2nd decade of life |
| | Swelling: Painless |
| | Bone: Skull, ribs, pelvis, upper end of femur, tibia, metatarsals, metacarpals, and phalanges |
| | Pathological fractures |
| | Deformities |
| | Skin: Brown pigmentation |
| | Precocious puberty in females: True sexual with early development of secondary sex characters and fast skeletal growth. |
| Investigation | CBC, ESR |
| | Serum calcium: Normal |
| | Serum phosphorus: Normal |
| | Alkaline phosphatase: Elevaterd |
| | Urinary hydroxyl proline: Elevated. |

| | X-rays show: Rarefaction and expansion of the affected bones or hyperostosis of bones esp. of base of skull; fractures and deformities may be seen |
|---|---|
| | Bone biopsy: Confirmatory. |
| D/d | Hyperparathyroidism |
| | Neurofibromatosis |
| | Bone cyst/s |
| | Bone tumors |
| | Paget's disease. |
| Complications | Shortening of limb |
| | Deformity of limb: For example, Shepherd's crook deformity of femur |
| | Blindness: Due to orbital involvement |
| | Thyrotoxicosis |
| Management | No specific treatment. |
| | Conservative treatment: |
| | Warm fomentation, SWD, or IR therapy |
| | Analgesics and NSAIDs |
| | Calcitonin: May be tried in acute disease, but results are unconclusive |
| | Surgicval treatment: |
| | Indication: Correction of deformities (fractures, expanding orbital cyst) |
| Prognosis | Mostly the lesions heal with slow progression. As precocity is of isosexual type, girls are prone to early pregnancy; and will be of short stature, rarely sarcomatous transformation of bone may occur. |

## Bibliography

1. Arnstein AR, et al. Recent progress in osteomalacia and rickets. Ann Int Med 67:1296, 1967.
2. Ashkar FS, et al. Thyroid storm treatment with blood exchange and plasmapheresis. J.A.M.A. 214:1275, 1970
3. Bailey and Love's Short Practice of Surgery (1965) Love M, Rains A.J. H., Capper W.M.; H.K. Lewis and Co., London.
4. Becker CE. Coma in myxedema. California Med 110:61, 1969.
5. Bell NH, et al. Effect of calcitonin in Paget's disease and polyostotic fibrous dysplasia. J Clin Endocrinol 31:283, 1970.
6. Bucker RH, Hughes FA Jr, Mashburn JD. Polyostotic fibrous dysplasia (Albrights syndrome). J Thoracic Cardiovas Surg 49:241, 1965.
7. Catt KJ. ABC of endocrinology. 1. Hormones in general. Lancet 1:763, 1970.
8. Catt KJ. ABC of endocrinology. 2. Pituitary function. Lancet 1:827, 1970.
9. Catt KJ. ABC of endocrinology. 3. Growth hormone. Lancet 1:933, 1970.
10. Catt KJ. ABC of endocrinology. 6. The thyroid glasnd. Lancet 1:1383, 1970.
11. Fraser SA, et. al. Osteoporosis and fractures following thyrotoxicosis. Lancet 1:981, 1971.
12. Gharib H. Triiodothyronine: Physiological and clinical significance. J.A.M.A. 227:302, 1974.
13. Haigler ED. Pituitary gigantism. Arch Int Med 132:588, 1973.
14. Kapoor PS. Accident and Emergency: Endocrine and Metabolic Emegencies, 2nd Ed. CBS, New Delhi, 2016.
15. Katz FH. Laboratory aids in the diagnosis of endocrine disorders. M Clin North. America 53:79, 1969.
16. Khairi MRA, et al. Paget's disease of bone (osteitis deformans): Symptomatic lesions and bone scan. Ann Int Med 79:348, 1973.

17. Kolb FO. Endicrine Disorders: Current Medical Diagnosis and Treatment. Maruzen, Tokyo, 1975.

18. Lawrence AM. Immunoassays in the diagnosis of endocrine disorders. S Clin North America 49:3, 1969.

19. Medina RG, Elliot DW. Thyroid carcinoma. Arch Surg 97:239, 1968.

20. Moe PJ. Hypopituitary dwarfism: The importance of early therapy. Acta paediat scandinav 57:300, 1968.

21. Parfitt AM. The spectrum of hypoparathyroidism. J Clin Endocrinol 34:152, 1972.

22. Raisz LG. The diagnosis of hyperparathyroidism. New England J Med 285:1006, 1971.

23. Riggs L, et al. Treatment for postmenopausal and senile osteoporosis. M Clin North America 56:989, 1972.

24. Rosenberg IN. Evaluation of thyroid function. New England J Med 286:924, 1972.

25. Roth J, et al. Acromegaly and other disorders of growth hormone secretion. Ann Int Med 66:760, 1967.

26. Samson Wright's Applied Physiology: Endocrine Glands, 10th Ed., Oxford University Press, London, 1963.

27. Sir Astley Cooper. Surgical anatomy of thyroid gland: Bailey and Love's Short Practice of Surgery, ed. 13th, H.K. Lewis and Co., London, 1965.

28. Smith R. The pathophysiology and management of rickets. Orthop Clin North America 3:601, 1972.

29. Yen SSC, et al. Effect of somatostatin in pastients with acromegaly. New England J Med 290:935, 1974.

# 20

# General Diseases of Bones and Joints

- Achondroplasia
- Osteitis fibrosa cystic
- Leontiasis ossea
- Solitary bone cyst
- Aneurysmal bone cyst
- Nonosteogenic fibroma

## Achondroplasia

| | |
|---|---|
| Definition | It is defined as a familial condition due to maldevelopment of bones of cartilage origin; characterized by markedly diminished stature, with the limbs in particular are stunted; obviously the legs are short, and the fingertips reach only to the greater trochanters (arms resembling the flippers); fingers diverge to resemble the spokes of a wheel. |
| Etiology | Unknown. |
| Pathogenesis | Maldeveloped cartilaginous bones; stunted limbs; short legs; fingers diverge; fingertips reaching only greater trochanters. |
| Diagnosis | Deformity: |

- Stature: Diminished
- Legs: Shortened
- Arms: Flippers like
- Fingers: Diverge like spokes of a wheel
- Skull: Base (cartilaginous) smaller than the vertex; prominent forehead; deprerssed nose

Muscles: Weakened

Gait: Short steps

Mental: Development normal

Occupation: Usually employed in circuses.

| | |
|---|---|
| Investigation | CBC, ESR |
| | X-rays skull, spine, pelvis, and limbs. |
| Management | Symptomatic |
| | Surgical treatment: |
| | Indication: Shortened legs |
| | Surgery: Leg lengthening. |

## Osteitis Fibrosa Cystic (Syn. Recklinghausen's Disease of Bone

| | |
|---|---|
| Definition | It is defined as generalized active bone resorption that results in diffuse cystic lesions, widely scattered throughout the skeleton; usually involve the long bones and the skull. |
| Etiology | Hyperparathyroidism (primary) |
| Factors | Chronic renal disease. |
| | Rickets |
| | Osteomalacia |
| | Acromegaly |
| | Adenomas: Thyroid, pituitary, pancreas |
| Pathogenesis | Bone destruction associated with the development of fibrous tissue; may be development of 'brown tumors' structurally similar to giant cell tumors of bone; bones deformed and fractured (pathological). |

Diagnosis    Skeletal S/S:
- Backache
- Arthralgia
- Pathological fracture: Spine, ribs, long bones
- Deformity: Kyphosis, bone bending, loss of stature
- Brown tumor: Jaw epulis
- Clubbing of fingers

Urinary tract S/S:
- Polydipsia
- Polyuria
- Urinary stones: Calcium oxalate or phosphate
- UTI
- Renal failure
- Uremia

Hypercalcemia S/S:
- Nausea, vomiting, thirst, anorexia, constipation, asthenia
- Muscular weakness, fatigue
- Hypertension

Investigation    Serum calcium: High (> 15 mg/dl)
Serum phosphate: Normal or low
TRP: < 80%
Alkaline phosphatase: Elevated
Serum chloride: High
Uric acid: Elevated
X-ray:
- Bone: May show demineralization; subperiosteal resorption of bone; multiple cystic lesions in the bones; mottling of the skull; may be pathological fracture/s; calcified articular cartilage
- KBU: May show urinary calculi; or nephrocalcinposis (diffuse stippled renal calcifications; extra-articular soft tissue calcifications.

ECG: May show a short Q-T interval
Eye: Band keratopathy (corneal calcification) seen by slit-lamp.

| Complications | Pathological fracture |
| --- | --- |
| | Renal damage |
| | Renal stones |
| | UTI |
| | Renal failure |
| | Uremia |
| | Cardiac failure |
| D/d | Multiple myeloma |
| | Metastatic carcinoma (thyroid, kidney, bladder) |
| | Idiopathic hypercalciuria with renal stones |
| | Osteoporosis. |
| Management | Conservative treatment: |
| | Fluids intake: PO |
| | Sod. Chloride, sulfate, phosphate, potassium phosphate IV infusions |
| | Reduce calcium intake |
| | Phosphate orally |

Drugs:
- Furosemide
- Calcitonin

Hemodialysis: life-saving in renal failure

Surgical treatment:

Surgery: Removal of parathyroid tumor

Indication:
- Parathyroid tumor
- Hyperplasia of all parathyroid glands (3) with subtotal resection of 4th

Postoperatively: Magnesium salts intake.

## Leontiasis Ossea

| Definition | It is defined as an enlargement of the facial bones and jaws; resulting in grossly altered facial shape and the air sinuses diminished in size; is a localized form of fibrous dysplasia. |
| --- | --- |
| Etiology | Unknown. |
| Pathogenesis | Enlarged facial bones and jaws; altered facial shape; diminished size of air sinuses; localized fibrous dysplasia. |
| Diagnosis | URC: |

- Nasal obstruction, DNS
- Lacrimal duct obstruction
- Headache

Deformity: Hideous:
- Enlarge facial bones; increased pressure on the eyes, brain, and cranial nerves.

| Investigation | X-rays skull—AP and LAT views |
| --- | --- |
| D/d | Sarcoma of maxillary antrum |

| | |
|---|---|
| Management | Symptomatic: |
| | Conservative treatment: |
| | Analgesics |
| | Nasal decongestants |
| | Eye drops |
| | Antibiotics |
| | Surgical treatment: |
| | Indication: Deformity. |
| | Surgery: |

- Correction of deformity
- Correction of DNS
- Opening of blocked lacrimal duct

## Solitary (Unicameral) Bone Cyst

| | |
|---|---|
| Definition | It is defined as a solitary bone cyst (in reality a separate condition, i.e. usually classified under the heading of cystic diseases of bone); usually appears at the end of 1st decade; fairly frequent; in incidence their rank second to enchondroma (solitary benign lesions of bone; usually occur in the long tubular bones (humerus, tibia, and fibula); is the residue of an abnormal phase of activity affecting one epiphyseal line in a growing child. |
| Etiology | It is obscure; possibly more than one factor responsible: |

- Localized failure of metaphyseal ossification at the time of rapid growth
- Infrequent occurrence in the flat bones and small tubular bones may be significant.

| | |
|---|---|
| Pathogenesis | Originate in the metaphysis adjacent to the epiphyseal plate; with growth of the bone, the epiphysis moves away from the lesion, that is then located in the metaphysis at a distance from the plate or in the diaphysis; referred to as latent (when at a distance) while referred to as active (adjacent to the plate); sclerosed walls at each ends of the cyst. |
| Investigation | X-rays show: Clear cavity in the bone; thin walled; may show tissues in it—angiomatous, myxomatous, fatty, and fibrous; ossification of varying degree may be seen; pathological fracture may be seen. |
| | Needle aspiration of any cystic fluid (usually clear amber). |
| Complications | • Pathological fracture |
| | • Coxa vara |
| | Malignant transformation: Unknown |
| Management | Surgical treatment of choice: |
| | Surgery: |

- Curettage and bone grafting: To be thorough (to avoid recurrences); sclerotic wall at each end of the cyst to be removed to expose normal medullary bone
- Resecting a nonessential bone

Precaution: To avoid injuring the epiphyseal plate, surgery to be delayed, until the epiphysis has migrated away from the cyst.

RT: Contraindicated, as not only ineffective, but may also induce malignant change or may damage the epiphyseal plate.

## Aneurysmal Bone Cyst

| | |
|---|---|
| Definition | It is defined as a localized bulging mass covered with a thin and often incomplete shell of bone; lesions that usually occur in older children and young adults; most often in the large long bones, and may also involve the flat bones and vertebrae; lesion may be considered as clinical and radiological, and not a pathological entity; in a tubular bone, the lesion is located nearer to one end than to the middle of the shaft. |
| Etiology | Uncertain |
| | Vascular disorders: Hemorrhage, venous dilatations |
| | Traumatic: Parosteal myositis ossificans |
| Pathogenesis | Grossly: A thin shell of bone forms the outer surface, while interior is loculated by a number of connective tissue septa—forming lakes filled with dark blood, that oozes profusely minus pulsation; lesions variable markedly in their gross structure; some are entirely vascular, while others contain connective tissue that is markedly ossified. |
| | Histologically: No characteristic tissue; principal features are connective tissue septa with adjoining large unlined spaces; varying ossification; and localized giant cell reaction within septa; pathological fracture. |
| Diagnosis | Bone: Large long bones, flat bones, and vertebrae |
| | Pain |
| | Swelling |
| | Local tenderness |
| | Movements of adjoining joint/s painful and restricted |
| | Muscular: Weakness; wastings |
| | Pathological fracture |
| Investigation | X-rays show: Localized bulging mass covered with a thin shell of bone; striking, heavy trabeculations or loculation; slight irregular cortical erosion. |
| | Needle aspiration biopsy to rule out malignancy |
| D/d | Giant cell tumor |
| | Chondromyxoid fibroma |
| Management | Conservative treatment: |
| | Analgesics and NSAIDs |
| | Warm fomentation, SWD, or IR therapy |
| | Surgical treatment: |
| | Indication: Failure of conservative treatment. |
| | Surgery: |
| | Curettage of lesions in long bones |
| | Excision of expanded vertebral lesions + adjoining involved tissue. |
| | After care: Physiotherapy: exercises. |

## Fibrous Metaphyseal Defect and Nonosteogenic Fibroma

| | |
|---|---|
| Definition | It is defined as lesions clubbed together; that when a metaphyseal defect fails to follow its usual evolutionary course, it forms a nonosteogenic fibroma; usually metaphyseal defects are small, innocuous, and asymptomatic; usually occur in children during 1st decade; exist for about 2–3 years and then disappear gradually; the occupied areas ossify and resume a normal trabecular pattern; occurring most often in distal femoral metaphysic; unlike metaphyseal defects, nonosteogenic fibromas are rarely multiple. |
| Etiology | Developmental defects<br>Localized and temporary cessation of ossification<br>Abnormal periosteal growth |
| Pathogenesis | Grossly: Lesional tissue highly characteristic: friable, vividly rusty colored, containing discrete bright yellow foci<br>Histologically: These central lesions are cellular fibromas containing a varying number of giant cells, clusters of macrophages containing lipid or iron; nonosteogenic fibromas rarely multiply; the nonosteogenic fibromas are developmental defects or hamartomas. |
| Diagnosis | Age:<br>• Metaphyseal defects: Usually in 1st decade,<br>• Nonosteogenic fibromas: Usually 2nd decade<br>Bone:<br>• Metaphyseal defects: Usually in distal metaphysic<br>• Nonosteogenioc fibromas: Usually in long bones of lower limbs (tibia and fibula)<br>Pain<br>Swelling<br>Local tenderness<br>Movements of adjoining joint/s painful and restricted<br>Muscular: Weakness; wastings<br>Pathological fracture. |
| Investigation | X-rays show:<br>• Metaphyseal defects: Small bowl shaped defects located eccentrically; sclerosed and scalloped bony margins and absent cortex peripherally<br>• Nonosteogenic fibromas: Bony margins sclerotic and scalloped; lesions trabeculated or loculated. |
| Management | Conservative treatment:<br>Analgesics and NSAIDs<br>Warm fomentation, SWD, or IR therapy<br><br>Surgical treatment:<br>Indication: Failure of conservative treatment.<br><br>Surgery:<br>Curettage of lesions in long bones<br>Excision of expanded vertebral lesions + adjoining involved tissue.<br>After care: Physiotherapy: Exercises. |

## Bibliography

1. Arnstein AR, et al. Recent progress in osteomalacia and rickets. Ann Int Med 67:1296, 1967.
2. Aurbach GD, et al. Hyperparathyroidism: Recent studies. Ann Int Med 79:566, 1973.
3. Barnes R. Aneurysmal bone cyst, J. Bone and Joint Surg. 38-B:301, 1956.
4. Beeler JW, et al. Aneurysmal bone cysts of s, J.A.M.A. 163:914, 1957
5. Campbell CJ, Harkess J. Fibrous metaphyseal defect of bone, Surg., Gynec. and Obst. 104:329, 1957.
6. Canale S Terry, Daugherty K, Jones Linda. Mosby Campbell's Operative Orthopaedics 9th Ed. Vol I-IV, 1998.
7. Charnley J. Achondroplasia 13:261, Bailey and Love's Short Practice of Surgery H.K. Lewis and Co., London, 1965.
8. Charnley J. Osteitis Deformans 13:255, Bailey and Love's Short Practice of Surgery H.K. Lewis and Co., London, 1965.
9. Charnley J. Osteitis Fibrosa Cystica 13:257, Bailey and Love's Short Practice of Surgery, H.K. Lewis and Co., London, 1965.
10. Clark JMP. Modern Trends in Orthopedics Fracture Treatment, Butterworths, London, 1962.
11. Cohen J. Simple bone cysts. Studies of cyst fluid in six cases with a theory of pathogenesis, J. Bone and Joint Surg. 42-A:609, 1960.
12. Compere EL, Coleman SS. Nonosteogenic fibroma of bone, Surg., Gynec. and Obst. 105:588, 1957.
13. Crooks F, Birkett AN. Fractures and Fracture-dislocations of the Cervical Spine. Brit. J. Surg 31: 252, 1944.
14. Cruz M, Coley BL. Aneurysmal bone cyst, Surg., Gynec. & Obst. 103:67, 1956.
15. Cunningham JB. Ackerman LV. Metaphyseal fibrous defects, J. Bone and Joint Surg. 38-A:797, 1956.
16. Fraser SA, et al. Osteoporosis and fractures following thyrotoxicosis. Lancet 1:981, 1971
17. Garceau GJ, Gregory CF. Solitary unicameral bone cyst, J. Bone and Joint Surg. 36-A:267, 1954.
18. Goldenberg RR. Nonosteogenic fibroma of bone, Bull. Hosp. Joint Dis. 17:230, 1956.
19. Kapoor PS. Accident and Emergency: Etiology, Diagnosis and Management 2nd Ed., CBS, New Delhi, 2016.
20. Kolb FO. Osteitis fibrosa cystica: Current Medical Diagnosis and Treatment, Maruzen Asean Edition, Bombay, 1975
21. Love M, Rains AJH, Capper WM. Disease Bailey and Love's Short Practice of Surgery H.K. Lewis and Co., London, 1965.
22. McRae R. Practical Fracture Treatment (1981) 1st Ed. Churchill Livingstone, 1981.
23. Rasz LG. The diagnosis of hyperparathyroidism. New England J Med 285:1006. 1971.
24. Riggs L, et al. Treatment for postmenopausal and senile osteoporosis. M Clin North America 56:989, 1972.
25. Smith R. The pathophysiology and management of rickets. Orthop Clin North America 3:601, 1972.

# 21

# Degenerative Diseases of Bones and Joints

**Osteoarthritis**
- Definition
- Etiology
- Pathogenesis
- Diagnosis
- Investigation
- Management

**Surgical procedures**
- Knee
- Hip
- Spine
- Shoulder
- Elbow
- Wrist
- Hand

**Charcot's joint**
- Definition
- Etiology
- Pathogenesis
- Diagnosis
- Investigation
- Management

## OSTEOARTHRITIS (SYN. DEGENERATIVE JOINT DISEASE; HYPERTROPHIC ARTHRITIS)

| | |
|---|---|
| Definition | It is defined as a chronic, progressive, arthropathy, characterized by the degeneration of articular cartilage (architectural deterioration) and by formation (hypertrophy) of bone at the articular margins, and without systemic manifestations. It is the commonest type of arthritis the world over. |
| Etiology | Primary or Idiopathic (syn. polyarticular degenerative) of unknown etiology; usually active in some joints at the same time; rarely occurs in younger age (< 40 years); commonly affecting the DIP joints. Secondary (syn. monarticular degenerative) affecting any joint due to pre-existing joint disorders: Congenital: Anomaly |

|  | Traumatic: Injury to articular cartilage due to: |
|---|---|
|  | • Intra-articular causes, e.g. intra-articular fracture or dislocation |
|  | • Extra-articular causes, e.g. bony block, torn muscle/or tendon |
| MOI | Direct trauma, RSA, sports injury, fall from a height |
|  | Inflammatory: Rheumatoid arthritis |
|  | Infective: Septic arthritis, tuberculosis |
|  | Endocrinal: Diabetes mellitus |
|  | Metabolic: Hyperparathyroidism |
|  | Neuropathic: Tabes dorsalis |
| Risk factors | Advancing age: > 60 years |
|  | Sedantary life |
|  | Overweight |
|  | Wrong posture and misuse of the joint |
|  | Strenuous exercises includes regular use of stairs. |
| Pathogenesis | (Table 21.1) |
|  | Synovitis: Hypersecretion of synovial fluid (SF), synovial membrane inflammed, e.g. thickened, hypertrophied |
|  | Articular cartilage: Softened, roughened, worned |
|  | Synovial membrane: Inflammed, e.g. thickened, hypertrophied |
|  | Subchondral bone: Sclerosis, ebunation, cysts formation |
|  | Articular surfaces: Osteophytes |
|  | Ankylosis: Bony. |
| Diagnosis | • Age > 60 years |
|  | • Onset–insidious |
|  | • Morning stiffness of joints |
|  | • Pain: Presenting symptom: Dull aching, aggravated by joint use, weight bearing, relieved by rest |
|  | • Systemic manifestations—absent |

**Table 21.1:** Pathogenesis of osteoarthritis

| Stage | Pathogenesis | Effects | Clinical (S/s) |
|---|---|---|---|
| I A | Synovitis | Hypersecretion—SF, Joint distension | Joint swelling, pain |
|  |  | Synovium—thickened, hypertrophied | Disabilty |
| I B | Joint capsule, burse, ligaments ligaments | Capsulitis, bursitis, tendinitis, muscle spasm | Movements painful, local tenderness |
| II | Cartilage | Roughened, worning | Movements painful and restricted |
| III | Bone (subchondral) | Sclerosis, eburnation, cysts and osteophytes | Pain, disability, |
| IV | Joint | Ankylosis (bony) | Movements restricted or absent |

- Swelling, or deformity
- Muscular wasting
- Crepitus
- Movements: Painful and restricted.

**Investigation**    X-Ray shows:
- Asymmetric narrowing of the joint space
- Osteophytes at joint margins

MRI studies: May reveal early changes, missed in X-rays

CT scan: Indicated in cervical or lumbar spondylosis associated with neurologic manifestation.

**Management:**    Aims:
- To relieve pain
- To improve joint function
- To prevent deformities.

Preventive treatment:

Occupational therapy: Joint protection and conservation by:

Avoiding joint stress, e.g. squatting, ascending/descending stairs, prolonged standing, long walks.

**Conservative treatment**

Physiotherapy:
- Exercises: Muscle strengthening exercises: active and passive
- Traction
- Heat, e.g. Infrared, short wave diathermy
- Massage, e.g. stroking, compression
- Aid devices for ambulation, e.g. a walking stick or a walker, crutches, braces/belts, cervical collars
- Accupuncture and acupressure
- Yoga therapy.

**Medical treatment:**

Drugs:

Analgesics and Nonsteroidal Anti-inflammatory drugs (NSAID)

Caution: Elderly patients are esp. vulnerable to NSAID toxicity

I/A Injection: Intra-articular steroids—for relief of pain:
- Hydrocortisone acetate 25 mg/mL + Lignocaine plain 1% 1 mL, Alt:
- Triamcinolone acetonide 40 mg/mL + Lignocain plain 1% 1 mL + Sodium hyaluronate 20 mg (2 mL) I/A repeat b.i.w.

Caution: Not to be used frequently.

**Surgical treatment:**

Indication:
- Persistent pain
- Reduction of activity
- Deformities

Surgery: Various procedures:
- Excision of osteophytes
- Excision of loose bodies
- Arthroscopic debridement
- Synovectomy
- Reconstruction (debridement of joint)
- Arthroplasty: Joint replacement
- Arthrodesis.

## SURGICAL PROCEDURES FOR REGIONAL OSTEOARTHRITIS

### Osteoarthritis of Knee

Surgery                Various procedures:
- Excision of osteophytes
- Excision of loose bodies
- Arthroscopic debridement
- Synovectomy
- Reconstruction (debridement of joint)
- Arthroplasty: Joint replacement
- Patellectomy
- Arthrodesis.

### Excision of osteophytes

Indication
- Persistent pain
- Reduction of activity
- Deformities

Postoperatively: Range of mobility increased, while pain and disability  may continue because of degenerative changes of articular surfaces.

### Excision of loose bodies

Preface                Osteophytes in osteoarthritis knee may get detached and form loose bodies in the joint, resulting in:
- Persistent pain
- Reduction of activity
- Deformities

Surgery: Excision of loose bodies

### Arthroscopic dèbridement

Indication
- Persistent pain
- Reduction of activity
- Deformities

Surgery: Debridement of joint

## Synovectomy

**Preface**    Usually severe and persistent proliferative synovitis occurs in osteoarthritis of knee, resulting in:

- Persistent pain
- Reduction of activity
- Deformities

Synovectomy is the procedure of choice for synovial pathogenesis only; Synovectomy + debridement of fibrillated cartilage + articular surface to be levelled, for fibrillated cartilage and irregular articular surfaces. Synovectomy + patellectomy, for severe pain deeper to the patella and chondromalacic articular surface of patella.

## Reconstruction (dèbridement of joint)

**Preface**    Usually of value in managing painful osteoarthritis of knees in overweight, but healthy women post 40 years of age

Indication:

- Persistent pain
- Reduction of activity
- Deformities

Surgery: Debridement of joint.

For osteoarthritis of both knees:

- Debridement of less severely affected knee + arthrodesis of more severely affected knee

Technique:

- Incision: Anteromedial
- Exposure: Anterior surface of distal femur and a portion of articular surface of proximal tibia, by retracting patella laterally
- Excision: Exostoses from both femoral condyles
- Denude: Degenerated cartilage of femoral condyles
- Narrowing: Patella to free its gliding proximally and distally without any mechanical obstruction
- Denude: Degenerated cartilage from tibial articular surface
- Spare: Menisci unless degenerated.

After care: Exercises post 1/52; flexion to be increased gradually.

## Arthroplasty

**Preface**    Arthroplasty of the knee joint not recommended unless the arthritis is monarticular; best suitable for young patients esp. for osteoarthritis post intra-articular fractures of the joint.

Indication:

- Persistent pain
- Reduction of activity
- Deformities

Surgery: Arthroplasty of the joint.

## Arthrodesis

**Preface**    Indicated in marked changes in bone and cartilage beside synovium involvement; usually more effective when knee in varus or valgus, with its relaxed ligaments; in bilateral knees involvement, then the more severe knee to be managed by arthrodesis, while the less severe one to be managed by synovectomy; results of fusion excellent: pain relieved with improved function.

Indication:

- Persistent pain
- Reduction of activity
- Deformities

## Patellectomy

**Preface**

The main disability of knee osteoarthritis may be roughened contiguous articular surfaces of patella and femur, caused by trauma, osteochondritis dissecans, or bipartite patella

Indication:

- Persistent osteoarthritis for yurts.
- Failure of conservative treatment
- X-ray: Suggestive of osteoarthritis
- Arthritis quiescent at time of surgery knee extension within 20 degree of normal

Surgery:

- Patellectomy
- Patellectomy + excision of osteophytes

Technique:

- Incision: Anteromedial from 2.5 cm proximal to 2.5 cm distal to patellar borders
- Incise: Quadriceps and patellar tendons and quadriceps expansion over the patella midline longitudinally
- Divide: Patella longitudinally and enucleate two halves of patella
- Repair: Quadriceps by placating lateral edge over the medial one.

Postopertively: Immobilization of joint with Buck's traction for 1/52.

After care: Exercises ASAP till restoration of quadriceps power.

## Osteoarthritis of Hip (Syn. Coxa Magna)

Surgery: Various procedures:

- Excision of osteophytes
- Arthroscopic debridement
- Reconstruction (debridement of joint)
- Arthroplasty (joint replacement)
- Acetabuloplasty
- Prosthetic replacement
- Osteotomy (proximal femur)
- Arthrodesis
- Neurectomy.

## Excision of osteophytes

**Indication**

- Persistent pain
- Reduction of activity
- Deformities

Surgery: Excision of large osteophytes obstructing mobility and impinging upon the acetabulum

Postoperatively: Results poor because the procedure fails to correct the degeneration of the articular surfaces.

### Arthroscopic dèbridement

Indication
- Persistent pain
- Reduction of activity
- Deformities

Surgery: Arthroscopic debridement of irregular articular cartilage

### Reconstruction (dèbridement of joint)

Indication
- Persistent pain
- Reduction of activity
- Deformities

Surgery: Reconstruction (debridement) of joint

### Arthroplasty

Indication
- Persistent pain
- Reduction of activity
- Deformities

Surgery: Arthroplasty is procedure of choice when sufficient head and neck available to make procedure feasible; exception: persons engaged in hard labor, e.g. mine workers.

### Acetabuloplasty

Indication
- Persistent pain
- Reduction of activity
- Deformities

Surgery: Acetabuloplasty.

### Prosthetic replacement

Preface
It is not a substitute for all disorders of the hip; never to be considered lightly; results of this procedure for osteoarthritis remain unsatisfactory as compared to that for fresh fractures or for nonunion of femoral neck, because of acetabular changers and remoddled acetabulum; reserved for those with marked cystic changes in femoral head, and for those with failed arthroplasty and remnant inadequate head and neck for revised arthroplasty.

Indication:
- Persistent pain
- Reduction of activity
- Disability

Surgery: Prosthetic replacement

Types:
- Medullary prosthesis (Moore and Thompson)
- Stem prosthesis (Judet): Frequently breaks or gets loosen in the bone.

## Osteotomy (proximal femur)

Preface
The beneficial effects of the osteotomy may be biological or mechanical; that no one type of osteotomy is suitable for every patient of osteoarthritis; that osteotomy results in partial increase in the width of joint space and clearance of cystic and sclerosed areas from the femoral head and acetabulum; usually all osteotomies to be internally fixed (fragments position maintained; risk of restricted mobility of hip and knee lowered; early mobilization, and few operative complications).

Indication:
- Persistent pain
- Reduction of activity
- Deformities

Surgery: Osteotomy (proximal femur).

Types:
Abduction (valgus) osteotomy:

Indication:
- Limp: Trendelenberg
- Deformity: Adduction
- Mobility: Hyperadduction
- Painful abduction

Adduction (varus) osteotomy:
- Limp: Antalgic abductor
- Deformity: Abduction
- Mobility: Hyperabduction
- Painful adduction.

Fixation:
- Internal fixation:

Advantages:
- Maintain: Fragmentism proper position
- Reduce: Restriction of hip and knee mobility
- Mobilization: Early
- Reduce: Medical complications.

## Arthrodesis

Preface
Procedure of choice in younger persons, esp. those requiring hard labor, e.g. mine workers; usually undertaken in monarticular osteoarthritis, and in severely destroyed joint surfaces; contraindicated in polyarticular osteoarthritis.

Indication:
- Persistent pain
- Reduction of activity
- Deformities

Surgery: Arthrodesis.

## Neurectomy (Syn. denervation of joints)

Preface        Anatomical pattern of joints innervation reveals limitations of this procedure utilized alone; may relieve pain partially; may be used as adjunct to procedures like arthroplasty; may be beneficial in the reconstruction procedures for knee and hip (supplied by well-defined articular branches), thus peripheral denervation in the knee, hip, and elbow, can be achieved more systemically than in other joints.

Indication:
- Persistent pain
- Reduction of activity
- Deformities

Surgery: Neurectomy (denervation of joint).
Regional:
Hip: Supplied by femoral, obturator, and sciatic nerves.
Surgery: Denervation of branches of all these nerves + arthroplasty of the hip joint
Limitations: Inaccessible branches directly from the lumbar plexus and those accompanying blood vessels to be considered precisely.
Knee: Supplied by posterior tibial, femoral, and obturator nerves.
Surgery: Denervation of branches of all these nerves + patellectomy.
Elbow: Supplied by a fairly constant and easily exposed nerve supply.
Surgery: Denervation.
Results: Best available, because of fairly constant and easily exposed nerve supply besides being a nonweight bearing joint.

## Osteoarthritis of Spine

Preface        Usually part of generalized osteoarthritis; entire spine and sacroiliac joints may be involved
Conservative treatment of choice
Surgery: Arthrodesis rarely indicated.

## Osteoarthritis of Shoulder (Syn. Periarthritis Shoulder)

Indication
- Persistent pain
- Reduction of activity
- Deformities
Conservative treatment of choice:
- Physiotherapy: SWD or IR therapy, exercises
Surgery: Rarely indicated.

## Osteoarthritis of Elbow

Indication
- Persistent pain
- Reduction of activity
- Deformities
Conservative treatment of choice:
Physiotherapy: SWD or IR therapy, exercises.
Surgery: Rarely indicated
Exception: Loose bodies that interfere with joint functioning.

## Osteoarthritis of Wrist

Indication
- Persistent pain
- Reduction of activity
- Deformities

Conservative treatment of choice

Surgical treatment: Rarely indicated for severe pain and disability:

Surgery: Arthrodesis of the wrist

Osteoarthritis of radio-scaphoid joint alone:

Surgery: Styloidectomy

## Osteoarthritis of Joints of Hand

Indication
- Persistent pain
- Reduction of activity
- Deformities

Conservative treatment of choice

Surgical treatment: Rarely indicated for severe pain and disability:

Surgery: Arthrodesis.

## CHARCOT'S JOINT

Definition | It is defined as the trophic affection of joints, that developed frequently in weight-bearing joints

Etiology | Tabes dorsalis, syringomyelia
Diabetic neuropathy
Alcoholic neuropathy.

Pathogenesis | Trophic changes in weight bearing joints; joints destruction.

Diagnosis | Genitourinary: Dysuria, pyouria,

Investigation | X-ray shows marked destruction of joints, sclerosis, fragmentation.

Management | Conservative treatment: Symptomatic.
Rest
Analgesics and NSAIDs
Antibiotics
Surgical treatment:
Surgery: Arthrodesis.

**Regional:**

Hip | Surgery:
Osteotomy: Indicated in destroyed femoral head and neck
Reconstruction
Artthrodesis

Knee | Surgery:
Arthrodesis is the surgical procedure of choice

Technique:

Charnley compression (modified) arthrodesis (most reliable):
- Insertion: Additional Steinmann pins inserted obliquely through medial tibial condyle and proximally into femoral medullary canal
- Arthrodesis: Knee in neutral position (most stable)

Postoperatively: Immobilization: in a POP spica for 2–3/12.
After care: Walking with knee support (brace) for a year.

**Ankle**      Surgery:
Arthrodesis is the surgical procedure of choice
Talectomy + tibiocalcaneal arthrodesis: Indicated in an case of talus
markedly destroyed and avascular

**Spine**      Surgery:
Arthrodesis.

## Bibliography

1. Adam A, Spence AJ. Intertrochanteric osteotomy for osteoarthritis of the hip. A review of fifty-eight operations. J. Bone and Joint Surg. 40-B:219, 1958.
2. Allison N, Coonse GK. Synovectomy in chronic arthritis. Arch. Surg. 18:824, 1929.
3. Anderson LD. Osteoarthritis. Campbell's Operative Orthopaedics, ed. 4th, Vol II, C.V. Mosby Co., Saint Louis, 1998.
4. Batchelor JS. Excision of the femoral head and neck in cases of osteoarthritis of the hips, Proc. Roy. Soc. Med. 38:689, 1945.
5. Bateman JE. Denervation of joints. Campbell's Operative Orthopaedics, ed. 4th, Vol II, C.V. Mosby Co., Saint Louis, 1998.
6. Blount WP. Proximal osteotomies of the femur, American Academy of Orthopedic Surgeons Instructional Course Lectures, Vol. IX, Ann Arbor, J.W. Edwards, p.1, 1952.
7. Boyd HB, Hawkins BL. Patellectomy: a simplified technique. Surg., Gynec. and Obst. 86:357, 1948.
8. Boystone BF, Stephensen CR. The surgical treatment of Charcot's spine: reversal of Charcot's arthropathy of the spine with complete bone and joint healing after solid extra-articular fusion, am. Surgeon 24:896, 1958.
9. Brown A. Arthrodesis of the hip. Guy's Hosp. Rep. 103:13, 1954.
10. Campbell JP, Jackson JP. Treatment of osteoarthritis of the hip by osteotomy. J. Bone and Joint Surg. 38-B:468, 1956.
11. Canale ST, et al. Campbell's Operative Orthopaedics, ed. 9th, Vol I-IV. C.V. Mosby Co., Saint Louis, 1998.
12. Charnley J. Arthrodesis of the knee. In De-Palma A.F., editor: Clinical orthopaedics, vol. 18, p. 37, J.B. Lippincott Co., Philadelphia, 1960.
13. Charnley J. Compression arthrodesis. E. and S. Livingstone Ltd., Edinburgh and London, 1953.
14. Cleveland M, Smith Alan deF. Fusion of the knee joint in cases of Charcot's disease. Report of four cases. J. Bone and Joint Surg. 13:849, 1931.
15. Crenshaw AH. Tuberculosis. Campbell's Operative Orthopaedics, ed. 4th, Vol II, C.V. Mosby Co., Saint Louis, 1998.
16. Crooks F, Birkett AN. Fractures and Fracture-dislocations of the Cervical Spine. Brit. J. Surg 1944: 31: 252.
17. Isserlin B. Joint debridement for osteoarthritis of the knee. J. Bone and Joint Surg. 32-B:302, 1950.
18. Kapoor PS. Osteoarthritis. Accident and Emergency, ed. 2nd, Part I, CBS, New Delhi, 2016.
19. Key JA. The treatment of tabetic arthrtopathies (Charcot's joints), Urol. and Cutan. Rev. 49:161, 1945.
20. Love M, et al. Bailey and Love's Short Practice of Surgery, ed. 13th, H.K. Lewis and Co., London, 1965.
21. Magnuson PB. Technique of debridement of the knee joint for arthritis. S. Clin. North America 26:249, 1946.
22. McMurray TP. A practice of orthopaedic surgery, ed. 2nd, Williams and wilkins Co., Baltimore, 1943.
23. McMurray TP. Osteoarthritis of the hip joint. Brit. J. Surg. 22: 716, 1935.
24. Nicoll EA, Holden NT. Displacement osteotomy in the treatment of osteoarthritis of the hip. J. Bone and Joint Surg. 43-B:50, 1961.
25. Steindler A. The tabetic arthropathies, J.A.M.A. 96:250, 1951.

# 22

# Affections of Nervous System

- Cerebral palsy
- Obstetric paralysis
- Spina bifida
- Filum terminale syndrome
- Pott's paraplegia
- Anterior poliomyelitis

## Cerebral Palsy

Definition    It is defined as disturbed muscular function caused by an intracranial lesion of the central nervous system; may occur to the baby in the womb or postdelivery; characterized by poor muscular coordination, weakness and muscular spasms that interfere with the movements, and speech disturbances; the disordered child is generally mentioned as spastic, although clinically spastic paralysis is one of various types:

Types    Spastic paralysis
Ataxia
Athetosis
Tremor
Rigidity.

Etiology    Perinatal:

- Traumatic (cause intracranial hemorrhage): Forceps injury (applied incorrectly or failure to use forceps in obstructive labor); or forced traction on the neck
- Anoxiatic: Anoxia caused by injudicious use of analgesics and anesthetics in the 2nd stage of labor; cerebral congestion caused by fetus neck encircled by the cord; or by inadequate resuscitation of the infant postnatal
- Jaundice: From erythroblastosis fetalis may damage the basal ganglia (may cause athetosis).

Prenatal:

- Congenital defects of brain: From viral infections, e.g. rubella, during 1st trimester of pregnancy (may cause ataxia and athetosis).

Postnatal:
- – Infective: Encephalitis
- – Convulsive: Cause intracranial hemorrhage

**Pathogenesis**     Based on the site of the intracranial lesion:

A. Lesions of cerebral cortex:
- • Muscle spasticity: Caused by lesions of premotor area or combined lesion of premotor area + motor area of anterior central gyrus
  Example: Spastic quadriceps: Involuntary contraction of quadriceps occurs on flexing the knee actively; hyperactive deep tendon reflexes (stretch) of spastic muscles; clonus may be present
- • Muscle flaccidity: Caused by lesions of main motor area
- • Muscle spasticity and muscle flaccidity: Caused by lesions of multiple motor areas.

B. Lesions of base of brain:
- • Athetosis or tremor: Casused by lesions of basal ganglia (esp. of caudate nucleus and putamen)
  Athetosis: May involve part or whole of limbs and muscles supplied by cranial nerves.
  Example: Facial palsy (constant grimacing and twitching with normal mental state).
  Tremor: Usually infective (encephalitis); tremor sensitives to antibiotics.
  Rigidity: May be caused by lesion of globus pallidus.

C. Lesions of cerebellum:
- • Ataxia: Caused by lesions of cerebellum (congenital or hemorrhagic); characterized by loss of sense of posture and of balance; muscles nonresponsive to changes in position; muscles of speech, trunk, and of limbs involved; nystagmus, nausea, dizziness on reading.

D. Diffuse lesions:
- • Rigidity: Caused by prolonged anoxia postobstructed labor (venous stasis caused by cord strangulation); rigidity may be intermittent (may improve with relaxation and medication) or constant (less chances of improvement); impaired mental status because of diffused brain damage.

**Diagnosis**     Intelligence: About half of spastic children have normal intelligencer
Deformity
Muscle spastic
Muscle flaccid
Muscle spastic and flaccid
Nystagmus
Speech: Disturbed
Facial palsy
Convulsions

**Investigation**     CBC, ESR
Blood sugar

Serum electrolytes

Mental testing: Based on motor activity and verbal responses

X-rays skull; cervical spine; of affected part

MRI brain

CT scan brain.

**Management**    Aim: To help the patient physically independent, emotionally healthy, socially competent and mentally alert. Trteatment varies with the severity and type of cerebral palsy. In severe cases, surgery may be used to treat some of the physical aspects of the disease; convulsions are controlled with barbiturates or other drugs.

Tests: To measure level and progress of development in cerebral palsy.

### Conservative treatment

Psychologic:

Mental strategy: Unless a severe defective mental capacity proved, the child with cerebral palsy are not to be deprived of treatment simply because of his/her abnormal motor and verbal responses

Training schedule: Directed toward developing: speech, mobility, self dependency, and learning.

Schedule: Includes psychotherapy, speech therapy, occupational therapy, physiotherapy, education, medical treatment including and orthopedic procedures when indicated.

Medical: Drugs:

A. Sedatives and tranquilisers:

Phenothiazines: Actions: Antipsychotic and anxiolytic actions

Drugs: Chlorpromazine, haloperidol, trifluperazine

Benzodiazepines: Actions: Anxiolytic, muscle relaxant, anticonvulsant

Drugs: Chlordiazepoxide, alprazolam, diazepam, oxazepam, loraxepam.

B. Anticonvulsants:

Barbiturates: Actions: Anticonvulsants, muscle relaxant

Drugs: Phenobarbitone, methylphenobarbitone

Succinimides: Action: Depressant motor cortex and to elevate threshold to convulsive stimuli

Drugs: Lamotrigine, topiramate.

Surgical treatment:

Indications: Spastic paralysis and athetosis (to help in correcting local physical disorders that impair patient's rehabilitation and nursing care)

Preoperative: Completely evaluated and undergone conservative care.

### Surgery

Soft tissues:

- Tendons: Tendon transfers, tenotomies, and Z-plastic lengthening (to correct deformity and to improve muscle power)
- Periarticular structures (to correct fixed deformities of joints).

Bones:
- Tarsal joints arthrodesis (to correct deformity and instability)
- Femur or tibia osteotomy (to correct angulation or torsion deformity).

Peripheral nervous system:
- Neurectomy of nerve branches (to improve muscle balance in spastic)

Paralysis

Caution: It is a destructive operation (to be used with no alternative)
- Local block: Infiltration with lignocaine (to paralyze branches for hours).

After care: Physiotherapy: exercises.

Regional
Lower limb
Foot

Deformities: Cerebral palsy spastic paralysis may cause deformities:
- Equinus, valgus, varus, talipes calcaneus, and clawing of toes.

Equinus deformity:
Etiology:
- Spastic triceps surae vs dorsiflexors (spastic, normal, flaccid
- Normal triceps surae vs flaccid dorsiflexor
- Flaccid triceps surae vs flaccid dorsiflexor.

### Management
Conservative treatment:
Indication: For mild deformity in young children
Measures: Stretching triceps surae manually or by using a caliper brace.

### Surgical treatment:
Indication: Failure of conservative treatment and for severe deformity
Surgery:
- Neurectomy of one or more branches of tibial nerve to the gastro-cnemius or soleus
- Release of triceps surae by distal transplantation of heads of origin of the gastrocnemius, lengthening of tendon of gastrocnemius, or lerngthening of tendocalcaneus.

Valgus/or varus deformity:

Etiology: Medial or lateral instability of foot caused by the imbalance between invertors and evertors.

### Management:
Conservative treatment:
Indication: Initial correction of deformity
Measures: Correcting deformity by wedging casts

Surgical treatment:
Indication: Failure of conservative measures and for severe deformities.

Surgery:
- Tenotomies or tendon lengthening, followed by wedging casts.

### Talipes calcaneus:

Etiology: Excessive or repeated lengthening of tendocalcaneus; spastic dorsiflexors of foot and the flaccid triceps surae.

### Management:

Conservative treatment:

Indication: Initial correction of deformity

Measures: Correcting deformity by wedging casts

Surgical treatment:

Indication: Failure of conservative measures and for severe deformities.

Surgery:

- Tenotomies or tendon lengthening, followed by wedging casts.

### Claws toes:

Antomy: Motor branch of lateral plantar nerve innervates all interossei (except those between 4th and 5th metatarsals, being supplied by plantar digital branch of 5th toe), 2nd, 3rd, and 4th lumbricals, and adductor hallucis; 1st lumbrical and flexor hallucis brevis, innervated by branches of medial plantar nerve.

Etiology: Imbalanced intrinsic muscles of foot because of the spastic paralysis.

Deformities: Spastic paralysis causes flexion of MTP joints of toes and extension or hyperextension of IP joints; greater toe flexed at MTP joint by pull of flexor hallucis brevis and hyperextended at IP joint.

### Management:

Conservative treatment:

Indication: Initial correction of deformity

Measures: Correcting deformity by manipulations and casts

Surgical treatment:

Indication: Failure of conservative measures and for severe deformities.

Surgery:

- Neurectomy of motor branch of lateral plantar nerve and supply to the interossei in 4th interosseous space
- Plantar capsulotomy of 1st MTP joint
- Division of heads of insertion of flexor hallucis brevis.

Knee

Deformities: Cerebral palsy spastic paralysis may cause deformities:

- Equinus, valgus, varus, talipes calcaneus, and clawing of toes.

### Equinus deformity

Etiology:

- Flexion contracture of knee
- Elongated patellar tendon
- Disabled hip or ankle, or both
- Imbalanced flexors and extensors of knee
- Knee recurvatum.

## Management
Conservative treatment:

Indication: Initial correction of deformity

Measures: Correcting deformity by repeated manual stretchings and bracing

Surgical treatment:

Indication: Failure of conservative measures and for severe deformities.

Surgery:
- Flexion deformity of hip, weakened gluteus maximus, triceps surae, or talipes calcaneus: To be corrected prior to any surgery on knee
- Flexion contracture of knee to be corrected fully by: Lengthening of tendons or by transferring tendons to femoral condyles.

Postoperative: Bracing.
- Elongated patellar tendon: To be corrected by division of the patellar retinacula and transferring hamstring tendons to the femoral condyles.
- Imbalanced flexors and extensors of knee: To be corrected by transferring insertions of hamstrings to the posterior supracondylar aspect of femur (improves functioning of hamstrings in hip extension, and reduces primary flexed position of hip and secondary flexed position of knee; Z-plasty lengthening of hamstring tendons, or biceps femoris and semimembranosus proximal to knee by dividing their tendons while leaving their muscular parts intact.
- Severe spasticity of hamstrings: To be corrected by neurectomy of some branches of sciatic nerve that innervate these muscles.
- Recurvatum of knee: Caused by contracture of tendocalcaneus and severe spasticity of knee extensors and deformed proximal end of tibia; to be corrected by tibial osteotomy; neurectomy of branches of femoral nerve to control spasticity of quadriceps, and stretching of tendocalcaneus with a brace.

Hip

Deformities: In cerebral palsy usually deformities of the hip caused by contracture or muscular imbalance:

Types: Flexion, flexion and internal rotation, or adduction
- Flexion and internal rotation deformity: More frequent, caused by spastic internal rotators vs flaccid external rotators:

  Example: Spatic tensor fasciae latae.
- Adduction deformity: Less frequent, caused by spastic adductors vs flaccid abductors.

## Management:
Conservative treatment:

Indication: Initial correction of deformity

Measures: Correcting deformity by manipulations and casts

Surgical treatment:

Indication: Failure of conservative measures.

**Surgery:**

- Soutter operation, followed by immobilization in external rotation.
  Example: Tensor fasciae latae main cause of deformity.
  Indication: Deformity—mild to moderate.
- Osteotomy (rotational) of femur, at subtrochanteric or supracondylar level
  Indication: Rotational imbalance deformity
  Postoperative: Range of internal rotation to be equal that of external rotation.
- Neurectomy (obturator) and adductor tenotomy: Neurectomy of both branches of obturator nerve (sparing supply from sciatic nerve and pectineus supplied by femoral nerve).

  Indications:
  - Servere scissors gait caused by adduction contracture of hip in a child, retaining sense of balance
  - Subluxated or dislocated hip.

**Upper limb**

In the upper limb paralysis is frequently diffuse than selective of any specific group of muscles:

Spastic paralysis: Deformities usually are of position: flexed fingers, flexed thumb with or without adduction, flexed wrist, pronated forearm, flexed elbow, and adducted and internally rotated shoulder

Aim of surgery: To retain functional mobility and painless stability (poor results compared to that in lower limb).

**Shoulder**

Deformities: In cerebral palsy usually deformities of the shoulder caused by spastic paralysis of muscles.

Types: Adduction and internal rotation.

**Management:**

Conservative treatment:

Indication: Initial correction of deformity

Measures: Correcting deformity by manipulations and braces

Surgical treatment:

Indication: Failure of conservative measures.

Surgery:

- Rotational osteotomy of humerus at the level of deltoid tubercle
- Fairbank; Sever modified operations.

**Elbow**

Deformity: In cerebral palsy usually deformities (mild to moderate) of the elbow caused by contracture or spasticity of flexor group of elbow; not severe enough to justify surgical treatment.

Management:

Conservative treatment:

Indication: Initial correction of deformity

Measures: Correcting deformity by manipulations and braces.

Surgical treatment:

Surgery: Not severe enough to justify surgical treatment.

Forearm wrist, hand

**Deformities:** In cerebral palsy a disabled hand is difficult to evaluate and treat than one due to motor and sensory deficits; spastic muscles and contracted joints are troublesome; muscle balancing difficult because of weakness and spasticity; intermittent spasticity or there may be athetosis.

## Management:
Conservative treatment:

Indication: Initial correction of deformity

Measures: Correcting deformity by manipulations, braces, and splints.

Surgical treatment:

Aims:

- To enable the thumb out of palm; and to help in the opening or releasing fingers grasp
- Thumb in the palm, unable to move out of it
- Deformed hand and wrist
- To provide grasp and release postsurgery
- Failure of conservative measures (braces and splints).

Conservative treatment:

Indication: Initial correction of deformity

Measures: Correcting deformities by stretching and splintage.

## Surgical treatment:
Indication:

- Loss of opening land closing hand to grasp objects
- Failure of conservative treatment.

Contraindications: Severe emotional disturbance and child < 8 years old.

## Surgery:
Thumb deformities:

- Thumb-in-palm deformity: Corrected by transferring flexor carpi radialis tendon to the extensor pollicis longus, rerouted from Lister's tubercle toward radial aspect of 1st metacarpal
- Deformed thumb: Corrected by arthrodesis of 1st MCP joint
- Opposition deformity: Corrected by tendon transferring.

Finger deformities:

A. Flexed MCP and proximal IP joints, and distal IP joint in extension: Corrected by:
   - Transferring a spastic wrist flexor to the common finger extensors
   - Releasing tendons of sublimi in case of functioning profundi
   - Arthrodesis of PIP joints for persisting severe flexion deformities

B. Flexed MCP and distal IP joints, and proximal IP joints in extension: Corrected by Littler's technique of intrinsic release.

Wrist deformities:

- Flexed wrist: To be corrected first by tendon transfer to balance wrist extensors vs flexors, followed by arthrodesis of the wrist later on

- Pronated wrist: To be corrected by transferring flexor carpi ulnaris tendon to the radius, and transferring pronator teres to the abductor pollicis longus or to a radial wrist extensor.

## Obstetric Paralysis

| | |
|---|---|
| Preface | Obstetric paralysis usually caused by delivery trauma (brachial plexus injury); shoulder joint may also got injured simultaneously; initially it may be flaccid paralysis involving the entire limb; later on until and unless all roots of the brachial plexus damaged severely, the paralysis subsides partially; finally a fixed deformity develops because of unopposed contracted muscles that pulled the limb into specific positions 9 shoulder abducted and internally rotated, elbow flexed, forearm pronated, and wrist palmar flexed. |
| Definition | It is defined as the upper lesion of brachial plexus, due to involvement of C5 and C6 nerve roots. |
| MOI | Obstructed labor—traction force |
| Mechanism of injury | The injury is due to increased angle between the neck and shoulder, as may occur during forced delivery of fetus, in obstructed labor; and also by fall of a heavy weight over the shoulder. |
| Pathogenesis | Shoulder subluxated posteriorly: Later on osseous changes develop in the humeral head and glenoid (small head, flattened glenoid, rotated and elevated scapula). |
| Diagnosis | Deformity: Because of muscle imbalance; prolonged immobilization in an abnormal position: |
| | Arm—hanging by side of body and internally rotated |
| | Elbow—fully extended |
| | Forearm—fully pronated |
| | Muscular wasting in lesions of long duration |
| | Loss of muscle power |
| | Loss of sensations and reflexes. |
| Investigation | X-ray of shoulder joint—AP and LAT views humeral head misshapen (post couple of months due to impaired blood supply); head displaced posteriorly |
| D/d | Fracture dislocation of shoulder |
| Management | Conservative treatment: |
| | Indication: May be justified within few days/or weeks post birth: |
| | Immobilization of arm in relaxation position, by use of splints (shoulder moderately abducted and externally rotated, elbow extended, forearm in neutral position |
| | Physiotherapy: Active and passive exercises |
| | Surgical treatment: |
| | Indication: |

- Failure of conservative measures
- In neurotmesis lesions.

Surgery:
- Exploration of brachial plexus; justified esp. in the complete brachial plexus type of paralysis: neurolysis alone may be advisable; suturing difficult.
- Osteotomy: Through proximal third of ulna
- Excision of radial head—deferred until growth is complete.

**Regional**

**Shoulder**

Surgical treatment:

Indication:
- Failure of conservative measures
- Movements: Restricted abduction and external rotation/or should joint subluxated posteriorly.

Surgery:
- Exploration of brachial plexus; justified esp. in the complete brachial plexus type of paralysis: Neurolysis alone may be advisable; suturing difficult.
- Reconstruction: Tendon transfers and releases indicated for increasing the abduction and external rotation provide the shoulder joint is normal.
- Osteotomy: Indicated in subluxated, displaced, or deformed shoulder joint.

Reconstruction (correcting internal rotation and adduction contracture):

Technique:
- Incision: (Deltopectoral approach) from acromion tip, distally to the point of tendinous insertion of pectoralis major muscle; divide this tendon
- Exposure: Coracobrachialis muscle by retracting deltoid laterally and the pectoralis major medially
- Exposure: Coracoid process by externally rotating and abducting shoulder
- Divide: Tip of coracoid process along with inserted muscles (coracobrachialis, short head of biceps, and pectoralis minor):
  - Exposure: Subscapularis tendon insertion at lesser tuberosity of humerus; divide it
  - Results: In increased range of external rotation and abduction movements
  - Acromionectomy: To remove any obstruction.

Postoperatively: Immobilization: with a shoulder POP spica with shoulder abducted and externally rotated, elbow flexed, forearm supinated, and wrist extended, for 2/52.

After care: Support with a brace and physiotherapy (exercises).

**Elbow**

Surgical treatment: Usually restricted mobility and deformity in obstetric paralysis not considered for treatment.

Indication:

- Failure of conservative measures
- Deformity: Dislocated radial head: anteriorly or posteriorly; flattened capitulum
- Movements: Severely restricted.

Preoperatively:

Immobilization: In a splint with shoulder abducted and externally rotated, elbow extended > 90 degree, and the forearm in midpronation; splint to be removed regularly and often; exercises (active and passive) of the limb

Surgery: Excision of radial head + osteotomy though proximal 1/3rd of ulna postoperatively: Immobilization: in a splint with shoulder abducted and externally rotated, elbow flexed, forearm supinated, and wrist extended, for 2/52

After care: Support with a brace and physiotherapy (exercises).

## Forearm, Wrist, Hand

Surgical treatment:

Preface      Paralyzed muscle causes loss of power to perform any particular function resulting in impaired hand balance, disturbed stable positions, and difficult coordination; any muscle with paralyzed antagonist, contracts unopposed, finally contracted; ligaments of immobilized joint contracted too; contractures may increase the stability of the hand at the sake of increased disability.

Example: Clawhand deformity (intrinsic minus position with subluxation):
Fingers:

- Paralyzed lumbricals and other intrinsic muscles; unopposed long flexors of fingers flex the IP joints of the fingers; unopposed long extensors of fingers extend the MCP joints; IP joints remain flexed.

Wrist: Flexed by strong finger flexors (tenodesign effect on long finger extensors that hyperextends the MCP joints further).

Thumb: Adducted by its unopposed long extensor (paralyzed intrinsic and abductor); extended CPM joint; flexed IP joint by unopposed long flexor (paralyzed adductor pollicis and abductor pollicis brevis).

MOI      Dynamic muscle imbalance by trauma, spasm, or disease.

Indication:

- Failure of conservative measures
- Movements: Restricted
- Severe deformity

Surgery: Tendon transfers and correction of deformity

Thumb:

A. To restore opposition of thumb:

Aim: Pinch function of the hand

Method:

Tendon transfer: Transferred tendons to be inserted into tendon of the abductor pollicis brevis.

Correction of deformity: Fixed adduction and external rotation of thumb to be corrected by dividing the fascia in the web between the index and thumb metacarpals; or a Z plasty of the web; by osteotomy or arthrodesis for very severe deformity.

Postoperatively: Immobilization: with a dorsal POP splint with wrist in flexion, thumb in opposition with extended distal phalanx, for 3/52.

After care: Support with a brace and physiotherapy (exercises).

## Spina Bifida

| | |
|---|---|
| **Definition** | Spina bifida (split spine) is defined as a congenital deformity present at birth, characterized by spinal vertebrae not properly developed to form the normal vertebral canal that protects the spinal cord; cord itself may be malformed and lacking in nerves that control the bladder and limb muscles. |
| **Preface** | Surgical procedures for spina bifida are in the domain of the neurosurgeon, while surgical procedures to correct deformities of the lower limb are in the domain of an orthopedic surgeon; deformities of the lower limb need correction alone; spina bifida of the upper spine is usually fatal. |
| **Etiology** | Muscle imbalances secondary to flaccidity or spasticity |

**Types**

- Spina bifida occulta: Commonest type; due to failure of fusion of neural arches, without protrusion of spinal cord of membranes, usually affecting a single vertabra in the lumbosacral region.
- Meningocele: Protrusion of meninges through defective spino-laminar segment.
- Meningomyelocele: Normally developed spinal cord or cauda equina, may lie adherent to the posterior aspect of the sac.
- Syringomyelocele: Rarest type, characterized by dilated central canal of the spinal cord, and the sac contains spinal cord along with nerves originating from it.
- Myelocele: Characterized by an elliptical raw surface (ununited groove), CSF discharging from central canal at its upper end;

Commonest type of spina bifida second to spina bifida occulta.

**Pathogenesis**

- Spina bifida occulta: A fibrous band—membrane reunions, connecting skin to the spina theca, growth of body yields pulling of spinal theca and nerve roots by the membrane.
- Meningocele: Contains CSF only.
- Meningomyelocele: Spinal cord or cauda equine adherent to sac.
- Syringomyelocele: Dilated central canal of spinal cord.
- Myelocele: Discharging CSF from spinal central canal.

**Diagnosis**

Spina bifida:

Deformity:

- Usually equinovarus deformity of foot
- Flexion contracture of hip
- Flexion contracture of knee

Skin: Swelling over lumbosacral region; or depression in the skin, patch of hair, trophic ulcer

Loss of sensation: In myelomeningocele or syringomyelocele

Discharging sinus: CSF discharge

Muscular weakness, paralysis of legs (advance case)

Incontinence of urine and feces.

Spina bifida occulta:
- Skin: Over midline of lumbosacral region shows cicatricial thickening, dimpling, dilated vessels, a tuft of hair/or a fibrofatty tumor
- Muscular weakness or paralysis of lower limbs.

| | |
|---|---|
| Investigation | Transillumination test: Cord and nerves seen as dark shadows; to distinguish meningocele from meningomyelocele.<br>X-ray lumbosacral spine: Reveals bony deficiency. |
| Complications | Meningitis<br>Paraplegia |
| Management | Surgical treatment of choice; to be provided ASAP, by a team of neurosurgeon (for spina bifida repair) and the orthopedic surgeon (for lower limb deformities correction) |

Preoperative:

Mandatory neurological examination to detect any area of anesthesis.

## Filum Terminale Syndrome (Syn. Cord-traction Syndrome)

| | |
|---|---|
| Definition | Filum terminale syndrome is defined as a congenital deformity present at birth, characterized by an abnormally thick and firm filum terminale that fails to lengthen in pace with vertebral column growing longer; prevents normal cephalad migration of the spinal cord, thereby exerting traction on it, that results in progressive paresthesia, deformities of the feet, faulty gait, deformity of spine (kyphoscoliosis). |
| Preface | Surgical procedures for spina terminale are in the domain of the neurosurgeon, while surgical procedures to correct deformities of the lower limb are in the domain of an orthopedic surgeon; deformities of the lower limb need correction alone. |
| Etiology | Specific entity (an abnormally thick and firm filum terminale that fails to lengthen in pace with vertebral column growing longer; prevents normal cephalad migration of the spinal cord, thereby exerting traction on it, causing disability. |
| Pathogenesis | Tight filum terminale (the dura tented posteriorly like a pole stretching the canvas of a tent). |
| Diagnosis | Deformity: |

- Usually pes cavus and claw toe
- Kyphoscoliosis

Muscular tightness: Hamstrings and triceps surae

Deep tendon reflexes: Weak

Incontinence of urine and feces.

Gait: Faulty

| Investigation | X-ray lumbosacral spine: Reveals bony deficiency. |
|---|---|
| | Myelography: Dural sac displaced posteriorly. |
| Management | Surgical treatment of choice; to be provided ASAP, by a team of neurosurgeon (for spinal surgery) and the orthopedic surgeon (for lower limb deformities correction). |
| | Preoperative: |
| | Mandatory neurological examination to detect any area of anesthesis. |
| | Surgery: Exploration |

- Exposure: Filum terminale by opening the dura
- Divide: Tight filum terminale ligated and divided

Postoperatively: S/S disappear or decrease.

## Pott's Paraplegia

| Preface | Pott's paraplegia, as a result of interference with the conductivity of the spinal cord; most often associated with tuberculosis of the dorsal spine (because of tuberculosis more prevalent in the dorsal spine; spinal cord terminates below level of 1st lumbar vertebra; the spinal canal narrowest in the dorsal region; the anterior ligament in the dorsal region loosely confines the cold abscess) |
|---|---|
| Etiology | Direct trauma: Mechanical compression by an extradural abscess or by a sequestrum |
| | Inflammatory: Active disease |
| | Vascular: Thrombosis in the spinal cord |
| Pathogenesis | Mechanical compression by extradural abscess, inflammatory tissue, or a caseating mass, sequestra, loose fragments of dead bone or disk pressing cord; neural arch lesion; infective thrombosis; pathological dislocation—bony ridge pressing cord. |
| Diagnosis | Clonus: Most prominent early sign |
| | Paraplegia: Varying rapidly through stages: muscular weakness, spasticity, and incoordination, leading to paraplegia in extension (cord not fully involved), and later onto paraplegia in flexion (cord fully involved); finally flaccid paralysis. |
| | Urinary: Incontinence |
| | Fecal: Incontinence. |

Types of Pott's Paraplegia

- Paraplegia of early onset: Occurring in florid phase of spinal disease (usually within 2 years)
- Paraplegia of late onset: Occurring many years post disease become (quiescent post many years).

| Investigation | CBC, ESR |
|---|---|
| | X-ray—AP and LAT views: |
| | Early sign: Reduced intervertebral space; hazy outline of the adjoining vertebral surfaces; may show an abscess |
| | Later sign: Wedging and gross destruction |
| D/d | Pott's fracture: Wedged verterbrae, with normal intervertebral spaces |

Secondary carcinoma: Osteolytic changes in the vertebral bodies, with normal intervertebral spaces

Prostatic carcinoma: Increased vertebral density

Spondylitis deformans: Peripheral lipping of vertebrae.

**Management** Aim: Postclinical diagnosis, treatment to start ASAP; status of spinal cord function to be observed carefully.

Conservative treatment:
- Immobilization

**Surgical treatment:**

Indications:

Absolute:
- Paraplegia with onset during conservative treatment (surgery delayed until muscular weakness occurs
- Paraplegia static or worsened during conservative treatment
- Loss of muscular power completely
- Severe paraplegia: Flaccid paraplegia, paraplegia in flexion, complete sensory loss, complete loss of muscular power for > 6/12.

Relative:
- Recurrent paraplegia
- Paraplegia: Onset in old age
- Painful paraplegia
- Complicated paraplegia.

Surgery: Procedures:
- Decompression: Anterolateral
- Costotransversectomy
- Laminectomy
- Arthrodesis.

Costotransversectomy:

Indication: Paravertebral abscess under pressure

Anterolateral decompression:

Indication: Failure of costotransversectomy

Laminectomy:

Indication: Paralysis secondary to cervical disease; spinal tumor syndrome; paraplegia secondary to posterior spinal disease

Posterior arthrodesis (Bosworth) + laminectomy:

Indication: Paralysis secondary to cervical disease; spinal tumor syndrome; paraplegia secondary to posterior spinal disease

Anterior arthrodesis + debridement:

Indication: Paralysis secondary to cervical disease; spinal tumor syndrome

Lumbar transversectomy:

Indication: Paraplegia causded by cauda equina.

**Prognosis** About 50% of Pott's paraplegics recovered spontaneously without antibiotics; and 50% got worst and eventually died.

## Anterior Poliomyelitis

| | |
|---|---|
| Preface | Poliomyelitis is an acute infectious disease caused by polioviruses (type I, II, and III); primarily an infection of the gastrointestinal tract.; while in serious form affects the central nervous system; destroys the motor neurons of the anterior horn cells of the spial cord that results in flaccid paralysis. |
| Epidemiology | worldwide problem; since 1988 cases of paralytic polio decreased worldwide (despite this, polio remains highly endemic throughout the Indian subcontinent (India, Pakistan, and Bangladesh) because of the inadequate three doses of vaccines, inadequate vaccine coverage, unvaccinated children amongst vaccinated children, overcrowded and unhygeinic conditions of poor dwellings.<br>Incidence; frequently in children of 2–15 years age. |
| Risk factors | Trauma<br>Fatigue<br>Intramuscular injections<br>Operative procedures. |
| Season | Throughout year—esp. during summer. |
| Incubation period | 1–2/52. |
| Transmission | Orofecal mainly. |
| Pathogenesis | Oral entry; replication of virus in oropharynx and intestines; entry blood circulation; to CNS—spinal cord and brain (anterior horn cells of lower motor neurons, grey ganglia, posterior horn cells and dorsal root ganglia up to thalamus and hypothalamus)—spinal cord or brain; lower motor neurons destroyed; in the brain (reticular formation, vestibular nuclei, cerebellar vermi, and deep cerebellar nuclei destroyed; motor cortex of precentral gyrus affected; finally flaccid paralysis occurs. |

## *Poliomyelitis Skeletal Deformity*

| | |
|---|---|
| Definition | It is defined as a deformity caused by anyone or a combination of any of the factors: Muscle imbalance, muscle spasm, faulty posture, impaired dynamics of activity, and growth. |
| Etiology | • Muscular imbalance<br>• Muscle spasm<br>• Postural default<br>• Impaired dynamics of activity and growth. |
| Types | Type I, Type II, and Type III. |
| Pathogenesis | |
| Diagnosis | • Deformities<br>• Muscle power: Imbalance, muscle weakness<br>• Joints: Flail<br>• Shortening of leg or arm. |
| Investigation | X-ray |
| Management | Convalescent period (16–24 months postacute febrile illness): orthopedic surgery contraindicated. |

Residual period (postconvalescent period): Orthopedic surgery plays an important role in rehabilitating the patient:

- To prevent/correct deformities
- To restore muscle power
- To stabilize flail joints
- To eliminate requirement of braces/corsets.

Aim: To help the patient become self-sufficient

Prevention/correction of deformity:

Conservative measures:

- Braces, splints, plaster casts, dynamic splinting
- Regular evaluation of muscle power.

Surgical measures:

Indication: Failure of conservative measures.

Preoperative: Age consideration:

- Progressive deformities: Scoliosis, pelvic obliquity require early definitive intervention
- Arthrodesis of tarsus, shoulder, knee deferred until skeletal maturity
- Tendon transferring: To eliminate dynamic force or to supplement power of paralyzed muscle(s): Deferred until skeletal maturity
- Discrepancy in leg lengthening: Deferred until skeletal maturity

Re-establishment of muscle power:

Surgical measures:

Tendon transfer:

Indications:

- To eliminate a dynamic force
- To supplement power of paralyzed muscle(s)

Principles:

- Transferred muscle to be strong enough
- Transferred tendon to be attached near the insertion of the paralyzed endon
- Transferred tendon to be either retained in its own sheath/or into another's tendon sheath
- Transferred muscle's vascular and nerve supply not to be impaired
- Contracted structures to be released prior to tendon transfer, i.e. to keep involved joint in normal position transferred muscle's tension to be re-established.

Muscle transplantation:

Indications:

- To replace power of paralyzed muscle(s).

Principles:

- Transplanted muscle to be large and strong enough
- Transplanted musculotendinous to work in straight line
- Transplanted muscle to be firmly attached to its new site

- Transplanted muscle essential to body dynamics, never to be transplanted
- Transferred musculotendinous to be under suffice tenson
- Transferred muscle's neurovascular supply not to be impaired.

Stabilization of Flail joint(s):

Surgical measures:

Soft tissue operations: Tenodesis, ligaments fixation, constructing artificial check ligaments (silk/or facia lata).

Drawbacks:

- Occurrence of deformity in the opposite direction
- Artificial check ligament may overstretch, thus loose its role.

Bone operations:

- Bone block: Preserves some movement
- Arthrodesis: Totally fixes joint in one functional position

Indications:

- To eliminate an abnormal movement
- To eliminate the provision of a brace.

Principles:

Upper limbs:

To require more mobility than stability: Grasp, reach, pinch and release

Arthrodesis:

- Shoulder: Limitations (cosmetic and functional)
- Elbow: Rarely indicated
- Wrist: Rarely indicated (limitations)
- Fingers and thumb: Rarely indicated.

Lower limbs:

- To require more stability than mobility: To support weight of the body.

Regional:

Lower limbs:

Foot and ankle: Tripple arthrodesis

Postoperative: A long leg plaster cast above knee applied with the foot is molded to the correct position, and knee at 20 degree flexion.

## Claw foot

Claw toes: (Modified Jones operation) correction of the deformity, tendon transferring, and arthrodesis of the interphalangeal joints

Cavus deformity: (Steindler operation) stripping of long plantar ligament and origins of short plantar muscles; (Dwyer operation) osteotomy of calus.

Talipes equinus: Tendocalcaneus lengthening, posterior capsulotomy of ankle joint, arthrodesis of ankle joint.

Bone block: Posterior bone block combined with triple arthrodesis, to stabilize foot against medial and lateral movements, while preserving the dorsiflexion of the ankle.

Postoperative: A long leg cast with ankle in neutral position and knee in 20 degree flexion.

Knee: disabilities:
* Flexion contracture of knee: Caused by contracture of the iliotibial band: corrected by division of the band and of the lateral intermuscular septum.
* Flexion contracture of knee: Caused by paralysis of the quadriceps muscle: corrected by conservative measures, or posterior capsulotomy and lengthening of hamstring the tendons, transferring tendons (biceps femoris and semitendionosus) supracondylar osteotomy of femur.
* Genu recurvatum: Caused by inadequate quadriceps power and relaxed soft tissues on back of knee: corrected by the reconstruction of soft tissues, and osteotomy of tibia.
* Flail knee: Corrected by a long leg brace, or arthrodesis of the knee in functional position.

Hip: Disabilities:
* Contracture of hip: Caused by contracture of iliotibial band: corrected by division of the band, and fasciotomy of hip and knee.
* Contracture of hip: Caused by paralysis of gluteus maximus and medius muscles: corrected by transferring erector spinae and tensor fasciae latae, and by transferring external oblique or iliopsoas tendon for the paralyzed gluteus medius muscle.
* Dislocation (posterior) of hip: Coxa valgum deformity, caused by the paralysis of gluteus medius and maximus muscles, and flexion and adduction contracture: corrected by open reduction and femoral shortening, varus osteotomy, arthrodesis (shelf operation) of hip.

Trunk: Disabilities:
* Pelvic obliquity: Caused by abduction contracture of hip, depressing pelvis on that side, altered symmetry of pelvis relative to the weight bearing thrust from above, trunk muscles affected, disrupting walking mechanics, fixed pelvic obliquity corrected by releasing flexion and abduction contractures of hip, followed by correction of lumbar curve by applying a turnbuckle cast, valgus osteotomy to shift weight bearing from adducted limb.
* Pelvic obliquity: Caused by paralysis of muscles of abdomen, back, and neck: corrected by fascial transplants, transferring iliotibial band and tensor fasciae latae.
* Paralytic scoliosis: Caused by long recumbency: corrected by the Milwaukee brace, fascial transplants, muscle transfers, athrodesis.

Upper limbs:
Shoulder: Disabilities:
* Disability caused by paralysis of shoulder: Corrected by the tendon and muscle transferring, or by the arthrodesis of the shoulder joint, after correction of hand, forearm, and elbow deformities, by reconstructive procedure.

Elbow: Disabilities:

- Disability caused by paralysis of elbow: Corrected by: the tendon and muscle transferring: to restore elbow flexion:
- Flexor plasty (Steindler, Bunnell's and Eyler's modifications)
- Triceps's anterior transferring (Bunnell and Carrol)
- Pectoralis minor transferring (Spira)
- Pectoralis major tendon transferring (Brooks and Seddon)
- Or rarely by the posterior bone block or arthrodesis.

Forearm disabilities:

- Disability caused by paralysis of elbow: Corrected by: tenotomy, fasciotomy, and osteotomy to correct deformities
- Osteoclasis to correct supination deformity.

Wrist and hand disabilities:

- Disability caused by paralysis of elbow: Corrected by: tendon transferring (Bunnell) after correcting the deformity.

Inequality of limb's length:

Lower limb:

- Disability caused by paralysis corrected by:
  - Limb shortening of longer limb by: Epiphyseal arrest by: epiphysiodesis (Phemister, Abbott and Gill) techniques, or stapling (Blount); resection of tibia or femur (Blount, White).
  - Limb lengthening of shorter limb by: Stimulating epiphyseal growth by: stripping periosteum, drilling metaphysic, curetting the metaphysis' medullary canal, implanting metals, ivory chips (Carpenter and Dalton), osteotomy and distraction.

Complications of leg lengthening:

- Deformities of foot: Valgus, equinovalgus, calcaneovagus
- Deformities of knee: Genu valgum, flexion contracture
- Deformities of tibia: Bowing of fragments, malunion or nonunion
- Restricted ankle movements.

## Bibliography

*Cerebral palsy*

1. Blumel J, Eggers GWN, Evans EB. Genetic, metabolic, and clinical study on one hundred cerebral palsied patients, J.A.M.A. 174:860, 1960.
2. Bost FC, Ashley RK, Kelley WJ. Role of the orthopedic surgeon in treatment of cerebral palsy, J.A.M.A. 160:256, 1956.
3. Burman MS. The spastic hand, J. Bone and Joint Surg. 20:133, 1938.
4. Eggers GWN. Surgical division of the patellar retinacula to improve extension of the knee joint in cerebral spastic paralysis, J. Bone and Joint Surg. 32-A:80, 1950.
5. Eggers GWN. Transplantation of hamstring tendons to femoral condyles in order to improve hip extension and to decrease knee flexion in cerebral spastic paralysis, J. Bone and Joint Surg. 34-A:827, 1952.
6. Goldner JL. Reconstructive surgery of the hand in cerebral palsy and spastic paralysis resulting from injury to the spinal cord, J. Bone and Joint Surg. 37-A:1141, 1955.
7. Ingram AJ. Cerebral Palsy, Campbell's Operative Orthopaedics, 4th Ed., Vol II:961, C.V. Mosby Co. Tokyo, 1965.

*Obstetric paralysis*

1. Kapoor PS. Accident and Emergency: Etiology, Diagnosis and Management, 2nd Ed., CBS, New Delhi, 2016.
2. Sever JW. Obstetric paralysis, J.A.M.A. 85:1862, 1925.
3. Thomas TT. Obstetrical or brachial birth palsy, Am. J. Obst. 73:577, 1916.

*Spina bifida*

1. Bailey and Love's Short Practice of Surgery, ed 13,H.K. Lewis and Co., London, 1965.
2. Bosworth DM, Della PA, Rahilly G. Paraplegia resulting from tuberculosis of the spine, J. Bone and Joint Surg. 35-A:735, 1953.
3. Campbell's Operative Orthopaedics, ed 9, Vol I-IV, C.V. Mosby Co. Tokyo, 1965.
4. Crenshaw AH. Pott's paraplegia, Campbell's Operative Orthopaedics, ed 4, Vol II:961, C.V. Mosby Co. Tokyo, 1965.
5. Garceau GJ. Filum terminale syndrome (cord traction syndrome), J. Bone and Joint Surg. 35-A: 711, 1953.
6. Girdlestone GR, Somerville EW. Tuberculosis of bone and joint, ed. 2, Oxford University Press, 1952.
7. Griffiths DL. Pott's paraplegia and its operative treatment, J. bone and Joint Surg. 35-B:487, 1953.
8. James JIP. Pott's paraplegia, ed 13:9, Med. Pregl. 1960.
9. Jones PH, Love JG. Tight filum terminale, A.M.A. Arch. Surg. 73:556, 1956 Pott's paralysis.
10. Knight G. Spina bifida, Bailey and Love's Short Practice of Surgery, ed 13, H.K. Lewis and Co., London, 1965.
11. Mercer W. Orthopaedic surgery, 4th ed, William and Wilkins Co, Baltimore, 1950.
12. Seddon HJ. Pott's paraplegia. In Platt, Sir Harry, editor: Modern Trends in Orthopedics, series 2, chap. 8, Butterworth and Co., Ltd., London, 1956.

*Anterior poliomyelitis*

1. Abbott LC, Gill GG. Surgical approaches to the epiphyseal cartilages of the knee and ankle joint, Arch. Surg. 46:591, 1943.
2. Bailey and Love's Short Practice of Surgery. Love M, Rains A.J. H., Capper W.M.; H.K. Lewis and Co., London, 1965.
3. Blount WP. Unequal leg length, American Academy of Orthopedic Surgeons Instructional Course Lectures, vol. XVII, St. Louis, 1960, pp. 218–45, The C.V. Mosby Co., St. Louis, 1960.
4. Brooks DM, Seddon HJ. Pectoral transplantation for paralysis of the flexors of the elbow. A new technique, J. Bone and Joint Surg. 41-B:36, 1959.
5. Bunnell S. Tendon transfers in the hand and forearm, American Academy of Orthopedic Surgeons Instructional Course Lectures, vol. VI, Ann Arbor, p. 106, J.W. Edwards, 1949.
6. Carpenter EB, Dalton JB. Jr. A critical evalution of epiphyseal stimulation, J.Bone and Joint Surg. 38-A:1089, 1956.
7. Ingram AJ. Campbell's Operative Orthopaedics, ed. 9th, Vol I-IV. C.V. Mosby Co., Saint Louis, 1998.
8. Kapoor PS. Accident and Emergency: Etiology, Diagnosis and Management, 2nd Ed., CBS, New Delhi, 2016.
9. Kapoor PS. Osteoarthritis. Accident and Emergency, ed. 2nd, Part I, CBS, New Delhi, 2016.
10. Steindler A. Muscle and tendon transplantation at the elbow, American Academy of Orthopedic Surgeons Instructional Course Lectures, vol. VII, Ann Arbor, J.W. Edwards, 1944.

# 23

# Neoplastic Affections of Bones and Joints

## Primary

| | | |
|---|---|---|
| Osteoblastic | Osteoma | Benign |
| | Osteoid osteoma | Benign |
| | Osteoblastoma | Benign |
| | Osteogenic sarcoma | Malignant |
| | Juxtacortical osteosarcoma | Benign/malignant |
| Osteoclastic | Osteoclastoma | Locally malignant |
| Cartilaginous | Chondroma (enchondroma) | Benign |
| | Chondroblastoma | Benign |
| | Chondrosarcoma | Malignant |
| Hematopoietic | Multiple myeloma | Malignant |
| | Leukemia | Malignant |
| | Reticulum cell sarcoma | Malignant |
| | Hodgkin's disease | Malignant |
| | Lymphosarcoma | Malignant |
| Vascular | Hemangioma | Benign |
| | Lymhangioma | Benign |
| | Glomus | Benign |
| | Angiosarcoma | Malignant |
| Neural | Neurofibroma | Benign |
| | Neurilemmoma (Schwannoma) | Benign/malignant |
| Nonosteogenic somatic tissue | Myxoma | Benign |
| | Myxosarcoma | Malignant |
| | Fibrosarcoma | Malignant |
| Unknown origin | Ewing's tumor | Malignant |
| Fatty | Lipoma | Benign |
| | Liposarcoma | Malignant |
| Mesenchymal | Myxoma | Benign |
| | Myxosarcoma | Malignant |
| Fibrous | Bone cyst | Benign |
| | Fibrous dysplasia | Benign |
| | Fibrosarcoma | Malignant |
| **Secondary** | Carcinoma | Malignant |

Preface

Various types of bone tumors are the neoplastic counterparts of the different tissue components that constitute bone; various groups of bone tumors are not to be regarded as absolutely clearly defined, and that an individual tumor may on occasions show features of more than one of these types; however accuracy depends on meticulous care and experienced collaboration (all clinical, radiological, and pathological data) to be carefully analyzed and adequately managed. Precise diagnosis and proper management can be made by adopting orderly methods and incorporating knowledge—freely interchanged amongst all the participating specialists.

Classification: A systematic classification mutually understood and accepted is essential of diagnosis; many classifications of bone tumors are available, e.g. Tables 23.1 and 23.2, all based on histogenesis; differ in details; and are modifications and refinements of that of the registry of Bone sarcoma of the American College of surgeons published by Codman in 1925, revised by Ewing's in 1939. As these classifications not suitable to all clinical entities, because many non-neoplastic lesions may be mistaken for tumors, thereby to be considered in differential diagnosis and for that includes in the classification.

Provisional diagnosis

Based on detailed history (patient's age, sex, race, and the occupation; lesion's site, size, duration, and mode of growth), physical examination; clinical evaluation of bone involved, site of the lesion within the bone (epiphyseal, metaphyseal, or diaphyseal): central, eccentric, or peripheral; periosteal reaction stimulated or not; the laboratory investigations (routine laboratoty profile not to be endorsed, e.g. estimation of serum alkaline phosphatase may be final in D/d of Paget's disease vs metastatic carcinoma, or osteosarcoma from osteomyelitis X-ray, ultrasound, MRI, CT scan, skeletal survey including.

BMR; and biopsy.

Biopsy (needle or aspiration) is the confirmatory diagnostic procedure, mostly recommended for the possibility of existence of a somatic tissue tumor, prior to surgery. Technique of a frozen section interpretation by an expert pathologist is very helpful in confirming the clinical diagnosis.

However accurate diagnosis depends upon histologic study.

X-rays: Provide one of the most important information (bone involved; number of lesions; site of lesion within bone—epiphyseal, metaphyseal, or diaphyseal; central, eccentric, or peripheral; periosteal reaction; and bone destruction; evidence of aggressiveness) for clinical diagnosis.

Management

Alternative and preferred methods of treatment for specific tumors and tumorlike lesions mentioned accordingly:

General measures: To build up the patient's health

CT: Greatly helpful in treating malignant tumors of somatic tissue

HT: Helpful in treating metastatic carcinoma

RT: Helpful in treating benign and malignant tumors of bone and somatic tissues; palliative for certain malignant tumors of bone, while

**Table 23.1:** Classification of bone tumors

| Derivation | Tumor | Biology |
|---|---|---|
| **Primary:** | | |
| Osteoblastic | Osteoma | Benign |
| | Osteoid osteoma | Benign |
| | Osteoblastoma | Benign |
| | Osteogenic sarcoma | Malignant |
| | Juxtacortical osteosarcoma | Benign/malignant |
| Osteoclastic | Osteoclastoma | Locally malignant |
| Cartilaginous | Chondroma (enchondroma) | Benign |
| | Chondrosarcoma | Malignant |
| Hematopoietic | Multiple myeloma | Malignant |
| | Leukemia | Malignant |
| | Reticulum cell sarcoma | Malignant |
| | Hodgkin's disease | Malignant |
| | Lymphosarcoma | Malignant |
| Vascular | Hemangioma | Benign |
| | Lymhangioma | Benign |
| | Glomus | Benign |
| | Angiosarcoma | Malignant |
| Neural | Neurofibroma | Benign |
| | Neurilemmoma (Schwannoma) | Benign/malignant |
| Nonosteogenic | Myxoma | Benign |
| somatic tissue | Myxosarcoma | Malignant |
| | Fibrosarcoma | Malignant |
| Unknown origin | Ewing's tumor | Malignant |
| Fatty | Lipoma | Benign |
| | Liposarcoma | Malignant |
| Mesenchymal | Myxoma | Benign |
| | Myxosarcoma | Malignant |
| Fibrous | Bone cyst | Benign |
| | Fibrous dysplasia | Benign |
| | Fibrosarcoma | Malignant |
| Secondary | Carcinoma | Malignant |
| to Primary | Sarcoma | Malignant |

the reticulum cell sarcoma may be cured by it; treatment of choice for the inaccessible malignant sarcomas, and for those debilitated elderly patients not withstanding major surgery; may control local lesions of Ewing's sarcoma and lymphomas, but fails to affect course of lesions; pain may be alleviated in myeloma or metastatic carcinoma.

ST: Includes following surgical procedures:
- Curettage and bone grafts
- Local excision

**Table 23.2:** Classification of tumors and tumorlike lesions of bone

| Tissue of derivation/or differentiation | Benign | Malignant |
| --- | --- | --- |
| Osseous | Osteoma | Osteosarcoma: |
| | Osteoid osteoma | • Central |
| | Osteoblastoma | • Juxtacortical |
| Cartilaginous | Chondroma (enchondroma) | Chondrosarcoma |
| | Osteochondroma | • Primary |
| | Chondroblastoma | • Secondary |
| | Chondromyxoid fibroma | |
| Reticuloendothelial | Eosinophilic granuloma | Multiple myeloma |
| | Hand Schuller Christian | Leukemia |
| | Letterer Siwe | Ewing's sarcoma |
| | | Malignant lymphoma: |
| | | • Hodgkin's disease |
| | | • Lymphosarcoma |
| | | • Reticulum cell sarcoma |
| Fibrous | Giant cell tumor (benign) | Giant cell tumor (malignant) |
| | Nonosteogenic fibroma | Fibrosarcoma |
| | Fibrous dysplasia | • Central (medullary) |
| | Bone cyst | • Periosteal |
| | Aneurysmal bone cyst | |
| Vascular | Hemangioma | Angiosarcoma |
| | Glomus | Angioblastoma |
| | Aneurysmal boner cyst | |
| Fatty | Lipoma | Liposarcoma |
| Neural | Neurofibroma | Neurosarcoma |
| | Neurilemmoma | |
| Notochordal | Chordoma | Chordoma |
| Mesenchymal | Myxoma | Myxosarcoma |
| | Ganglion | |
| Parosteal | Aneurysmal bone cyst | Juxtacortical sarcoma |

- Segmental resection/or total excision of bone
- Amputation
- Disarticulation.

## Curettage and Bone Grafts

Indication     Fibrous lesions of bone:
- Solitary (unicameral) bone cyst
- Fibrous dysplasia
- Nonosteogenic fibroma
- Aneurismal bone cyst
- Giant cell tumor

- Chondroblastoma
- Osteoblastoma
- Chondromyxoid fibroma.

Central cartilaginous tumors in small bones

Similar tumors in children

Recurrent tumors post curettage and graft

C/I:
- Recurrent giant cell tumor; recurrent lesion in the proximal femur or pelvis (fibrous and cartilaginous tumors).

## Segmental Resection/or Total Excision of Bone

Principle   Confirmed diagnosis to be made prior to segmental resection, considered for any bony lesion (history, examination, X-ray, and biopsy)

Indication:

Benign tumors of bone

Tumors of unknown potential:

Giant cell tumors

Central cartilaginous tumors

Tumors of suspected malignancy (knee or elbow)

Juxtacortical osteosarcomas

C/I: Malignant sarcomas of bone.

Technique of segmental resection:

Excision of calcaneus: Post excision

- TA lengthening, and its distal end sutured to the posteroinferior part of talus, Alt:
  - Plantar fascia mobilization, and its proximal end sutured to TA
  - Prosthetic calcaneus replacement + TA lengthening and suturing
  - Immobilization: In a long leg POP cast, with foot in equines and knee in 20 degree flexion for 2/12.

After care: Brace with a spring.

Resection of distal third of fibula + substituted fibular graft

Resection of distal femur + substituted tibial graft

Resection of pubis and ischium

Resection of sacrum (partial)

Resection of clavicle (partial or entire)

Resection of scapula (partial or entire)

Resection of proximal humerus + substituted fibular graft

Resection of humeral shaft

Resection of distal radius + substituted fibular graft

Resection of distal ulna

Resection of metacarpal + substituted tibial/fibular graft.

## Amputation

Indication
- Primary malignant tumors except Ewing's sarcoma
- Metastases in bone: Solitary, severely painful, destructive/or deforming

- Benign but aggressive neoplasms that cannot be removed locally
- Lesions causing major deformities.

Level:

- To be selected preoperatively (proximal to nearest joint proximal to the neoplasm, i.e. for tumors of leg or forearm level to be proximal to knee or elbow).

Exception: Osteogenic sarcoma or fibrosarcoma of distal femoral metaphysic treated by high thigh amputation

Forequarter amputation:

Indication:

- Malignant tumors in the proximal part of humerus (neck, glenoid, or body of scapula, or clavicle)
- Carcinoma breast metastasizes into axillary lymph glands, vessels, or brachial plexus.

Hindquarter amputation:

Indication:

- Malignant tumors in the proximal part of femur metastasizing into soft tissues
- Malignant tumors in the acetabulum, ilium, or ischium.

## Disarticulation of Limb

Indication          Fibrosarcoma (Multifocal) of midshaft femur or humerus.

## OSTEOBLASTIC

### Osteoma

Preface            True osteomas occur rarely and almost never except in the bones of the   face (maxillary paranasal sinuses, orbit, and middle ear's bones; term   osteoma has been applied indiscriminatory to unrelated lesions of congenital, traumatic, and inflammatory origin (exostoses and enostoses)—are basically heterotopic bone formation; osteomas of facial bones may impair function and endanger life by involving a vital structure.

Definition         Osteomas are defined grossly as dense masses that resemble ivory in texture and are sharply demarcated from the adjoining bone; may be entirely medullary or may project into a cavity; osteoblastic connective tissue origin.

                   Types: True osteomas, subungal osteoma, parosteal or juxtacortical

Etiology           Unknown.

Pathogenesis       Dense masses of bone with fibrous or vascular components

Diagnosis          Age: Older children and adolescents

                   Sex: M/F  2:1

                   Pain

                   Local tenderness

                   Bone: More often in femur and tibia

Investigation      X-rays show dense sclerotic lesion with radiolucent center.

| Management | Rest |
|---|---|
| | Warm fomentation and massage |
| | Analgesics/NSAIDs |
| | Surgical treatment of choice |
| | Surgery: Removal (curettage or local resection) is curative. |
| Prognosis | Good |

## Osteoid Osteoma

| Definition | Osteoid osteoma is defined as a small single benign lesion that forms osteoid and bone; usually occurs either in the femur or tibia; probably the most chronic of all the solitary tumorlike lesions of bone; origin-osteoblastic connective tissue. |
|---|---|
| Etiology | Unknown. |
| Pathogenesis | Small lesion consisting of a nidus or core of osteoid and bone, surrounded by a zone of sclerosis that is more striking when lesion in cortical than in cancellous bone; some lesions consist mostly of delicate streamers of new osteoid, others of large masses of mature osteoid, and still others of dense spongy bone; prominent osteoblasts. |
| Diagnosis | Age: Older children and adolescents |
| | Sex: M/F 2:1 |
| | Pain: Vague in the beginning, gradually increases in severity (Boring) |
| | Local tenderness |
| | Bone: More often in femur and tibia |
| Investigation | X-rays show dense sclerotic lesion with radiolucent center |
| Management | Rest |
| | Warm fomentation and massage |
| | Analgesics/NSAIDs |
| | Surgical treatment of choice |
| | Surgery: Removal (curettage or local resection) is curative. |
| Prognosis | Good |

## Osteoblastoma

| Definition | Osteoblastoma is a rare benign lesion, found usually in children and adolescents, most often in the spine or small bones of the hands or feet, rarely in large long bones; osteoblastomas are defined grossly as granular, friable, grey or red to brown, and vascular; osteblastic connective tissue origin. |
|---|---|
| Etiology | Unknown. |
| Pathogenesis | vascular fibroblastic lesion; bone formation; pattern of regular irregularity in the form and distribution of the neoplastic trabeculae of bone; giant cells predominate in certain areas. |
| Diagnosis | Age: Older children and adolescents |
| | Sex: M/F 2:1 |
| | Pain |
| | Local tenderness |
| | Bone: More often in femur and tibia |

| | |
|---|---|
| Investigation | X-rays show a lytic but well-circumscribed expanded lesion; may be radiolucent, or may be radiopaque mottling within it dense sclerotic lesion with radiolucent center. |
| Management | Rest: |
| | Warm fomentation and massage |
| | Analgesics/NSAIDs |
| | Surgical treatment of choice |
| | Surgery: Removal is curative. |
| Prognosis | Good |

## Osteogenic Sarcoma (Malignant)

| | |
|---|---|
| Definition | It is defined as the most frequent primary highly malignant tumor of the bone that occurs most often during 2nd and 3rd decades; affects mainly the large tubular bones (most often the distal femur, then the proximal tibia, then the proximal humerus, in terms of descending frequency), but may affect any bone in the body; originates from osteoblastic cells of bone. |
| Site | Metaphysis of long bone, growth being checked by the epiphyseal plate from spreading to epiphysis. Post fusion, the growth spreads to the epiphysis and articular cartilage. |
| Spread | Tumor may be central or commonly eccentric, destroys the cortex and produces marked periosteal reaction. An early systemic spread to lungs—causes blood stained pleural effusion. |
| Properties | Osteogenic or osteolytic. |
| Etiology | Unknown. |
| Possibility | May be related to the sites of growth. |
| Pathogenesis | Neoplastic bone and osteoid within a definitely malignant tumor of connective tissue. |
| Diagnosis | Pain—precedes swelling |
| | Swelling: Palpable bony hard fusiform, commonly seen in the region of knee or shoulder |
| | Hot |
| | Venous engorgement: Visible distended skin veins |
| | Local tenderness |
| | Weight loss |
| | Anemia |
| | Movements: Painful and restricted |
| | Fractures: Pathological. |
| Investigation | CBC, ESR |
| | X-ray—diagnostic. The lesions variable from sclerotic to lytic, are fairly large, located in the metaphysis, abolishing bone architecture, and new bone formation (sub-periosteally)—resulting in stripping of periosteum (Codman's triangle and Sun-rays appearance). |
| | PET-CT Scan |
| | CXR—pleural effusion |
| | Biopsy—to be performed with great care (risk of dissemination). |

| | |
|---|---|
| Management | Surgical: Amputation (as high as possible) is the treatment of choice. Femur/Tibia—hind-quarter amputation or disarticulation through hip Humerus—fore-quarter amputation or disarticulation through shoulder joint. Radiotherapy—controversial. Radiotherapy to both lungs along with amputation may affect survival rate. Chemotherapy—in combination with amputation may be beneficial Agents<br>• Methotrexate 12–15 g/m$^2$ PO or IM<br>• Doxorubicin 60–75 mg/m$^2$ IV Rept. Every 3/52. |
| Prognosis | Poor—mortality rate > 90% (death within two years post diagnosis). |

## Juxtacortical Osteosarcoma

| | |
|---|---|
| Definition | Juxtacortical osteosarcomas are comparatively rare tumors resulting from progressive proliferation and ossification of the periosteum or of the parosteal connective tissues or of both; develop in juxtaposition to or in continuity with a bone; affects mainly the large tubular bones (most often the distal femur), but may affect flat bones also; originates from osteoblastic cells of bone. |
| Etiology | Unknown. |
| Pathogenesis | Mass composed mainly of mature lamellar bone; disoriented bone—composed of large trabeculae or solid in some areas; sheets of dense connective tissue separating parts of the tumor; tissue with subtle malignant changes, while large parts of lesion benign. |
| Diagnosis | Diagnosis: Pain—precedes swelling<br>Swelling: Palpable bony hard fusiform, commonly seen in the region of knee or shoulder<br>Hot<br>Venous engorgement: Visible distended skin veins<br>Local tenderness<br>Weight loss<br>Anemia<br>Movements: Painful and restricted<br>Fractures: Pathological. |
| Investigation | CBC, ESR<br>X-ray—diagnostic. The lesions variable from sclerotic to lytic, are fairly large, located in the metaphysis, abolishing bone architecture, and new bone formation (subperiosteally)—resulting in stripping of periosteum (Codman's triangle and Sun-rays appearance).<br>PET: CT Scan<br>CXR: Pleural effusion<br>Biopsy: to be performed with great care (risk of dissemination). |
| Management Surgical | Amputation (as high as possible) is the treatment of choice.<br>Femur/Tibia—hind-quarter amputation or disarticulation through hip |

Humerus—fore-quarter amputation or disarticulation through shoulder joint

Radiotherapy—controversial. Radiotherapy to both lungs along with amputation may affect survival rate.

Chemotherapy—in combination with amputation may be beneficial

Agents

- Methotrexate 12–15 g/m$^2$ PO or IM
- Doxorubicin 60–75 mg/m$^2$ IV Rept. Every 3/52.

| | |
|---|---|
| Prognosis | Usually favorable post adequate treatment. |

## OSTEOCLASTIC

## Osteoclastoma (Giant Cell Tumor)

| | |
|---|---|
| Definition | Osteoclastoma (Giant cell tumor) is a rare primary benign (50%), a third aggressive (recur), and rest frankly malignant tumor, that occurs most often in adults; affects mainly the large tubular bones, most often near knee and distal radius, but may affect any bone of limbs and spine; originates from nonosteoblastic connective tissue derivation. |
| Etiology | Unknown. |
| Pathogenesis | No bone formation within tumor; trabeculae thin and separated widely; subchondral bone destroyed; collapsed articular surface. |
| | Histologically: Tumor is highly vascular, stromal cells—plump, round, or oval, nuclei vesicular, prominent nucleoli; multinucleated giant cells; |
| Diagnosis | Pain: Initially painless; pain appears later on (malignancy supervenes) |
| | Swelling: At ends of long bones (near knee and distal radius) |
| | Local tenderness |
| | Pathological fractures |
| | Movements of adjoining joints painful and restricted. |
| Investigation | X-ray shows: Eccentrically located osteolytic focus with expansion and cortical erosion; roughly spherical foamlike areas in cancellous ends of femur and tibia, or distal radius; loss of trabeculae and destroyed bony shell (malignancy). |
| Management | Surgical treatment: |
| | Surgery: Pocedures: |

- Complete curettage + bone grafting, Alt:
- Local resection: If feasible
- Amputation: For recurrent or aggressive lesions:

Technique: (As high as possible)—treatment of choice.

- Femur/Tibia: Hind-quarter amputation or disarticulation through hip
- Humerus—fore-quarter amputation or disarticulation through shoulder joint

Radiotherapy—controversial. Radiotherapy to both lungs along with amputation may affect survival rate.

Chemotherapy—in combination with amputation may be beneficial

Agents:

- Methotrexate 12–15 g/m$^2$ PO or IM
- Doxorubicin 60–75 mg/m$^2$ IV Rept. Every 3/52.

| Prognosis | About 50% are benign: Favorable outcome, regardless of treatment |
|---|---|
| | About a third are aggressive: Require further treatment |
| | Rest are: Frankly malignant with poor prognosis. |

## CARTILAGINOUS LESIONS

### Enchondromas (Syn. Chondromas)

| Definition | Enchondromas are defined as benign central cartilaginous tumors that are found mainly from the 2nd through the 5th decades as single lesions; derived from displaced epiphyseal cartilage, or from the connective tissue of bone marrow; usually expansile that cause thinning of the cortex with little periosteal reaction. |
|---|---|
| Etiology | Unknown. |
| Pathogenesis | Grossly tissue of lesion appears to be cartilage like, gray, cortex thinned from within; diffusely cellular; uniformed cell structure; calcified. |
| Diagnosis | Pain |
| | Local tenderness |
| | Swelling |
| | Fracture: Pathological (bones of hands or feet, long bones, flat bones) |
| | Lesions: May be multiple, gray. |
| Investigation | X-ray shows: Discrete foci of radiolucency with mottling; cortical expansile lesions without extensive erosion (phalangeal shaft lesions: central or eccentric; long bones: central) |
| Management | Rest |
| | Warm fomentation and massage |
| | Analgesics/NSAIDs |
| | Surgical treatment of choice |
| | Surgery: Curettage + bone graftingor. |
| Prognosis | Good. |

### *Osteochondromas (Syn. osteocartilaginous Exostoses)*

| Definition | Osteochondromas are defined as benign cartilaginous tumors that are confused with primary bone tumors; by far the most frequent of tumors and tumorlike lesions of bone; not true tumors but are developmental defects or malformations; found mainly durting 1st and 2nd decades as single or multiple lesions; derived from cartilaginous bones. |
|---|---|
| Etiology | Unknown. |
| Pathogenesis | Grossly tissue of lesion appears to be cartilage like, gray, cortex thinned from within; diffusely cellular; uniformed cell structure; calcified; originate within periosteum as a small cartilaginous nodule; grows by process of enchondral bone formation that results in a stalk of cancellous bone surrounded by thin cortex and covered on its free end by cartilaginous cap; both cortical and cancellous components develop in continuity with analogous components of parent bone. |
| Types | • Stalked |
| | • Sessile |

| | |
|---|---|
| Diagnosis | Pain |
| | Local tenderness |
| | Swelling |
| | Fracture: Pathological (bones of hands or feet, long bones, flat bones) |
| | Lesions: May be multiple, gray. |
| Investigation | X-ray shows: Discrete foci of radiolucency with mottling; cortical expansile lesions without extensive erosion (phalangeal shaft lesions: central or eccentric; long bones: central). |
| Management | No treatment reqduired for an osteochondroma, until and unless reveals spurt of growth in a child or reactivation of growth in an adult |
| | Rest |
| | Warm fomentation and massage |
| | Analgesics/NSAIDs |
| | Surgical treatment: |
| | Indication: No treatment required for an osteochondroma, until and unless reveals spurt of growth in a child or reactivation of growth in an adult |
| | • Symptoms: Because of pressure on adjoining structures (severe). |
| | Surgery: |
| | • Curettage + bone grafting |
| | • Excision of osteochondromas. |
| Prognosis | Good |

## Chondromyxoid Fibroma

| | |
|---|---|
| Definition | Chondromyxoid fibroma defined as a benign (may be potentially malignant) tumor of cartilaginous derivation; most often occur in the 2nd and 3rd decades, and in the bones of lower limbs (femur, tibia, fibula, tarsals, and metatarsals), occasionally in long or flat bones; usual eccentrically in the metaphysis of long bones, while involving the entire width of smaller bones. |
| Etiology | Unknown. |
| Pathogenesis | Massive trabeculation/or loculation; subperiosteal or perosteal lesion covered by a thin shell of bone. |
| Diagnosis | Age: Young adults (2nd and 3rd decades) |
| | Sex: M = F |
| | Pain |
| | Swelling |
| | Local tenderness |
| | Movements of adjoining joints painful and restricted |
| Investigation | X-rays show radiolucent lesions with thinned and bulged cortices; marginal sclerosis; may be multiple foci of osteolysis. |
| Management | Rest |
| | Warm fomentation and massage |
| | Analgesics/NSAIDs |
| | Surgical treatment of choice |
| | Surgery: Curettage or excision. |
| Prognosis | Good |

## Chondroblastoma (Epiphyseal Giant Cell Tumor)

| | |
|---|---|
| Definition | Chondroblastoma is defined as a benign (may be potentially malignant) tumor; most often occur in young adults (< 20 years), and in the epiphysis of major tubular and in flat bones of lower limbs (femur, tibia, fibula, tarsals, and metatarsals), and flat bones. |
| Etiology | Unknown. |
| Pathogenesis | Ovoid areas of mottled translucency in epiphyses; massive trabeculation/or loculation; rarefaction and cortical expansion with erosion. |
| Diagnosis | Age: Young adults (< 20 years)<br>Sex: Predominantly male<br>Pain<br>Swelling: Epiphyseal areas of major tubular bones, and flat bones<br>Local tenderness<br>Movements of adjoining joints painful and restricted. |
| Investigation | X-rays show radiolucent lesions with thinned and bulged cortices; marginal sclerosis; may be multiple foci of osteolysis. |
| Management | Rest<br>Warm fomentation and massage<br>Analgesics/NSAIDs<br>Surgical treatment of choice<br>Surgery: Curettage or excision. |
| Prognosis | Good |

## Chondrosarcoma

| | |
|---|---|
| Definition | It is defined as the frequent primary or secondary malignant tumor of the cartilage that occurs most often in adults (30–60 years of age); affects mainly the large tubular bones (most often the proximal femur and pelvis), but may affect any bone preformed in cartilage in the body; originates from cartilaginous derivation. |
| Site | Metaphysis of long bone, growth being checked by the epiphyseal plate from spreading to epiphysis. Post fusion, the growth spreads to the epiphysis and articular cartilage. |
| Spread | Tumor may be central or commonly eccentric, destroys the cortex and produces marked periosteal reaction. An early systemic spread to lungs—causes blood stained pleural effusion. |
| Properties | Primary chondrosarcomas are rare, fulminating; secondary chondro-sarcomas are frequent, indolent, grow slowly, tend to recur locally post excision |
| Etiology | Unknown. |
| Possibility | May be related to the sites of growth. |
| Pathogenesis | Hypercellularity; absent cells polarity; hyperchromic nuclei and of multinucleation; occasional binucleate cell; crowding of cells. |
| Diagnosis | Pain—precedes swelling<br>Swelling: Palpable bony hard fusiform, commonly seen in the region of knee or shoulder |

|  | Hot |
|---|---|
|  | Venous engorgement: Visible distended skin veins |
|  | Local tenderness |
|  | Weight loss |
|  | Anemia |
|  | Movements: Painful and restricted |
|  | Fractures: Pathological. |
| Investigation | CBC, ESR |
|  | X-ray—diagnostic: Show an irregular dissolution of bone, often without significant new bone formation; usually cortex expanded and thinned; may be irregularly mottled and calcified interior of long bones with fuzzy localized destruction of cortex. |
|  | PET—CT Scan |
|  | CXR—pleural effusion |
|  | Biopsy—to be performed with great care (risk of dissemination). |
| Management | Surgical: Amputation (as high as possible)—treatment of choice. |
|  | Femur/Tibia—hind-quarter amputation or disarticulation through hip |
|  | Humerus—fore-quarter amputation or disarticulation through shoulder joint |
|  | Radiotherapy—controversial. Radiotherapy to both lungs along with amputation may affect survival rate. |
|  | Chemotherapy—in combination with amputation may be beneficial |
|  | Agents: |
|  | • Methotrexate 12–15 g/m² PO or IM |
|  | • Doxorubicin 60–75 mg/m² IV Rept. Every 3/52. |
| Prognosis | • Excellent: For complete excision |
|  | • Recurrence and progression: For incomplete excision. |

## LESIONS OF UNKNOWN ORIGIN

### Ewing's Sarcoma

| Definition | Is defined as a rare primary malignant tumor, originating from the mesenchymal connective tissue derivation; that occurs most often in childhood (5–15 years); affects mainly the large tubular bones of the lower limbs or the pelvis, but may affect any bone, occasionally even the skull or a facial bone. |
|---|---|
|  | Site: Diaphysis of long bones. |
|  | Properties: Tumor may be osteolytic or osteoblastic. |
| Etiology | Unknown. |
| Pathogenesis | Osteolytic lesions; mottled destruction of the cancellous bone; reactive endosteal and periosteal new bone formed; soft tissue infiltration of the tumor. |
|  | Histologically: Variable changes because of extensive hemorrhage and necrosis; highly cellular, without a visible stroma; typical cell with round or oval nucleus and no nucleolus; cells loosely arranged or closely packed. |

| | |
|---|---|
| Metastasis | Potential for hematogenous metastasis and most common sites of metastases are lungs, bones, and bone marrow. |
| Diagnosis | Pain: Increases progressively |
| | Fever: Low grade |
| | Anemia |
| | Local tenderness |
| | Swelling: Palpable bony hard swelling |
| | Movements: Painful and restricted. |
| Investigation | CBC: Leukocytosis; ESR: increased |
| | X-ray—diagnostic. Marked diffuse rarefaction of the shaft, with the subperiosteal deposition of bone in layers (onion effect); occasionally periosteal reaction (Sunburst) and medullary destruction evidenced by diffuse rarefaction or mottling. |
| | PET: CT Scan |
| | CXR |
| | Biopsy: Diagnostic |
| D/d | Chronic osteomyelitis. |
| | Reticulum cell sarcoma |
| | Metastatic neuroblastoma |
| | Lymphoma |
| | Metastatic carcinoma. |
| Management | It is highly unsatisfactory. |
| | Radiotherapy: Highly sensitive to RT. Little effect on distant metastasis. RT in combination with CT yields better result. |
| | Surgical: Amputation—rarely indicated in failure cases of RT and CT. |
| Prognosis | Very poor. Most lethal of all primary tumors of bone. |
| | Mortality rate > 95% despite treatment (palliative). |

## Reticuloendothelial (Syn. Hematopoietic) Lesions

### Multiple Myeloma (Plasma Cell Myeloma)

| | |
|---|---|
| Definition | Multiple myeloma is defined as the frequent primary malignant tumor of hematopoietic origin that occurs most often in adults over 40 years of age; affects mainly the spine, ribs, skull, and femora, but may affect any bone in the body; malignant proliferation of plasma cells that involves > 10% of bone marrow. |
| Etiology | Unknown. |
| Pathogenesis | Grossly the tumor is soft, purple to red in color, necrotic in parts; highly vascular. |
| | Histologically: Immature plasma cells; frequent binucleate cells; cells as compact masses, or arranged in distinct cords |
| Diagnosis | Age—usually appears in 6th and 7th decades of life and is rare in < 40 years. |
| | Race—seen in all races. |
| | Sex—twice common in males |
| | Severe bone pain—aggravated by motion |

|   |   |
|---|---|
|   | Bones are involved in 90% of patients—skull, pelvis, spine, ribs and femurs |
|   | Pathological fractures |
|   | Fever |
|   | Fatigue, thirst, loss of weight, anemia. |
| Investigation | CBC |
|   | Anemia—normocytic, normochromic type |
|   | Rouleau formation—marked |
|   | ESR—greatly elevated |
|   | TLC and Platelet count—normal |
|   | Serum alkaline phosphatase—elevated |
|   | Serum protein total—elevated |
|   | Serum globulin—elevated |
|   | Urine—appearance of Bence-Jones proteose—precipitates on addition of nitric acid and disappears on warming |
|   | X-ray—diagnostic, e.g. shows multiple punched out areas |
|   | MRI—highly accurate in detecting an early epidural involvement |
|   | Bone marrow (aspiration) biopsy—shows sheets of plasma cells with large nuclei and nucleoli. |
| D/d | Connective tissue disorders. |
|   | Chronic infections. |
|   | Skeletal metastasis. |
|   | Amyloidosis—always associated with plasma cell neoplasia. |
|   | Abnormal gamma globulin products, esp. those of Bence Jones type, are directly involved in these tissue (amyloid) infiltrates. |
| Management | No effective treatment known and the disease is always fatal. |
|   | General measures: |
|   | Aims: |

- To relieve pain and reduce tumor masses
- To ambulate patient to combat negative calcium balance
- To prevent exposure to trauma to avoid occurrence of the pathological fractures.

Conservative treatment:

Blood transfusion: To combat anemia

Analgesics: For control of pain

Chemotherapy (CT):

Alkylating Agents:

- Melphalan (Alkeran)—most effective agent available.
  Dose: 6 mg o.d. PO, for 2–3 weeks
  Maintenance dose: 1–4 mg o.d. every 4 weeks along with
- Prednisone 2 mg/kg
- Cyclophosphamides 50–100 mg PO 1–3 times o.d. along with Vincristine 1.4 mg/sq.m weekly.

Radiotherapy (RT):
- For control of pain and for reducing tumor mass

Surgical therapy (ST):
Surgery:
* Decompression with radiotherapy—for cord compression
* Stem cell transplantation (SCT)—for selective patients.

**Prognosis**     Average survival time after diagnosis is 2 years. Occasionally a patient may live for many years in apparent remission.

# Leukemia

**Definition**     It is defined as highly malignant tomor characterized by skeletal changes that are caused by an enormous proliferation of marrow cells affecting mature and growing bone in separate ways; in adults these changes occur fairly late and are usually unmarked; diffuse osteoporosis or focal areas of bone destruction; pathological fractures may occur (vertebrae and ribs); in children profound changes in bones may occur (diagnostic).

**Etiology**     Unknown.

**Pathogenesis**     Depressed bone growth because of disability; usually caused by the proximal humerus); severe form: rarefied metaphysic; eroded cortex from within; reactive periosteal bone formed on long bones shafts; rarely increased; pathological fracture may occur.

**Diagnosis**     Pain
Swelling
Local tenderness
Movements: Painful and restricted

**Investigation**     X-ray show: Narrow bands of increased radiolucency in metaphyses adjoining the epiphyseal plates; rarely an increased periosteal bone density (osteoporosis).

**Management**     General measures:
Aims:
* To relieve pain and reduce tumor masses
* To ambulate patient to combat negative calcium balance
* To prevent exposure to trauma to avoid occurrence of the pathological fractures.

Conservative treatment:
Blood transfusion: To combat anemia
Analgesics for control of pain

Chemotherapy (CT):
Alkylating Agents:
* Melphalan (Alkeran)—most effective agent available.
  Dose: 6 mg o.d. PO, for 2–3 weeks
  Maintenance dose: 1–4 mg o.d. every 4 weeks along with
* Prednisone 2 mg/kg
* Cyclophosphamides 50–100 mg PO 1–3 times o.d. along with
Vincristine 1.4 mg/sq.m weekly.

Radiotherapy (RT):
- For control of pain and for reducing tumor mass

Surgical therapy (ST):

Surgery:
- Decompression with radiotherapy—for cord compression
- Stem cell transplantation (SCT)—for selective patients.

**Prognosis**     Average survival time after diagnosis is 2 years. Occasionally a patient may live for many years in apparent remission.

## Lymphomas

**Preface**     Lymphomas are complex tumors with multiple manifestations; are mostly generalized; while often involve bone, they usually do so only secondarily; rarely cause a primary tumor of bone.

## Hodgkin's Disease

**Definition**     Hodgkin's disease is defined as malignant tumor differentiated from other lymphomas because of varying reactions it produces in the bone; lesions may be osteoblastic or osteolytic or both (in long bones and pelvis are usually osteolytic, while in vertebrae usually osteoblastic or both); most often occur in vertebrae and iliac bones by direct invasion from lymph nodes.

**Etiology**     Unknown.

**Pathogenesis**     Lesions may be osteoblastic or osteolytic or both (in long bones and pelvis are usually osteolytic, while in vertebrae usually osteoblastic or both); most often occur in vertebrae and iliac bones by direct invasion from lymph nodes, less often spread by metastasis.

**Diagnosis**     Pain

Swelling

Local tenderness

Movements: Painful and restricted

**Investigation**     X-ray

**Management**     General measures:

Aims:
- To relieve pain and reduce tumor masses
- To ambulate patient to combat negative calcium balance
- To prevent exposure to trauma to avoid occurrence of the pathological fractures.

Conservative treatment:

Blood transfusion: To combat anemia

Analgesics: For control of pain

Chemotherapy (CT):

Alkylating Agents:
- Melphalan (Alkeran)—most effective agent available.
  Dose: 6 mg o.d. PO, for 2–3 weeks
  Maintenance dose: 1–4 mg o.d. every 4 weeks along with

- Prednisone 2 mg/kg
- Cyclophosphamides 50–100 mg PO 1–3 times o.d. along with Vincristine 1.4 mg/sq.m weekly
  Radiotherapy (RT):
  – For control of pain and for reducing tumor mass

Surgical therapy (ST):
Surgery:

- Decompression with radiotherapy—for cord compression
- Stem cell transplantation (SCT)—for selective patients.

Prognosis     Average survival time after diagnosis is 2 years. Occasionally a patient may live for many years in apparent remission.

## Lymphosarcoma

Preface        Lymphosarcoma usually includes all malignant lymphomas except the Hodgkin's disease, includes. Reticulum cell sarcoma; bone involvement; bone involvement occurs less often in lymphosarcoma (10%) than in Hodgkin's disease; most often occur in vertebrae and iliac bones by direct extension from lymph nodes; less often occur in long bones (femur, tibia, and humerus) spread by metastasis or as multifocal origin.

Etiology       Unknown.

Pathogenesis   Lesions are totally osteolytic and may cause periosteal reaction esp. of reticulum cell sarcoma, as they grow rapidly and markedly raise the medullary pressure.

Diagnosis      Pain
               Swelling
               Local tenderness
               Movements: Painful and restricted

Investigation  X-ray show: Lesions resembling metastatic carcinoma or reticulum cell sarcoma of bone.
               Biopsy: Diagnostic

D/d            Ewing's tumor: Easy to differentiate clinically.

## Management

General measures:

Aims:

- To relieve pain and reduce tumor masses
- To ambulate patient to combat negative calcium balance
- To prevent exposure to trauma to avoid occurrence of the pathological fractures.

Conservative treatment:
Blood transfusion: To combat anemia
Analgesics: For control of pain

Chemotherapy (CT):
Alkylating Agents:

- Melphalan (Alkeran)—most effective agent available.

Dose: 6 mg o.d. PO, for 2–3 weeks

Maintenance dose: 1–4 mg o.d. every 4 weeks along with

- Prednisone 2 mg/kg
- Cyclophosphamides 50–100 mg PO 1–3 times o.d. along with Vincristine 1.4 mg/sq.m weekly

Radiotherapy (RT):

– For control of pain and for reducing tumor mass

Surgical therapy (ST):

Surgery:

- Decompression with radiotherapy—for cord compression
- Stem cell transplantation (SCT)—for selective patients.

| | |
|---|---|
| Prognosis | Average survival time after diagnosis is 2 years. Occasionally a patient may live for many years in apparent remission. |

## Reticulum Cell Sarcoma

| | |
|---|---|
| Definition | Reticulum cell sarcoma of bone is defined as a solitary lesion, different from the generalized/disseminated type that is highly malignant (invades the viscera and other tissues; often fatal within 2 years); most frequent in the patients post 4th decade; usually affects shaft of a long tubular bone (femur, tibia, or humerus) or the pelvis, and occasionally a vertebra; origin within bone. |
| Etiology | Unknown. |
| Pathogenesis | Osteolytic entirely, involving a large area of the bone; there may be a pathological fracture frequently. |
| Diagnosis | Pain |
| | Swelling |
| | Local tenderness |
| | Movements: Painful and restricted |
| Investigation | X-ray show: Large area of destruction, shading into irregular mottled bone; tubular bones may show a rough reticular pattern; bone unexpanded, without any periosteal reaction. |
| | Biopsy: Histologically: highly cellular and pleomorphic, non-anaplastic; type cell (large reticulum cell, with oval/kidney shaped nucleus within cytoplasm containing cell debris; many lymphocytes and normal reticulum cells may be visible; complex reticular stroma embedded with single cell or cells in clusters form surrounded by fibers. |
| D/d | Ewing's tumor: Easy to differentiate clinically |
| Management | General measures: |
| | Aims: |

- To relieve pain and reduce tumor masses
- To ambulate patient to combat negative calcium balance
- To prevent exposure to trauma to avoid occurrence of the pathological fractures.

Conservative treatment:

Blood transfusion: To combat anemia

Analgesics: For control of pain

Chemotherapy (CT):

Alkylating Agents:

- Melphalan (Alkeran)—most effective agent available.
  Dose: 6 mg o.d. PO, for 2–3 weeks
  Maintenance dose: 1–4 mg o.d. every 4 weeks along with
- Prednisone 2 mg/kg
- Cyclophosphamides 50–100 mg PO 1–3 times o.d. along with
  Vincristine 1.4 mg/sq.m weekly
  Radiotherapy (RT):
  – For control of pain and for reducing tumor mass

Surgical therapy (ST):

Surgery:

- Decompression with radiotherapy—for cord compression
- Stem cell transplantation (SCT)—for selective patients.
- Amputation

| | |
|---|---|
| Prognosis | Average survival time after diagnosis is 2 years. Occasionally a patient may live for many years in apparent remission. |

## VASCULAR LESIONS OF BONE

### Hemangioma

| | |
|---|---|
| Definition | Hemangiomas are defined as benign tumors of vascular origin; that may occur usually in the vertebrae or skull; may also occur in the pelvis, or bones of hand and feet; multiple hemangiomas of the bone are rare; symptomatic hemangiomas of the bone are extremely rare. |
| Etiology | Unknown. |
| Pathogenesis | Osteolytic lesion. Histologically: Large closely packed vascular channels with thin walls encased in radiating trabeculae of heavy bone |
| Diagnosis | Pain Backache Headache Swelling |
| D/d | Hemolytic anemia Aneurysmal bone cyst |
| Investigation | X-ray show focal areas of low density and vertical striations within vertebral body; skull: may show a circumscribed area of rarefaction with bulging outer table, and radiating trabeculae. Biopsy: Aspiration biopsy |
| Management | Based upon its size and severity of symptoms. RT: For small lesions, and those confined to a vertebral body Dose: Usually 2–4 K roentgen units ST: Laminectomy. |

### Lymphangioma

| | |
|---|---|
| Definition | Lymphangiomas are defined as rare benign tumors of vascular origin; that may occur usually in the skin or subcutaneous tissue; that cystic |

hygromas are large lymphangiomas consisting of the large coalescing locules, that are found usually in the neck, axilla, or groin; mostly seen in children; mortality rate high because of difficulty in excision of tumor.

| | |
|---|---|
| Etiology | Unknown. |
| Pathogenesis | Osteolytic lesion. |
| | Histologically: Capillary or cavernous; large closely packed vascular channels with thin walls. |
| Diagnosis | Pain |
| | Backache |
| | Headache |
| | Swelling |
| D/d | Hemolytic anemia |
| | Aneurysmal bone cyst |
| | Hemangioma |
| Investigation | X-ray show focal areas of low density and vertical striations; may show a circumscribed area of rarefaction, and radiating trabeculae. |
| | Biopsy: Aspiration biopsy |
| Management | Based upon its size and severity of symptoms. |
| | RT: For small lesions |
| | Dose: Usually 2–4 K roentgen units |
| | ST: Excision. |

## Glomus Tumor

| | |
|---|---|
| Definition | It is defined as a rare benign tumor of vascular origin; usually seen in the skin and subcutaneous tissues of the limbs, esp. of hands and feet, particularly in the nail bed; small pin head size; highly tender. |
| Etiology | Unknown |
| Pathogenesis | Glomus tumor originates in a glomus body (arteriovenous shunt consisting of an afferent arteriole connected to a venuole by canal/s (Sucquet-Hoyer); hypertrophic and hyperplastic glomus cells (normally present in the arteriole muscle encircling the canal/s) forming glomus tumor. |
| | Histologically: Variable from large compact sheets of uniform glomus cells (small spindle/or large polyhedral) with few vascular channels, to an aggregated vascular channels cuffed by the multiple layers of polyhedral glomus cells. |
| Diagnosis | Pain: Excruciating, burning or lancinating type |
| | Lesion: Small, bluish red, discolored skin |
| | Local tenderness: Exquisitely tender |
| | Site: Nail bed of hands and feet |
| Investigation | X-ray shows: Erosion caused by pressure from the tumor, causing discrete area of cortical destruction and varying area of medullary destruction. |
| Management | Excision of the tumor. |

## Angiosarcoma

| | |
|---|---|
| Definition | Angiosarcoma of vascular origin is defined as the frankly malignant tumor that has the potential to metastasize; grows rapidly; occurs rarely, most often in young adults; affects men and women equally; affects mainly head, neck, and paranasal sinuses; frequently affects the limbs. |
| Etiology | Unknown |
| Pathogenesis | Grows rapidly; invades the adjoining structures and metastasizes. |

Grossly: The tumor is circumscribed and encapsulated; firm and rubbery; cut surface trbeculated or matted with small cystic areas; edematous; calcified; ossified tissues; in highly cellular lesion—tumor appears soft, cut surface hemorrhagic and necrotic; in subperiosteal lesion – bone eroded, saucerlike.

Histologically: Difficult to diagnose; variable (from markedly well differentiated ones to markedly anaplastic ones).

| | |
|---|---|
| Diagnosis | Pain: Very severe |
| | Swelling |
| | Pathological fracture: May be found. |
| Investigation | CBC |
| | Serum acid phosphatase estimation |
| | X-ray—diagnostic. Shows irregular destruction of bone without surrounding reaction, while sclerosis in case of metastasis from carcinoma prostate |
| | CXR |
| | Mammography CT scan |
| | US abdomen and pelvis |
| | Biopsy. |
| Management | No effective treatment known and the disease is always fatal. |

## *General Measures*

Aims
- To relieve pain and reduce tumor masses
- To ambulate patient to combat negative calcium balance
- To prevent exposure to trauma to avoid occurrence of the pathological fractures.

Conservative treatment:

Blood transfusion: To combat anemia

Analgesics: For control of pain

Chemotherapy (CT):

Alkylating Agents:
- Melphalan (Alkeran)—most effective agent available.
  Dose: 6 mg o.d. PO, for 2–3 weeks
  Maintenance dose: 1–4 mg o.d. every 4 weeks along with
- Prednisone 2 mg/kg
- Cyclophosphamides 50–100 mg PO 1–3 times o.d. along with Vincristine 1.4 mg/sq.m weekly

Radiotherapy (RT): palliative value only.
  – For control of pain and for reducing tumor mass.

Surgical therapy (ST):
Surgery:
- Local resection: unsatisfactory.

Amputation of the affected limb + lymphadenectomy.

Prognosis      Average survival time after diagnosis is 2–3 years.

## NEURAL LESIONS OF BONE

### Neurofibroma

| | |
|---|---|
| Definition | It is defined as a benign tumor of neural origin, characterized by the proliferation of all elements of a peripheral nerve; rarely develops as a solitary lesion; may occur anywhere in the body, but frequently found in the subcutaneous or deeper fibrous tissues. |
| Etiology | Unknown. |
| Pathogenesis | Proliferated Schwann cells of fibroblastic tissue (often of neurons). Histologically: Proliferated fibroblastic tissue with variable amounts of collagenization. |
| Diagnosis | Pain Swelling Local tenderness Numbness: by nerve compression. |
| Investigation | X-ray show bone destruction by pressure from the neurofibroma; bone may be osteoporotic |
| Management | Symptomatic Conservative treatment: Analgesics and NSAIDs SWD or IR therapy |
| | Surgical treatment: Indication: Relief from pain or numbness Surgery: Excision. |

### Neurofibromatosis (Multiple Neurofibromatosis or von Recklinghausen's Disease)

| | |
|---|---|
| Definition | It is defined as a symptom complex comprising development of multiple neurofibromas; is a malformation of nervous system with hereditary linkage. Lesions: Neurofibromas and secondary lesions |
| Etiology | Unknown |
| Pathogenesis | Many forms of neurofibromas develop in subcutaneous areas: |

- Small nonencapsulated nodules covered by abnormally pigmented skin, at the nerve endings in the skin, or as large infiltrative growths accompanied by marked thickened skin and subcutaneous tissues (elephantiasis neuromatosa)
- Tangled wormlike masses of nerve fibers developed within nerves (plexiform neurofibroma).

| | Bone destruction by a neurofibroma of periosteal nerve |
|---|---|
| Diagnosis | Pain |
| | Swelling |
| | Local tenderness |
| | Skin: pigmented (café-au-lait) spots |
| | Deformity: Tibial bowing; pseudarthrosis of tibia; scoliosis |
| | Numbness: By nerve compression |
| Investigation | X-ray show bone destruction by pressure from the neurofibroma; bone may be osteoporotic; destroyed epiphyseal plates; deformed. |
| Management | Symptomatic: |
| | Conservative treatment: |
| | Analgesics and NSAIDs |
| | SWD or IR therapy |
| | Surgical treatment: |
| | Indication: Relief from pain or numbness |
| | Surgery: Excision. |

## Neurosarcoma (Syn. malignant Schwannoma)

| | |
|---|---|
| Definition | Neurosarcoma of neural origin is defined as the frankly malignant tumor that has the potential to metastasize; grows rapidly; occurs rarely, most often in elderly; affects men and women equally; affects mainly head, neck, and paranasal sinuses; frequently affects the limbs. |
| Etiology | Unknown |
| Pathogenesis | Grows rapidly; invades the adjoining structures and metastasizes. |
| | Grossly: The tumor is circumscribed and encapsulated; firm and rubbery; cut surface trabeculated or matted with small cystic areas; edematous; calcified; ossified tissues; in highly cellular lesion—tumor appears soft, cut surface hemorrhagic and necrotic; in subperiosteal lesion—bone eroded, saucerlike. |
| | Histologically: Difficult to diagnose; variable (from markedly well differentiated ones to markedly anaplastic ones). |
| Diagnosis | Pain: Very severe |
| | Swelling |
| | Local tenderness |
| | Numbness |
| | Pathological fracture: May be found. |
| Investigation | CBC, ESR |
| | Serum acid phosphatase estimation |
| | X-ray—diagnostic. Shows irregular destruction of bone without surrounding reaction, while sclerosis in case of metastasis from carcinoma prostate. |
| | CXR |
| | Biopsy. |
| Management | No effective treatment known and the disease is always fatal. |
| | General measures. |

Aims
- To relieve pain and reduce tumor masses
- To ambulate patient to combat negative calcium balance
- To prevent exposure to trauma to avoid occurrence of the pathological fracture.

Surgical treatment: May be curative
Surgery: Based upon the site of the tumor:
- Local resection
- Amputation.

## Fibrous Lesions of Bone

Definition | Defined as lesions of bone that are originated from/or differentiated as fibrous tissue; also including fibrous lesions having bone as an occasional or constant feature; spontaneous malignant transformation unknown.

Lesions | Fibrous dysplasia, solitary bone cyst, aneurysmal bone cyst, non-osteogenic fibroma, giant cell tomor, osteoblastoma, chondroblastoma, and chondromyxoid fibroma; only first six are basically fibrous lesions, and out of these only giant cell tumor is a true neoplasm (osteoblastoma, chondroblastoma and the chondromyxoid fibroma); the six basically fibrous lesions of bone usually occur in children or young adults.

Pathogenesis | Histologically: Multinucleated giant cells are constant features of most of these lesions, though these cells are transient (post-trauma) in bone cysts and in fibrous dysplasia.

## Solitary (Syn. Unicameral) Bone Cyst

Definition | It is defined as lesions that are frequent; rank second to enchondram; occur usually in the 1st or 2nd decade of life; most often result in pathological fracture; usually involve the long tubular bones (femur, tibia, and the humerus) and flat bones (iliac).

Predisposing factors:
- Localized failure of metaphyseal ossification at time of fast growth
- Encapsulated medullary hemorrhage
- Dysplastic tissue
- Blocked drainage of interstitial fluid in fast growing and remodeled cancellous bone

Etiology | Obscure.

Pathogenesis | Fibrous lesions originated in metaphysis adjoining epiphyseal plate (latent); with bone growth, the epiphysis moves away from the lesion; then found in the metaphysic or in the diaphysis (active); resulting in expansion and thinning of the cortex; usually a distinct sclerotic margin; without any periosteal reaction; pathological fracture.

Histologically: Large closely packed vascular channels with thin walls encased in radiating trabeculae of heavy bone.

Diagnosis | Pain
Backache
Headache

|            | Swelling |
|            | Pathological fracture. |
| D/d        | Hemolytic anemia |
|            | Aneurysmal bone cyst |
| Investigation | X-rays show: Characteristic appearance: lesion expansile; thinning of cortex; usually a distinct sclerotic margin without any periosteal reaction except that in pathological fracture; trabeculations formed. |
| Management | Conservative treatment: |
|            | Indication: Young children (active bone cyst) surgery to be delayed. |
|            | Analgesics |
|            | SWD or IR diathermy |

Surgical treatment:
- Curettage + bone grafting
- Resecting a nonessential bone.

## Fibrous Dysplasia

| Definition | Fibrous dysplasia defined as lesions that originate as developmental defect, a hamartoma; extent of skeletal involvement variable, i.e. (monostotic, monomelic, and polyostotic); occur usually in the 1st or 2nd decade of life; most often result in pathological fracture; usually involve the long tubular bones ends (femur, tibia, and the humerus), flat bones (iliac, ribs); females affected more than males. |
| Etiology | Uncertain. |
| Predisposing factors | • Localized failure of metaphyseal ossification at time of fast growth |
|          | • Encapsulated medullary hemorrhage |
|          | • Dysplastic tissue |
|          | • Blocked drainage of interstitial fluid in fast growing and remodeled cancellous bone. |
| Pathogenesis | Fibrous dysplasia lesions originate from proliferation of moderately cellular and vascular fibrillar connective tissue embedded with bony spicules (metaplastic resulting from collagenous osteogenesis); the monostotic (commonest) lesion usually affects proximal femur, but may involve any bone in the body most pathological fracture. |
|          | Histologically: Large closely packed vascular channels with thin walls encased in radiating trabeculae of heavy bone. |
| Diagnosis | Pain |
|          | Backache |
|          | Headache |
|          | Swelling |
|          | Deformity: Shepherd's crook |
|          | Pathological fracture |
| D/d      | Hemolytic anemia |
|          | Aneurysmal bone cyst |
| Investigation | X-rays show: Rarefaction of bones; formation of bone cysts; lesions ill defined; gradual shading of lesion into normal bone; cortex expansile and thinned without any periosteal reaction except that in case of the |

pathological fracture; pattern of trabeculations variable; initially lesions appear like ground glass, but later on irregular calcification visible; skull and bones of hand sclerosed.

| | |
|---|---|
| Management | Conservative treatment: |
| | Indication: Young children (active bone cyst) surgery to be delayed. |
| | Analgesics |
| | SWD or IR diathermy |

Surgical treatment:
- Curettage + bone grafting
- Osteotomy: To correct any existing deformity
- Resecting a nonessential bone.

## NONOSTEOGENIC FIBROMA

| | |
|---|---|
| Definition | Defined as lesions characterized by failure of a metaphyseal defect to follow its normal evolutionary course, resulting in formation of a nonosteogenic fibroma that behaves like a tumor; usually these lesions are small, innocuous, asymptomatic, and are frequent; occur usually in during the 1st and 2nd decades of life; most often result in pathological fracture; usually involve the metaphysic of long tubular bones (femur, tibia, and the humerus). |
| Etiology | Obscure. |
| Predisposing factors | • Localized failure of metaphyseal ossification at time of fast growth |
| | • Encapsulated medullary hemorrhage |
| | • Dysplastic tissue |
| | • Blocked drainage of interstitial fluid in fast growing and remodeled cancellous bone. |
| Pathogenesis | The lesional tissue is highly characteristic, i.e. friable, rusty colored |
| | Histologically: The lesions are cellular fibromas consisting of variable number of multinucleated giant cells; clusters of macrophages with iron or lipid seen; containing fewer giant cells and are more fibroblastic. |
| Diagnosis | Pain |
| | Backache |
| | Headache |
| | Swelling |
| | Pathological fracture |
| D/d | Fibrous dysplasia |
| | Aneurysmal bone cyst |
| Investigation | X-rays shows a distinctive appearance of fibrous metaphyseal defect. |
| | Biopsy: Indicated in case of a large lesion. |
| Management | Conservative treatment: |
| | Indication: Young children (active bone cyst) surgery to be delayed. |
| | Analgesics |
| | SWD or IR diathermy |

Surgical treatment:
- Curettage + bone grafting
- Local resection.

## Aneurysmal Bone Cyst

| | |
|---|---|
| Definition | It is defined as benign lesions that are frequent; usually occur in older children and young adults; usually involve the long tubular bones (femur, tibia, and humerus), flat bones (iliac), and vertebrae. |
| Etiology | Uncertain. |
| Predisposing | • Localized failure of metaphyseal ossification at time of fast growth |
| | • Encapsulated medullary hemorrhage |
| | • Dysplastic tissue |
| | • Blocked drainage of interstitial fluid in fast growing and remodeled cancellous bone. |
| Pathogenesis | Grossly: Intact lesions: Outer surface like a thin shell of bone, while interior one loculated by connective tissue septa, forming likes filled with dark blood that oozes heavily; lesion having variable structure, i.e. vascular or those containing heavily ossified connective tissue. |
| | Histologically: Large closely packed vascular channels with thin walls encased in radiating trabeculae of heavy bone. |
| Diagnosis | Pain |
| | Backache |
| | Headache |
| | Swelling |
| | Pathological fracture |
| D/d | Giant cell tumor |
| | Chondromyxoid fibroma |
| | Nonosteogenic fibroma |
| | Fibrous dysplasia |
| Investigation | X-rays shows a distinctive appearance of fibrous metaphyseal defect; Lesion nearer to bone end than to the middle of bone shaft; localized bulging mass covered with a thin bony shell; central lesion may show a striking and heavy trabeculation/or loculation. |
| | Biopsy: Indicated in case of a suspected lesion. |
| Management | Conservative treatment: |
| | Indication: Young children (active bone cyst) surgery to be delayed. |
| | Analgesics |
| | SWD or IR diathermy |
| | RT: Indicated in vertebral lesions. |
| | Surgical treatment: |
| | • Curettage + bone grafting |
| | • Local resection. |

## SYNOVIAL LESIONS

### Ganglion

| | |
|---|---|
| Definition | Is defined as a cystic or partially cystic lesion that originates from or related to the synovial membrane, thereby found near a tendon sheath or joint capsule; most frequent on the dorsal or volar surface of the wrist; may also be found in the foot, ankle, and knee; firm, fluctuant |

cystic masses; movable (related to tendon sheaths) or fixed to the surrounding structures.

Etiology            Traumatic: Herniation of synovial membranes

Pathogenesis        Variable gross and microscopic features:

- Discrete cysts often multilocular, lined with synovium, filled with clear mucinous fluid; often having a pedicle attached to a synovial sheath; found on dorsum of hand and feet.

- Poorly circumscribed; merged into surrounding tissue; containing masses of sticky mucin that infiltrated and separated bundles of connective tissue; rarely having well defined lining; found on large joints; originate mostly from proliferative reaction caused by the traumatised synovial tissues (myxoma and mucinous cysts), or displaced synovial tissue or extravasated mucin into para-articular tissues. Diagnosis: Pain

Disability

Cosmetic stigma

Investigation       X-ray wrist: AP and LAT views

Management          Conservative treatment:

Strapping

Inj. Hydrocortisone with lignocaine 2% into the ganglion

Threading: A corrugated silken thread passed through ganglion: to be removed marginally daily till end of the week.

Analgesics and NSAIDs

Surgical treatment of choice

Surgery: Excision.

Recurrences: Fairly common, esp. of poorly excised ones.

## Pigmented Villonodular Synovitis

Definition          It is defined as benign lesion that may develop in any synovial space, synovial joints, i.e. knee, hip, ankle, shoulder, or elbow; also seen in synovium of the tarsal, carpal, and phalangeal joints; usually occurs in young adults causing pain and swelling increased in severity with each exacerbation.

Etiology            Obscure.

Pathogenesis        Variable gross and microscopic features:

Grossly: Reddish or rusty brown synovium with interspersed areas of fresh hemorrhage and large yellowish areas of accumulated lipid; exaggerated villous pattern; long tangled villi; strands of synovial tissue matted together or floating within the joint synovial fluid; firm nodules scattered within synovium; generalized synovitis; extra-articular structures (muscles) may be involved.

Histologically: Synovium markedly thickened by proliferated large polyhedral cells, containing varying amounts of fibrous tissue based upon lesion duration; frequent multinucleated giant cells with large masses of iron pigment in stroma and cells.

| Diagnosis | Pain |
|---|---|
| | Swelling: Swollen boggy joint |
| | Skin: Temperature raised |
| | Local tenderness |
| | Disability |
| | Loss of function: Partial |
| Investigation | X-ray AP and LAT views |
| D/d | Synovioma: Contains no giant cells |
| | Malignant tumor |
| | Hemophilia |
| Management | Conservative treatment: |
| | Strapping |
| | Inj. Hydrocortisone with lignocaine 2% into the ganglion |
| | Threading: A corrugated silken thread passed through ganglion: to be removed marginally daily till end of the week. |
| | Analgesics and NSAIDs |
| | Surgical treatment of choice |
| | Surgery: Excision. |
| | Recurrences: Fairly. |

## Synovial Chondromatosis

Common, esp. of poorly excised ones.

| Definition | Defined as an affection, characterized by multiple cartilaginous nodules that develop and grow within the synovial membrane of a joint, a bursa, or a tendon sheath; is a rare lesion. |
|---|---|
| Etiology | Obscure |
| Pathogenesis | Grossly: Synovium thickened, containing multiple small cartilaginous or partially ossified cartilaginous masses (1–4 mm) spread throughout the synovium underneath surface. |
| | Histologically: Apparent masses evolution; focal proliferations of mesenchymal cells embedded in a mucinous or chondroid matrix; hyaline cartilage nodules formation; pedunculated nodules hanging into the joint cavity. |
| Diagnosis | Pain |
| | Swelling |
| | Disability |
| D/d | • Traumatic arthritis: Detached fragments of articular cartilage and bone embedded in the synovium |
| | • Osteoarthritis. |
| Investigation | X-ray joint: AP and LAT views: unusual extensive ossification; multiple small irregular opacities; thickened synovium; increased synovial fluid; subchondral bone plate changes; narrowing of joint space. |
| Management | Surgical treatment of choice. |
| | Surgery: Synovectomy. |

## Synovial Sarcoma

| | |
|---|---|
| Definition | It is defined as the highly malignant tumor (usually always fatal) originating from the synovial tissue; develops exclusively in the limbs, most often in the lower limb, esp. around the knee, that is most frequent site; other frequent sites are foot, ankle, wrist, and forearm; usually occurs in the adults; grows slowly; remnant for long-time. |
| Etiology | Unknown. |
| Pathogenesis | Grossly: Firm, except for rapidly growing tumors; originate from mesenchymal tissue appropriately stimulated into synovial tissue. |
| | Histologically: Variable: irregular clefts and glandlike spaces lined by cuboidal or columnar pseudoepithelial cells a fibrosarcomatous stroma; usually the tumor may be composed of a single cell responsible for the behavior of tumor; spindle cell or fibrosarcomatous component is the highly malignant part, while pseudoepithelial cell component is less malignant. |
| Diagnosis | Pain: May or may not be present |
| | Swelling of joint |
| | Movements: Painful and restricted. |
| D/d | Ewing's tumor |
| | Reticulum cell sarcoma |
| | Carcinoma |
| | Periosteal fibrosarcoma |
| Investigation | X-ray AP and LAT views. |
| Management | Surgical treatment: |
| | Amputation + lymphadenectomy of regional lymph nodes: |
| | Amputation: At a level much higher than the tumor. |
| | Indications: |
| | • For foot or ankle: Through proximal tibia |
| | • For knee: Through middle or proximal femur |
| | Wide local resection + lymphadenectomy of regional lymph nodes: |
| | Indication: For less malignant and more indolent tumors. |

## MESENCHYMAL LESIONS

## Myxoma

| | |
|---|---|
| Definition | Myxomas are defined as rare benign tumors that originate from the mesenchymal tissue; usually lesions are small, well encapsulated, cystic or fluctuant; while large ones, are poorly encapsulated, lobulated or polypoid, and may ooze along planes of tissue. |
| Etiology | Obscure. |
| Pathogenesis | Grossly: Lesions are soft, mucoid, and sometimes their contents ooze from the cut surface |
| | Histologically: Sparse cellular element, composed of spindle shaped and stellate cells, spread irregularily in a loose myxoid or myxomatous matrix that contains only fine fibrils, thus related to ganglia. |

| Diagnosis | Pain |
| --- | --- |
| | Swelling |
| | Disability |
| Investigation | X-ray AP and LAT views |
| Management | Surgical treatment of choice |
| | Surgery: Enucleation |
| | Indication: Small myxomas |
| | Surgery: Wide local resection |
| | Indication: Large ruptured myxomas. |

## Myxosarcoma

| Definition | Myxosarcomas are defined as rare malignant tumors that originate from the mesenchymal tissue; usually bulky pseudoencapsulated infiltrating myxomatous masses; usually develop about the pelvis or in the lower limbs; clinical course may be protracted, resecting them locally is difficult, and lesions often recur. |
| --- | --- |
| Etiology | Obscure. |
| Pathogenesis | Grossly: Lesions usually are bulky pseudoencapsulated infiltrating myxomatous masses |
| | Histologically: Sparse cellular element, composed of spindle shaped and stellate cells, spread irregularly in a loose myxoid or myxomatous matrix that contains only fine fibrils. |
| Diagnosis | Pain |
| | Swelling |
| | Disability |
| | Movements: Painful and restricted. |
| Investigation | X-ray AP and LAT views |
| Management | Surgical treatment of choice |
| | Surgery: Amputation |
| | Indication: Protracted clinical course |
| | Surgery: Radical local resection |
| | Indication: Ruptured lesions. |

## FATTY LESIONS

### Lipoma

| Definition | Lipoma is defined as the most frequent benign tumor of connective tissue; occurs mostly in women during 5th decade; usually originates subcutaneously, while sometimes in more deeper sites; occasionally involves synovium (lipoma arborescens), and rarely the periosteum or the bony medullary canal; usual sites are neck, axilla, shoulder, back, arm, and rarely the lower limbs: groin and upper thigh. |
| --- | --- |
| Etiology | Obscure. |
| Pathogenesis | Grossly: Well encapsulated fatty benign tumor; containing variable quantities of connective tissue lodged in strands that demarcate the lesion into lobules. |

|   | Histologically: Frequently contain mature fat cells; while in some cases predominant cells are granular (xanthoma), in others predominant tissue is fibrous or vascular (telangiectatic); no metastasis. |
|---|---|
| Diagnosis | Swelling: Soft, circumscribed, semi-fluctuant, movable mass that grows slowly |
|   | Painless: Usually |
|   | Cosmetic stigma. |
| Investigation | X-ray show: Lipoma as distinctive as it appears as a discrete radiolucent area within soft tissue. |
| D/d | Neurofibromatosis: Hereditary, associated cutaneous pigmentation |
|   | Liposarcoma |
| Management | Surgical treatment of choice |
|   | Surgery: Enucleation |
|   | Indication: Superficial lipomas |
|   | Surgery: Wide excision |
|   | Indication: Deep-seated lipomas. |

## Liposarcoma

| Definition | Liposarcoma is defined as the most frequent differentiated somatic soft issue sarcoma; occurs in men and women with equal frequency; usually occurs post 4th decade, but may occur in infants and children; occurs most often in the limbs esp. in the thigh. Usually originates subcutaneously, while sometimes in more deeper sites; occasionally involves synovium (lipoma arborescens), and rarely the periosteum or the bony medullary canal; usual sites are neck, axilla, shoulder, back, arm, and rarely the lower limbs: groin and upper thigh. |
|---|---|
| Etiology | Unknown. |
| Pathogenesis | Grossly: Encapsulated and lobulated; soft and gelatinous or mucoid, or greasy and fatty, or firm and fibrous; usually contain different types of tissue within same tumor; cut surface may show patches of varying colors due to hemorrhage and necrosis. |
|   | Histologically: Bariable: |
|   | • Well-differentiated (capillaries arranged characteristically; rather indolent); growth slow; metastasizes rarely. |
|   | • Poorly differentiated (besides above, contains large bizarre lipoblasts with atypical nuclei); metastasizes frequently. |
|   | • Adenoid/or round cell (highly cellular; large, oval or polyhedral cells with foamy cytoplasm and central nuclei); metastasizes frequently. |
|   | • Undifferentiated (mixed); metastasizes frequently. |
| Diagnosis | Swelling: Firm, fixed mass in the deeper tissues |
|   | Painless: Initially, becomes painful later on |
|   | Cosmetic stigma. |
| Investigation | X-ray show: Decreased density, though the radiolucency character of lipoma absent as the tumor possess well differentiated fatty tissue. |
| D/d | Neurofibromatosis: Hereditary, associated cutaneous pigmentation lipoma |

| Management | Surgical treatment of choice |
|---|---|
| | Surgery: Amputation |
| | Indication: Recurrences post local resection |
| | Surgery: Wide local excision |
| | Indication: Initial stage, as in advance cases recurrences are high. |
| | RT: Liposarcomas are radiosensitive, but RT cannot destroy them |
| | Indication: As palliative treatment for inoperable tumors, or to reduce size of large ones prior to surgery. |

## Tumors and Tumorlike Lesions of Soft Tissues

| Preface | Tumors and tumorlike lesions of soft tissues are more frequent than those of bone; includes most lesions encountered clinically, while many lesions of the soft tissue are not true tumors; classification (Table 23.3) of these lesions based upon clinical evaluation (history and physical examination); in majority of these lesions the X-rays play a little diagnostic role (exceptions are synovioma, liposarcoma, and myositis ossificans), but valuable in determining the extent of a tumor and about bone's involvement; biopsy is mandatory for confirming diagnosis. |
|---|---|

**Table 23.3:** Classification of tumors and tumorlike lesions of somatic soft tissue

| Tissue of derivation/ or differentiation | Benign | Malignant |
|---|---|---|
| Fibrous | Fibromatoses:<br>• Keloid<br>• Desmoid tumor<br>• Palmar and plantar<br>• Sternocleidomastoid tumor<br>Reactive proliferations:<br>• Myositis ossificans<br>Fibroma | Differentiated fibrosarcoma<br>Dermatofibrosarcoma<br>Kaposi's sarcoma<br>Fibrosarcoma |
| Vascular | Hemangioma<br>Lymphangioma<br>Glomus tumor | Hemangiopericytoma<br>Angiosarcoma |
| Neural | Neuroma<br>Neurofibroma<br>Neurilemmoma | Neurofibrosarcoma<br>Neuroepithelioma |
| Muscular | Leiomyoma<br>Granular cell myoblastoma | Leiomyosarcoma<br>Rhabdomyosarcoma |
| Fatty | Lipoma<br>Lipogranuloma | Liposarcoma |
| Mesenchymal | Myxoma<br>Mesenchymoma | Myxosarcoma<br>Mesenchymoma malignant |
| Synovial | Ganglion<br>Nodular synovitis<br>(Giant cell tumor of tendon sheath)<br>Synovial osteochondromatosis<br>Pigmented vilonodular synovitis | Synovial sarcoma |

## Fibromatoses

| | |
|---|---|
| Definition | Fibromatoses are defined as lesions that tend to grow by an invasive proliferation of fibroblasts, develop to be nodular or infiltrative, recur post removal; not to metastasize. |
| Lesions | Keloid |
| | Desmoid tumors |
| | Palmar and plantar fibromatosis |
| | Sternocleidomastoid fibromatosis |
| | Myositis ossificans. |

## Keloid

| | |
|---|---|
| Definition | It is defined as a localized lesion of connective tissue characterized by post traumatic massive, highly collagenized overgrowth + of fibrous tissue that infiltrates adjoining normal tissue; differentiated from the simple hypertrophic scar by the cauliflowerlike projections caused by the lesional tissue; usually occur in front of chest wall, arm, buttock, thigh |
| Etiology | Traumatic: Direct violence—blow or hit by a stick |
| | Indirect violence: Post injection prick |
| Pathogenesis | Grossly: Cauliflowerlike/clawlike projections of lesional tissue (massive collagenized overgrowth of fibrous tissue infiltrating adjoining normal tissue). |
| | Histologically: Massive proliferation of fibroblasts |
| Diagnosis | Pain |
| | Swelling: Overgrowth |
| | Itching |
| | Cosmetic stigma |
| Investigation | X-rays—AP and LAT views. |
| Management | Conservative treatment: |
| | Anlgesics and NSAIDs |
| | Antiallergics |
| | Lignocaine gel application |
| | Local injection hydrocortisone + hyalase + lignocaine |
| | Surgical treatment of choice |
| | Surgery: Excision. |

## Desmoid Tumors

| | |
|---|---|
| Definition | It is defined as benign but locally aggressive and infiltrating fibroblastic lesions that may occur in muscle anywhere in the body; usually seen in the anterior abdominal wall of child borne women of 40 years age; does not metastasize. |
| Etiology | Traumatic: Direct violence—blow or hit by a stick |
| | Indirect violence: Post injection prick |
| Pathogenesis | Grossly: Circumscribed lesion; usually infiltrates tissue diffusely; skin spared; though adherent to bone without its erosion. |

Histologically: Sparsely cellular, collagenized fibroblastic lesion that infiltrates muscle; muscle bundles destroyed or undergo proliferative reaction characterized by formation of giant cells.

| | |
|---|---|
| Diagnosis | Female: Male (2:1) |
| | Pain |
| | Swelling |
| | Itching |
| | Cosmetic stigma |
| Investigation | X-rays—AP and LAT views. |
| Management | Conservative treatment: |
| | Anlgesics and NSAIDs |
| | Antiallergics |
| | Lignocaine gel application |
| | Local injection hydrocortisone + hyalase + lignocaine |
| | RT: Beneficial. |
| | Surgical treatment of choice |
| | Surgery: Wide local excision. |

## Palmar and Plantar Fibromatosis (Syn. Dupuytren's Contracture)

| | |
|---|---|
| Definition | It is defined as benign lesions of connective tissue characterized by massive, contractures of palmar or plantar fascia; second most frequent of the fibromatoses; palmar ones occur more in men than women; of plantar fascia are relatively rare; usually occur in the palm or sole. |
| Etiology | Unknown. |
| Pathogenesis | Palmar fibromatosis: Appears as a painless subcutaneous nodule in the palm, mostly in line with the ring finger at the distal palmar crease, later on more nodules appear and form bands; finally MP joints become flexed; lesions may become quiescent at any stage. |
| | Grossly: Hard, firm nodules and bands of thickened tissue found superficially in the palmar fascia; skin adherent to the fascia; later on entire fascia densely thickened and yellowish. |
| | Histologically: Early lesion shows massive proliferation of fibroblasts; cells arranged in a distinct pattern; later on cells more oriented with increased collagen; finally thickened acellular mass of disorganized fascial tissue with multiple cells; no encapsulation. |
| | Plantar fibromatosis: Usually affects the medial half of plantar fascia; finally a hammer toe may form; its pathogenesis identical with that of palmar fibromatosis. |
| Diagnosis | Pain |
| | Deformity: Palmar—flexed MP joints; plantar—hammer toe |
| | Itching |
| | Cosmetic stigma |
| | Disability. |
| Investigation | X-rays—AP and LAT views. |
| Management | Conservative treatment: |
| | Anlgesics and NSAIDs |

Antiallergics

Lignocaine gel application

Local injection hydrocortisone + hyalase + lignocaine

Surgical treatment of choice

Surgery: Reconstruction.

## Sternocleidomastoid Fibromatosis (Syn. congenital Muscular Torticollis)

| | |
|---|---|
| Definition | It is defined as benign fibromatosis, distinct from desmoid tumor both morphologically and clinically; usual occurs within 2/52 post child's birth; may involve the sternocleidomastoid muscle diffusely; usually disappears within a year.; does not metastasize. |
| Etiology | Unknown. |
| Pathogenesis | Grossly: Sternocleidomastoid muscle swollen partly/or completely; tumors within muscle smooth, firm, and freely mobile. |
| | Histologically: Muscle fibers replaced by diffuse infiltrated fibroblasts; fairly cellular and oriented, or acellular and similar to a desmoid. |
| Diagnosis | Pain |
| | Swelling |
| | Deformity: Torticollis |
| | Cosmetic stigma. |
| Investigation | X-rays—AP view. |
| Management | Conservative treatment: |
| | Anlgesics and NSAIDs |
| | Antiallergics |
| | Lignocaine gel application |
| | Local injection hydrocortisone + hyalase + lignocaine |
| | RT: Beneficial. |
| | Surgical treatment of choice |
| | Surgery: Wide local excision. |

## Myositis Ossificans

| | |
|---|---|
| Definition | It is defined as benign fibromatosis, characterized by a localized lesion of heterotopic non-neoplastic cartilage and bone caused by trauma (sum of all reactions of somatic soft tissue that follow trauma, resulting in formation of cartilage and bone); lesion usually forms in or adjacent to muscle with proximity to bone; usual occurs in children and young adults; does not metastasize. |
| Etiology | Traumatic: Crush injuries |
| | Fall from a height |
| | RSA |
| | Sports injury |
| Pathogenesis | Grossly: Crush injury resulting in compressed muscle and adjoining soft tissue structures against a bone; may also develop post avulsion of tendinous or fascial attachments, e.g. brachialis muscle post elbow dislocation. |

|  | Histologically: Muscle fibers replaced by diffuse infiltrated fibroblasts; fairly cellular and oriented, or acellular; proliferated connective tissue of fascia and related structures; bone appears in the matured lesion |
| Diagnosis | Pain |
|  | Swelling |
|  | Deformity: Flexed elbow |
|  | Cosmetic stigma |
|  | Movements: Painful and restricted |
| Investigation | X-rays show: Lesion progressively ossifying and maturing |
| Management | Conservative treatment: |
|  | Anlgesics and NSAIDs |
|  | Antiallergics |
|  | Lignocaine gel application |
|  | Local injection hydrocortisone + hyalase + lignocaine |
|  | RT: Beneficial. |

Surgical treatment:

Indication: To be excised only for:

- Severe enough symptoms
- Mature lesion (usually 6–12/12 post-trauma, because excising premature lesion may cause extensive recurence

Surgery: To be excised intact.

## Kaposi's Sarcoma (Syn. Idiopathic Hemorrhagic Sarcoma)

| Definition | Kaposi's sarcoma is defined as a rare, highly malignant tumor of the fibroblastic origin that has the potential to metastasize; occurs most often in men over 40 years of age; affects mainly limbs, and paranasal sinuses but may form wherever fibrous tissue available; rarely affects the hands and feet; most often involves the shoulders and interscapular region. |
| Etiology | Unknown |
| Pathogenesis | Grossly: The tumor develops as a reddish purple macule or nodule in the skin of the limb, that enlarges and blackens; adjoining lesions develop and enlarge, fuse to form dark reddish blue plaques; both limbs may be involved symmetrically; lesion may extend toward trunk Histologically: initially lesion resembles a granulomatous inflammatory reaction; later on proliferated fibroblasts, collagen formation, and proliferated vascular elements (mixed picture of fibrosarcoma with the fibrosarcoma). |
| Diagnosis | Pain |
|  | Swelling |
|  | Skin: Reddish purple macule or nodules, ulceration |
|  | Death may occur from infection or hemorrhage. |
| Investigation | CBC |
|  | Serum acid phosphatase estimation |
|  | X-ray—diagnostic. Shows irregular destruction of bone without surrounding reaction. |

CXR

Mammography CT scan

US abdomen and pelvis

Biopsy.

| | |
|---|---|
| Management | No effective treatment known and the disease is always fatal. |
| General measures | Aims |

- To relieve pain and reduce tumor masses
- To ambulate patient to combat negative calcium balance
- To prevent exposure to trauma to avoid occurrence of the pathological fractures.

Conservative treatment:

Blood transfusion: To combat anemia

Analgesics for control of pain

Chemotherapy (CT):

Alkylating Agents:

- Melphalan (Alkeran)—most effective agent available.
  Dose: 6 mg o.d. PO, for 2–3 weeks
  Maintenance dose: 1–4 mg o.d. every 4 weeks along with
- Prednisone 2 mg/kg
- Cyclophosphamides 50–100 mg PO 1–3 times o.d. along with

Vincristine 1.4 mg/sq.m weekly

Radiotherapy (RT):

- For control of pain and for reducing tumor mass
- For diffuse lesions

Surgical therapy (ST):

Surgery: Wide local excision

Indication: Early lesions.

| | |
|---|---|
| Prognosis | Average survival time after diagnosis is 2 years. Occasionally a patient may live for many years in apparent remission. |

## Fibrosarcoma

| | |
|---|---|
| Definition | Fibrosarcoma of bone is defined as the frankly malignant tumor of the fibroblastic origin that has the potential to metastasize; occurs rarely; occurs most often in young adults; affects men and women equally; affects mainly limb, but may form wherever fibrous tissue available; rarely affects the hands and feet; most often involves the shoulders and interscapular region. |
| Etiology | Unknown |
| Pathogenesis | Grossly: The tumor is circumscribed and encapsulated; firm and rubbery; cut surface trabeculated or matted with small cystic areas; edematous; calcified; ossified tissues; in highly cellular lesion—tumor appears soft, cut surface hemorrhagic and necrotic; in subperiosteal lesion—bone eroded, saucerlike. |
| | Histologically: Variable (from markedly well differentiated ones to markedly anaplastic ones). |

| | |
|---|---|
| Diagnosis | Pain—very severe |
| | Swelling |
| | Pathological fracture: may be found. |
| Investigation | CBC |
| | Serum acid phosphatase estimation |
| | X-ray—diagnostic. Shows irregular destruction of bone without surrounding reaction, while sclerosis in case of metastasis from carcinoma prostate |
| | CXR |
| | Mammography CT scan |
| | US abdomen and pelvis |
| | Biopsy. |
| Management | No effective treatment known and the disease is always fatal. |
| General measures | |
| Aims | • To relieve pain and reduce tumor masses |
| | • To ambulate patient to combat negative calcium balance |
| | • To prevent exposure to trauma to avoid occurrence of the pathological fractures. |

Conservative treatment:

Blood transfusion: To combat anemia

Analgesics: For control of pain

Chemotherapy (CT):

Alkylating Agents:

• Melphalan (Alkeran)—most effective agent available.
  Dose: 6 mg o.d. PO, for 2–3 weeks
  Maintenance dose: 1–4 mg o.d. every 4 weeks along with

• Prednisone 2 mg/kg

• Cyclophosphamides 50–100 mg PO 1–3 times o.d. along with Vincristine 1.4 mg/sq.m weekly
  Radiotherapy (RT):
  – For control of pain and for reducing tumor mass

Surgical therapy (ST):

Surgery:

• Decompression with radiotherapy—for cord compression

• Stem cell transplantation (SCT)—for selective patients.

| | |
|---|---|
| Prognosis | Average survival time after diagnosis is 2 years. Occasionally a patient may live for many years in apparent remission. |

## MUSCULAR LESIONS

### Leiomyosarcoma

| | |
|---|---|
| Definition | Leiomyosarcoma is defined as the rare malignant tumor that originates In the smooth muscle of a blood vessel; that has the potential to metastasize early; aggressive locally; occurs most often in young adults; affects men and women equally; usually develops in the deep soft tissues; affects mainly limb, but may form wherever fibrous tissue |

available; rarely affects the hands and feet; most often involves the thighs, legs, shoulders and upper arm.

Etiology          Unknown

Pathogenesis      Grossly: Within a muscle; firm, grayish white, encapsulated; often soft, hemorrhagic, necrotic, and noncapsulated; may result in coalescence of multiple tumors.

Histologically: Variable (pleomorphic, alveolar, or embryonal); the pleomorphic type (markedly well differentiated) composed of spindle and strap-shaped cells with large bizarre nuclei, usually seen in limbs; the alveolar type (carcinomatous type) composed of cells grouped along septa in an alveolar form; the embryonal type composed of round cells of spindle cell tumor.

Diagnosis         Pain—very severe

Swelling

Pathological fracture: may be found.

Investigation     CBC

Serum acid phosphatase estimation

X-ray—diagnostic. Shows irregular destruction of bone without surrounding reaction, while sclerosis in case of metastasis from carcinoma prostate

CXR

Mammography CT scan

US abdomen and pelvis

Biopsy.

Management        No effective treatment known and the disease is always fatal.

General measures

Aims
- To relieve pain and reduce tumor masses
- To ambulate patient to combat negative calcium balance
- To prevent exposure to trauma to avoid occurrence of the pathological fractures.

Conservative treatment:

Blood transfusion: To combat anemia

Analgesics: For control of pain

Chemotherapy (CT):

Alkylating Agents:
- Melphalan (Alkeran)—most effective agent available.
  Dose: 6 mg o.d. PO, for 2–3 weeks
  Maintenance dose: 1–4 mg o.d. every 4 weeks along with
- Prednisone 2 mg/kg
- Cyclophosphamides 50–100 mg PO 1–3 times o.d. along with

Vincristine 1.4 mg/sq.m weekly

Radiotherapy (RT):

– For control of pain and for reducing tumor mass

Surgical therapy (ST):

Surgery: Radical surgery:

- Amputation
- Disarticulation.

| | |
|---|---|
| Prognosis | Average survival time after diagnosis is 2 years. Occasionally a patient may live for many years in apparent remission. |

## Rhabdomyosarcoma

| | |
|---|---|
| Definition | Rhabdomyosarcoma is defined as the frankly malignant tumor of the fibroblastic origin that has the potential to metastasize; occurs most often in 4–7th decades; affects mainly head and neck, pelvis, and limbs (lower limbs > upper limbs). |
| Etiology | Unknown |
| Pathogenesis | Grossly: Within a muscle; firm, grayish white, encapsulated; often soft, hemorrhagic, necrotic, and noncapsulated; may result in coalescence of multiple tumors. |
| | Histologically: Variable (pleomorphic, alveolar, or embryonal); the pleomorphic type (markedly well differentiated) composed of spindle and strap-shaped cells with large bizarre nuclei, usually seen in limbs; the alveolar type (carcinomatous type) composed of cells grouped along septa in an alveolar form; the embryonal type composed of round cells of spindle cell tumor. |
| Diagnosis | Initially symptomless; later on: |
| | Pain |
| | Swelling: Deep seated, fusiform mass, movable (with relaxed muscle), while fixed (with contracted muscle) |
| | Local tenderness |
| | Pathological fracture: May occur |
| Investigation | CBC |
| | Serum acid phosphatase estimation |
| | X-ray—diagnostic. Shows irregular destruction of bone without surrounding reaction, while sclerosis in case of metastasis from carcinoma prostate |
| | CXR |
| | Mammography CT scan |
| | US abdomen and pelvis |
| | Biopsy. |
| D/d | Reticulumm cell sarcoma |
| | Lymphomas |
| | Ewing's sarcoma |
| | Neuroblastoma |
| Management General measures | No effective treatment known and the disease is always fatal. |
| Aims | • To relieve pain and reduce tumor masses |
| | • To ambulate patient to combat negative calcium balance |

- To prevent exposure to trauma to avoid occurrence of the pathological fractures.

Conservative treatment:

Blood transfusion: To combat anemia

Analgesics: For control of pain

Chemotherapy (CT):

Alkylating Agents:

- Melphalan (Alkeran)—most effective agent available.
  Dose: 6 mg o.d. PO, for 2–3 weeks
  Maintenance dose: 1–4 mg o.d. every 4 weeks along with
- Prednisone 2 mg/kg
- Cyclophosphamides 50–100 mg PO 1–3 times o.d. along with Vincristine 1.4 mg/sq.m weekly
  Radiotherapy (RT):
  – For control of pain and for reducing tumor mass

Surgical therapy (ST):

Surgery:

- Amputation
- Disarticulation (for lesions of limbs).

Prognosis    Average survival time after diagnosis is 2 years. Occasionally a patient may live for many years in apparent remission.

## METASTATIC LESIONS

### Metastatic Carcinoma

Definition    Metastatic carcinoma is defined as the most frequent malignant tumor of bone; while metastatic sarcoma occurs rarely; metastatic carcinoma occurs most often post 40 years of age; affects mainly the large bones (most often the pelvis, femur, tibia, skull, spine, sternum, ribs, humerus, skull, ribs, and pelvis), but may affect any bone in the body; commoner than the primary bone tumor; occurs either by direct extension or by metastasis.

Properties    Tumor may be osteolytic (majority) or osteoblastic (minority).

Etiology    Metastasis from primary growth in breast, bronchus, thyroid, prostate, and kidney.

Pathogenesis    slowly growing tumors stimulating more osseous reaction than a rapidly growing, highly anaplastic type. Carcinomas of the breast and of prostate are the most frequent tumors to metastasize. Secondary deposits liable to occur esp. as a result of a primary growth in breast, bronchus, thyroid, prostate, uterus—cervical, and kidney:

- Breast: Commonest source of secondary carcinoma of bone (spine, pelvis, proximal ends of femur and humerus)
- Bronchus: Commonest source of secondary carcinoma of bone (spine, pelvis, and proximal ends of humerus)
- Thyroid: Commonest source of secondary carcinoma of bone (flat bones of vertex of the skull).

- Prostate commonly associated with osseous dissemination; common manifestation is diffuse sclerosis of the pelvis and lumbosacral spines; osteoblastic type of metastasis (peculiar)
- Uterine cervix: Commonest source of secondary carcinoma of bone (spine, pelvis, and proximal ends of femur)
- Kidney: Commonest source of secondary carcinoma of bone (pelvis, spine, and proximal end of femur).

| | |
|---|---|
| Diagnosis | Pain—very severe |
| | Swelling |
| | Pathological fracture: May be found. |
| Investigation | CBC |
| | Serum acid phosphatase estimation |
| | X-ray—diagnostic. Shows irregular destruction of bone without surrounding reaction, while sclerosis in case of metastasis from carcinoma prostate |
| | CXR |
| | Mammography CT scan |
| | US abdomen and pelvis |
| | Biopsy. |
| Management | It is highly unsatisfactory. |
| | Radiotherapy (RT): Sensitive to radiotherapy |
| | RT in combination with CT yields better result. |
| | Surgical: |

- Mastoidectomy combined with testosterone—in case of secondary deposits from carcinoma breast
- Thyroidectomy combined with radioactive iodine—in case of secondary deposits from carcinoma thyroid
- Orchidectomy combined with estrogen therapy—in case of secondary deposits from carcinoma prostate.

| | |
|---|---|
| Prognosis | Poor. |

## Bibliography

1. Ackerman LV, del Regato JA. Cancer; diagnosis, treatment and prognosis, ed. 2, C.V. Mosby Co., St. Louis, 1954.
2. Aegerter E, Kirkpatrick JA. Ortopedic diseases: physiology, pathology, radiology, W.B. Saunders Co., Philadelphia, 1958.
3. Agarwal M, et al. Limb salvage surgery for osteosarcoma: effective low-cost treatment. Clin Orthop Relat Res: 459:82–91, 2007.
4. Anderson KJ. Synovial sarcoma, West. J. Surg. 59:141, 1951.
5. Barnes R. Aneurysmal bone cyst, J. Bone and Joint Surg. 38-B:301, 1956.
6. Bate TH. Hemangioma of the tendon sheath, J. Bone and Joint Surg. 36-A:104, 1954.
7. Bauer WH, Harell A. Myxoma of bone, J. Bone and Joint Surg. 36-A:263, 1954.
8. Bennett GA. Reactive and neoplastic changes in synovial tissues, Proc. Inst. Med. Chicago 18:26, 1950.
9. Bingold AC. Joint changes in neurofibromatosis, J.Bone and Joint Surg. 34-B:76, 1952.
10. Brailsford JF. The radiology of bones and joints, ed. 5, Williams and Williams Co., Baltimore, 1954.

11. Bremner RA, Jelliffe AM. The management of pathological fracture of the major long bones from metastatic cancer, J. Bone and Joint Surg. 40-B: 652, 1958.

12. Cade S. Primary malignant tumors of bone, Brit. J. Radiol. 20:10, 1947.

13. Caffey J. Pediatric x-ray diagnosis, ed. 3, The Yearbook Publishers, Inc. Chicago, 1956.

14. Campanacci M. Bone and Soft tissue tumors.Ney York: Springer: p. 455–63, 1990.

15. Campbell CJ, Harkess J. Fibrous metaphyseal defect of bone, Surg., Gynec. and Obst. 104:329, 1957.

16. Campbell WC. Osteogenic sarcoma, J. Bone and Joint Surg. 17:827,1935.

17. Carrol RE. Osteoid osteoma in the hand, J. Bone and Joint Surg. 35-A:888, 1953.

18. Cobey MC. Hemangioma of joints, Arch. Surg. 46:465, 1943.

19. Coley BL. Neoplasms of bone and related conditions. Their etiology, pathogenesis, diagnosis, and treatment, ed 2, Hoeber Medical Division, Harper and Row, Publishers, Inc., New York, 1960.

20. Coley BL. Resection: A conservative measure in the treatment of bone tumors, Am., Surgeon 23:13, 1957.

21. Compere EL, Coleman SS. Nonosteogenic fibroma of bone, Surg., Gynec. and Obst. 105:588, 1957.

22. Compere EL. The diagnosis and treatment of giant-cell tumors of bone, J. Bone and Joint Surg. 35-A:822, 1953.

23. Crtuz M, Coley BL. Aneurysmal bone cyst, Surg., Gynec. and Obst. 103:67, 1956.

24. Cunningham JB, Ackerman LV. Metaphyseal fibrous defects, J. Bone and Joint Surg. 38-A:797, 1956.

25. Dahlin DC, et al. Chodromyxoid fibroma of bone, J. Bone and Joint Surg. 35-A: 831, 1953.

26. Desai SS, Jambhekar NA. Pathology of Ewing's sarcoma/PNET: current opinion and emerging concepts, Indian Journal of Orthopaedics vol 44, 4:363, 2010.

27. Dwinnell LA, et al. Parosteal (juxtacortical osteogenic sarcoma, J.Bone and Joint Surg. 36-A:732, 1954.

28. Ferguson AB Sr. The present trend in treatment of osteogenic sdarcoma. In DePalma, A.F., editor: Clinical Othopedics, vol. 14 p. 63, J.B. Lippincott Co., Philadelphia, 1959.

29. Fitts WT, et al. Fractures in metastatic carcinoma, Am. J. Surg. 85:282, 1953.

30. Frankle CJ. Aspiration biopsy of the spine, J. Bone and Joint Surg. 36-A:69, 1954.

31. Garceau GJ, Gregory CF. Solitary unicameral bone cyst, J. Bone and Joint Surg. 36-A:267, 1954.

32. Gee VR, Push DG. Giant cell tumor of bone, Radiology 70:33, 1958.

33. Ghormley RK. Chondromas and chondrosarcomas of the scapula and the innominate bone, A.M.A. Arch. Surg. 63:48, 1951.

34. Gilmer WS Jr, MacEwen GD. Central (medullary) fibrosarcoma of bone, J. Bone and Joint Surg. 40-A:121, 1958.

35. Gilmer WS Jr. Tumors and tumorlike lesions of somatic tissue, Campbell's Operative Orthopaedics, ed. 9th, Vol I-IV. C.V. Mosby Co., Saint Louis, 1998.

36. Haggart GE, Capel JW. Early diagnosis of primary malignant bone tumors, J.A.M.A. 152:883, 1953.

37. Iwamoto Y. Diagnosis and treatment of Ewing's sarcoma. Jpn J Clin Oncol 37:79–89, 2007.

38. Jaffe HL. Benign osteoblastoma, Bul. Hosp. Joint Dis. 17:141, 1956.

39. Jaffe HL. Tumors and timorous conditions of the bones and joints, Lea and Febiger, Philadelphia, 1958.

40. Jain S, Kapoor G. Chemotherapy in Ewing's sarcoma, Indian Journal of Orthopaedics vol 44, 4:369, 2010.

41. Jenkin RD. Ewing's sarcoma a study of treatment methods, Clin Radiol 17: 97–106, 1966.

42. Kapoor PS. Oncological Emergencies, Accident and Emergency: Etiology, Diagnosis and Management, 2nd Ed., CBS, New Delhi, 2016.

43. Lansche WE, Spjut HJ. Chondrosarcoma of the small bones of the hand, J. Bone and Joint Surg. 40-A:1139, 1958.

44. Larsen RD, Posch JL. Dupuytren's contracture. With special reference to pathology, J. Bone and Joint Surg. 40-A:773, 1958.

45. Lawson TL. Fibular transplant for osteoclastoma of the radius, J. Bone and Joint Surg. 34-B:74, 1952.

46. Lichtenstein L. Bone tumors, ed. 2, The C.V. Mosby Co, St. Louis, 1959.

47. Lichtenstein L. Pathology: diseases of bone, New England J. Med. 255:427, 1956.

48. Lipscomb PR. Tumors of the tendons and tendons and tendon sheaths including ganglia and xanthomas, American Academy of Orthopaedic Surgeons Instructional Course, Lectures, vol. XI, Ann Arbor, p. 50, J.W. Edwards, 1954.

49. Lumb G, Prossor TM. Plasma cell tumors, J. Bone and Joint Surg. 30-B:124, 1948.

50. McLeod JJ, et al. Fibrosarcoma of bone, Am. J. Surg. 94:431, 1957.

51. Medina RG, Elliot DW. Thyroid carcinoma. Arch Surg 97:239, 1968.

52. Mercer W. Orthopedic Surgery, 4th Ed., Williams and Wilkins Co., Baltimore, 1950.

53. Morton JJ. Giant cell tumor of bone, Cancer 9: 1012, 1956.

54. Ottolenghi CE. Diagnosis of orthopedic lesionsdd by aspiration biopsy. Results of 1061 punctures, J. Bone and joint Surg. 37-A:443 1955.

55. Platzer RF. Treatment of multiple myeloma, New York J. Med. 54: 103, 1954.

56. Stewart MJ, et al. Fibrous dysplasia of bone, J. Bone and Joint Surg. 44-B:302, 1962.

57. Tiwari A, et al. Outcome of multimodality treatment of Ewing's sarcoma of the extremities, Indian Journal of Orthopaedics vol 44, 4:378, 2010.

58. Tracey JF, et al. Primary malignant tumors of bone, J. Bone and Joint Surg. 39-A:554, 1957.

59. Tudway RC. Radiotherapy for osteogenic sarcoma, J. Bone and Joint Surg. 43-B:61, 1961.

60. Vieta JO, et al. Survey of Hodgkin's disease and lymphosarcoma in bone, Radiology 39:1, 1942.

61. Vincent RG. Malignant synovioma, Ann. Surg. 152:777, 1960.

62. Wildermuth O, et al. Management of diffuse metastasis from carcinoma of the prostate, J.A.M.A. 172:1607, 12960.

# Index